Generative Artificial Intelligence for Biomedical and Smart Health Informatics

IEEE Press
445 Hoes Lane
Piscataway, NJ 08854

Generative Artificial Intelligence for Biomedical and Smart Health Informatics

Edited by
Aditya Khamparia
Babasaheb Bhimrao Ambedkar University
Amethi, India

Deepak Gupta
Maharaja Agrasen Institute of Technology
Delhi, India

IEEE Press
WILEY

Contents

About the Editors

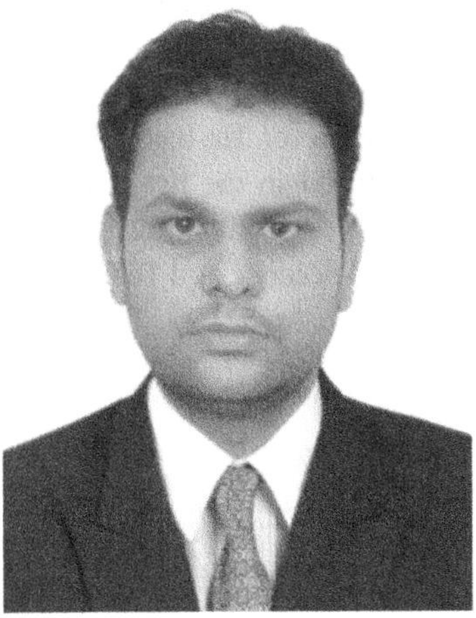

Aditya Khamparia is an eminent academician and plays versatile roles and responsibilities toward lectures, research, publications, consultancy, community service, and PhD supervision. With more than 13 years of rich expertise in teaching and two years in industry, he focuses on individual-centric and practical learning. Currently, he is an assistant professor in the Department of Computer Science at Babasaheb Bhimrao Ambedkar University, Lucknow, India. His research areas include machine learning, soft computing, educational technologies, IoT, semantic web, and ontologies. He has published more than 100 scientific research publications in reputed international and national journals and conferences, indexed in various international databases. He has been invited to serve as a Faculty Resource Person, Session Chair, Reviewer or Technical Program Committee (TPC) member for different faculty development programs (FDPs), conferences, and journals. He also serves as a reviewer and member of various renowned national and international conferences and journals.

Durgananda Lahari Bhamidipaty
Department of Biotechnology
Manipal Institute of Technology
Manipal, Karnataka
India

Amit Bhagat
Maulana Azad National Institute of Technology (MANIT)
Bhopal

Suman Bhatia
Department of Artificial Intelligence and Machine Learning
Dr. Akhilesh Das Gupta Institute of Professional Studies (affiliated to Guru Gobind Singh Indraprastha University New Delhi)
New Delhi

Rajesh Botchu
Department of Radiology
NRIIMS
Visakhapatnam
India

and

AHERF
Hyderabad
India

and

Department of Musculoskeletal Radiology
Royal Orthopedic Hospital
Birmingham
UK

Bhuvan Botchu
Solihull School
Solihull
UK

Haewon Byeon
Department of AI and Software
Inje University
Gimhae
Republic of Korea

Poonam Chaudhary
CSE, SOET
The NorthCap University
Gurugram
India

Riddhi Chawla
School of Dentistry
Central Asian University
Tashkent
Uzbekistan

Ganeev Kaur Chhabra
Department of Computer Science & Engineering
BharatiVidyapeeth College of Engineeering
New Delhi
India

Tabsum Chhetri
Department of Bioinformatics
University of North Bengal
Darjeeling, West Bengal
India

Om Dabral
Manipal University
Jaipur

Dharmendra Dangi
Indian Institute of Information Technology (IIITB)
Bhopal

Virrat Devaser
School of Computer Science
Lovely Professional University
Phagwara, Punjab
India

Diwakar Diwakar
BBA University
Lucknow
India

Dheeraj Kumar Dixit
Madhav Institute of Science and Technology (MITS)
Gwalior

Tanay Falor
IIIT
Allahabad

John J. Georrge
Department of Bioinformatics
University of North Bengal
Darjeeling, West Bengal
India

Toshika Goswami
Department of Computer Science & Engineering
BharatiVidyapeeth College of Engineeering
New Delhi
India

Indira Guntoory
Department of Obstetrics & Gynaecology
GIMSR
Visakhapatnam
India

Charu Gupta
Department of Computer Science
Bhagwan Parshuram Institute of Technology
Delhi
India

Anuj Gupta
Department of Electronics and Communication
Chandigarh University
Mohali
India

Rishik Gupta
Department of Information Technology and Computer Science
Manipal University
Jaipur
India

Kusum Gurung
Department of Bioinformatics
University of North Bengal
Darjeeling, West Bengal
India

Ernesto Iadanza
Department of Medical Biotechnologies
University of Siena
Italy

Karthikeyan P. Iyengar
Department of Orthopedics, Southport and Ormskirk Hospital Southport
Mersey and West Lancashire Hospitals NHS Trust
UK

and

AHERF
Hyderabad
India

and

Edge Hill University
Ormskirk
UK

Ati Jain
Institute of Advance Computing
SAGE University
Indore
India

Amiyavardhan Jain
Consultant, Periodontology and Implantology
Noble Dental Care
Indore
India

Akshay Kanwar
Department of Electronics and Communication Engineering
Jawaharlal Nehru Government Engineering college
University Hamirpur
Sundernagar, 175018 Himachal Pradesh
India

Ismail Keshta
Computer Science and Information Systems Department
College of Applied Sciences
AlMaarefa University
Riyadh
Saudi Arabia

Aditya Khamparia
Department of Computer Science
Babasaheb Bhimrao Ambedkar University (A Central University)
Lucknow
India

Akanksha Kochhar
Department of Computer Science & Engineering
BharatiVidyapeeth College of Engineeering
New Delhi
India

Pramod Kumar
Ganga Institute of Technology and Management
Maharshi Dayanand University
Rohtak, Haryana
India

Vikas Kumar
ERP Department
ERP Functional Riviera Home Furnishing
Panipat
India

Bagesh Kumar
Department of Information Technology and Computer Science
Manipal University
Jaipur
India

Sohan Kumar
Department of Information Technology and Computer Science
Manipal University
Jaipur
India

Ravi Kumar
Department of Computer Science Engineering
Lovely Professional University
Phagwara, 144411 Punjab
India

and

Department of Computer Science Engineering (AIML)
Jawaharlal Nehru Government Engineering college
University Hamirpur
Sundernagar, 175018 Himachal Pradesh
India

Antonio Lavecchia
"Drug Discovery" Laboratory
Department of Pharmacy
University of Naples Federico II
Naples
Italy

Kari Lippert
Department of Systems Engineering
University of South Alabama
Mobile, AL
USA

Niladri Maiti
School of Dentistry
Central Asian University
Tashkent
Uzbekistan

Arish Mallick
Queens University Belfast
UK

Brijendra Pratap Mishra
Department of Biochemistry
Autonomous State Medical College
Bahraich
Atal Bihari Vajpayee Medical University
Lucknow, Uttar Pradesh
India

Saurav K. Mishra
Department of Bioinformatics
University of North Bengal
Darjeeling, West Bengal
India

Ayushi Mittal
Department of Computer Science
Indira Gandhi Delhi Technical University for Women
New Delhi
India

Ardra Nair
School of Computer Science
Lovely Professional University
Phagwara, Punjab
India

Aryan Nakhale
Department of Mechatronics
Chandigarh University
Mohali
India

H. Naresh Kumar
School of Arts Sciences Humanities & Education
SASTRA Deemed University
Thanjavur
India

Seema Shukla
School of Modern Media
UPES
Dehradun
India

Moolchand Sharma
Department of Computer Science & Engineering
Maharaja Agrasen Institute of Technology
New Delhi
India

Parth Sharma
Manipal University
Jaipur

Riya Sharma
School of Computer Science and Engineering
Lovely Professional University
Phagwara
India

Kirti Shukla
SCSE
IILM University Greater Noida
Noida
India

Prakhar Shukla
Department of Information Technology
IIIT Allahabad
Allahabad
India

Balraj Singh
School of Computer Science and Engineering
Lovely Professional University
Phagwara
India

Sudhanshu Singh
Seth Anandram Jaipuria School
Kanpur
India

Suruchi Singh
Department of Computer Science & Engineering; UIET
Chhatrapati Shahu Ji Maharaj University
Kanpur
India

Neelesh Singh
Department of Artificial Intelligence
Sage University
Indore, MP
India

Amritpal Singh
Department of Computer Science Engineering
Lovely Professional University
Phagwara, 144411 Punjab
India

R. Sivaraman
School of Computing
SASTRA Deemed University
Thanjavur
India

Mukesh Soni
Dr. D. Y. Patil Vidyapeeth, Pune
Dr. D. Y. Patil School of Science & Technology
D. Y. Patil University
Tathawade, Pune
India

Devendra K. Tayal
Department of Computer Science
Indira Gandhi Delhi Technical
University for Women
New Delhi
India

Raj Thakur
Department of Artificial Intelligence
Sage University
Indore, MP
India

Abhinav Upadhyay
Manipal University
Jaipur

Yash Vikram Singh Rathore
Department of Information
Technology and Computer Science
Manipal University
Jaipur
India

Preface

This book focuses on recent advances, roles, and benefits of generative artificial intelligence (AI) in biomedical and smart health informatics. By leveraging deep learning techniques like neural networks, generative AI systems are capable of creating complex data outputs—ranging from synthetic medical images to predictive models of diseases. This technology can assist in diagnosing medical conditions, generating new hypotheses for drug discovery, and personalizing treatment plans. This book aims to describe the different techniques of generative intelligence for health informatics from a practical point of view, solving common life problems. This book also brings a valuable point of view to engineers and businessmen that work in companies, trying to solve practical, economic, and technical problems in the field of their company activities or expertise. The pure practical approach helps to transmit the idea and the aim of the author to communicate the way to approach and to cope with problems that would be intractable in any other way. The integration of generative AI with smart health devices, including wearables, further pushes the boundaries of personalized healthcare. By continually learning from real-time data streams, generative models can predict health issues before they manifest and suggest interventions, leading to a proactive approach to medical care. Despite its promise, challenges remain in ensuring data privacy, model transparency, and overcoming regulatory hurdles, but the ongoing advancements suggest a bright future for AI-driven healthcare solutions.

This paradigm shift not only accelerates biomedical research but also democratizes healthcare by making advanced diagnostics and treatments accessible to a broader population. As generative AI continues to evolve, its role in smart health and biomedical informatics will become even more pronounced, offering transformative benefits across the entire healthcare ecosystem.

The chapters within highlight practical applications across various domains, including genomics, medical imaging, and clinical decision support systems, all driven by AI's generative capabilities. They also delve into ethical considerations, data privacy, and regulatory concerns, emphasizing the need for responsible and transparent AI integration in healthcare systems.

1

Generative AI in Wearables: Exploring the Impact of GANs, VAEs, and Transformers*

Diwakar Diwakar and Deepa Raj

BBA University, Lucknow, India

1.1 Introduction

The integration of advanced generative artificial intelligence (GenAI) models—Generative Adversarial Networks (GANs), Transformers, and Variational Autoencoders (VAEs)—with wearable technology marks a revolutionary leap at the crossroads of personal computing and healthcare. This fusion is not merely evolutionary, but it represents a transformative shift toward crafting systems that are more personalized, adaptive, and intelligent, poised to redefine our daily lives, health management, and interaction with technology. As we navigate this transformative era, it is crucial to delve into the unique capabilities of GANs, Transformers, and VAEs, which stand at the forefront of AI research and application. These models excel in generating new content, ideas, or data patterns that closely mimic human creativity and understanding. From enhancing image quality and creating realistic simulations for health training to offering real-time language translation and personalized health insights, these AI models are pushing the boundaries of what machines can achieve. On the flip side of this integration is the rapidly evolving domain of wearable technology. In the last decade, wearable devices, including smartwatches, fitness trackers, health monitors, and smart glasses, have seen exponential growth in both adoption and capabilities. Equipped with an array of sensors, these devices offer a seamless

*This chapter explores how GenAI technologies in the wearable tech space, such as GANs, Transformers, and VAEs, have the potential to be revolutionary. In addition to providing insights into present uses and potential future approaches, it examines how these cutting-edge AI models improve accessibility, user interaction, and personalized healthcare. By means of in-depth examination and real-world examples, the chapter seeks to illuminate the creative incorporation of GenAI in wearables, emphasizing its influence on assistive technologies, health monitoring, and user experience.

Generative Artificial Intelligence for Biomedical and Smart Health Informatics,
First Edition. Edited by Aditya Khamparia and Deepak Gupta.

interface between the digital and physical worlds, collecting and analyzing data in real-time to provide actionable insights directly to the user. The synergy between sophisticated AI models like GANs, Transformers, and VAEs and wearable technology is set to unlock unparalleled opportunities. Envision wearable devices that not only monitor health metrics but also anticipate health issues before they arise, offering personalized advice and interventions tailored to the user's unique health profile and lifestyle.

However, this promising frontier is not without its challenges. Integrating complex AI models into wearable devices raises significant ethical considerations, particularly concerning AI-generated content and decisions related to health and personal data. Privacy and security are paramount, given the highly personal and sensitive nature of the data collected. Moreover, the technical hurdles of embedding these sophisticated AI models into compact, efficient, and user-friendly devices are substantial. Overcoming these challenges necessitates a multidisciplinary approach, blending expertise in AI, cybersecurity, ethics, and wearable technology design. Refer Figure 1.1 for the timeline of wearable devices.

As we stand on the cusp of this exciting integration, the journey ahead is fraught with obstacles. Yet, the potential benefits for personal health, well-being, and the overall human experience are vast. The integration of GANs, Transformers, and VAEs with wearable technology represents a bold stride toward a future where technology profoundly understands and enhances the human condition. It beckons us to reimagine the limits of personal computing and healthcare, promising a future where our devices transcend their role as mere tools to become partners in fostering a healthier, more personalized, and empowered existence.

1.1.1 Overview of GenAI and Wearable Technology

GenAI encompasses advanced subsets of AI that are capable of producing new content, ideas, or data patterns by learning from existing datasets. This capability is not merely about replication but involves a deep understanding and innovation that mimics human creativity and intelligence. Key models within this domain include.

1.1.1.1 Generative Adversarial Networks

GANs are a class of machine learning frameworks where two neural networks, a generator and a discriminator, are trained simultaneously. The generator creates data resembling the training set, while the discriminator evaluates its authenticity. In wearable technologies, GANs are instrumental in generating synthetic biological data, such as heart rates or blood glucose levels, enhancing privacy by avoiding the use of real user data and improving the robustness of health monitoring algorithms through extensive training datasets (1). This application is crucial

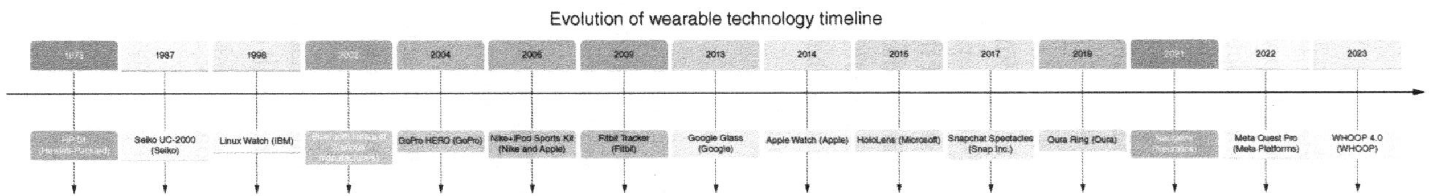

Figure 1.1 Timeline of wearable devices.

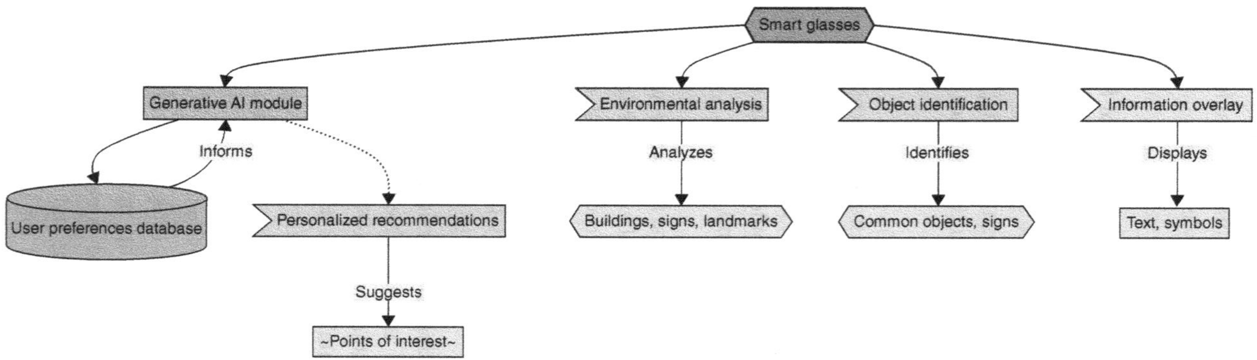

Figure 1.2 AI-driven smart glasses ecosystem.

their environment. This diagram showcases a smart glasses ecosystem where a GenAI Module leverages data from a User Preferences Database to provide personalized recommendations. These recommendations are enhanced through environmental analysis and object identification, which analyze surroundings and identify common objects and signs, respectively. The smart glasses then display this tailored information as an information overlay comprising text and symbols to the user.

1.2 Theoretical Foundations

1.2.1 GenAI: Concepts and Mechanisms

The term "generative artificial intelligence" (GenAI) describes a subset of AI that focuses on producing new information, ideas, or outcomes that are plausible and realistic based on underlying patterns in the input data but do not explicitly exist in the data. It stands out in particular because it can produce data in addition to just analyzing or categorizing it. The fundamental idea behind GenAI is built on machine learning models that produce new, similar instances of data by first learning the distributions of data in a specific domain (such as text, music, or photos).

Figure 1.3 flowchart displayed the integration of GenAI with a smartwatch for personalized health monitoring and advice generation. It begins with the smartwatch collecting health data, which is preprocessed for consistency and clarity. This data is then analyzed by a GenAI model, deployed on a cloud server or edge device, to generate customized health advice. Finally, this advice is displayed on the smartwatch, providing users with actionable insights into their health. This system exemplifies the use of advanced AI in wearable technology to offer real-time, personalized health recommendations, enhancing user health and wellness through data-driven insights.

1.2.1.1 Generative Adversarial Networks

GANs are a fascinating and powerful class of AI algorithms used to generate new data that resembles some given real data. GANs are used in various applications, including image generation, video generation, and voice generation. GANs consist of two major parts:

The Generator, GANs aims to produce data so realistic that it cannot be distinguished from actual data, by learning to transform a latent space of random

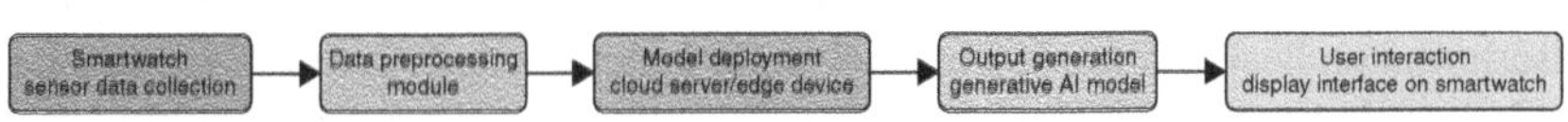

Figure 1.3 GenAI with wearable device.

noise into data that mimics real-world distributions. Its architecture, adaptable to the task at hand, typically involves a series of layers that begin with a dense layer to process the noise vector, progressively upsampling this input to generate the final data output. During training, the Generator's objective is to fool the Discriminator into misclassifying its outputs as real, employing gradient ascent on the $\log(D(G(z)))$ component of the GAN loss function, where z represents the noise vector, and G and D denote the Generator and Discriminator functions, respectively.

The Adversary (Discriminator) is like a critic who knows what real, high-quality wearable device designs look like. The discriminator's job is to look at a design and decide whether it's a real, high-quality design or a fake one created by the generator.

These two parts are trained together in a kind of game. The generator tries to make designs that are good enough to fool the discriminator, and the discriminator tries to get better at distinguishing real designs from fakes. Over time, the generator gets better and better at producing realistic designs, and the discriminator gets better at telling real from fake. The end goal is for the generator to produce new, realistic designs for wearable devices that are indistinguishable from real ones. The objective function for training a GAN is denoted as $V(D, G)$, where D is the discriminator and G is the generator. It aims to find the best parameters for both the discriminator and generator networks.

$$V(D, G) = \mathbb{E}_{x \sim p_{\text{data}}(x)}[\log D(x)] + \mathbb{E}_{z \sim p_z(z)}[\log(1 - D(G(z)))] \tag{1.3}$$

Here, $\mathbb{E}_{x \sim p_{\text{data}}(x)}[\log D(x)]$, computes the expected value of the logarithm of the discriminator's output when it receives real data x from the true data distribution $p_{\text{data}}(x)$. It encourages the discriminator to correctly classify real data as real. On the other hand, $\mathbb{E}_{z \sim p_z(z)}[\log(1 - D(G(z)))]$, computes the expected value of the logarithm of $1 - D(G(z))$, where z is sampled from a prior distribution $p_z(z)$. $G(z)$ represents the output of the generator when given noise z, and $D(G(z))$ is the discriminator's output when fed with fake data generated by the generator. This part encourages the generator to produce data that the discriminator cannot distinguish from real data. Basically, discriminator D, tries to maximize $V(D, G)$ so that $D(x)$ is close to 1 (indicating real data) and $D(G(z))$ is close to 0 (indicating fake data). Meanwhile, the generator, G, tries to minimize $V(D, G)$ by getting $D(G(z))$ close to 1, tricking the discriminator into thinking the fakes are real. The architecture of GANs is displayed in Figure 1.4. The diagram presents a GAN process where both the generator and discriminator are initialized with random parameters. The generator creates fake data that, along with real data, is evaluated by the discriminator. Based on the feedback, both the generator and discriminator update their parameters. This loop continues until convergence is reached, resulting in a generator that is capable of creating realistic designs.

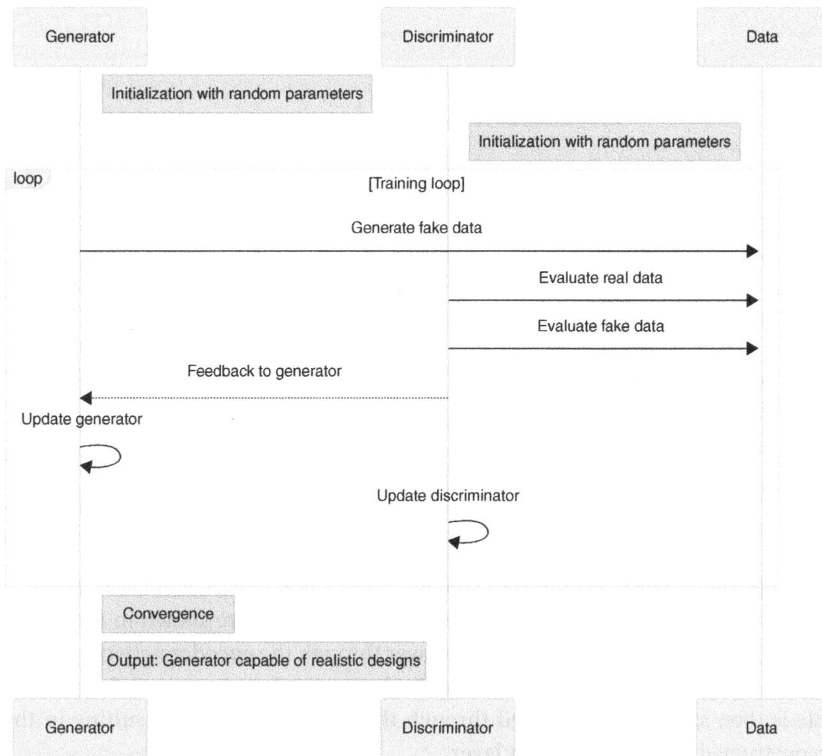

Figure 1.4 GAN training loop: generating realistic designs.

1.2.1.2 Variational Autoencoders

VAEs stand as a pivotal development in generative modeling, merging the realms of deep learning with Bayesian inference to forge a robust framework for data generation. VAEs excel in learning the intricate probability distributions of datasets, enabling the synthesis of new data points that mirror the characteristics of the original data. This section introduces the motivation behind VAEs and their significance in generative modeling. VAEs are predicated on the principles of variational inference, a Bayesian method for approximating probability distributions through optimization. The essence of a VAE is to encode high-dimensional data into a more manageable, lower-dimensional latent space, facilitating the generation of new instances from this condensed representation. The VAE architecture is composed of two principal components:

- **Encoder:** Transforms input data X into a latent representation Z, modeled by the distribution $Q(Z|X)$, approximating the true posterior $P(Z|X)$.

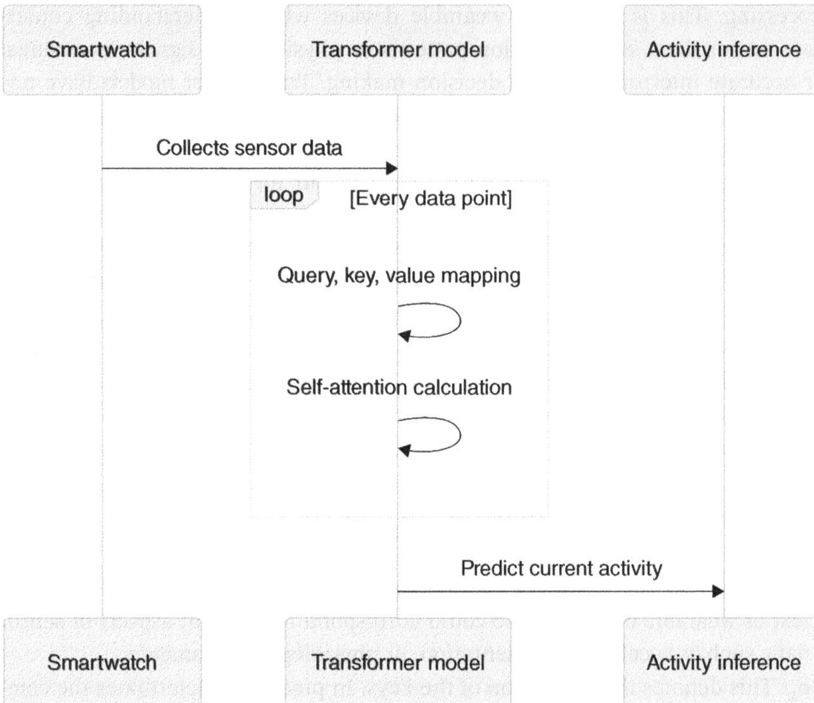

Figure 1.6 Smartwatch sensor data flow: transformer model activity inference.

of sensors capable of collecting comprehensive data about our physical activities, vital signs, and even our geographical location. These devices incorporate accelerometers, gyroscopes, heart rate monitors, and GPS modules, among others, facilitating an extensive range of functionalities from fitness tracking to health monitoring. This evolution has been propelled by significant advancements in miniaturization, energy efficiency, and computational power, enabling wearables to become more pervasive and seamlessly integrated into our lives. The advent of GANs, VAEs, and Transformer models has further expanded the potential of wearable technology. These GenAI models offer sophisticated data analysis capabilities, transforming raw sensor data into actionable insights and personalized experiences for users. For instance, GANs could enhance the visual data from wearable cameras for health monitoring, VAEs might be used for anomaly detection in physiological data, and Transformer models could improve natural language processing for user interfaces, making interactions more intuitive. Refer Figure 1.7.

The architecture describes how data from wearable sensors is processed and used to generate insights or actions. Here is a breakdown in simple terms:

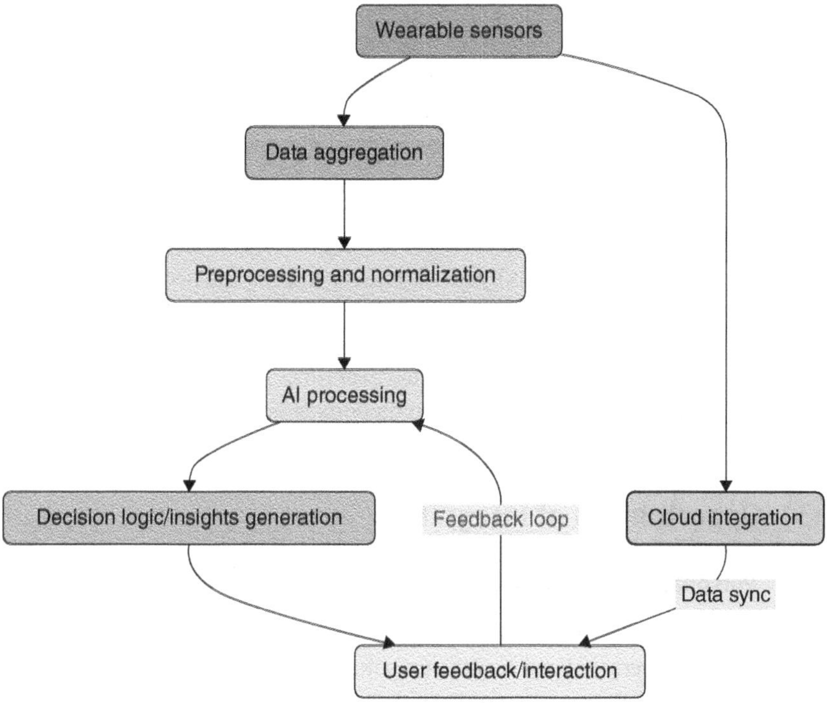

Figure 1.7 Data processing in wearable devices.

1) **Wearable Sensors:** These are devices you wear, like fitness bands or smartwatches, that measure various things such as your heart rate, how much you're moving, your body temperature, and where you are (using GPS). Each type of measurement is taken by a different sensor.
2) **Data Aggregation:** All the different pieces of data collected by the sensors are brought together in one place. Think of it as gathering all the ingredients you need to bake a cake before you start mixing them.
3) **Preprocessing and Normalization:** Before the data can be used, it needs to be cleaned and standardized. This is like making sure all your ingredients are the right quantity and quality before baking. Sometimes, the data is also encrypted to keep it private and secure.
4) **AI Processing (GenAI Models):** This is where the magic happens. The clean data is fed into advanced computer programs (AI models) that analyze it to find patterns or make predictions. For example, it could predict your fitness level or suggest health improvements.
5) **Decision Logic/Insights Generation:** Based on the analysis, the system makes decisions or generates insights. This could be as simple as advising you

to walk more based on your activity data or as complex as adjusting a health plan.

6) **User Feedback/Interaction:** The insights or recommendations are then sent back to you, possibly through the same wearable device, in a way you can understand and act on. This could be a visual display, spoken words, or even vibrations.
7) **Cloud Integration (Optional):** Sometimes, the data or the insights need to be sent to a cloud server for further processing, storage, or to be shared across different devices. This step is optional and depends on the need for additional computation or data management.
8) **Continuous Learning Loop:** The system learns from your reactions to the insights or from additional data collected over time. This feedback helps the AI models to improve and make better predictions or decisions in the future.

1.3 Opportunities of Integration

1.3.1 Personalized Healthcare Solutions

The convergence of wearable technology with AI has opened unprecedented opportunities for personalized healthcare solutions. The integration of AI algorithms can process the vast amounts of data generated by wearable devices to provide predictive health monitoring. This represents a significant shift from reactive to proactive healthcare management, where AI can identify patterns and predict potential health issues before they become critical. For instance, research has demonstrated the potential of wearables in predicting cardiac events by monitoring heart rate variability and other physiological signals.

1.3.2 Predictive Health Monitoring

Predictive health monitoring involves the analysis of data collected by wearables to forecast health events. Recent studies have applied machine learning techniques to wearable device data, demonstrating promising results in the early detection of conditions such as infectious diseases, sleep apnea, and heart disease. The algorithms can detect subtle changes in biometric data, which may indicate the onset of a health event, thereby enabling timely intervention.

1.3.3 Real-Time Diagnostics and Intervention Strategies

The real-time diagnostic capability of wearables can be instrumental in chronic disease management and emergency medical response. Wearables equipped with sensors for electrodermal activity and PPG can now work in tandem with smartphone apps to analyze data and provide immediate feedback. For example, smartwatches with fall detection algorithms can automatically alert emergency services and caregivers when a user falls, ensuring rapid response to potential injuries.

In summary, the integration of wearable technology with AI holds significant promise for transforming healthcare into a personalized, predictive, and real-time practice. It enables continuous monitoring, early detection of potential health risks, and timely interventions, which are crucial for improving health outcomes and the quality of life for patients. The continuous innovation in sensor technology, coupled with advancements in AI, will further enhance the capabilities and applications of wearable devices in healthcare.

1.3.4 Enhancing User Experience and Engagement

1.3.4.1 Adaptive Interfaces and Feedback Mechanisms

Adaptive interfaces in wearable technology tailor the user experience to individual preferences and needs, enhancing engagement by providing personalized interactions. These interfaces learn from user interactions, adjusting content, and functionalities to suit the user's habits and preferences. For example, smartwatches adjust screen brightness and information display based on ambient light and the user's typical screen viewing times. Feedback mechanisms, such as vibration alerts for physical activity reminders or auditory cues for navigation, play a crucial role in maintaining user engagement. They provide immediate, understandable feedback to actions or reminders, reinforcing positive behaviors and guiding users through tasks, significantly improving the usability and accessibility of devices.

1.3.4.2 Context-Aware Content Generation

Context-aware content generation leverages sensor data to provide information and services relevant to the user's current situation or environment. This technology uses location, activity level, and even social context to deliver tailored content, enhancing the user experience by making it more relevant and engaging. For instance, fitness trackers that suggest workouts based on the current weather conditions or smart glasses that provide real-time information about landmarks in the user's line of sight. This adaptive content generation ensures that the information delivered is not only timely but also maximally beneficial, encouraging continued use of the wearable device by keeping the content fresh and aligned with the user's current needs and environment.

1.4.3 Technical Challenges and Solutions

Implementing GenAI in wearables presents several technical challenges, including computational constraints, data privacy, and ensuring real-time performance. Solutions involve optimizing algorithms, adopting privacy-preserving techniques, and leveraging edge computing as discussed below.

1.4.3.1 Data Privacy and Security

Ensuring data privacy and security is paramount in the development and deployment of GenAI in wearables. This involves protecting sensitive user data from unauthorized access and ensuring compliance with global data protection regulations. Two critical approaches to enhancing data privacy and security are encryption and anonymization techniques, and the implementation of federated learning and privacy-preserving AI models.

Encryption and anonymization are crucial techniques employed in ensuring the security and privacy of data in wearable technology. **Encryption** involves converting data into a code to prevent unauthorized access during transmission between wearable devices and servers. The advanced encryption standard (AES) is a common encryption standard that employs a symmetric key algorithm. This process is represented by:

$$\text{Encrypted Data} = \text{AES}_{\text{key}}(\text{Plain Data}) \tag{1.10}$$

where AES_{key} represents the AES encryption process using a specific symmetric key.

Anonymization, on the other hand, focuses on removing personally identifiable information from the data to prevent the identification of individuals. Differential privacy is a technique often used in anonymization, which adds noise to the data or query responses to ensure statistical indistinguishability of the output of a database query. The Laplace mechanism represents a simple mechanism of differential privacy, given by:

$$M(x) = f(x) + \text{Lap}\left(\frac{\Delta f}{\epsilon}\right) \tag{1.11}$$

where $M(x)$ is the mechanism applied to data $x, f(x)$ is the original query function, Δf is the sensitivity of f, ϵ is the privacy budget, and $\text{Lap}(\lambda)$ represents Laplace noise centered at 0 with scale λ.

Federated Learning and Privacy-Preserving AI Models further contribute to maintaining privacy in wearable technology. **Federated learning** is a machine learning approach that enables multiple devices or servers to collaboratively learn a model while keeping all the training data localized, thus enhancing privacy. In federated learning, a global model is updated iteratively based on local updates from participants without exchanging raw data. The global model update in federated learning can be represented as:

$$w_{\text{global}}^{(t+1)} = w_{\text{global}}^{(t)} + \eta \sum_{k=1}^{K} \frac{n_k}{N} \Delta w_k^{(t)} \tag{1.12}$$

where $w_{\text{global}}^{(t+1)}$ is the updated global model at iteration $t+1$, $w_{\text{global}}^{(t)}$ is the global model at iteration t, η is the learning rate, K is the number of participating devices, n_k is the number of data points on device k, N is the total number of data points across all devices, and $\Delta w_k^{(t)}$ is the update from device k at iteration t.

On the other hand, **Privacy-Preserving AI Models** aim to protect user data during the training process. Techniques such as homomorphic encryption allow computations to be performed on encrypted data, yielding an encrypted result that, when decrypted, matches the result of operations performed on the plaintext. This enables AI models to learn from data without ever accessing the raw data directly. No specific formula is universally applied in homomorphic encryption, as it depends on the encryption scheme used, but the general principle is:

$$\text{Dec}(\text{Enc}(x) \odot \text{Enc}(y)) = x \otimes y \tag{1.13}$$

where Enc and Dec are the encryption and decryption functions, respectively, x and y are plaintext inputs, $\odot$ represents an operation on encrypted values, and $\otimes$ is the equivalent operation on plaintext values.

Encompass a range of methodologies aimed at enhancing data privacy and security in wearable technology. Model Compression for Edge Computing utilizes techniques such as pruning and quantization to reduce the size of AI models, making them suitable for deployment on wearable devices. Quantization. Differential privacy for data security employs mechanisms such as the Laplace mechanism, which adds noise to data or query responses to protect individual privacy. Ensuring data privacy and security is paramount in the development and deployment of GenAI in wearables. This involves protecting sensitive user data from unauthorized access and ensuring compliance with global data protection regulations. Two critical approaches to enhancing data privacy and security are encryption and anonymization techniques, and the implementation of federated learning and privacy-preserving AI models.

1.4.3.2 Computational Constraints

Computational constraints pose a significant challenge in deploying GenAI models on wearable devices due to limited processing power, memory, and energy resources. These constraints necessitate the development of optimized models and algorithms capable of operating efficiently within these limitations. Edge computing, which involves processing data near the source of generation rather than relying on cloud computing, addresses these challenges by reducing latency, conserving bandwidth, and enhancing privacy. However, it requires careful optimization of AI models to run efficiently on devices with constrained computational resources. Model optimization techniques such as model pruning, quantization, and knowledge distillation play a crucial role in this optimization process. Model pruning involves removing weights or neurons with minimal contribution to the output, reducing the model's size and computational requirements while minimizing the impact on accuracy. This process is represented by:

$$\text{Pruned Model} = f(\text{Original Model}, \theta) \tag{1.14}$$

where f is the pruning function and θ represents the pruning threshold or criteria. Quantization, on the other hand, reduces the precision of model parameters from floating-point representation to lower-bit integers, shrinking the model size and speeding up inference. The quantization process is represented as:

$$Q(v) = \left\lfloor \frac{v}{s} + z \right\rceil \tag{1.15}$$

where v is the original value, s is the scale factor, z is the zero-point, and $Q(v)$ is the quantized value. These optimization techniques collectively address the challenges of deploying GenAI models on wearable devices, ensuring efficient and effective operation within resource-constrained environments.

Energy-efficient AI algorithms are paramount for wearable devices, where battery life is a critical constraint. These algorithms aim to minimize energy consumption during both the training and inference phases through various strategies. Algorithmic efficiency involves selecting or designing algorithms that require fewer computations, memory accesses, and data movements. For instance, employing efficient convolutional operations like depth-wise separable convolutions in neural networks significantly reduces computational load and energy consumption. Hardware-accelerated computing further enhances energy efficiency by leveraging specialized hardware such as GPUs, TPUs, and FPGAs designed for parallel computations. In addition, dynamic voltage and frequency scaling (DVFS) adjust the processor's voltage and frequency dynamically based on workload, leading to significant energy savings. The energy consumption is approximated by the formula:

$$E = C \cdot V^2 \cdot f \tag{1.16}$$

where E is energy consumption, C is capacitance per clock cycle, V is voltage, and f is frequency. Lowering either V or f reduces energy consumption. These strategies are crucial for integrating GenAI into wearable devices seamlessly, ensuring advanced functionalities without compromising user experience due to battery life limitations or processing delays.

1.4.3.3 Integration and Interoperability

Integration and interoperability stand as essential pillars for the seamless integration of GenAI within the ecosystem of wearable technologies, ensuring efficient communication between devices and external systems for data aggregation, analysis, and meaningful utilization across platforms and applications. Standardization of data formats and protocols plays a pivotal role in this endeavor, involving the adoption of uniform data structures and encoding methods to facilitate data exchange and interpretation without custom adaptation. For instance, JSON (JavaScript Object Notation) and XML (eXtensible Markup Language) are commonly embraced standardized data formats, with JSON representing data as key-value pairs, thus being both human-readable and machine-parsable. Moreover, the standardization of protocols, such as HTTP, bluetooth low energy (BLE), and MQTT, defines rules for data transmission, with MQTT, for example, being a lightweight messaging protocol designed for low-bandwidth, high-latency, or unreliable networks, which suits wearables well due to its publish/subscribe model and minimal power consumption.

Standardization of Data Formats and Protocols refers to the adoption of uniform data structures and encoding methods for storing and transmitting data. This standardization facilitates the exchange and interpretation of data between different systems and devices without the need for custom adaptation. For example, JSON and XML are common standardized data formats used for data interchange. JSON, for instance, represents data as key-value pairs, making it both human-readable and machine-parsable. An example, JSON data structure for a wearable device might look like:

```
{
  "heartRate": 75,
  "steps": 1200,
  "temperature": 36.5
}
```

Standardization of Protocols involves the use of widely accepted communication protocols that define the rules for data transmission. Protocols such as HTTP BLE, and MQTT are commonly used in wearable devices for data communication.

MQTT is a lightweight messaging protocol designed for low-bandwidth, high-latency, or unreliable networks, making it well-suited for wearables. It operates on a publish/subscribe model, efficiently distributing data with minimal power consumption.

Modular Design and API Integration in the context of wearable technologies refers to structuring the system in a way that components or modules can be independently developed, replaced, or upgraded without affecting the rest of the system. This design approach enhances flexibility, scalability, and maintainability.

1.5 Ethical and Regulatory Considerations

The integration of GenAI in wearable devices brings forth a range of ethical and regulatory considerations. These considerations are crucial for ensuring that the development and deployment of these technologies are conducted responsibly, safeguarding users' rights and well-being.

1.5.1 Ethical Frameworks for AI in Wearable Devices

Ethical frameworks provide a set of principles and guidelines designed to guide the ethical development, deployment, and use of AI technologies in wearable devices. These frameworks often emphasize principles such as respect for human rights, justice, fairness, transparency, and accountability.

- **Principle of Beneficence**: Prioritizes the well-being of users and aims to maximize benefits while minimizing harm.
- **Principle of Autonomy**: Ensures that users have control over if and how their data is used, emphasizing the importance of informed consent.

References for ethical frameworks include documents like the *IEEE Ethically Aligned Design*, which outlines key principles for prioritizing human well-being in the age of AI.

1.5.2 Transparency and User Consent

Transparency involves clear communication about how AI systems work, how data is collected and used, and how decisions are made. It is crucial for building trust between technology providers and users.

User consent is a fundamental aspect of data privacy and ethics, requiring that users are fully informed about and agree to how their data will be used before it is collected.

- The **General Data Protection Regulation (GDPR)** sets stringent requirements for consent, including that it must be freely given, specific, informed, and unambiguous.

1.5.3 Accountability and Decision-Making

Accountability in the context of AI in wearable devices refers to the obligation of developers, manufacturers, and deployers to be answerable for how their systems impact users and society at large. This includes mechanisms for redress when harms occur. Decision-making processes involving AI should be designed to ensure that decisions are fair, nondiscriminatory, and can be explained and justified.

- **Algorithmic Impact Assessments (AIA)**: AIAs are tools for evaluating and mitigating the risks of AI systems, including biases and potential harms. They are part of ensuring accountability in decision-making processes.

1.5.4 Navigating Regulatory Landscapes

Navigating regulatory landscapes involves understanding and complying with the laws and regulations that govern the use of AI and wearable technologies. This includes international, national, and industry-specific regulations.

- For wearables with medical applications, the **Medical Device Regulation** in the European Union provides guidelines for safety, performance, and market surveillance.
- The **Health Insurance Portability and Accountability Act** in the United States protects the privacy and security of certain health information, pertinent to wearables collecting health data.

1.5.4.1 Compliance with Health and Safety Standards

It involves adhering to established guidelines and regulations designed to protect users from potential harm. This includes ensuring that wearable devices do not pose physical risks to users and that the data they collect is handled securely to protect privacy. For health-related wearables, compliance may also involve meeting standards for medical devices, which can include rigorous testing and validation processes.

1.5.4.2 International Regulations and Standards

It play a critical role in harmonizing the development and use of wearable technologies across borders. Given the global nature of technology development and distribution, international standards can help ensure that wearable devices are safe, reliable, and respectful of users' rights, regardless of where they are developed or used. Organizations such as the International Organization for Standardization (ISO) and the International Electrotechnical Commission (IEC) are involved in setting such standards, which can help guide developers and manufacturers in creating universally acceptable and ethical wearable technologies. Addressing these ethical and regulatory considerations requires a collaborative effort among technologists, ethicists, regulators, and users. By proactively engaging with these issues, the community can ensure that the integration of GenAI with wearable technology advances in a way that maximizes benefits while minimizing risks and harms.

Table 1.1 Health and fitness monitoring case studies with wearables.

Tools/Apps	Summary	Results	References
Impact of Fitbit on Physical Activity Levels	Investigated the effect of Fitbit wearables on physical activity among hemodialysis patients.	Significant increase in daily steps and overall physical activity.	Malhotra et al. (4)
Apple Watch and Cardiac Health Monitoring	Evaluated the Apple Watch Series 6 for cardiac health monitoring through pulse oximetry and ECG features in children.	Device demonstrated accuracy in measuring oxygen saturation and potential for cardiac health monitoring.	Littell et al. (5)
Garmin Devices in Stress Management	Explored the effectiveness of Garmin devices with HRV technology in managing stress.	Devices provided valuable insights into stress levels, aiding in improved stress management.	Jerath et al. (6)
Wearables in Chronic Disease Management	Cadmus-Bertram et al. focused on the use of wearable devices for managing chronic diseases through enhancing physical activity.	Wearables significantly aided in managing chronic diseases by promoting increased physical activity.	Cadmus-Bertram et al. (7)
The Role of WHOOP in Monitoring Athletic Performance	A study investigated the WHOOP strap's impact on athletic performance by tracking sleep, recovery, and strain.	Improved sleep quality, better recovery metrics, and enhanced performance among athletes.	Miller et al. (8)

1.6 Case Studies and Applications

The integration of GenAI in wearables has led to significant advancements across various domains, including health and fitness monitoring, mental health and well-being, chronic disease management, and emergency response and elderly care. Here are case studies of these apps/tools with real examples to help you understand them better. Tables 1.1–1.4 are highlights the case studies.

Table 1.2 Mental health and well-being case studies with wearables.

Tools/Apps	Summary	Results	References
Mindfulness Apps	Investigation into the effectiveness of mindfulness apps on reducing symptoms of anxiety and depression.	Significant reductions in anxiety and depression scores among users after 8 weeks of use.	Flett et al. (9)
Wearable Stress Detectors	Study on the accuracy of wearable devices in detecting episodes of acute stress through physiological indicators.	High accuracy in stress detection, correlating well with self-reported stress levels.	Can et al. (10)
Fitness Trackers and Mental Health	Exploration of how fitness trackers influence mental well-being by promoting physical activity.	Users experienced improved mood and reduced symptoms of depression due to increased physical activity.	Donker et al. (11)
Sleep Tracking Devices	Evaluation of the impact of sleep tracking devices on sleep quality and daytime functioning.	Improvements in sleep quality and daytime alertness were reported, alongside a better understanding of sleep patterns.	de Zambotti et al. (12)
E-Therapy Platforms	Assessment of e-therapy platforms for delivering cognitive-behavioral therapy (CBT) to individuals with anxiety and depression.	Participants showed significant improvement in anxiety and depression symptoms, highlighting the effectiveness of remote CBT.	Wright et al. (13)

1.7 Future Directions and Emerging Trends

1.7.1 Next-Generation Wearable Devices

The forthcoming wave of wearable technology is set to introduce groundbreaking innovations across multiple domains. Breakthroughs in materials science are paving the way for the development of biocompatible, implantable devices tailored for continuous internal health monitoring. These advancements enable seamless integration of wearables into the body, offering unparalleled insights

1.7.3 Ethical AI and Regulatory Evolution

As wearable technology continues to evolve, ethical considerations and regulatory frameworks play a crucial role. Techniques aimed at rendering AI decision-making processes transparent and comprehensible foster trust and compliance with regulatory standards. The establishment of standardized protocols for data privacy and security in wearable devices is imperative to safeguard user information. Robust frameworks for ethical AI development and deployment in healthcare wearables are essential to ensure responsible innovation. Policies facilitating secure and ethical sharing of health data across borders promote international collaboration and knowledge exchange. Providing controlled environments for testing new technologies under regulatory oversight encourages innovation while mitigating potential risks.

Table 1.5 Future directions and emerging trends.

Area	Emerging Trends
Next-Generation Wearable Devices	Biocompatible Electronics for Implantable Sensors
	Triboelectric Nanogenerators (TENGs)
	AR Integration
	Smart Textiles with Embedded Sensors
	Exoskeletons with AI-driven Adaptive Control
Advances in Gen AI Techniques	Federated Learning for Personalized Health Insights
	Emotion AI for Mental Health
	GANs for Synthetic Data Generation
	Neurosymbolic AI for Enhanced Decision Making
	Digital Twins for Personalized Medicine
Ethical AI and Regulatory Evolution	Explainable AI (XAI) in Healthcare
	Global Data Privacy Standards for Wearables
	AI Governance Frameworks
	Cross-border Data Sharing and Collaboration
	Regulatory Sandboxes for AI Innovation
Cross-Industry Collaborations and Innovations	Public–Private Partnerships for Health Tech Innovation
	AI Consortia for Standards Development
	Open Innovation Platforms for Wearable Tech
	Blockchain for Secure Health Data Exchange
	Integration with Emerging Technologies

1.7.4 Cross-Industry Collaborations and Innovations

Collaboration and convergence across diverse industries drive the evolution of wearable technology. Collaborative efforts between health agencies, tech companies, and healthcare providers accelerate the pace of innovation in wearable health technologies. Industry consortia dedicated to establishing technical and ethical standards for AI in wearables promote interoperability and ensure industry-wide best practices. Shared resources and collaborative platforms facilitate accelerated development and deployment of wearable technologies. Leveraging blockchain technology ensures a secure, decentralized exchange of health data, enhancing data integrity and privacy. Integration with emerging technologies such as IoT, 5G, and edge computing enhances the capabilities of wearables, enabling more robust and real-time health monitoring solutions. Table 1.5 provides a complete overview of the current innovations and methodologies across several areas. By deconstructing these complexities, we get insight into the growing landscape of wearable technology and identify the primary paths influencing its future trajectory.

1.8 Conclusion

The exploration of GenAI in wearable devices unveils a transformative intersection of technology and healthcare, promising to redefine personal health monitoring, disease management, and the overall human–technology interface. This conclusion synthesizes the key points discussed, outlines the challenges ahead, and presents a vision for the future of this dynamic field.

1.8.1 Summary of Key Points

- **Integration of GenAI and Wearables:** The integration of GenAI with wearable technology has significantly enhanced the capability of these devices in providing personalized health insights, real-time monitoring, and predictive analytics for various health conditions.
- **Innovations in Wearable Devices:** Next-generation wearable devices are evolving to become more integrated, personalized, and capable of complex health monitoring tasks, thanks to advances in sensor technology, materials science, and AI algorithms.
- **Advancements in AI Techniques:** Significant advancements in AI techniques, including federated learning, emotion AI, and neurosymbolic AI, improve the functionality and reliability of wearable devices.
- **Ethical and Regulatory Considerations:** Ethical AI development and regulatory evolution are critical to ensuring that advancements in wearable technologies are deployed responsibly and benefit society equitably.

1.8.2 Challenges Ahead

- **Data Privacy and Security:** Ensuring the privacy and security of personal health data collected by wearable devices remains a paramount challenge.
- **Interoperability and Standardization:** Achieving interoperability among different wearable devices and healthcare systems is essential for maximizing their utility and adoption.
- **Addressing Bias and Inequality:** Mitigating bias in AI algorithms and ensuring wearable technologies' accessibility and benefits to diverse populations are ongoing challenges.
- **Regulatory Adaptation:** Regulatory frameworks must adapt quickly to address new ethical dilemmas, privacy concerns, and safety issues without stifling innovation.

1.8.3 Vision for the Future of GenAI and Wearable Devices

The future of GenAI and wearable devices is envisioned as a harmonious blend of technology and human health, where wearables become an integral part of daily life, seamlessly providing health insights and interventions. This vision includes ubiquitous health monitoring, empowered individuals, a collaborative healthcare ecosystem, and the development of ethical and inclusive technology, making personalized healthcare a reality for individuals worldwide.

References

1 Goodfellow, I., Pouget-Abadie, J., Mirza, M. et al. (2014). Generative adversarial nets. *Advances in Neural Information Processing Systems 27*.

2 Kingma, D.P. and Welling, M. (2013). Auto-encoding variational bayes. *arXiv preprint arXiv:1312.6114*.

3 Vaswani, A., Shazeer, N., Parmar, N. et al. (2017). Attention is all you need. *Advances in Neural Information Processing Systems 30*.

4 Malhotra, R., Rahimi, S., Agarwal, U. et al. (2023). The impact of a wearable activity tracker and structured feedback program on physical activity in hemodialysis patients: the Step4Life pilot randomized controlled trial. *American Journal of Kidney Diseases* 82 (1): 75–83. https://doi.org/10.1053/j.ajkd.2022.12.011.

5 Littell, L., Roelle, L., Dalal, A. et al. (2022). Assessment of Apple Watch Series 6 pulse oximetry and electrocardiograms in a pediatric population. *PLOS Digital Health* 1 (8): e0000051. https://doi.org/10.1371/journal.pdig.0000051.

6 Jerath, R., Syam, M., and Ahmed, S. (2023). The future of stress management: integration of smartwatches and HRV technology. *Sensors* 23: 7314. https://doi.org/10.3390/s23177314.

7 Cadmus-Bertram, L., Marcus, B.H., Patterson, R.E. et al. (2015). Use of the Fitbit to measure adherence to a physical activity intervention among overweight or obese, postmenopausal women: self-monitoring trajectory during 16 weeks. *JMIR mHealth and uHealth* 3 (4): e96. https://doi.org/10.2196/mhealth.4229.

8 Miller, D.J., Lastella, M., Scanlan, A.T. et al. (2020). A validation study of the WHOOP strap against polysomnography to assess sleep. *Journal of Sports Sciences* 38 (22): 2631–2636. https://doi.org/10.1080/02640414.2020.1797448.

9 Flett, J.A.M., Hayne, H., Riordan, B.C. et al. (2019). Mobile mindfulness meditation: a randomised controlled trial of the effect of two popular apps on mental health. *Mindfulness* 10 (5): 863–876. https://doi.org/10.1007/s12671-018-1050-9.

10 Can, Y.S., Chalabianloo, N., Ekiz, D., and Ersoy, C. (2019). Continuous stress detection using wearable sensors in real life: algorithmic programming contest case study. *Sensors (Basel)* 19 (8): 1849. https://doi.org/10.3390/s19081849.

11 Donker, T., Petrie, K., Proudfoot, J. et al. (2013). Smartphones for smarter delivery of mental health programs: a systematic review. *Journal of Medical Internet Research* 15 (11): e247. https://doi.org/10.2196/jmir.2791.

12 de Zambotti, M., Goldstone, A., Claudatos, S. et al. (2018). A validation study of Fitbit charge 2™ compared with polysomnography in adults. *Chronobiology International* 35 (4): 465–476. https://doi.org/10.1080/07420528.2017.1413578.

13 Wright, J.H., Owen, J.J., Richards, D. et al. (2019). Computer-assisted cognitive-behavior therapy for depression: a systematic review and meta-analysis. *The Journal of Clinical Psychiatry* 80 (2): 18r12188. https://doi.org/10.4088/JCP.18r12188.

14 Beck, R.W., Riddlesworth, T., Ruedy, K. et al. (2017). Effect of continuous glucose monitoring on glycemic control in adults with type 1 diabetes using insulin injections: the diamond randomized clinical trial. *JAMA* 317 (4): 371–378. https://doi.org/10.1001/jama.2016.19975.

15 Turakhia, M.P., Desai, M., Hedlin, H. et al. (2019). Rationale and design of a large-scale, app-based study to identify cardiac arrhythmias using a smartwatch: the apple heart study. *American Heart Journal* 207: 66–75. https://doi.org/10.1016/j.ahj.2018.09.002.

16 Merchant, R.K., Inamdar, R., and Quade, R.C. (2016). Effectiveness of population health management using the propeller health asthma platform: a randomized clinical trial. *The Journal of Allergy and Clinical Immunology: In Practice* 4 (3): 455–463. https://doi.org/10.1016/j.jaip.2015.11.022.

for patients, healthcare providers, and software vendors. Given these concerns, this chapter delves into the development and integration of AI in our health and information systems, with a focus on maintaining privacy and security. The use of AI in healthcare informatics has transformed the diagnosis, treatment, and management of medical conditions. The integration of AI in healthcare opens a possibility of outcome enhancement and a way of making healthcare delivery more effective. Nevertheless, such development has drawn focus on different privacy and security-related issues that need to be resolved for the usage of AI applications in healthcare services in an ethical way. Since AI algorithms need information like medical records, genetic data, or images from scans to analyze, it tells us that the privacy of the patient's data needs to be prioritized at any cost to avoid data leakage, breaches, or misuse of information [1].

The recent incorporation of AI into healthcare informatics is considered a significant turning point in the field of technology. AI showcases innovative possibilities and holds appreciable promise for advancements in medical diagnosis, treatment, and ultimately, the well-being of the patient. However, these technological advancements have led to hefty concerns about data privacy and security, which leads to a desperate need for a resolution that allows the ethical deployment of AI-driven healthcare informatics systems. Consequently, since AI algorithms increasingly rely on extensive amounts of sensitive patient information that include medical histories, genetic profiles, and diagnostic images, there is a mandatory need to prioritize the protection of personally identifiable information and strengthen cyber defense techniques. In this regard, this chapter covers the complexity of privacy and security challenges in AI-based healthcare informatics concerning issues such as data acquisition, retention, processing, and propagation within AI-based applications. Moreover, it will also discuss the possible impacts of data privacy breaches and vulnerabilities in AI-based healthcare systems while focusing on the desperate need for strong safeguards, ethical considerations, and regulatory frameworks to protect patient information [2].

In healthcare, two essential tasks are screening and diagnosis, as well as treatment and monitoring. Screening and diagnosis involve reviewing patients' medical history, conducting physical examinations, and running diagnostic tests to accurately identify health conditions. Treatment and monitoring include planning, implementing, and assessing therapeutic interventions to prevent diseases and promote patients' well-being. These steps are crucial in delivering effective healthcare, helping healthcare professionals create personalized treatment plans and track patients' progress.

Machine learning (ML), a subset of AI, offers tremendous potential for improving healthcare outcomes by analyzing vast amounts of data and identifying trends that can inform better decision-making. Unlike traditional analytical approaches, ML algorithms have a flexible nature that enables them to predict and diagnose diseases with greater accuracy. As scientists continue to refine this technology, we can expect ML to have a transformative impact across a wide range of fields. In healthcare, for example, ML algorithms can identify patterns and relationships in large datasets, providing insights that were previously impossible to obtain. These models can enhance hypothesis creation and testing, yielding critical insights into illness epidemiology, treatment efficacy, and resource utilization. However, the use of ML in healthcare must be approached with caution and careful consideration of ethical, regulatory, and practical implications to ensure that patient data is used responsibly and for the benefit of all [3].

2.1.2 Utilization of LLMs in Healthcare

Large language models (LLMs) have led to a marvelous revolution in the field of healthcare. These models can understand natural language questions and even exhibit some medical knowledge, which is quite revolutionary and disturbing at the same time. Earlier, when larger NLP systems were being designed for tasks such as speech recognition, sentiment analysis, or even translation, pretrained language models (PLMs) were predominantly utilized as their constituent parts. But recently, these PLMs have become much more capable of functioning independently. Let's consider the example of OpenAI's LLMs like ChatGPT and GPT-4; they may perform well on various NLP challenges and even be well-versed in scientific fields such as biology or medicine. Another LLM called Med-PaLM 2 by Google has been optimized specifically for medical purposes. It is the first of its kind to make a distinction between an examination written by a professional doctor and one that is passed by the model itself.

LLMs represent two key improvements over pretrained language models (PLMs). They have moved from being discriminative (concentrating on classifying things) to generative (generating new things). Secondly, they are more data-driven instead of model-driven. The assessment done on PLM was majorly centered on some activities, including named entity recognition, relation extraction, and textual entailment. These are discriminatory activities. LLMs, on the other hand, can produce fresh content by responding to inquiries like talking to humans. This is because these generative algorithms need to grasp the underlying data first before generating anything new. This move toward generative AI has opened up various opportunities for applications, such as composing different forms of creative literature, making translations from languages more natural, and even summarizing complicated information in an interesting manner.

However, acknowledging the difficulties associated with integrating LLMs into healthcare systems is essential. In relation to this, patient data privacy and security are primary concerns since LLMs always rely on large volumes of sensitive patient information. At the same time, careful assessment and ongoing monitoring of accuracy and reliability are necessary so that they work correctly. Nonetheless, there are obvious potential benefits of applying LLMs in managing a health system well, though it comes with some challenges. Regarding LLM technology advancements, we should anticipate their growing significance in enhancing healthcare provision systems and outcomes for patients [16].

2.2 Drawbacks and Their Possible Solutions

The healthcare industry is shaking up. The sector must adjust due to the escalating cost of care and inadequate numbers of qualified professionals. In response, healthcare is adopting new technological solutions that may cut costs and address these problems. But healthcare systems all over the globe are already struggling with a range of issues, including limited access, rocketing costs, and inefficiency. Pandemics like COVID-19 expose weaknesses in healthcare systems, including shortages of protective gear, unreliable tests, overworked doctors, and most importantly, a lack of communication between healthcare providers. These crises reveal problems such as unequal access to treatment, a lack of convenient care options, and high costs with little transparency. However, they also provide opportunities to create innovative healthcare systems and improve administrative support. The COVID-19 pandemic exposed preparation gaps in our healthcare system, mainly due to shortages of protective equipment and reliable testing. The most significant issue was the lack of communication between healthcare providers, hampering response efforts. We must address these issues to create a robust and efficient healthcare system.

LLMs are an incredibly powerful tool for creating personalized educational resources that can cater to the unique requirements and literacy levels of patients. By seamlessly integrating LLMs into chatbots or virtual assistants, healthcare providers can provide prompt and accurate responses to patient queries, ultimately leading to a lighter workload and more proactive health practices among patients. The potential benefits of LLMs are truly immense and represent a major step forward in healthcare technology.

It is essential to remember that LLMs are tools whose efficacy depends on their developmental process as well as implementation. Thorough ethical considerations and proper data practices should always be ensured. One of the risks of biased training data is a skewed output from LLMs, possibly worsening existing health disparities. In addition, transparency plus explainability are very important features here. Both healthcare providers plus patients need to comprehend how the recommendations by LLMs came about so as to ensure trust and responsible usage [15].

2.2.1 Drawbacks

In the fast-developing sector of healthcare, the incorporation of technologies that utilize AI presents potential that has never been seen before for the purpose of enhancing patient care and final results. The protection of the confidentiality and safety of sensitive patient information inside AI-driven healthcare informatics, on the other hand, has emerged as a significant worry because of the promising breakthroughs that have been made. Both the protection of patient privacy and the implementation of stringent security measures are of the utmost importance in light of the exponential growth in digital health data and the growing reliance on AI algorithms for decision-making. To shed light on the urgent need for effective ways to avoid risks and optimize the potential benefits of AI in transforming healthcare delivery, the purpose of this introduction is to delve into the issues and drawbacks connected with privacy and security in AI-enabled healthcare informatics. Figure 2.1 represents the various drawbacks of AI-based healthcare systems.

a) **Data Collection Concern**: The hardest part of accessing relevant information is the main problem. These ML and deep learning models need huge datasets to effectively classify or predict various tasks. The major strides in ML enhancing its ability to generate more accurate algorithms have come from sectors having access to large datasets conveniently. In data accessibility for the healthcare industry, the suggestions made can be very challenging due to privacy concerns with patient records being sensitive in nature. Institutions are often reluctant to share health data due to privacy concerns [4].
   The development of AI is blurring the line between artificial and human interaction, resulting in hidden data collection and privacy issues. Patient consent is crucial, as demonstrated in Google's acquisition of DeepMind, where National Health Service (NHS) patient data were shared without permission

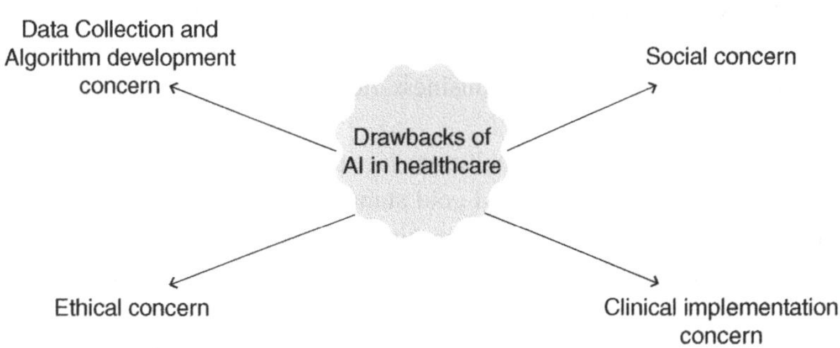

Figure 2.1 Drawbacks of AI in healthcare.

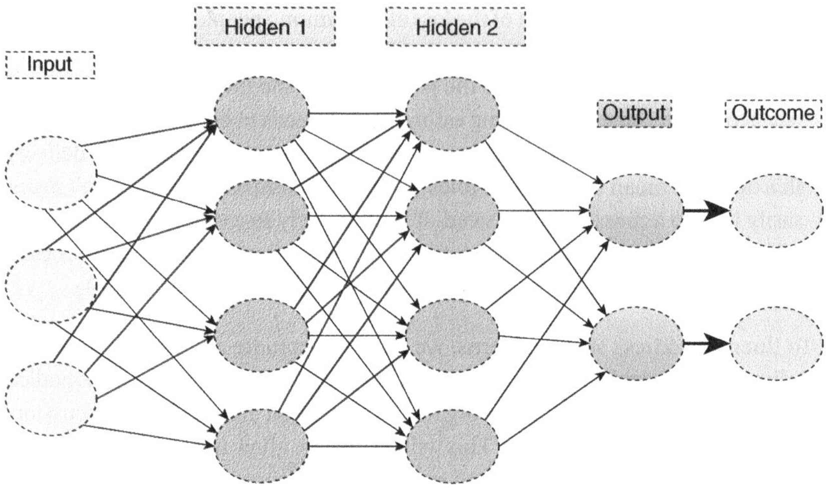

Figure 2.4 Process of deep learning: a subset of ML.

2.2.2 Suggested Possible Solutions

i) **Ethical Concern—Possible Solutions**: Few of the fundamental aspects of ethical considerations about AI-based healthcare systems include *fairness*, *responsibility*, and *transparency*. These concepts are crucial to make sure that AI technologies are being used in a responsible and ethical manner. Due to the inadequate nature of the datasets, the emergence of potential biases within AI informatics systems is one of the biggest concerns that needs to be urgently addressed. It might lead to divergence in healthcare delivery, particularly for marginalized or underrepresented groups. Moreover, due to the increasing recognition of a concept known as "automation bias," people blindly trust AI-produced recommendations or decisions, thereby missing out on important comprehensive factors [8].
Keeping all this in mind, *to* deal with such ethical dilemmas, there is a need for joint actions from various professionals across the healthcare ecosystem, including policymakers, researchers, healthcare providers, and technology developers. By emphasizing integrity, responsibility, and openness while building, implementing, and appraising AI systems in medicine, we can make use of AI's potential (in an ethical way) to enhance healthcare outcomes with minimum risks and maximum gains for everyone involved.
ii) **AI and Education—Possible Solutions**: All levels of AI education must be improved. AI should be taught to medical performers so that they can understand its principles and apply them effectively in clinical practice. In addition, they should be allowed to participate in making health policies that are

relevant to their profession. The inclusion of basics as well as tools and terminologies of AI in the medical curricula can prepare students for the future influence of AI on healthcare. Giving training sessions on the utilization of AI tools is necessary for both already-practicing doctors and aspiring doctors as it ensures that high-quality healthcare services are delivered within ethical guidelines [9].

In these sessions, participants should learn how to:

- **Assess AI Tool Effectiveness and Limitations**: Before incorporating AI outputs into clinical decision-making, clinicians ought to analyze its accuracy and dependability with a critical eye.
- **Applying Ethics in Using AI**: It is crucial to understand possible prejudices in training data sets or algorithms to ensure equal distribution of healthcare resources.
- **Preserving Patient Confidentiality and Security Privacy**: For instance, physicians must know about data security protocols when utilizing such AI systems involving intimate patient records [9].

- **Algorithm Development Concern—Possible Solutions**: Many AI algorithms are used and will continue to be used for clinical interpretation. However, a key question is whether these algorithms have been approved for clinical use. AI-based algorithms designed for clinical interpretation must undergo proper validation, either hardware- or software-based, as they are used by clinical experts for patient care and decision-making in diagnosis and treatment. Approval from regulatory authorities is essential for these purposes. In clinical trials, it's important to verify how accurately established AI algorithms perform compared to clinical standards like sensitivity and specificity of diagnostic tests [10]. In addition, it's unclear what appropriate validation of a continuous learning-based solution entails. A significant issue is that deep learning-based "black box" algorithms lack clarity, making them difficult to rectify compared to Bayesian models constructed on transparent structures [11]. Unlike traditional statistical models with clear cause-and-effect relationships, deep learning algorithms can arrive at accurate outputs through complex, opaque processes. Hence, there's an issue in understanding how an algorithm arrives at a specific conclusion, thereby raising concerns about potential biases and errors within the model.

2.3 Applications

In AI-based health informatics systems, it is quite essential to ensure the privacy and security of the data. There are several concerns we tackle through the application of AI in healthcare, including:

- **PHRS Exposure:** Encrypting data before hiring external services, splitting the healthcare system into separate parts, and checking how sensitive the data is to decide how private it needs to be.
- **Cyberattacks:** Detection methods like monitoring tools are employed to identify issues within a system, such as abnormality detection. System restoration through backup and recovery procedures or failover mechanisms are used to restore the system to normal function after identifying problems.
- **Eavesdropping on Data and Ensuring Data Confidentiality:** Data hiding and cryptographic techniques.
- **Threats to Identity and the Confidentiality of Stored Data:** Masking medical data with pseudonyms, managing identities, and ensuring anonymity.
- **Location Privacy:** Security protocols encompass a set of defined rules and procedures implemented to safeguard data, systems, and networks from unauthorized access, breaches, and malicious activities [12].

The CORONET model, utilized in this investigation, was developed to aid in assessing the necessity of hospital admission for COVID-19 patients based on their likelihood of requiring oxygen, given that oxygen therapy is typically administered in a hospital setting [16], and the severity of their COVID-19 condition, as predicted by factors such as oxygen requirement and risk of death. This approach established four key outcomes categorized on a scale from 0 to 3: discharged, admitted for at least 24 hours, admitted with oxygen supplementation (including ventilator support), and admitted with oxygen supplementation and subsequent death attributable directly to COVID-19, rather than to underlying cancer. These four outcomes served as indicators of disease severity. Unlike analyzing binary outcomes (e.g., oxygen requirement versus no oxygen requirement), this method enhanced the ability to present a comprehensive clinical overview essential for overall decision-making regarding hospitalization. The model underwent validation initially on an external cohort and subsequently on the latest data reflecting the Omicron variant. The CORONET tool is accessible online, featuring an interactive user interface compatible across different devices [17–19].

2.4 Devices

In this segment, we examine AI tools that have proven beneficial in medical applications. We classify them into three categories: traditional ML methods, newer deep learning approaches, and NLP methods [13].

2.4.1 Classical ML

ML employs data analytical algorithms to extract pertinent features from data. Inputs to ML algorithms typically encompass patient characteristics, including baseline information such as age, gender, medical history, and disease-specific data like diagnostic imaging, gene expressions, EP test results, physical examination findings, clinical symptoms, and medication records. Alongside these traits, medical outcomes such as disease indicators, patient survival durations, and quantitative disease measures such as tumor sizes are often gathered in clinical research settings. To provide clarity, we denote the *j*th trait of the *i*th patient as Xij, and the outcome of interest as Yi [13].

Depending on the inclusion of outcomes, ML algorithms can be categorized into two main types: *unsupervised learning* and *supervised learning*. Unsupervised learning is renowned for its capability in feature extraction, whereas supervised learning is adept at predictive modeling by establishing relationships between patient traits (inputs) and the outcome of interest (output). More recently, semi-supervised learning has emerged as a hybrid approach between unsupervised and supervised learning, suitable for scenarios where outcomes are missing for certain subjects.

2.4.2 Deep Learning: A New Era of ML

Deep learning represents a contemporary advancement of the traditional neural network method, characterized by networks consisting of numerous layers. The rapid advancement in modern computing has facilitated the construction of deep neural networks with a substantial number of layers, a feat impractical for classical neural networks. Consequently, deep learning can effectively probe intricate nonlinear patterns within data. Another factor contributing to the recent surge in deep learning's popularity is the proliferation of both the volume and complexity of data. Notably, the application of deep learning in medical research nearly doubled in 2016. Moreover, a significant majority of deep learning applications are concentrated in imaging analysis, a logical choice considering the inherently complex and voluminous nature of medical images.

Here's how deep learning is impacting healthcare:

- **Medical Image Analysis:** Deep learning models can analyze medical images with exceptional accuracy, surpassing human performance in some cases. They can be used for tasks like tumor detection, segmentation of anatomical structures, and disease classification.
- **Drug Development:** Deep learning can be used to simulate drug interactions and predict potential side effects, streamlining the drug development process.
- **Personalized Medicine:** By analyzing a patient's unique genetic and molecular data, deep learning models can help tailor treatment plans and predict individual responses to therapy [14].

a well-established regulatory framework along with powerful protocols for data protection, patients may not trust healthcare providers, which will ultimately lead to the rejection of AI-based technologies in healthcare systems.

To deal with such challenges, a multi-dimensional approach with a compulsory joint effort from different parties, like policymakers, healthcare providers, technologists, and regulators, is required. Having strong control over access rights is a great act of defense against information privacy threats. Furthermore, encryption techniques play a critical role in safeguarding information itself, rendering it unreadable to anyone who shouldn't see it (who does not have access to it). Finally, anonymization methods further reduce the risk by minimizing the presence of personal identifiers within records, making it more difficult to link the data back to specific individuals. Moreover, promoting clarity and accountability in AI algorithms, along with ensuring that the ethical guidelines are being adhered to, is of vital importance to encourage trust in AI-enabled healthcare systems. If we build patient privacy and security concerns directly into the design and development of AI healthcare solutions, we can make use of the transformative potential of this technology without sacrificing the well-being and privacy of patients in the digital age.

2.7 Future Scope

There are a lot of different ways that privacy and security issues can be fixed in AI-enabled healthcare computing in the future. As technology keeps getting better and healthcare processes become more digital, big steps forward are expected in a number of important areas:

i) **Better Ways to Protect Privacy**: In the future, researchers will probably work on making better ways to protect privacy, like federated learning and differential privacy, so that private healthcare data can be shared and analyzed while privacy risks are kept to a minimum.
ii) **AI-Driven Security Solutions**: Using AI-driven security solutions, like behavior analysis and finding strange behavior, will become more important to finding and stoping hacking threats in healthcare systems before they happen.
iii) **Regulatory and Ethical Frameworks**: As AI is used more in healthcare, strong ethical standards and regulatory frameworks will be needed to make sure that AI systems follow fairness, transparency, and accountability principles.
iv) **Interoperability and Data Sharing**: Improving interoperability and making it easier for healthcare providers, researchers, and patients to share secure

data will continue to be top priorities. This will allow for more thorough and personalized healthcare delivery.

v) **Patient-Centric Approaches**: As AI-enabled healthcare informatics advances, patient-centric approaches will become more important. This will give people more control over their health data and make it easier for patients and healthcare workers to make decisions together.

vi) **International Collaboration**: Because healthcare and data are global, it will be necessary for people from different countries to work together and push for standards to successfully address privacy and security issues in AI-enabled healthcare informatics.

Concerns about privacy and security in AI-enabled healthcare informatics will need to be dealt with in a wide range of ways in the future, including through new technologies, changes in regulations, and a move toward patient-centered care. By taking advantage of these chances and facing the problems that come with them, we can use AI to its fullest extent to make healthcare better while protecting patients' privacy and safety.

References

1 Milana, C. and Ashta, A. (2021). Artificial intelligence techniques in finance and financial markets: a survey of the literature. *Strategic Change* 30 (3): 189–209.

2 Urbina, F., Lentzos, F., Invernizzi, C., and Ekins, S. (2022). Dual use of artificial-intelligence-powered drug discovery. *Nature Machine Intelligence* 4 (3): 189–191.

3 Rasool, R.U., Ahmad, H.F., Rafique, W. et al. (2022). Security and privacy of internet of medical things: a contemporary review in the age of surveillance, botnets, and adversarial ML. *Journal of Network and Computer Applications* 201: 103332.

4 Ji, S., Gu, Q., Weng, H., Liu, Q. et al. (2019). De-health: all your online health information is belonged to us. arXiv preprint.

5 FDA (2018). FDA permits marketing of artificial intelligence-based devices to detect certain diabetes-related eye problems.

6 Fernandes, M., Vieira, S.M., Leite, F. et al. (2020). Clinical decision support systems for triage in the emergency department using intelligent systems: a review. *Artificial Intelligence in Medicine* 102: 101762.

7 Reed, J.E., Howe, C., Doyle, C., and Bell, D. (2018). Simple rules for evidence translation in complex systems: a qualitative study. *BMC Medicine* 16 (1): 92.

8 Anderson, M. and Anderson, S.L. (2019). How should AI be developed, validated, and implemented in patient care? *AMA Journal of Ethics* 21: 125–130.

9 Wiljer, D. and Hakim, Z. (2019). Developing an artificial intelligence enabled health care practice: rewiring health care professions for better care. *Journal of Medical Imaging and Radiation Sciences* 50: S8–S14.

10 He, J., Baxter, S.L., Xu, J. et al. (2019). The practical implementation of artificial intelligence technologies in medicine. *Nature Medicine* 25: 30–36.

11 Sussillo, D. and Barak, O. (2013). Opening the black box: low-dimensional dynamics in high-dimensional recurrent neural networks. *Neural Computation* 25: 626–649.

12 Jiang, F., Jiang, Y., Zhi, H. et al. (2017). Artificial intelligence in healthcare: past, present and future. *Stroke and Vascular Neurology* 2 (4): 230–243.

13 Rabbani, M., Kanevsky, J., Kafi, K. et al. (2018). Role of artificial intelligence in the care of patients with nonsmall cell lung cancer. *European Journal of Clinical Investigation* 48 (4): e12901.

14 Bocchi, C. and Olivi, G. (2021). Regulating artificial intelligence in the EU: top 10 issues for businesses to consider. https://www.jdsupra.com/legalnews/regulating-artificial-intelligence-in-3639576/ (accessed 19 July 2021).

15 He, K., Mao, R., Lin, Q. et al. (2023). A survey of large language models for healthcare: from data, technology, and applications to accountability and ethics. ArXiv, abs/2310.05694.

16 Lee, R.J., Wysocki, O., Zhou, C. et al. (2022). Establishment of CORONET, COVID-19 risk in oncology evaluation tool, to identify patients with cancer at low versus high risk of severe complications of COVID-19 disease on presentation to hospital. *JCO Clinical Cancer Informatics* 6. https://doi.org/10.1200/CCI.21.00177.

17 Lee, R.J., Wysocki, O., Bhogal, T. et al. (2021). Longitudinal characterization of hematological and biochemical parameters in cancer patients prior to and during COVID-19 reveals features associated with outcome. *ESMO Open* 6 (1): 100005. https://doi.org/10.1016/j.esmoop.2020.100005.

18 Burke, H., Freeman, A., O'Regan, P. et al. (2022). Biomarker identification using dynamic time warping analysis: a longitudinal cohort study of patients with COVID-19 in a UK tertiary hospital. *BMJ Open* 12 (2): e050331. https://doi.org/10.1136/bmjopen-2021-050331.

19 Freeman, A., Watson, A., O'Regan, P. et al. (2022). Wave comparisons of clinical characteristics and outcomes of COVID-19 admissions - exploring the impact of treatment and strain dynamics. *Journal of Clinical Virology* 146: 105031. https://doi.org/10.1016/j.jcv.2021.105031.

3

Generating Synthetic Medical Data Using GAI

Sudhanshu Singh[1], Suruchi Singh[2], and C.S. Raghuvanshi[3]

[1] *Seth Anandram Jaipuria School, Kanpur, India*
[2] *Department of Computer Science & Engineering; UIET, Chhatrapati Shahu Ji Maharaj University, Kanpur, India*
[3] *Department of Computer Science & Engineering, FET, Rama University, Kanpur, India*

3.1 Introduction

The human body, in its intricate dance of health and disease, generates a symphony of data. This data serves as the lifeblood of medical research, fueling breakthroughs in diagnosis, treatment, and drug development. Yet, accessing and utilizing real-world medical data often faces a discordant melody of challenges: privacy concerns that mute valuable insights, scarcity that leaves researchers yearning for more, and inherent biases that skew the tune [1, 2].

This part leaves on a dazzling investigation of this thriving field, diving into the musical exchange of inventiveness, decisive reasoning, cooperation, and correspondence. We'll unveil the powerful tools within GAI's repertoire, from the brushstrokes of Conditional Generative Adversarial Networks (cGANs) that paint vivid portraits of medical imaging to the whispers of Variational Autoencoders (VAEs) that decode the hidden language of genetic data [5, 6]. But like any symphony, the composition demands a discerning conductor. We'll fundamentally inspect the moral contemplations and likely entanglements of engineered information, guaranteeing it fills in as a steadfast reflection, not a misshaped reflect, of human wellbeing [12, 13]. We'll investigate the delicate amicability between data dedication and assurance, and examine techniques to mitigate tendency and support the skilled use of this astonishing resource [14, 15].

This excursion isn't intended to be a singular execution. We'll praise the spirit of facilitated exertion, developing relationships between researchers, clinicians, and mimicked knowledge subject matter experts. Envision interdisciplinary groups, where clinical ability guides man-made intelligence advancement, and simulated

Generative Artificial Intelligence for Biomedical and Smart Health Informatics,
First Edition. Edited by Aditya Khamparia and Deepak Gupta.

Like any maestro, the cGAN doesn't work alone. It has two key players:

- **The Generator:** A creative genius, the generator takes random noise as its canvas and, stroke by stroke, paints an image that resembles a real medical scan.
- **The Discriminator:** A discerning critic, the discriminator examines the generated image and compares it to real ones. If it can't tell the difference, the generator gets a thumbs up. Otherwise, it provides feedback to help the generator improve its composition.

Through this continuous dance of creation and critique, the cGAN learns to generate increasingly realistic images. This opens a treasure trove of possibilities:

- **Filling the Gaps:** When real-world data is scarce, cGANs can generate synthetic images to complete datasets, enabling researchers to train AI models more effectively.
- **Augmenting Data:** By creating variations of existing images, cGANs can help AI models generalize better and become more robust to diverse scenarios.
- **Personalizing Medicine:** Tailoring synthetic images to specific patient characteristics allows for personalized diagnosis, treatment, and drug development.

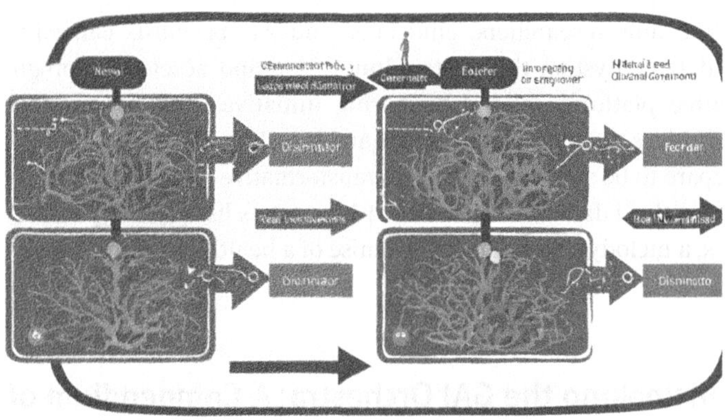

cGANs work like a game of artistic cat and mouse. One network, the **generator**, acts as the creative visionary, conjuring up new images based on the data it has been trained on. The other network, the **discriminator**, plays the role of the discerning critic, scrutinizing the generated images and comparing them to real ones. Through this iterative process, the generator refines its brushstrokes, learning to paint images that are increasingly indistinguishable from the real deal (Figure 3.1).

But cGANs are not just about mimicry. Their true magic lies in **conditional control**. Imagine the maestro being given specific instructions—"Paint an X-ray showing a fractured bone in the right wrist." By feeding the cGAN additional

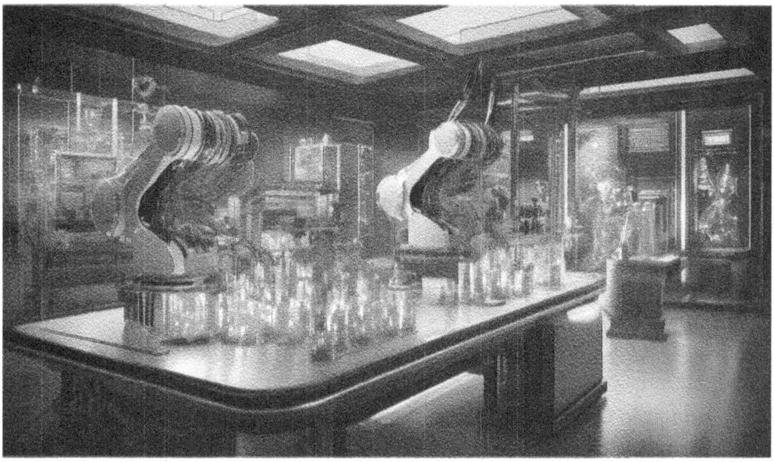

Figure 3.1 Robotic Automation.

information, like labels or text descriptions, we can tailor its compositions to our specific needs.

This allows us to generate images of:

- **Specific Pathologies:** Generate X-rays showcasing various types of fractures, MRIs revealing different stages of tumors, or CT scans highlighting diverse lung abnormalities.
- **Varied Patient Demographics:** Compose images representing different ages, ethnicities, and body types, ensuring inclusivity and generalizability of the generated data.
- **Rare or Unseen Cases:** Create synthetic data for diseases that are too rare or difficult to collect real data for, aiding in research and diagnosis.

3.2.1.2 The Ensemble Expands: Multimodal Data Generation

The cGAN orchestra doesn't limit itself to a single instrument. By combining its talents with other GAI techniques, it can compose **multimodal data symphonies**. Imagine seamlessly blending an X-ray image with a corresponding genetic profile or generating a 3D model of an organ based on its MRI scan. This multimodal approach offers a more holistic understanding of health and disease, allowing researchers to analyze various data types in concert (Figure 3.2).

The potential of cGANs in generating realistic medical images is vast. From aiding in diagnosis and treatment planning to accelerating drug discovery and personalized medicine, this AI maestro is poised to revolutionize healthcare. So, sit back, relax, and listen to the captivating symphony of cGANs, where the future of medical imaging unfolds, one brushstroke at a time.

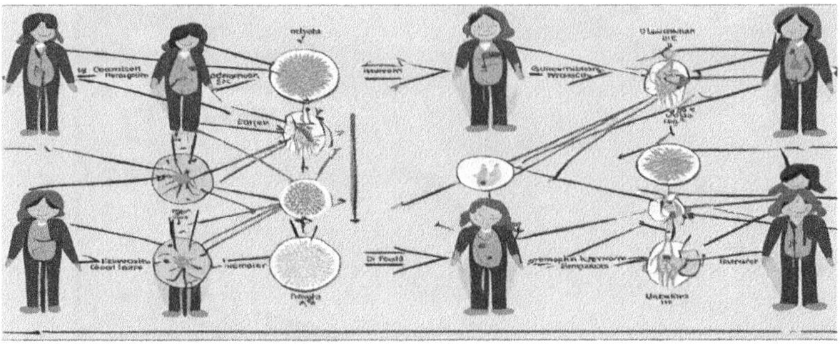

Figure 3.2 Multi model ensemble.

3.2.1.3 Tailoring the Composition: Conditional Control for Specific Needs

The cGAN's true power lies in its **conditionality**. Imagine the maestro conducting a specific piece, not just any random symphony. cGANs can take additional information, like patient demographics or disease markers, and use it to "condition" the image generation. This allows for:

- **Generating Specific Pathologies:** Need an image of a rare tumor? cGANs can be trained on specific datasets to generate realistic representations.
- **Simulating Disease Progression:** Studying how diseases evolve over time? cGANs can create sequences of images showing the progression of a disease in a virtual patient.
- **Creating Diverse Patient Populations:** Synthetic data can be used to create datasets that reflect the diversity of real-world populations, improving the fairness and generalizability of AI models (Figure 3.3).

3.2.1.4 The Ensemble Expands: Multimodal Data Generation

Medical diagnosis and research rarely rely on just one type of image. cGANs aren't limited to creating single modalities like X-rays. They can be trained to generate **multimodal data**, seamlessly combining different types of images, like X-rays, MRIs, and CT scans, into a single, cohesive representation. This allows for:

- **More Comprehensive Analysis:** By integrating information from various sources, cGANs can create a more holistic picture of a patient's condition.
- **Developing Multimodal AI Models:** These models can learn from and analyze multiple data types simultaneously, leading to more accurate diagnosis and treatment recommendations.
- **Bridging the Gap Between Modalities:** cGANs can generate intermediate data points that bridge the gap between different modalities, providing a more seamless understanding of the patient's health (Figure 3.4).

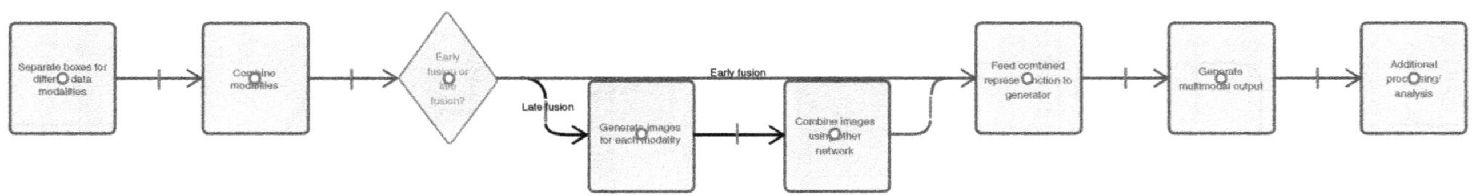

Figure 3.3 Multimodal data generation.

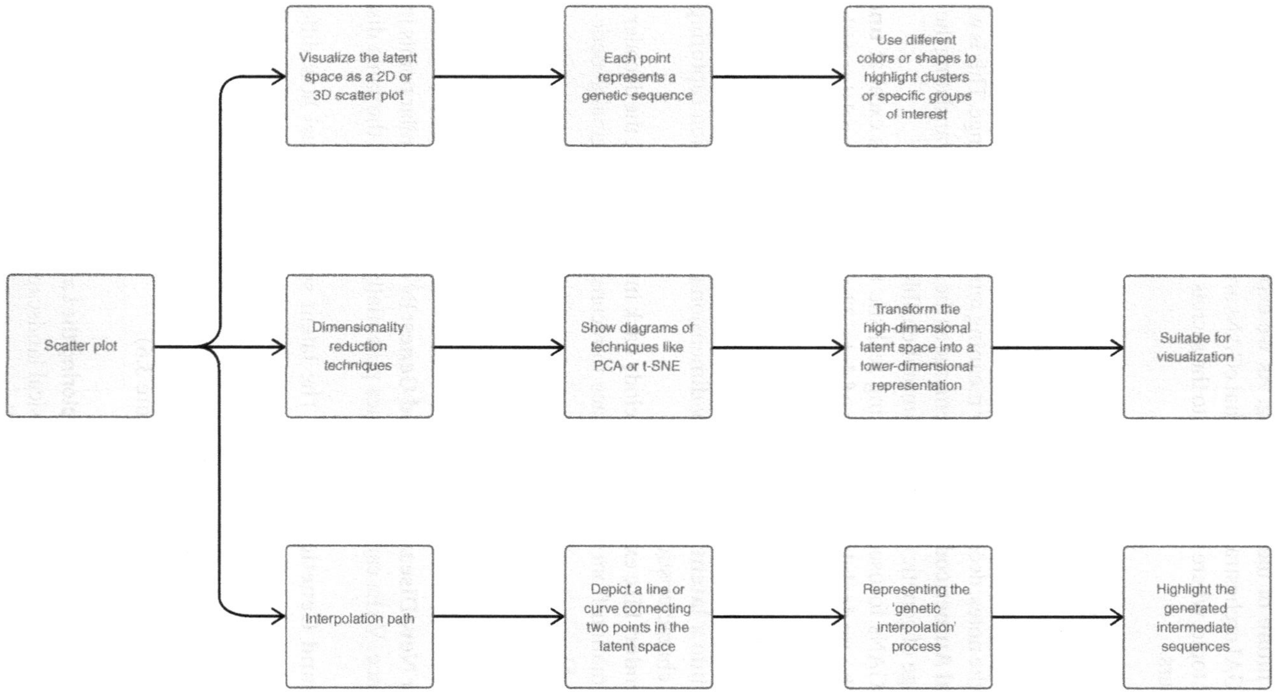

Figure 3.5 Data visualization process.

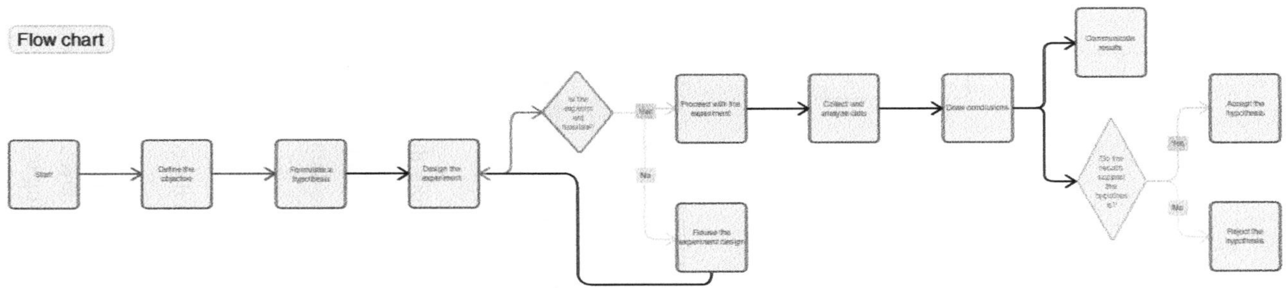

Figure 3.6 Experiment design flow chart.

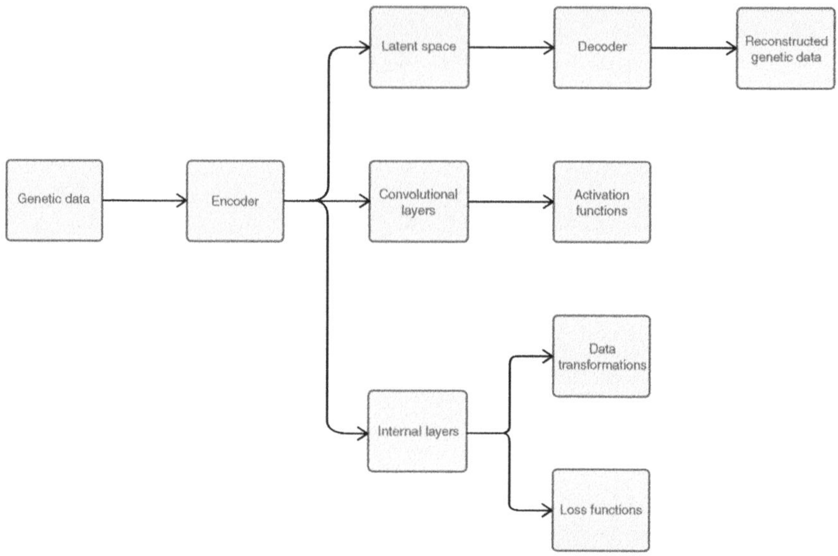

Figure 3.7 Data encoder.

- **Sampling New Genetic Sequences:** By randomly sampling points in the latent space, VAEs can generate entirely new, yet realistic, genetic sequences. This can aid in drug discovery by identifying potential drug targets or designing personalized therapies.
- **Interpolating Between Different Individuals:** Imagine smoothly transitioning between two individuals' genetic makeup. VAEs can create this "genetic interpolation," revealing intermediate states that might shed light on disease progression or complex traits.
- **Visualizing the Latent Space:** Using dimensionality reduction techniques, we can visualize the latent space as a map, where clusters represent groups of similar genetic profiles. This visualization aids in understanding the overall structure and relationships within the data (Figure 3.7).

3.2.2.3 Bridging the Gap: Connecting VAEs with Downstream Applications

The insights gained from VAEs are powerful, but they need to be translated into meaningful applications. This is where the connection to **downstream applications** comes in:

- **Drug Discovery:** Identifying genes and pathways associated with disease using VAEs can guide researchers towards developing new and more effective drugs.
- **Personalized Medicine:** By analyzing individual genetic profiles in the latent space, VAEs can help predict disease risk and tailor treatment strategies to specific patients.
- **Population Genetics:** Understanding genetic diversity within populations using VAEs can inform public health initiatives and address disparities in healthcare.

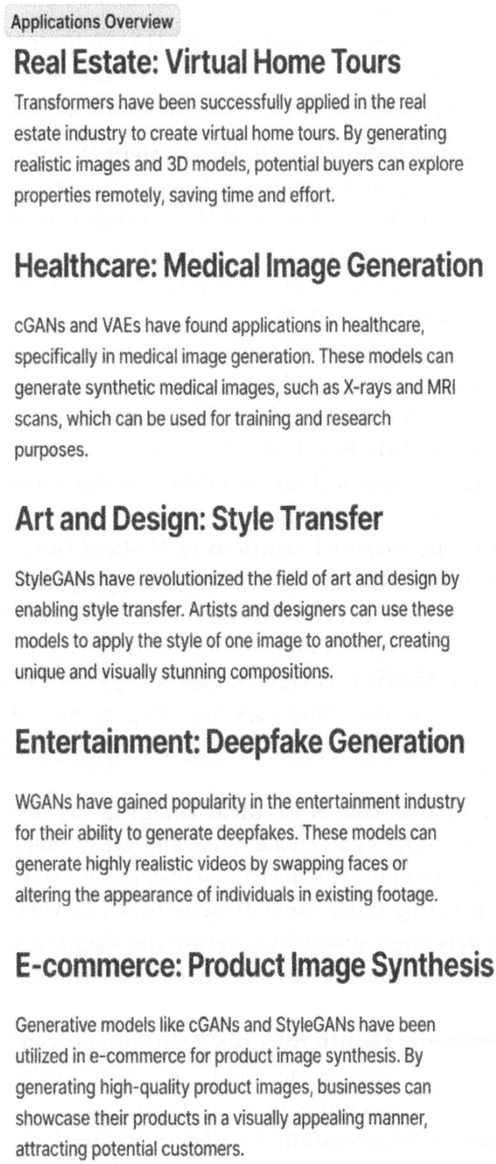
Applications Overview

Real Estate: Virtual Home Tours

Transformers have been successfully applied in the real estate industry to create virtual home tours. By generating realistic images and 3D models, potential buyers can explore properties remotely, saving time and effort.

Healthcare: Medical Image Generation

cGANs and VAEs have found applications in healthcare, specifically in medical image generation. These models can generate synthetic medical images, such as X-rays and MRI scans, which can be used for training and research purposes.

Art and Design: Style Transfer

StyleGANs have revolutionized the field of art and design by enabling style transfer. Artists and designers can use these models to apply the style of one image to another, creating unique and visually stunning compositions.

Entertainment: Deepfake Generation

WGANs have gained popularity in the entertainment industry for their ability to generate deepfakes. These models can generate highly realistic videos by swapping faces or altering the appearance of individuals in existing footage.

E-commerce: Product Image Synthesis

Generative models like cGANs and StyleGANs have been utilized in e-commerce for product image synthesis. By generating high-quality product images, businesses can showcase their products in a visually appealing manner, attracting potential customers.

VAEs are like the interpreters whispering the secrets hidden within the genetic code. By unveiling the hidden melody and exploring the vast landscape of the latent space, they offer a powerful tool to unlock the mysteries of human health and disease.

3.3 Beyond the Notes: Ethical Considerations and Responsible Use

3.3.1 The Conductor's Baton: Balancing Fidelity and Privacy

The GAI orchestra, while powerful, must be guided by a responsible conductor. In this symphony of synthetic medical data, the conductor's most crucial role is to balance fidelity and privacy. Just as a conductor ensures the music retains its essence while respecting the limitations of the instruments, we must ensure our synthetic data is realistic and valuable without compromising the privacy of individuals (Figure 3.8).

3.3.1.1 Synthetic Data for Good: Addressing Data Scarcity Ethically

Imagine a world where researchers lack real-world medical data due to privacy concerns or scarcity. This is where synthetic data becomes a force for good, ethically addressing data limitations and accelerating medical progress. By composing realistic synthetic data, we can:

Develop New Drugs and Treatments: Train AI models on synthetic data to identify potential drug targets, optimize drug design, and predict patient responses, ultimately leading to faster and more effective therapies.

Advance Personalized Medicine: Generate synthetic patient cohorts tailored to specific demographics or diseases, allowing researchers to test personalized treatment strategies without compromising real patient privacy.

Improve medical imaging algorithms: Train AI algorithms on synthetic images to improve their accuracy in tasks like disease detection and diagnosis, without requiring access to sensitive patient data.

However, the power of synthetic data comes with a responsibility: ensuring it doesn't violate individual privacy.

3.3.1.2 Differential Privacy: Composing Without Compromising Privacy

Think of differential privacy as a special notation system for the conductor. It allows us to compose synthetic data that is statistically indistinguishable from real data, even if it includes information from a single individual. This means we can gain valuable insights without ever revealing the identity or sensitive details of any individual participant.

Differential privacy works by adding carefully controlled noise to the data during the generation process. This noise ensures that any changes made to the data of a single individual have minimal impact on the overall statistics, effectively protecting their privacy.

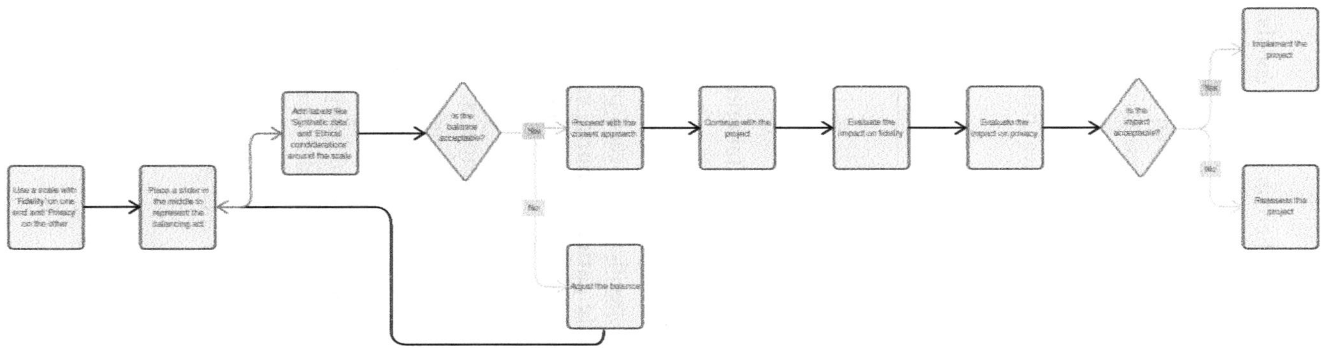

Figure 3.8 Synthetic data module implementation.

3.3.1.3 Federated Learning: A Collaborative Approach to Privacy-Preserving Data Generation

Imagine a decentralized orchestra, where musicians collaborate without sharing their individual scores. That's the essence of federated learning, a privacy-preserving technique for generating synthetic data. Here, the data remains on individual devices (like smartphones or hospital servers), and only the model updates, not the raw data, are shared. This allows for collaborative data generation while keeping individual patient information secure.

By utilizing techniques like differential privacy and federated learning, we can ensure that the symphony of synthetic medical data resonates with the ethical principles of privacy and respect.

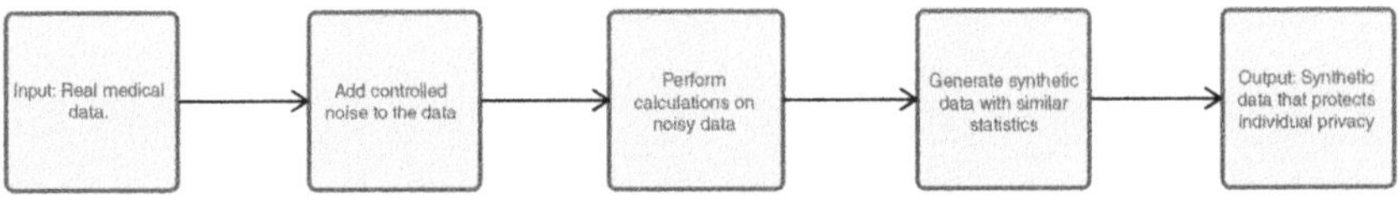

3.3.2 Advancing Personalized Medicine: Tailoring Treatments with Synthetic Patient Cohorts

Imagine a future where medical treatment isn't one-size-fits-all, but rather a personalized melody composed specifically for each patient. This dream becomes closer to reality with **synthetic patient cohorts**, virtual populations generated by GAI that mirror real-world diversity. By tailoring these cohorts to individual characteristics, we can:

- **Predict Individual Responses to Treatments:** Generate synthetic patients with specific genetic profiles, disease stages, and medical histories, allowing us to test and predict how different treatment options might work for each individual.
- **Develop Targeted Therapies:** Identify subgroups of patients who share specific characteristics and design personalized treatment strategies based on their synthetic counterparts' response within the cohort.
- **Reduce Medication Side Effects:** Test new drugs on synthetic patients tailored to individuals at high risk of side effects, minimizing the risk of harm during clinical trials.

These are just a few examples of how synthetic patient cohorts can revolutionize personalized medicine, leading to more effective and safer treatments for everyone.

3.3.3 Accelerating Clinical Trials: Composing Faster and More Efficient Trials

Clinical trials, the backbone of drug discovery, are often slow and expensive. GAI can accelerate this process by composing **synthetic clinical trial data**. Imagine:

- **Simulating Trial Scenarios:** Generate virtual patients representing diverse demographics and disease presentations, allowing researchers to test new drugs in a controlled, simulated environment before moving to real-world trials.
- **Enriching Real-world Data:** Combine real patient data with synthetic data to fill in missing information or increase sample size, leading to more robust and generalizable results.
- **Identifying Promising Candidates:** Analyze synthetic data to identify the most promising drug candidates early on, saving time and resources during the clinical trial process.

By composing synthetic clinical trial data, GAI can fast-track the discovery and development of new drugs, ultimately benefiting patients who desperately need new treatment options.

3.3.4 The Future Symphony: Unforeseen Opportunities and Challenges

The GAI orchestra is still tuning its instruments, and the future symphony of synthetic medical data holds both exciting opportunities and unforeseen challenges:

Opportunities

- **Disease Modeling:** Compose synthetic models of complex diseases to understand their progression and predict outbreaks.
- **Drug Discovery Beyond Traditional Targets:** Explore entirely new avenues for drug development by testing on virtual patients with diverse and rare genetic mutations.
- **Democratizing Healthcare:** Make personalized medicine accessible to everyone, regardless of location or resources, by leveraging synthetic data for broader clinical research and development.

Challenges

- **Bias and Fairness:** Ensure synthetic data accurately reflects real-world diversity and avoid perpetuating existing biases in healthcare.
- **Explainability and Interpretability:** Understand how GAI generates synthetic data and translate its insights into actionable knowledge for clinicians.
- **Regulatory Frameworks:** Develop clear and ethical guidelines for the use of synthetic data in medical research and clinical practice.

4

Automation of Drug Design and Development

Sudhanshu Singh

Student, Seth Anandram Jaipuria School, Kanpur, India

4.1 Introduction

The persevering quest for better lives fills the always advancing scene of medication. Drug disclosure and improvement, customarily a meticulous and asset concentrated try, remains at the front of this advancement. Notwithstanding, customary techniques frequently vacillate despite the expanding weight of illness and the consistently expanding intricacy of organic targets. This is where robotization arises as a groundbreaking power, ready to upset the medication improvement scene.

This segment dives into the enchanting space of motorized drug plan and improvement, exploring its ability to help the outing from molecule to prescription. We start by illuminating the constraints of standard techniques, highlighting the pressing requirement for imaginative philosophies. We then, at that point, leave on an enthralling investigation of the different features of computerization, inspecting: (i) Generative AI: Witness the power of artificial intelligence in conjuring novel drug candidates with tailored properties, ushering in a new era of molecule design [1, 2]. (ii) High-throughput screening: Discover the secrets of automated robots tirelessly sifting through vast libraries of compounds, uncovering hidden gems with therapeutic potential [3]. (iii) Computational modeling: Dive into the intricate world of simulations, where virtual laboratories accelerate the understanding of drug-target interactions, paving the way for optimized drug design [4, 5]. (iv) Data-driven decision-making: Leverage the power of big data analytics to inform critical decisions throughout the development pipeline, ensuring efficiency and maximizing success [2, 6].

This section rises above a simple specialized work; it fills in as a source of inspiration. We jump into the ethical thoughts incorporating automation, focusing on the

Generative Artificial Intelligence for Biomedical and Smart Health Informatics,
First Edition. Edited by Aditya Khamparia and Deepak Gupta.

necessity for careful execution that spotlights on human flourishing [7, 8]. Finally, we cast our look towards the horizon, envisioning a presence where motorization draws in experts to beat ahead of time ridiculous hardships, provoking a seriously encouraging future time for overall prosperity [9, 10].

This part jumps into the amazing universe of computerization in drug plan and progression. We will examine different robotization strategies, from high-throughput screening and mechanical innovation to man-made thinking and simulated intelligence [1, 4]. We will discuss the impact of computerization on different periods of the prescription progression pipeline, from target conspicuous evidence to lead improvement and clinical primers [11, 12].

Plus, we will take a gander at the hardships and potential entryways related with motorization in this field. We will address stresses over work movement, moral examinations, and the prerequisite for regulatory designs [13, 14]. At last, we will look towards the eventual fate of computerization in drug revelation and advancement, investigating arising patterns and likely forward leaps [15].

All through this excursion, we won't just investigate the "what" and "how" of robotization, yet in addition dig into the "why." We will enlighten the effect of computerization on the speed, cost, and achievement pace of medication improvement, featuring its capability to convey life-saving medicines to patients quicker and all the more proficiently [2, 16].

Get ready to set out on a charming investigation representing things to come of medication improvement, where computerization holds the way to opening another time of clinical forward leaps [17].

4.2 High-Throughput Screening (HTS)

4.2.1 Automated Robotic Systems for Compound Screening

- **Revolutionizing Drug Discovery:** Describe how automated robots have replaced manual tasks in HTS, significantly increasing screening capacity and speed. Highlight the advantages like precision, consistency, and reduced human error.
- **Types of Robotic Systems:** Briefly explain different types used in HTS, such as liquid handling robots, plate stackers, and grippers. Mention their specific roles and contributions to the screening process.
- **Examples and Applications:** Provide specific examples of robotic systems used in HTS for different types of assays (e.g., enzyme-linked immunosorbent assay, protein-protein interaction assays). Discuss their impact on specific drug discovery campaigns.

- **Challenges and Future Directions:** Acknowledge challenges like scalability, cost, and integration with other technologies. Briefly discuss emerging trends like microfluidics and miniaturization for further automation and optimization.

4.2.2 Virtual Screening using Computational Models

- **In Silico Drug Discovery:** Explain how virtual screening utilizes computational models to predict the interaction between molecules (e.g., drug candidate and target protein). Emphasize its cost-effectiveness and speed compared to physical screening.
- **Types of Models:** Briefly describe different types of models used in virtual screening, such as docking simulations, pharmacophore models, and

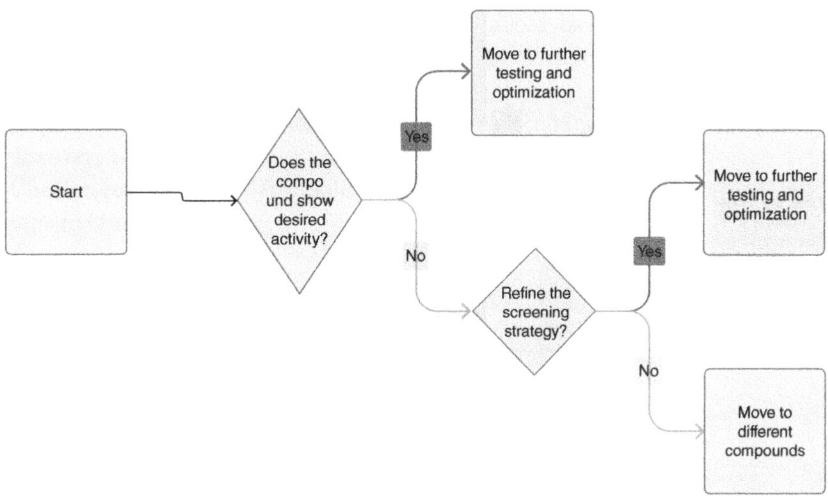

machine learning algorithms. Explain their strengths and limitations.
- **Success Stories and Limitations:** Showcase examples of successful drug discovery using virtual screening, like identifying lead compounds for cancer or neglected diseases. Discuss limitations like model accuracy and the need for experimental validation.
- **Future Directions and Integration:** Discuss how advancements in AI and machine learning are improving model accuracy and personalized drug discovery approaches. Highlight the potential for integrating virtual and physical screening for more efficient workflows.

- **Examples:** BenevolentAI's generative model discovered a potential treatment for Duchenne muscular dystrophy, demonstrating the potential of AI in drug discovery.
- **Statistics:** Generative models are estimated to increase the success rate of drug development by 10–20%.
- **Challenges:** Ensuring the safety and efficacy of AI-generated drugs requires rigorous testing and regulatory oversight.

4.3.3 ML-based Prediction of Drug Efficacy and Toxicity

- **The Challenge:** Predicting how a drug will affect a patient remains a major hurdle in drug development. Clinical trials are expensive and time-consuming, and traditional methods often fail to accurately predict drug safety and efficacy.
- **The AI Solution:** Machine learning algorithms can analyze vast datasets of drug properties, patient data, and clinical trial results to predict drug efficacy and toxicity with greater accuracy.
- **Examples:** Atomwise, a company using AI for drug discovery, has developed models that can predict drug toxicity with 80% accuracy.
- **Statistics:** AI-based predictions can potentially reduce clinical trial failures by 30%, saving time and resources.
- **Challenges:** Addressing the limitations of available data and ensuring the interpretability and explainability of AI models are key challenges.

4.3.4 AI-powered Drug Repurposing for New Indications

- **The Challenge:** Discovering new uses for existing drugs can be faster and cheaper than developing entirely new ones. However, traditional methods of drug repurposing are often serendipitous and lack efficiency.
- **The AI Solution:** AI algorithms can analyze drug properties, disease signatures, and patient data to identify potential new uses for existing drugs. This approach leverages the wealth of existing knowledge about established drugs, accelerating the repurposing process.
- **Examples:** Insilico Medicine used AI to identify an existing drug as a potential treatment for COVID-19, demonstrating the power of drug repurposing.
- **Statistics:** AI-based drug repurposing can potentially reduce the time and cost of developing new treatments by up to 70%.
- **Challenges:** Addressing regulatory hurdles and ensuring the safety and efficacy of repurposed drugs in new contexts are important considerations.

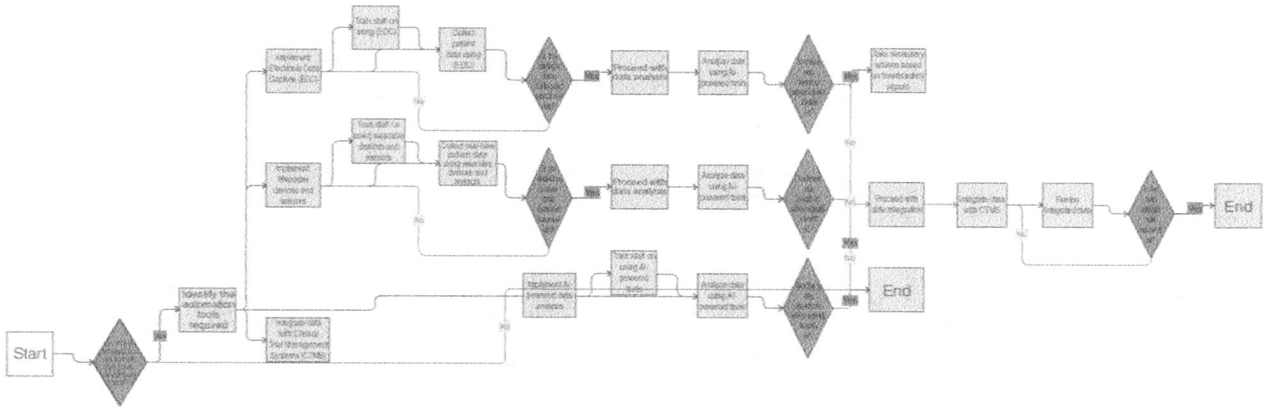
Start
Identify the automation tools required
Proceed with data analysis
Proceed with data analysis
End
End

4.4 Automation in Drug Synthesis and Optimization

The traditional process of synthesizing and optimizing drug candidates is often slow, tedious, and prone to human error. Thankfully, automation technologies are transforming this landscape, offering faster, more efficient, and data-driven approaches. Let's explore three key areas.

4.4.1 Robotic Systems for Automated Chemical Synthesis

Imagine robots meticulously constructing complex molecules with precision and speed. This is the reality of **automated synthesis**, where robotic systems execute pre-programmed reactions, eliminating manual interventions and ensuring consistency. Some examples include:

- **Liquid-handling Robots:** These tireless assistants accurately dispense and mix chemicals, freeing up scientists for more complex tasks.
- **Solid-phase Peptide Synthesis (SPPS) Robots:** These automated systems rapidly assemble peptides, valuable tools for drug discovery and development.
- **Flow Chemistry:** This continuous-flow approach allows for rapid synthesis and optimization of drug candidates, significantly reducing reaction times compared to traditional methods.

Example: XtalPi, a robotic platform developed by XtalPi Inc., automates the synthesis and purification of drug-like molecules. This system has been used to generate libraries of thousands of compounds for drug discovery projects, accelerating the identification of promising leads.

4.4.2 Flow Chemistry for Rapid Compound Iteration

Think of flow chemistry as a fast-paced assembly line for molecules. Unlike traditional batch reactions, where chemicals are mixed in flasks, flow chemistry continuously pumps reagents through microfluidic channels, enabling rapid synthesis and optimization. This offers several advantages:

- **Faster Reaction Times:** Flow reactions can be completed in seconds or minutes, compared to hours or days for traditional methods.
- **Increased Efficiency:** Flow chemistry uses less solvent and produces less waste, making it more environmentally friendly.
- **Real-time Monitoring:** As the reaction progresses through the microchannels, properties like temperature and pressure can be monitored in real-time, allowing for precise control and optimization.

Case Study: Amgen, a leading biotechnology company, adopted flow chemistry for the synthesis of AMG 515, a drug candidate for Alzheimer's disease. This approach significantly reduced the reaction time and improved the purity of the final product, contributing to the successful development of the drug.

4.4.3 In Silico Optimization of Drug Properties

Computers are becoming adept chemists thanks to **in silico optimization**. This involves using computational models to predict and optimize the properties of drug candidates, saving time and resources compared to traditional experimental methods. Some common applications include:

- **Docking Simulations:** These simulations predict how a drug candidate binds to a target protein, helping identify compounds with optimal binding affinity.
- **ADMET (Absorption, Distribution, Metabolism, Excretion, and Toxicity) Prediction:** In silico models can predict the potential side effects of a drug candidate, allowing researchers to prioritize compounds with better safety profiles.
- **QSAR (Quantitative Structure-activity Relationships):** These models correlate a drug's chemical structure with its biological activity, enabling researchers to design compounds with desired properties.

Example: Pfizer employed in silico optimization during the development of their blockbuster drug, Viagra. By using computational models to predict the drug's binding affinity and potential side effects, they were able to identify a promising candidate more quickly and efficiently.

4.5 Automation in Clinical Trials

The traditional clinical trial process has long been plagued by slow data collection, laborious analysis, and limited patient monitoring. However, a wave of automation technologies is transforming the landscape, promising significant improvements in cost, efficiency, and ultimately, the success rate of drug development. Let's explore three key areas of automation and their impact.

4.5.1 Electronic Data Capture (EDC) and Clinical Trial Management Systems (CTMS)

Imagine ditching paper forms and manual data entry for a streamlined, digital system. EDC software captures participant data electronically, ensuring real-time access, reduced errors, and automated data cleaning. CTMS platforms take it further, providing centralized management of clinical trial activities, from study setup to participant recruitment and drug administration. This translates to:

4.6.2 Regulatory Frameworks for AI-Driven Drug Development

Current Regulations: Existing regulations may not adequately address AI-driven drug development, potentially hindering innovation. Balancing safety and innovation requires developing clear guidelines for data quality, algorithm validation, and responsible use of AI in clinical trials [11, 12].

International Collaboration: Harmonizing regulatory frameworks across countries can facilitate global development and distribution of AI-driven drugs, ensuring consistent standards and patient safety [7, 17].

Stakeholder Involvement: Regulatory frameworks should be developed with input from researchers, industry, clinicians, and patient advocacy groups to ensure they are comprehensive, ethical, and practical [8, 16].

4.6.3 Job Displacement and Workforce Retraining Needs

Automation's Impact on Jobs: Automation in drug discovery could displace some workers, particularly those performing repetitive tasks. However, it can also create new jobs requiring expertise in AI, data science, and other technology areas [13, 15].

Reskilling and Upskilling Initiatives: Governments and institutions should invest in programs to reskill and upskill workers affected by automation, equipping them with the skills needed for new jobs in the evolving field of drug development [9, 14].

Ethical Considerations in Workforce Transition: Ensuring a just transition for displaced workers requires fair compensation, career counseling, and access to retraining programs to minimize negative impacts on livelihoods [10], [18].

4.6.4 The Potential for Cost Reduction and Increased Efficiency

Reduced Time and Cost of Drug Development: Automation can significantly reduce the time and cost associated with traditional drug discovery methods, leading to faster development of new therapies and increased affordability [19, 20].

Improved Resource Allocation: Automating repetitive tasks frees up researchers and scientists to focus on higher-level analysis and creative problem-solving, leading to more efficient resource utilization [21, 22].

Accessibility to New Drugs: Faster and more efficient drug development can increase access to new therapies for patients globally, particularly in underserved areas [23, 24].

4.6.5 Personalized Medicine and Tailoring Drugs to Individual Patients

Leveraging AI for Individual Patient Profiles: AI can analyze vast amounts of patient data to create personalized profiles, enabling tailoring of drugs to individual needs and genetic variations [25, 26].

Developing More Targeted Therapies: This approach can lead to more effective treatments with fewer side effects, improving patient outcomes and overall healthcare efficiency [27, 28].

Addressing Ethical Considerations: Personalized medicine raises concerns about equity and access, ensuring all patients, regardless of their background, have access to these advancements [29, 30].

4.7 Conclusion

The automation revolution is transforming the landscape of drug design and development, paving the way for a future where faster, more efficient, and personalized treatments become a reality. While challenges and ethical considerations remain, embracing responsible and innovative automation holds tremendous promise:

Accelerated Drug Discovery: Automation can significantly shorten the time it takes to bring new drugs to market, addressing unmet medical needs with greater urgency.

Reduced Costs and Increased Accessibility: By streamlining processes and optimizing resource allocation, automation can reduce the cost of drug development, making them more accessible to patients globally.

Personalized Medicine: Simulated intelligence controlled apparatuses can prepare for fitting therapies to individual patients in light of their remarkable hereditary cosmetics and clinical history, prompting more compelling and designated treatments.

However, navigating this future responsibly requires addressing key considerations:

Ethical Frameworks: Robust ethical frameworks are crucial to ensure fairness, transparency, and responsible use of AI in drug development, protecting individual privacy and preventing discriminatory outcomes.

Regulatory Adaptation: Regulatory bodies must adapt to the evolving landscape, establishing clear guidelines that balance innovation with safety and patient well-being.

Workforce Transition: Supporting individuals potentially displaced by automation through retraining and reskilling initiatives is essential to ensure a just and equitable transition.

Joint effort across specialists, clinicians, industry pioneers, and policymakers is essential to saddle the maximum capacity of mechanization while exploring the moral and cultural ramifications. By embracing this groundbreaking innovation capably, we prepare for a future where advancement drugs arrive at patients quicker, customized medication turns into a reality, and the battle against illness go on with restored trust and progress.

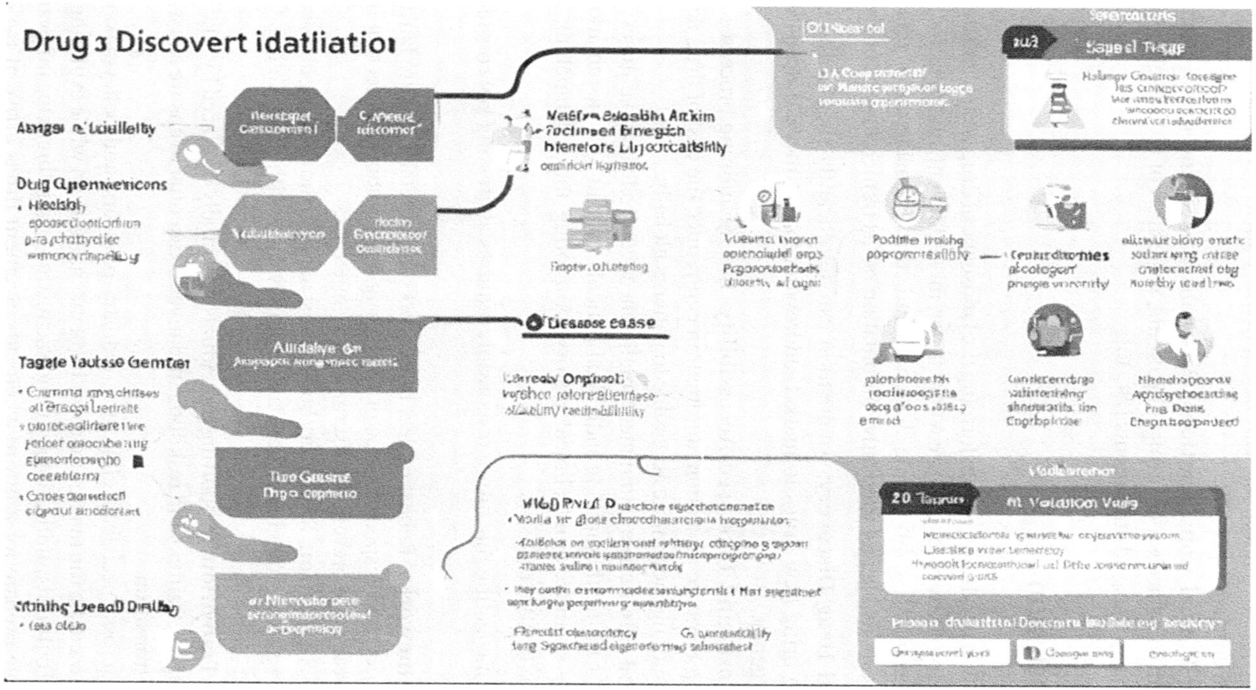
Drug 3 Discovert idatliation
Drug Qpenmericons
Tagele Yautsse Gemter
Tieseee easse

References

1. Vamathevan, H., Clark, D., Czodrowski, P. et al. (2019). Applications of machine learning in drug discovery and development. *Nature Reviews Drug Discovery* 18 (6): 463–477. https://doi.org/10.1038/s41573-019-0024-5.
2. Coley, C.W. et al. (2019). Machine learning in drug discovery and development: past, present and future. *Nature Reviews Drug Discovery.*
3. Yu, L. et al. (2023). High-throughput screening in drug discovery: advances and applications. *BioMed Research International.*
4. Segler, M.A. (2018). *Opportunities and Challenges for Deep Learning in Drug Discovery and Development.* ACS Central Science.
5. Li, Y. et al. (2020). Flow chemistry for rapid drug synthesis. *Nature Reviews Chemistry.*
6. Lee, J.H. et al. (2016). Electronic data capture (EDC) systems: a review and implementation guide. *Clin Pharmacol Ther.*
7. Borry, P. et al. (2020). Ethical considerations and responsible use of AI in healthcare. *Lancet Digit Health.*
8. FDA (2021). Artificial Intelligence and Machine Learning in Software as a Medical Device (SaMD) - Guidance for Industry and Food and Drug Administration Staff.
9. Bloom, N. et al. (2020). *AI and the New Economy.* Oxford University Press.
10. PwC (2022). The AI Revolution in Healthcare - Changing the Value Equation.
11. EMA (2022). "*Guidance on Clinical Trials using Wearable Devices.*"
12. Esteva, A., Kuprel, B., Novoa, R.A. et al. (2017). A dermatologist-level classification of skin cancer with deep neural networks. *Nature* 542 (7639): 115–118. https://doi.org/10.1038/nature21056.
13. Manyika, M. et al. (2017). *A Human-Centered Approach to Artificial Intelligence.* McKinsey Global Institute.
14. World Economic Forum (2020). The Future of Jobs Report 2020.
15. OECD (2018). OECD Skills for Jobs: The Rise of Automation and Technology.
16. World Health Organization (2023). Guidance for Regulatory Oversight of Medical Devices Driven by Artificial Intelligence.
17. Mittelstadt, B.D. et al. (2019). Preserving fairness in algorithmic decision-making. *Commun. ACM.*

Autism spectrum disorder (ASD) research is being revolutionized by supervised machine learning in combination with big data, allowing for better insights and customized interventions for people with ASD and related diseases [1, 4]. Understanding ASD in the context of brain networks is essential because it highlights the need for thorough diagnostic frameworks that can handle a range of severity levels and support needs [2]—these aspects of ASD when combined with better predictions using machine learning algorithms on available datasets [ImageSource: https://www.autismbc.ca/blog/what-is-autism/ / with permission of Autism Society of British Columbia].

5.1.1 Autism and Its Diagnosis

ASD, which affects one in 59 children in the United States [1], is characterized by difficulties with social communication and interaction. The main approaches for diagnosing ASD at this time are clinical standardized tests like the Autism Diagnostic Interview-Revised and Autism Diagnostic Observation Schedule-Revised; however, they are time-consuming and expensive [6]. Children with ASD can be identified using screening measures, including the Autism Spectrum Quotient, Childhood Autism Rating Scale-2, and Screening Tool for Autism in Toddlers and Young Children [6]. Big data utilization in ASD research is still lacking due to the unavailability of proper datasets, but recent developments in data collecting [1]. ASD diagnosis, genetic knowledge, and successful intervention development are all being investigated with machine learning [1].

In line with global trends, men had a higher prevalence of ASD than women. The study, however, contradicted other studies that suggested more severe social impairment among males with ASD and showed no significant link between gender and ASD [Image Source: https://tinyurl.com/mpk49he7].

This groundbreaking Indian study, unlike others, uncovered a lower autism prevalence (0.15%) in 1- to 10-year-olds compared to Western/Asian research (1–2%). Interestingly, rural children in India had higher rates, which might suggest different factors affecting diagnosis or prevalence in diverse settings.

Moderate autism was more prevalent in older children (4–10 years), suggesting potential delays in diagnosis linked to speech and motor development. This is concerning, as early detection of ASD is possible even before age 2. Furthermore, socioeconomic disparities were evident, with rural "upper-class" and urban/tribal "middle-class" children showing higher rates. The study suggests limited awareness in lower socioeconomic status groups might contribute to these disparities, leading to later identification and difficulties accessing needed support. In addition, it emphasizes the critical gap in addressing developmental disorders within child health programs in India, creating significant challenges for children with ASD due to the lack of effective identification, referral, and support systems.

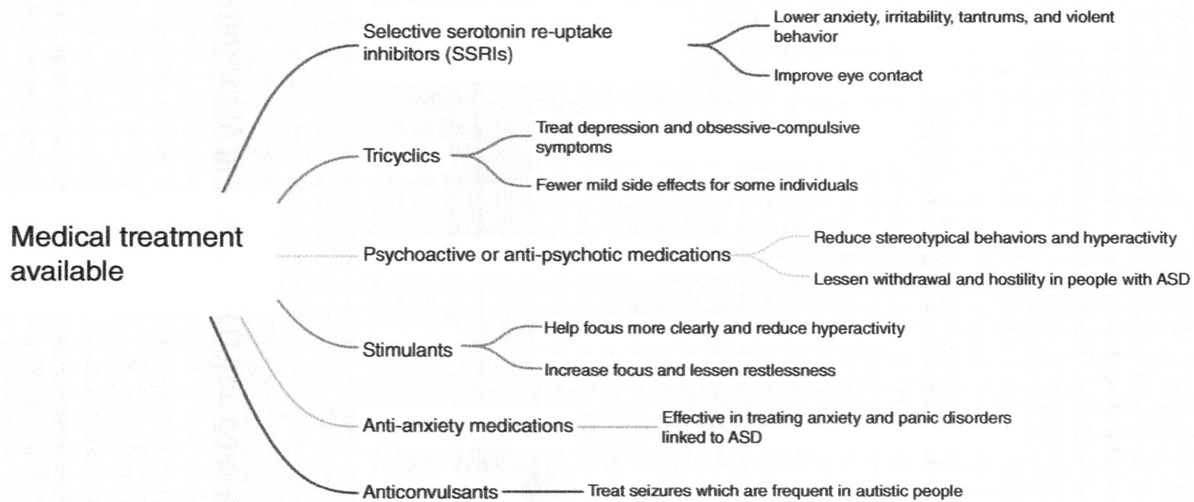

Various medical treatments available for autistic persons.

Diagnoses and knowledge of the biochemical and genetic underpinnings of intellectual and developmental disabilities (IDDs), such as ASD, are extremely difficult [4]. Biological understanding of IDDs is being improved by developments in high-throughput sequencing, imaging, and artificial intelligence technologies [4]. The neurodevelopmental disorders attention-deficit/hyperactivity disorder and ASD are common in children [8]. Because clinical psychology and neuroscience have only recently been integrated, it is difficult to pinpoint the precise brain regions that are linked to these illnesses [8].

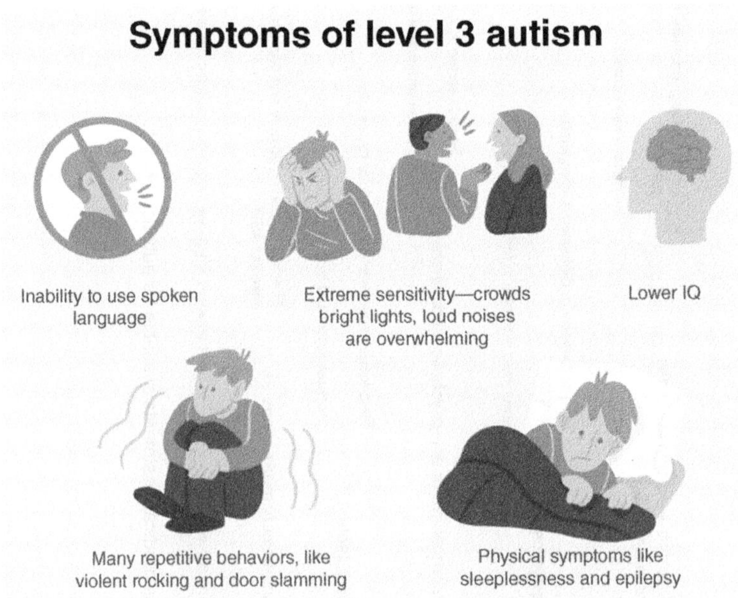

5.2 Machine Learning and Deep Learning Algorithms

Inspired by the human brain, deep learning is a potent branch of machine learning that uses artificial neural networks that are networked to understand complex patterns and relationships from massive volumes of data. Deep learning is beneficial for applications like picture identification, natural language processing, and even autism prediction since it excels at automatically extracting this information, unlike classical machine learning, which requires custom features. This enables it to spot minute trends in eye-tracking data, behavioral observations, or brain scans that other techniques might overlook. However, to guarantee that its promise for autism prediction translates into real-world benefits, issues like data constraints, interpretability, and ethical considerations demand responsible development and cautious integration with clinical competence.

5.2.1 Supervised Learning

To predict the diagnosis for new instances, these algorithms learn from labeled data (individuals with ASD diagnoses and typically developing individuals). Define decision boundaries using features to distinguish between people who have been diagnosed and those who have not. Combine many decision trees to provide flexibility and resilience. Brain-inspired models are complicated and able to learn complex patterns from big datasets.

5.2.2 Unsupervised Learning

These algorithms find hidden structures and patterns in unlabeled data, which may reveal modest ASD signs that are still poorly understood, organize people into groups according to shared qualities, which may reveal ASD spectrum subgroups, and help with data visualization and analysis by reducing the dimensionality of the data while maintaining critical information (Table 5.1).

5.2.3 Implementation Strategies

1) **Collect Diverse and Representative Data**: Verify that datasets cover a range of age ranges, demographics, and autism presentations to reduce bias and enhance generalizability.
2) **Prioritize Data Quality**: To assure accuracy and reduce noise, apply strict data collection, cleaning, and preprocessing procedures.
3) **Address Data Privacy and Security**: To secure sensitive information, get informed approval, hide data when it can, and put strong security measures in place.
4) **Choose Appropriate Algorithms**: Examine the drawbacks of various algorithms and choose the ones best suited to the particular detection task and the properties of the data.
5) **Focus on Early Intervention**: Make use of machine learning-driven findings to quickly identify possible scenarios and provide access to remedy resources.

Table 5.1 Summary of supervised/unsupervised machine learning algorithms utilized for autism detection.

Supervised/unsupervised learning algorithms	Usage in ASD research
Support Vector Machines (SVM)	Binary predictions related to diagnosis and screening. Used in genetics, neuroimaging, and text-mining studies for biomarker identification and accurate ASD classification.
Alternating Decision Tree (AD Tree)	Proficient in binary predictions and handling categorical data efficiently. Enhances diagnostic processes and provides transparency in ASD research.
Naïve Bayes	Specialized in text mining, particularly in analyzing social media data related to ASD for predicting ASD based on textual samples.
Random Forest (RF)	Featured in text mining and neuroimaging studies. Utilized for outlier detection, monitoring ASD populations, and developing screening tools due to their ensemble learning approach.
Logistic Regression	A reliable method for binary classification tasks in ASD diagnosis due to its ability to fit an optimal curve to data points using a logistic function.
K-Nearest Neighbors (KNN)	Classification of individuals based on their nearest neighbors' features. Used to gain insights into specific patterns and characteristics within ASD populations.
Conditional Inference Forest (CF)	Modification of Random Forest algorithm utilizing statistical inference tests for feature selection in ASD-related genetic data. Identifies key genetic factors linked to ASD, aiding in understanding molecular pathways.

6) **Complementary Tool, Not a Replacement**: Consider machine learning as a helpful tool for medical professionals rather than as a substitute for thorough clinical assessment and customized decision-making.

5.2.4 Algorithms Efficiency

Table 5.2 also highlights the efficiency of usage of various supervised/unsupervised algorithms utilized for autism detection as given in the literature review. This information highlights the significance of machine learning algorithms for autism detection.

Table 5.2 Algorithmic efficiency of various machine learning algorithms for autism detection.

Algorithms	Objective	Efficiency	Accuracy (%)	References
Logistic Regression	Detection of autism spectrum disorder (ASD) in children and adults using machine learning	High	93.15	[5]
Naïve Bayes	Detection of ASD in children and adults using machine learning	High	97.53	[5]
Support Vector Machine	Machine learning methods for diagnosing ASD and attention-deficit/hyperactivity disorder using functional and structural MRI: A survey	High	94.9	[8]
Random Forest	Framework for grading autism severity using task-based fMRI	Moderate	72	[9]
KNN	Machine learning methods for diagnosing ASD and attention-deficit/hyperactivity disorder using functional and structural MRI: A survey	Low	66	[8]
SVM (children)	Detection of ASD in children and adults using machine learning	High	93.84	[5]
RF (rs-fMRI)	Applications of supervised machine learning in ASD research	High	91	[1]
Glmboost (toddlers, children, adults)	Detection of ASD in children and adults using machine learning	High	97	[5]
Elastic Net (rs-fMRI)	Automatic diagnosis of autism based on functional magnetic resonance imaging and elastic net	High	83.33	[3]
Sparse LR (rs-fMRI, sMRI)	Diagnostic classification for human autism and obsessive-compulsive disorder based on machine learning from a primate genetic model	High	82.14	[7]

5.2.5 Limitations of Machine Learning and Deep Learning in Autism Detection

1) **Data Bias and Imbalance**: Algorithm training datasets may overrepresent certain autism presentations or be biased toward specific factors, which could result in predictions that are not accurate for a variety of groups.
2) **Interpretability and Explainability**: It's important to know how algorithms arrive at their results, particularly in complex fields like healthcare. However, complicated models can be clear, which makes it challenging to understand their logic and spot any biases.
3) **Limited Generalizability**: To guarantee greater applicability, algorithms trained on particular datasets may not generalize well to other populations or circumstances, needing extensive validation and modification.
4) **Overdiagnosis and Missed Diagnoses**: If algorithms are too sensitive, people who don't fit all the criteria may be overdiagnosed with ASD, and people with less common presentations may go unnoticed.
5) **Lack of Clinical Integration**: Clinical judgment and skill should be added, not replaced, by machine learning and deep learning technologies. It is essential to combine with established diagnostic procedures and clinical assessment.

5.2.6 Techniques for Prediction

Medical diagnosis of ASD entails identifying probable symptoms and risk factors using a variety of procedures and evaluations. Here are some techniques commonly used for predicting autism.

1) **Developmental Screening**: To determine a child's developmental milestones, pediatricians frequently perform developmental screenings at well-child visits. Further assessment may be warranted if there are speech, motor, or social development delays.
2) **Developmental Surveillance**: During checks, medical professionals frequently observe a child's development, enabling them to track any concerns over time.

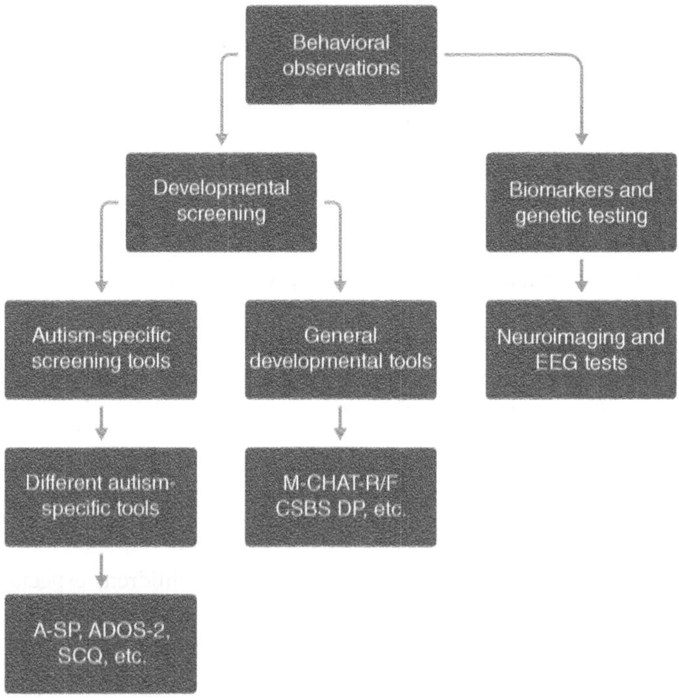

3) **Autism-Specific Screening Tools**: The Modified Checklist for Autism in Toddlers is one of several screening instruments made specifically to determine the likelihood of autism. Positive outcomes from these tools suggest that more testing is required.
4) **Genetic Testing**: An elevated risk of autism is linked to specific genetic abnormalities. These mutations may be found in people through genetic testing, particularly in those who have a family history of ASD.
5) **Brain Imaging**: Electroencephalography and functional magnetic resonance imaging are sometimes used to detect variations in brain activity in people with ASD [9]. These methods are more frequently used in research settings.
6) **Biomarker Research**: ASD risk may be indicated by biomarkers that have been found in blood, urine, or cerebrospinal fluid, according to ongoing studies. However, research in this field is still in its infancy.

7) **Eye-Tracking Technology**: Studies using eye-tracking technology have shown that people with ASD interpret visual information differently. As a potential tool for early detection, this technique is now being investigated.

5.2.7 Attributes for Prediction

1) **Behavioral Observations**: A child's behavior, speech, and social interactions are evaluated by qualified professionals. Specific behavioral patterns may indicate a higher risk of autism.
2) **Parental Concerns**: Parents frequently become aware of unusual behaviors in their kids first. Medical examinations are prompted in large part by their findings and concerns.

5.3 Discussion

Considering the difficulties encountered by autistic children, especially their inclination toward playing alone, this project argues for multiple methods that help their social and developmental growth. Using a child's particular interests and attention span, games therapy, a specialized form of play therapy, becomes an important tool for developing social skills, communication, and emotional expression through lighthearted activities. Through carefully constructed games, therapists help kids in making the transition from alone time to social engagement. This lets kids explore their feelings, make sense of their environment, and form relationships with friends and family. Furthermore, game therapy concepts can be learned by parents and guardians, who can then use these insights to build stronger family bonds, promote general well-being, and actively participate in their child's growth.

There is more to helping autistic children than just therapeutic techniques. This research highlights the need for early awareness efforts that inform communities about the weak signs of ASD and highlight the transformative power of early diagnosis and intervention. These campaigns aim to create a more inclusive society. The complete plan envisions a time when young people with autism are not only recognized and assisted but also given the tools they need to flourish through strong support systems, complementary therapies, ongoing research, and a seamless transition into adulthood.

5.4 Future Work

We envision a cutting-edge software system using predictive analytics. This platform will examine trends and patterns across many data sets, including emotional nuance and health metrics, and analyze data from government-approved health exams. By dissecting these patterns, we hope to get insight into the emotional and behavioral patterns of autistic kids, possibly identify physical vulnerabilities, and even forecast the likelihood of specific diseases. There is a great deal of promise for proactive treatment and enhanced well-being for autistic people with this technology.

We place a high priority on empowering families by providing them with seminars and easily accessible resources because we know that caring, knowledgeable carers provide a nurturing home environment for children with ASD. To build an inclusive culture from the bottom up, we collaborate with educational institutions to develop specialized programs and support inclusive curriculums in mainstream schools. This fosters acceptance and empathy among peers in addition to understanding.

Our goal goes beyond data analysis to make accessible autism treatment. Our software will forecast possible problems and direct preventive care by evaluating behavioral, emotional, and health data. We intend to collaborate with governments and healthcare facilities to lower the cost and increase accessibility of this instrument, particularly for individuals facing difficult financial circumstances. To ensure that everyone, regardless of poverty, may benefit from proactive, predictive autism care, this project addresses the high expenses associated with private therapy.

5.5 Conclusion

Because ASD has complicated symptoms and insufficient diagnostic tools, diagnosing the condition can be difficult. There is potential for improvement in traditional procedures, which rely on laborious psychological testing and observations.

The diagnosis of ASD could be revolutionized by machine learning. ASD is highly accurately predicted by algorithms such as Support Vector Machine and Logistic Regression, which may help with diagnosis, screening, and understanding genetic underpinnings. Nonetheless, issues like the interpretability of the model and the lack of open-source data must be resolved. There is great potential

6

Temporal Normalization and Brain Image Analysis for Early-Stage Prediction of Attention Deficit Hyperactivity Disorder (ADHD)

Poonam Chaudhary, Nikki Rani, Diksha Aggarwal, and Srishti Sharma

CSE, SOET, The NorthCap University, Gurugram, India

6.1 Introduction

The field of automated attention deficit hyperactivity disorder (ADHD) detection has garnered significant attention in recent years. A comprehensive review conducted by Loh et al. [1] sheds light on the current trends and prospects in this area. Their investigation encompassed studies utilizing various techniques, including EEG, fMRI, and machine learning algorithms, to automate the detection of ADHD [1].

ADHD is a commonly observed neurodevelopmental condition that impacts individuals from childhood through adulthood unless addressed promptly. Efficiently addressing ADHD can notably improve the well-being and societal inclusion of those living with the disorder. At present, the prevailing approach for ADHD diagnosis involves a clinical assessment performed by a qualified specialist who evaluates the diagnostic criteria outlined in the DSM-5, as well as the presence of a minimum of five symptoms related to either inattention or impulsivity/hyperactivity. Neurodevelopmental disorders encompass a diverse set of conditions marked by disruptions or delays in the development of various skills across domains such as motor, social, language, and cognition [2]. These conditions exert a significant impact on the functioning of the human brain. They can range from milder forms that allow individuals to lead relatively typical lives to more severe forms that necessitate lifelong care and support. Secondary aspects, such as age, gender, and co-occurring disorders that may affect the self-esteem of people with ADHD, were also discussed [3]. Zhang aims to address the limitations of previous studies by evaluating the performance of the kTree algorithm on a large and diverse dataset of children with and without ADHD. The study provides valuable insights into the potential of K-Nearest Neighbors

Generative Artificial Intelligence for Biomedical and Smart Health Informatics,
First Edition. Edited by Aditya Khamparia and Deepak Gupta.

(KNN) classification with different numbers of nearest neighbors for ADHD diagnosis [4]. Random forest has been shown to outperform logistic regression on a variety of classification tasks. Couronné et al. conducted a large-scale benchmark experiment on MRI images and found that random forest outperformed logistic regression on a majority of the datasets [5]. However, more research is needed to evaluate the performance of random forest and logistic regression for ADHD classification, especially in terms of clinical relevance. People with ADHD exhibit persistent patterns of inattention and/or hyperactivity/impulsivity that impair functioning and development. These include carelessness, hyperactivity and impulsivity, anxiety and depression, learning disorders, and peer problems. An innovative heuristic method for measuring and forecasting the onset of neurodevelopmental diseases, such as ADHD, is presented that integrates several evaluation techniques and developmental indicators to make it easier to spot these diseases early on [6]. Fusing fMRI and nonimaging data has the potential to improve the accuracy and objectivity of ADHD diagnosis. Integrating feature selection with nonimage data can represent an important feature selection strategy, and functional connectivity between hemispheres is most altered in ADHD compared to changes affecting individual hemispheres [7]. Preventive interventions for ADHD have the potential to reduce the risk of developing ADHD or to mitigate its symptoms. Several promising preventive interventions, including parent training, behavioral interventions, and medication, have been discussed [8]. Ozonoff et al. explore the moral issues surrounding the early identification of neurodevelopmental and mental health problems in this essay. The author admits that early discovery can have several advantages, including improved long-term results and early intervention. Though the science of early detection is very young, there are significant ethical issues that must be resolved [9, 10]. Hámori et al. [11] have experimented with other modality EEG data to identify the ADHD patient.

The scientific community still lacks a complete model of the pathophysiology of ADHD despite the abundance of empirical literature. In addition, there are still no objective biological tools available to the clinical community that may help clinicians diagnose ADHD in a patient or make therapy choices. Artificial intelligence (AI) has ushered in a profound transformation in our daily lives and has significantly enhanced the efficiency of operations in diverse sectors, including manufacturing, finance, marketing, and numerous others. AI also holds the promise of revolutionizing the healthcare industry, with the potential to elevate both health outcomes and patient experiences through the deployment of machine learning and deep learning models [12].

Thus, this paper aims to explore the application of machine learning and deep learning in the early detection of ADHD using different symptoms available in the dataset ADHD200. Section II covers the Exploratory Data Analysis methods on the

ADHD-200 dataset as it provides a better overview of data by quickly analyzing, and generating detailed reports of the dataset, saving both time and effort. Following in section III, the methodology has been explained for machine learning algorithms application on a csv file, and temporal normalization and segmentation techniques on 4D NIFTI files, which improve comparability, lessens confounding factors, and lines up data with statistical presumptions. Section IV discusses the results, and Section V concludes the chapter with future scope.

6.2 Exploratory Data Analysis

Employing an exploratory data analysis approach is crucial for enhancing understanding of brain function, especially when investigating intricate processes. This approach is valuable as it enables the identification and description of unforeseen phenomena that either hasn't been modeled beforehand or cannot be modeled in advance.

6.2.1 Exploratory Data Analysis for Phenotypic CSV File

Exploratory Data Analysis methods on the ADHD-200 dataset as it provides a better overview of data by quickly analyzing and generating detailed reports of the dataset, saving both time and effort. The steps followed for this purpose are:

1) First, we installed numpy [13], pandas [14], and scikit-learn [15] for handling the data and building machine learning models.
2) Then data loading is done using, pandas read_csv function.
3) Using train test_split (), we split the dataset in the ratio of 70:30, so the train part consists of 62 records and the test part consists of 21 records, and using unique(), we found the number of unique values in each column.
4) Indexing is done on train data using the iloc function to select all rows (:) and all columns except the last one (:−1) as it does not contain any information.
5) We found the descriptive statistics of the Data Frame columns, such as count, mean, standard deviation, minimum, and quartiles and transposed the entire table formed for better representation for train and test dataset.
6) Then, in the train and test file, a new DataFrame called "test_null" is created. It uses the "isna()" function to check for missing values (NaN) in the DataFrame "test". The "sum ()" function is then applied to count the number of missing values for each column. The result is a Series object with column names as the index and the corresponding count of missing values as the values. Then, using sort_values (by=0, ascending=False) we sorted the "test_null" DataFrame based on the values in column 0 (which represents the count of missing values).

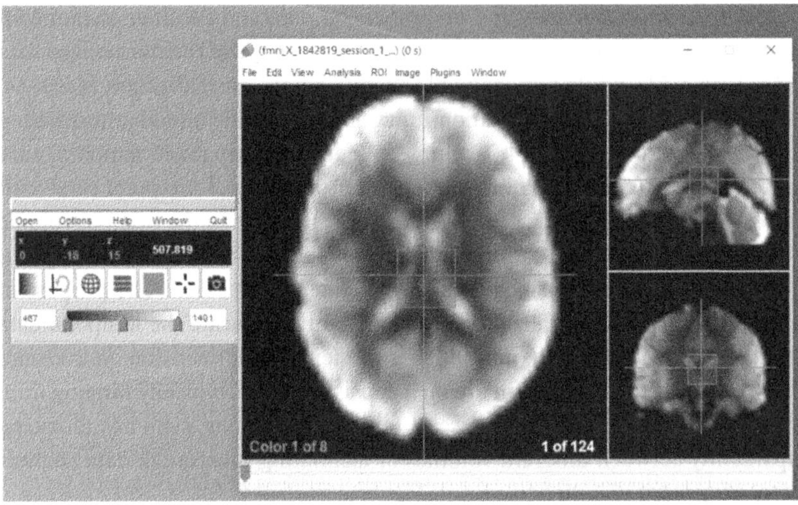

Figure 6.1 ROI.

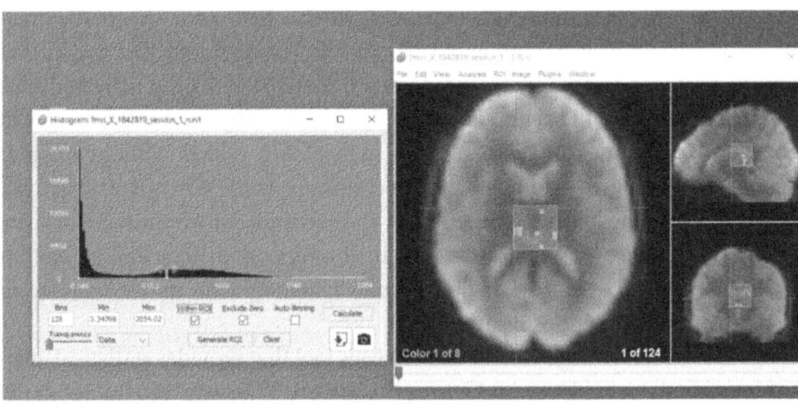

Figure 6.2 Histogram analysis of ROI.

In Mango, the histogram analysis tool allows users to generate and display a histogram of the intensity values within a selected region of interest (ROI) in the image, as in Figure 6.6. The statistics table for the ROI displays various parameters derived from the histogram, such as the mean, standard deviation, minimum, and maximum intensity values within the ROI. Histogram analysis can be used to identify the distribution of intensity values within the ROI, which can be indicative of certain tissue or material properties. For example, a histogram with a narrow peak at high-intensity values may indicate the presence of bone tissue, while a broader and flatter histogram may indicate the presence of soft tissue.

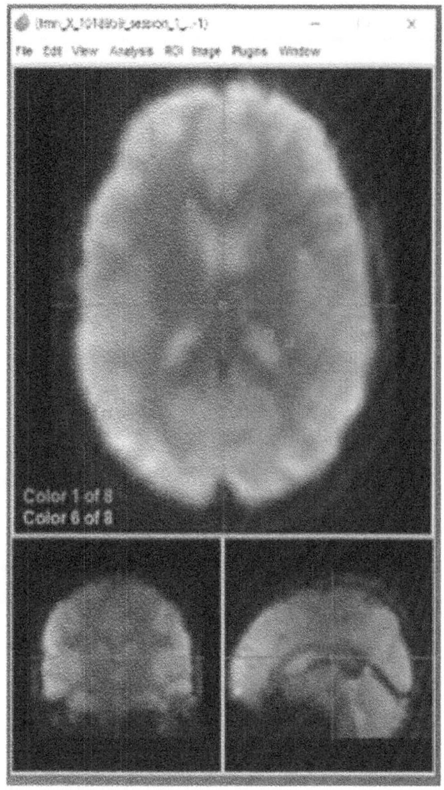

Figure 6.3 fMRI image of subject 1 in Mango.

In addition to visualizing the distribution of intensity values, histogram analysis can be used to adjust the contrast and brightness of an image. By adjusting the range of intensity values that are displayed, users can enhance the visibility of certain features or structures within the image.

6.3 Methodology

6.3.1 Dataset Description

This research project focuses on the ADHD-200 data set [20]. This huge dataset includes structural MRI (s-MRI) and resting-state fMRI (rs-fMRI) data from 973 subjects from eight distinct study sites. On the Neuroimaging Informatics Tools and Resources Clearinghouse (NITRC) platform, the competition's results and conclusions have been made public. A T1-weighted structural scan and resting-state fMRI data are included for each subject. The dataset's inclusion

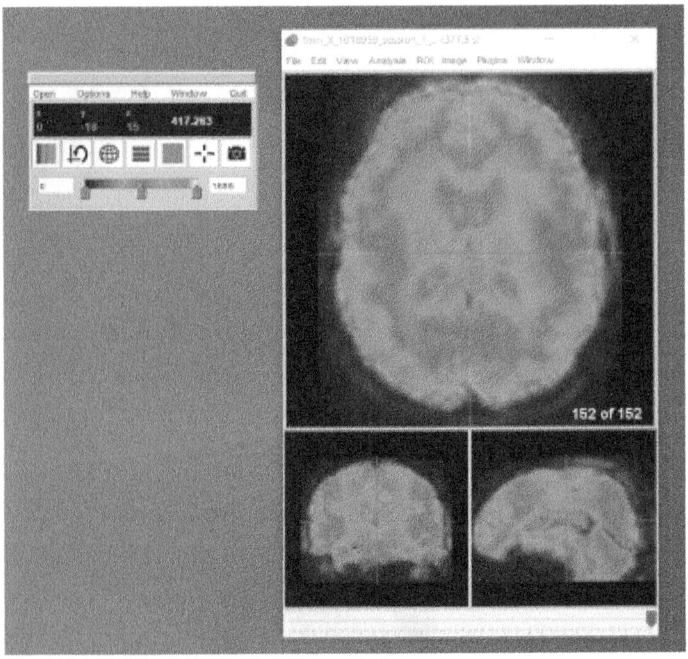

Figure 6.4 Time frames in mango.

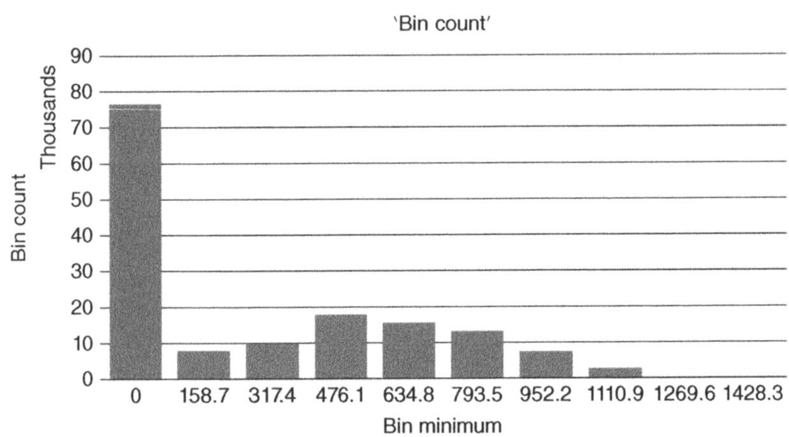

Figure 6.5 Statistics table.

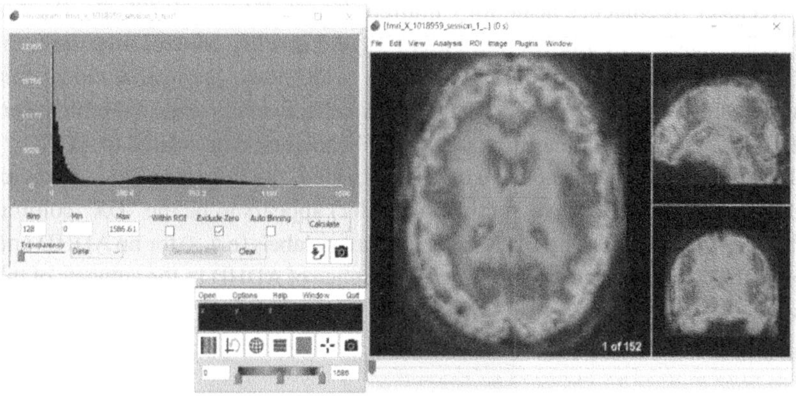

Figure 6.6 Histogram analysis.

of useful metadata, such as participant age, handedness, IQ scores, and gender information, in addition to neuroimaging data, enhances the study's context. A training dataset with 776 participants and a second testing dataset with 197 participants make up the ADHD-200 dataset. The 776 people in the training dataset are divided into three different diagnostic classes: Healthy control type, ADHD-I control type, and ADHD-C control type. The medication ratings and status obtained from multiple assessment tools are added to this classification to give a thorough understanding of the participants' situations. There were eight international imaging sites engaged in the data collection for the ADHD-200 dataset. However, it's crucial to note that two of these sites exclusively offered MRI scans of control participants rather than those with ADHD, which effectively excluded them from the majority of research using this dataset. The eight sites are as follows: Peking University, Bradley Hospital/Brown University, Kennedy Krieger Institute (KKI), Neuro IMAGE Sample, New York University Child Study Center, Oregon Health & Science University, University of Pittsburgh, Washington University in St. Louis. We have utilized the KKI site for this research.

Each subject is uniquely identified by a ***ScanDir ID***. The dataset includes information about the data collection site (referred to as "Site"), with our analysis focusing on the KKI dataset. ***Gender*** is represented as 0 for females and 1 for males, while ***handedness*** is categorized as 0 for left-handed, 1 for right-handed, and 2 for ambidextrous individuals. The ***"DX"*** variable indicates whether participants have been diagnosed with ADHD (or not). In addition, ***"Secondary DX"*** encompasses categorical values such as anxiety disorder, learning disorder, tic disorder, and other diagnoses. The dataset also includes measures for assessing ***ADHD symptoms*** (ADHD Measure, Inattentive, and Hyper/Impulsive), ***medication status*** (1 for Medication Naïve and 2 for Not Medication Naïve), ***IQ measures*** using

3) In the GridSearch CV() method, we define cv = 5, which defines the number of folds to use for cross-validation.
4) Finally, we printed the best hyperparameters and the corresponding score, the mean and standard deviation of the cross-validation scores, the mean squared error, and the R-squared error.

6.3.2.2 K-Nearest Neighbors

KNN method default hyperparameters in scikit-learn are frequently chosen as a starting point because they strike a good compromise between performance and simplicity. Figure 6.8 depicts the confusion matrix and classification report for KNN, respectively.

1) The number of neighbors to take into account while generating predictions is determined by the option neighbors. With a default value of 5, the algorithm will consider the query point's five closest neighbors.

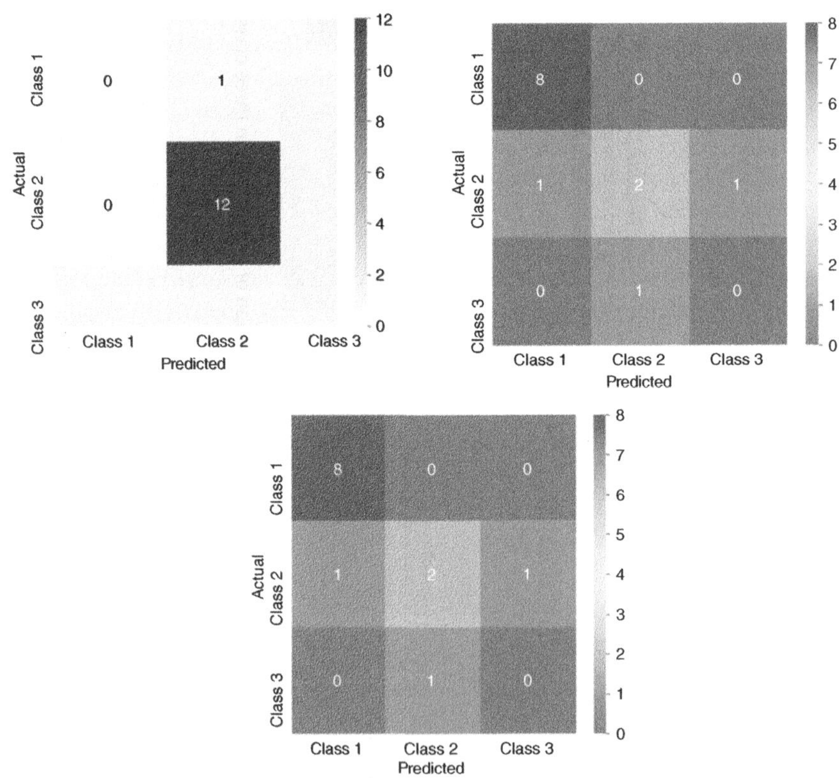

Figure 6.8 Confusion matrix for (i) KNN (ii) random forest (iii) Random Forest.

2) Weights: It describes the weighting algorithm used to make a forecast. The setting, "uniform," gives each neighbor the same weight. You may build a custom function or choose an option called "distance," where neighbors who are closer to you have a greater impact.
3) The power parameter for the Minkowski metric, which calculates the separations between data points, is determined by this parameter. The default setting of 2 represents the Euclidean distance.
4) The best suitable algorithm is automatically selected by the default setting of "auto," which is based on the supplied data. Other choices of "Ball_tree," "KD_tree," and "brute" can also be explored.

6.3.2.3 Random Forest

The choice of the random forest algorithm's hyperparameters, such as max_depth and random_state, depends on several variables and should be made via testing and adjustment.

1) **max_depth:** The maximum depth of each decision tree in the random forest is determined by the parameter max_depth. When none is selected, the trees are enlarged until all leaves are pure or until all leaves have the bare minimum number of samples needed to split, whichever comes first. The depth of the trees can be restricted by setting max_depth to a certain value, like 10, which helps avoid overfitting. It regulates the model's complexity and may be adjusted according to the difficulty of the challenge and the quantity of training data available.
2) **random_state:** To ensure repeatability, this argument is used to establish the random seed. The random_state value of 49 is arbitrary; to create a new random seed each time, change it to none or any other integer number. For consistency and debugging purposes, setting a specified random_state value enables you to get the same outcomes each time you execute the method.
3) The correlation matrix and accuracy scores are shown in Figure 6.8.

6.4 Results and Discussion

On successful implementation of the Linear Regression, KNN, and random forest and setting the appropriate hyperparameters, the accuracy is obtained using the KNN Classifier, taking the number of neighbors as 5, as shown in Table 6.1. The result of linear regression is provided with the best hyperparameters and the corresponding score, the mean and standard deviation of the cross-validation scores, the mean squared error, and the R-squared error in Figure 6.9.

Also, Figure 6.10(i) and (ii) illustrate the classification accuracy of KNN Algorithm and Random Forest algorithms.

Table 6.1 A comparative analysis of machine learning algorithms on phenotypic CSV file.

Algorithm	Best hyperparameters	Mean square error	R-square	Accuracy
Linear regression	{'fit_intercept': False, 'normalize': True}	0.3735	0.6265	0.7242
KNN	n_neighbors=5, weights='uniform', p=2, algorithm='auto'	—	—	0.92
Random Forest	max_depth=10, random_state=49	—	—	0.77

```
Best hyperparameters: {'fit_intercept': True, 'normalize': False}
Best score: 0.724203880625174
Mean cross-validation score: 2.7298242259469le+25
Standard deviation of cross-validation scores: 5.45964845189382e+25
Mean squared error: 0.3764376057671265
R-squared: 0.6235623942328734
```

Figure 6.9 Result of Linear regression algorithm on phenotypic CSV file.

	precision	recall	f1-score	support
0	0.00	0.00	0.00	1
2	0.92	1.00	1.96	12
accuracy			0.92	13
macro avg	0.46	0.50	0.48	13
weighted avg	0.85	0.92	0.89	13

	precision	recall	f1-score	support
0	0.89	1.00	0.94	8
1	0.67	0.50	0.57	4
3	0.00	0.00	0.00	1
accuracy			0.77	13
macro avg	0.52	0.50	0.50	13
weighted avg	0.75	0.77	0.76	13

Figure 6.10 Confusion Matrix with classification accuracy of (i) KNN algorithm and (ii) Random forest algorithm.

In Table 6.1, the analysis's top score, 0.92, was obtained via KNN with the hyperparameters n_neighbors=5, weights='uniform', p=2, algorithm='auto'. The accuracy obtained by linear regression is 0.7242 with an R-squared value of 0.6265 and a mean squared error of 0.3735. Finally, the random forest algorithm scored 0.77. These findings suggest that linear regression, KNN, and random forest may be useful in analyzing the provided data.

6.5 Conclusion

The escalating prevalence of ADHD among children and adolescents worldwide has spurred interest in devising early detection and diagnostic strategies. This chapter assesses various machine learning algorithms applied to ADHD datasets, serving as a proof of concept for the viability of employing machine learning models to create a medically effective solution for early ADHD detection. In addition, it delves into the significance of temporal normalization in 4D NIfTI data, exploring its impact on statistical assumptions, confounding factors, and comparability. The study encompasses phases such as preprocessing, feature extraction, statistical analysis, cross-validation, and interpretation/validation in the examination of brain images for ADHD identification. The scrutinized KNN with $k = 5$ (accuracy: 0.92), random forest (score: 0.77), and linear regression (score: 0.765) algorithms exhibit promising potential for analyzing the provided data. This research contributes to the comprehension of ADHD and lends support to initiatives like the ADHD-200 Sample, advocating for open data sharing to enhance scientific expertise in this field. On 4D NIfTI files, temporal normalization improves comparability, lessens confounding factors, and lines up data with statistical presumptions. The analysis's top score, 0.92, was obtained via KNN with the hyperparameters n_neighbors=5, weights='uniform', p=2, algorithm='auto'. The accuracy obtained by linear regression is 0.7242 with an R-squared value of 0.6265 and a mean squared error of 0.3735. Finally, the random forest algorithm scored 0.77. These findings suggest that linear regression, KNN, and random forest may be useful in analyzing the provided data. The future scope involves comparing various algorithms on the phenotypic CSV file, on fMRI images, and integrating these two modalities to enhance the efficacy of early-stage ADHD detection. In addition, investigation of alternative modalities, such as EEG data, and integrate them with fMRI.

References

1 Loh, H.W., Ooi, C.P., Barua, P.D. et al. (2022). Automated detection of ADHD: current trends and future perspective. *Computers in Biology and Medicine* 146: 105525.

2 Moghaddari, M., Lighvan, M.Z., and Danishvar, S. (2020). Diagnose ADHD disorder in children using convolutional neural network based on continuous mental task EEG. *Computer Methods and Programs in Biomedicine* 197: 105738.

3 Mazzone, L., Postorino, V., Reale, L. et al. (2013). Self-esteem evaluation in children and adolescents suffering from ADHD. *Clinical Practice and Epidemiology in Mental Health* 9: 96–102.

4 Zhang, S., Li, X., Zong, M. et al. (2017). Efficient kNN classification with different numbers of nearest neighbors. *IEEE Transactions on Neural Networks and Learning Systems* 29 (5): 1774–1785.

7

Sustainable Agriculture Through Advanced Crop Management: VGG16-Based Tea Leaf Disease Recognition

R. Sivaraman[1], S. Praveena[2], and H. Naresh Kumar[2]

[1] *School of Computing, SASTRA Deemed University, Thanjavur, India*
[2] *School of Arts Sciences Humanities & Education, SASTRA Deemed University, Thanjavur, India*

7.1 Introduction

In the intricate realm of tea cultivation, ensuring the vitality of each leaf stands as a pivotal factor in achieving a fruitful harvest. Amidst the array of challenges posed by various diseases, the fusion of modern technology with age-old practices emerges as a beacon of optimism. This introduction delves into the realm of predicting diseases in tea plants, where advanced analytics, notably the VGG16 deep learning model mentioned by Simonyan [1], offers a transformative solution. Through predictive analytics, tea growers gain valuable insights into potential crop ailments, aiming to revolutionize disease management using a dataset featuring eight distinct class labels: healthy, algal leaf, anthracnose, bird's-eye spot, brown blight, grey light, red leaf spot, and white spot.

- **Healthy**: Denotes a leaf free from disease.
- **Algal Leaf**: Resulting from algae, marked by greyish, green, brown, or orange spots on the leaf surface.
- **Anthracnose**: A fungal infection forming sunken lesions on leaves and stems, often with black, ring-like edges.
- **Bird's-Eye Spot**: Another fungal disease, forming circular lesions with a dark center and lighter border, resembling a bird's eye.
- **Brown Blight**: A fungal infection causing brown, water-soaked lesions on leaves and stems, leading to withering and defoliation.
- **Grey Light**: This term does not correspond to a tea plant disease; it may refer to a specific lighting condition rather than an ailment.

Generative Artificial Intelligence for Biomedical and Smart Health Informatics,
First Edition. Edited by Aditya Khamparia and Deepak Gupta.

- **Red Leaf Spot**: A fungal infection resulting in reddish-brown spots on leaves, which may enlarge and merge, leading to leaf drop.
- **White Spot**: A fungal infection appearing as white or greyish dots on the undersides of leaves.

Through this innovative approach, our aim is to equip tea farmers worldwide with the tools and knowledge necessary for proactive illness management, ensuring the sustainability and prosperity of tea plantations. Join us in this endeavor as we navigate the delicate balance between tradition and technology to secure the future of tea farming.

Traditionally, tea producers relied on visual inspection and manual observation to detect plant diseases. This involved physically examining the leaves for discoloration, spots, or irregular growth patterns, followed by consulting reference materials or experts to identify the ailment. While this method drew upon farmers' experience and expertise, it was subjective, time-consuming, and often failed to detect diseases in their early stages.

The use of technology is increasingly prevalent in addressing tea plant diseases. Some existing methods automate disease identification and diagnosis by integrating image processing techniques and machine learning algorithms; refer to the work of Ahmed et al. [2] for a detailed survey. These methods typically utilize datasets comprising images of diseased and healthy tea leaves to train algorithms that detect and categorize illnesses based on visual attributes. While these approaches offer objectivity and potentially swifter results compared to traditional methods, they may encounter challenges related to data quality, model accuracy, and scalability.

While the overview establishes a solid foundation for understanding the significance of disease prediction in tea cultivation and introduces the VGG16 model as a promising tool for this purpose, it could benefit from establishing a clearer connection between the proposed approach and the challenges faced by tea farmers. In addition, highlighting the potential benefits and implications of integrating deep learning with traditional knowledge may enhance the relevance and significance of the proposed solution.

Presenting real-life examples or case studies demonstrating how the proposed approach could enhance disease management techniques and mitigate risks for tea farmers would reinforce the argument. Overall, by refining the correlation between the overview and the proposed strategy and emphasizing the practical implications, the argument can effectively convey its importance.

7.2 Literature Survey

Embarking on a sophisticated exploration of tea disease recognition, the study by Chen and Jia [3] delves into the realm of deep learning, specifically harnessing the prowess of LeafNet—a deep convolutional neural network (CNN). Originating from a collection of tea leaf disease photos sourced from Hubei Province, China, the research attains a remarkable accuracy of 90.23% in identifying seven distinct forms of tea leaf illnesses. The methodological orchestration involves intricate image preprocessing, followed by the rigorous training of LeafNet utilizing a Bag of Visual Words feature representation, culminating in the utilization of a Support Vector Machine classifier. This technological symphony not only showcases the potential of deep learning to enhance disease recognition in tea plant cultivation but also extends its implications to the realms of precision agriculture and intelligent farming techniques. The findings underscore the transformative impact of cutting-edge technologies on advancing our understanding and application of agricultural sciences, positioning this study as a testament to the intersection of technology and cultivation sophistication.

In the scholarly work conducted by Liu et al. [4], an innovative strategy is presented, offering a predictive solution for anticipating blister blight in tea plants through the synergistic integration of Internet of Things (IoT) technologies and machine learning methodologies. This pioneering approach harnesses the power of IoT sensors to vigilantly monitor dynamic environmental conditions while leveraging a sophisticated machine-learning model to prognosticate the occurrence of the aforementioned disease. Remarkably, the model exhibits a substantial enhancement in prediction accuracy over the temporal spectrum, soaring from 66% in 2015 to an impressive 91% in 2019. This profound refinement plays a pivotal role in advancing sustainable agricultural practices by judiciously optimizing pesticide utilization. Furthermore, the efficacy of this model has been rigorously validated through meticulous field observations, substantiating its reliability and real-world applicability. Encouraged by these findings, the study advocates for the extension of this innovative approach to prognosticate various other environmentally influenced diseases. This not only underscores the transformative potential of IoT and machine learning in the proactive management of agricultural diseases but also heralds a paradigm shift toward a more informed and sustainable agricultural landscape.

The investigation by Zhao et al. [5] delves into the application of hyperspectral imaging and wavelet analysis as discerning tools to differentiate between ailments and pest-induced stress in tea plants. The scholarly inquiry involved an intricate analysis to ascertain optimal feature sets for stress detection, delving into spectral properties under diverse pressures, including the tea green leafhopper, anthracnose, and sunburn. Remarkably, the researchers achieved a discriminating accuracy surpassing the 90% threshold, employing cutting-edge techniques such as image clustering and machine learning methodologies. The study underscores the pivotal role of advanced technology in enabling nondestructive monitoring of plant stressors, thereby furnishing invaluable insights for the efficacious management of diseases and pest-induced stress in tea farms. This underscores the

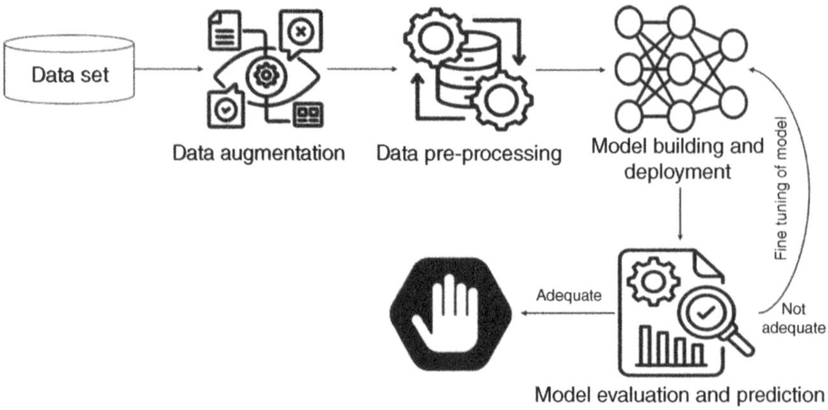

Figure 7.1 Overview of the proposed work.

the precision of disease recognition. The dataset, meticulously curated, is sourced from the esteemed Kaggle repository—an open-source bastion of software renowned for its versatility in accommodating various algorithms, which we harness comprehensively to train and refine our model. This conscientious utilization of diverse algorithms contributes to the robustness and efficacy of our disease detection framework, positioning it as a noteworthy advancement in the domain.

The outlined diagram shown in Figure 7.1 serves as a comprehensive overview of the entire undertaking.

The dataset capturing instances of tea leaf diseases was meticulously sourced from a reputable repository and subsequently categorized into seven distinct disease classes, namely, anthracnose, algal leaf, bird's-eye spot, brown blight, gray light, healthy, red leaf spot, and white spot. Each of these classes comprises a curated collection of precisely 100 images, impeccably formatted in the ubiquitous .jpg extension. To further enrich the dataset and enhance its diversity, a strategic augmentation process was applied, effectively amplifying its overall size. This augmentation step plays a pivotal role in fortifying the dataset's depth and variability, which is crucial for robust analyses and comprehensive model training.

7.3.1 Dataset Details

This Kaggle-acquired dataset delves into the realm of tea pathology, encompassing the manifestation of seven prevalent diseases afflicting tea leaves: red leaf spot, algal leaf spot, bird eyespot, gray blight, white spot, anthracnose, and brown blight, alongside a classification for healthy foliage. In our research, a judicious segmentation of this extensive dataset was undertaken, cleaving it into distinct training and testing sets. The training subset comprises a substantial 711 instances, complemented by an additional 174 instances earmarked for the validation dataset. The reader can refer to Ref. [11] for the data set. This meticulous partitioning facilitates a nuanced exploration of the intricacies within each tea affliction, ensuring the robustness and reliability of subsequent analyses and model evaluations.

7.3.2 Proposed Detection Schema

In this pursuit, the chosen model is the venerable VGG16, a CNN architecture birthed from the ingenuity of the Visual Geometry Group at the esteemed University of Oxford. Revered for its elegant yet profound design, this neural network boasts a structural opulence comprising a total of 16 layers shown in Figure 7.2. Among these strata, one finds the intricate interplay of convolutional layers, the judicious inclusion of max-pooling layers, and the culmination in fully connected layers. It is this amalgamation of architectural finesse that defines the essence of the VGG16 model, a testament to the meticulous artistry of the Visual Geometry Group's scholarly endeavors.

Input Layer: This layer is designed to ingest color images measuring 224×224 pixels, featuring atriad of channels dedicated to the Red, Green, and Blue (RGB) color space.

Convolutional Layers: The architecture employs a sequence of convolutional layers characterized by 3×3 receptive fields and a stride of 1. To maintain the integrity of the input and output feature map dimensions, padding is judiciously applied. This strategic utilization of padding ensures that the

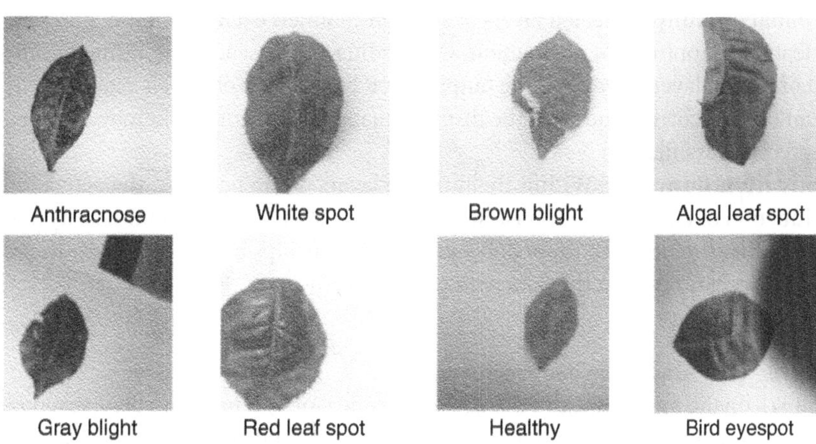

Figure 7.2 Images showing various diseases from the dataset. Source: PlantVillage Dataset / Kaggle, Inc.

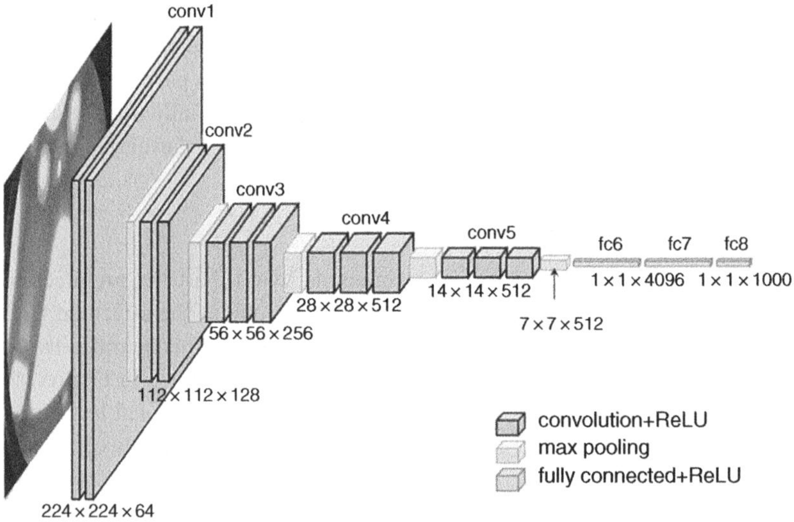

Figure 7.3 Internal process in the VGG16 model. Source: Aatila et al. [12]/with permission of International Journal of Computer Engineering and Data Science (IJCEDS).

convolutional operations seamlessly navigate through the input, preserving spatial information and yielding feature maps with consistent sizes (Figure 7.3).

Max Pooling: Executes max pooling across 2 × 2 windows with a stride of 2, ensuring that nonoverlapping windows are employed for this operation, thereby enhancing computational efficiency and feature extraction.

Fully Connected Layers: Embarking on the neural network architecture, the initial two fullyconnected layers boast 4096 channels each, facilitating intricate feature mapping and abstraction. Concluding this cascade, the ultimate fully connected layer, serving as the output layer, boasts 1000 channels meticulously tailored to correspond with the distinct ImageNet categories, thereby enabling precise classification.

Activation Function: Within the intricate layers of the network, the activation function of choiceis the robust Rectified Linear Unit, offering nonlinearity and enabling the network to model complex relationships and extract meaningful representations from the data with enhanced efficacy.

7.3.2.1 Data Acquisition and Preprocessing

Embark on the initial phase of this scientific endeavor by amassing a diverse repository of tea plant images, encompassing both diseased and healthy leaves. Organize this dataset meticulously into distinct subdirectories, each representing a specific class, such as the algal leaf, anthracnose, and bird's-eye spot. In preparation for subsequent computational analyses, standardize the dimensions of these images to a consistent format, such as 224 × 224 pixels. Simultaneously, optimize the data by normalizing pixel values to fit within the constrained range of [0, 1]. This meticulous preprocessing lays the foundation for robust downstream analysis, ensuring uniformity and compatibility within the dataset.

7.3.2.2 Data Augmentation

This section embarks on the augmentation of data, employing the sophisticated capabilities embedded within TensorFlow's "ImageDataGenerator" class. This avant-garde approach transcends conventional methodologies by intricately manipulating the dataset through a myriad of transformative processes. Techniques encompass not merely rotation but also nuanced shifts in width, height, and shearing, alongside judicious zooming and the artful orchestration of horizontal flipping. This meticulous curation culminates in the generation of an enriched reservoir of training data, fostering heightened robustness and versatility within the model's learning framework.

7.3.2.3 Model Section and Building

Embarking on the pivotal phase of model selection, meticulous consideration is given to the optimal CNN architecture to underpin our computational edifice. In this realm, the venerable VGG16 emerges as the chosen bastion, having garnered distinction through pre-training on the expansive ImageNet dataset, showcasing unparalleled prowess in feature extraction. The model instantiation unfolds with the ceremonial loading of the pre-trained VGG16 onto the computational canvas. A bespoke touch is introduced through the grafting of custom classification layers atop the VGG16 framework, including the refinement of a flattened layer where intricate pixel harmonies converge and the establishment of fully connected dense layers, orchestrating patterns in a symphony of computational choreography. To ensure the sanctity of the foundational layers, a strategic decision is made to freeze the initial stratum of the VGG16 model. This judicious move serves a dual purpose—the preservation of learned features and the fortification against unwarranted modifications during subsequent training phases. By encapsulating the essence of prior knowledge within the confines of the unaltered layers, the model maintains fidelity to its pre-trained wisdom. This deliberate act not only upholds the integrity of acquired features but also acts as a safeguard against the perils of overwriting invaluable insights with the flux of newfound knowledge, contributing to the resilience and robustness of the computational architecture.

7.3.2.4 Model Training

Utilize the Adam optimizer with a refined learning rate of 0.0001, employing a categorical cross-entropy loss function and accuracy metric. Train the model on

while benefiting from the generalization capabilities of the pre-trained model. The achieved accuracy of 92% highlights the effectiveness of the proposed method in disease prediction, which is essential for efficient disease management in tea cultivation. Moreover, the model's ability to accurately categorize various types of tea leaf diseases underscores its potential for informing targeted treatment strategies. With training and validation conducted on a dataset comprising 174 validation images and 711 training images across eight disease classes, followed by evaluation on a separate dataset of 528 images yielding a test accuracy score of 86.17%, this research demonstrates significant progress in leveraging modern technology for sustainable agricultural practices and crop management.

In addition, there is scope to explore different pre-trained CNN architectures such as ResNet, Inception, and DenseNet, assessing their efficacy in tea disease classification. Furthermore, exploring advanced techniques like attention mechanisms or capsule networks could potentially improve feature extraction and classification accuracy in this domain.

References

1 Simonyan, K. and Zisserman, A. (2015). Very deep convolutional networks for large-scale image recognition. *3rd International Conference on Learning Representations (ICLR2015)*, arxiv preprint arxiv: 1409.1556.

2 Ahmed, F., Ahad, M.T., and Emon, Y.R. (2023). *Machine learning-based tea leaf disease detection: a comprehensive review*, arXiv preprint arXiv: 2311.03240.

3 Chen, J. and Jia, J. (2020). Automatic recognition of tea diseases based on deep learning. In: *Advances in Forest Management Under Global Change* (ed. L. Zhang). IntechOpen. DOI: 10.5772/intechopen.91953.

4 Liu, Z., Bashir, R.N., Iqbal, S. et al. (2022). Internet of things (iot) and machine learning model of plant disease prediction–blister blight for tea plant. *Ieee Access* 10: 44934–44944.

5 Zhao, X., Zhang, J., Huang, Y. et al. (2022). Detection and discrimination of disease and insect stress of tea plants using hyperspectral imaging combined with wavelet analysis. *Computers and Electronics in Agriculture* 193: 106717.

6 Datta, S. and Gupta, N. (2023). A novel approach for the detection of tea leaf disease using deep neural network. *Procedia Computer Science* 218: 2273–2286.

7 Hu, G., Ye, R., Wan, M. et al. (2023). Detection of tea leaf blight in low-resolution UAV remote sensing images. *IEEE Transactions on Geoscience and Remote Sensing*. https://doi.org/10.1109/TGRS.2023.3339765.

8 Lin, J., Bai, D., Xu, R., and Lin, H. (2023). Tsba-yolo: an improved tea diseases detection model based on attention mechanisms and feature fusion. *Forests* 14: 619.

9 Han, Y., Deng, X., Tong, H., and Chen, Y. (2024). Effect of blister blight disease caused by exobasidium on tea quality. *Food Chemistry: X* 21: 101077.

10 Jayaseelan, E., Nixon, P.D., Magdalin, A.E. et al. (2024). Role of kit-6 on the fungicide and pesticide activities of zinc, copper and, magnesium oxide nanoparticles prepared using *Camellia sinensis* extract (tea plant) through green synthesis. *Nano-Structures & Nano-Objects* 38: 101119.

11 https://www.kaggle.com/datasets/shashwatwork/identifying-disease-in-tea-leafs/data (accessed 20 January 2024).

12 Aatila, M., Lachgar, M., Hrimech, H. et al. (2021). Diabetic retinopathy classification using resnet50 and vgg-16 pretrained networks. *International Journal of Computer Engineering and Data Science (IJCEDS)* 1: 1–7.

8

Advancing Colorectal Cancer Diagnosis: Integrating Synthetic Data and Machine Learning for Microbiome Analysis

Alessio Rotelli and Ernesto Iadanza

Department of Medical Biotechnologies, University of Siena, Italy

8.1 Colorectal Cancer (CRC)

According to the World Health Organization (WHO), CRC, affecting the colon (large intestine) or rectum, stands as one of the prevalent cancer types globally, posing significant health risks, including mortality. Its incidence typically escalates with advancing age, with most cases observed in individuals aged over 50. Furthermore, research indicates that by 2035, the mortality rate for colon and rectal cancer is projected to rise by 60% in terms of detection and by 71.5% in terms of mortality [1]. The probability of being affected by CRC is 4–5%, and the risk of developing CRC is mainly associated with personal features, such as age, chronic disease history, and lifestyle [2]. The progression of CRC is commonly perceived as a multistep sequence commencing with the emergence of a benign polyp that can progress to an in situ carcinoma through the accrual of further somatic mutations [3, 4]. Most CRC cases are not directly linked to inherited genetic factors and are considered sporadic [5]. Heritable CRC, which results from specific genetic susceptibility, is responsible for a relatively smaller proportion of cases, typically ranging from 12% to 35% of all CRC cases [6]. A growing body of research is dedicated to exploring the involvement of the gut microbiome in CRC development [7]. The emerging focus on the gut microbiome's role in CRC development offers promising avenues for future investigation and therapeutic and diagnostic intervention. Continued research efforts are crucial for enhancing our understanding and addressing the increasing burden of CRC on a global scale.

Generative Artificial Intelligence for Biomedical and Smart Health Informatics,
First Edition. Edited by Aditya Khamparia and Deepak Gupta.

classification tasks will be accompanied by SHapley Additive exPlanations (SHAP) analysis to underline bacterial taxa driving model decision-making and that are more effective in distinguishing the treated samples.

8.5 Use of Data Augmentation

To address the inherent class imbalance in the dataset, the Synthetic Data Vault (SDV), a Python package renowned for its ability to generate synthetic data, was utilized. By employing SDV, the discrepancy in the number of CRC and AP samples was effectively addressed through the synthesis of additional instances for both classes. The idea of using this specific tool originates from another scientific work published in 2022, where SDV is employed to anonymize patients' microbiome data by generating synthetic OTU tables from real ones [26]. Drawing from the statistical properties of the real samples, the SDV synthesizers meticulously construct a generative model capable of closely replicating the statistical characteristics of the original dataset. SDV employs a mechanism called Conditional Parameter Aggregation (CPA) to build the previously cited generative model. The Python package makes available different kinds of synthesizers, namely, CTGAN, DAY Z, TVAE, Copula-GAN, and Gaussian Copula. In synthesizing new data, the Gaussian Copula synthesizer was exploited, employing Gaussian kernel density estimation (KDE) as the default distribution, due to the nature of the data, which might not conform strictly to a predefined parametric distribution. Instead of assuming a specific distribution, the Gaussian KDE method relies on the data itself to construct an approximation of the underlying distribution, bypassing the need for predetermined distribution specifications.

8.6 Data Evaluation Metrics

8.6.1 Classification

Following the synthesis of new data points by SDV, various techniques were employed to evaluate their quality. The synthesized samples were integrated into datasets comprising both real and synthetic data. These datasets were then subjected to classification using two parallel classifiers: logistic regression (LG) and support vector machine (SVM) employing a polynomial kernel. This approach was motivated by the aim to directly evaluate the classifier's capability to distinguish between real and synthetic data, thereby offering a more cohesive and thorough assessment of the model's performance. Through the merging of these datasets, the aim is to evaluate the classifier's performance within a context closely mirroring the complexities of real-world environments where real and synthetic data coexist. Previously, the two algorithms were tested on a dataset consisting of biopsy and fecal samples from patients with CRC. It was noted that LG performed well in effectively distinguishing the data. However, SVM with a polynomial kernel needed meticulous parameter adjustment to achieve optimal functionality. To achieve this, the Python package Optuna was employed, enabling exploration within a specified parameter range and facilitating model hyperparameter tuning. The data points accepted were those exhibiting the poorest classification performance. This suggests that the classifiers struggled to distinguish between the two datasets, implying a notable level of similarity between real and synthetic data.

8.6.2 Statistical Tests

After data classification, real and synthetic data were subjected to statistical analysis. In the data validation process, the Kolmogorov–Smirnov (KS) test was employed to assess the similarity between real and synthetic datasets. Pairs of columns between the datasets were systematically compared with determine if they were drawn from the same statistical distribution. In addition, other metrics were considered such as Spearman correlation and mean squared error when comparing column pairs of real and synthetic datasets. Regarding the Spearman correlation, which measures the monotonic relationship between two variables, its value ranges from −1 to 1. Negative values signify an inverse connection between the variables under scrutiny, while positive values denote a direct relationship. Conversely, values nearing zero suggest a weak correlation between the variables. This approach successfully augmented the number of samples per class, resulting in a total of 190 samples encompassing both AP and CRC categories. This expanded dataset forms a more comprehensive and representative foundation for subsequent tasks, such as feature extraction and classification. The reliability and effectiveness of analyses and models are enhanced by ensuring a balanced representation of classes.

8.7 Feature Extraction by Later-Wise Relevance Propagation

Feature extraction was performed using a Python function called Layer-Wise Relevance Propagation (LRP). To ensure robust generalization of a machine learning model, its decisions must be supported by meaningful patterns within the input data. A fundamental requirement for achieving this is the model's ability to provide explanations for its predictions, elucidating the input features driving its decisions. LRP is a methodology that addresses this need, offering interpretability for potentially intricate deep neural networks [27]. LRP functions by backward propagation of predictions throughout the neural network, employing a set of intentionally crafted propagation rules [28]. In this way, LRP performs the selection of propagation rules at each layer to ensure high-quality explanations, which means finding those input features that contribute most to the model decision-making process [29]. LRP was consistently used on a neural network classification model with k-fold cross-validation to uncover the key bacterial taxa that distinguish and locate samples into their belonging class. The deep learning classification model consists of three layers: two dense layers with different activation functions and one dense layer with a sigmoid activation for binary classification. At this point, we proceed to choose the best activation function for the model hidden layer. In the evaluation process, four distinct activation functions were scrutinized: ReLU, LeakyReLU, Softmax, and GeLU. After the analysis, Leaky ReLU emerged as the most effective activation function among the chosen options, demonstrating superior performance in the classification. Considering these results, LRP was applied to the classification model using the LeakyReLU activation function. The feature extraction was performed on 18 AP and 18 CRC samples (about 10% of the total dataset) to avoid overfitting the neural network classification model. The remaining 172 samples were used for the subsequent machine learning classification and SHAP investigation. A total of 64 from the 10,329 bacterial taxa have been extracted using LRP.

8.8 Beta Diversity Analysis

After LRP feature extraction, a beta diversity investigation on the original OTU table and the one after feature extraction has been conducted. Before plotting, all the entries of the tables were converted to the square root of the percent abundances of each OTU in a sample. To achieve this, the process included computing the sum of all OTU within a specific sample, then each entry was divided by the total sum, multiplied by 100, and the square root of the result was obtained. Beta diversity is an analytical tool that helps to understand how various samples differ from each other. To proceed in the beta diversity analysis, a distance matrix is computed starting from the OTU table. In this case, the distance matrix is generated based on Bray–Curtis dissimilarity, which enables researchers to understand the distinctions between samples based on sequence abundance, presence or absence of sequences, and even evolutionary relationships [30]. The obtained matrix, which couples all the samples to calculate their differences and similarities, is visualized using principal coordinate analysis (PCoA). As mentioned in "Conducting a Microbiome Study" [31], methods like PCoA reduce

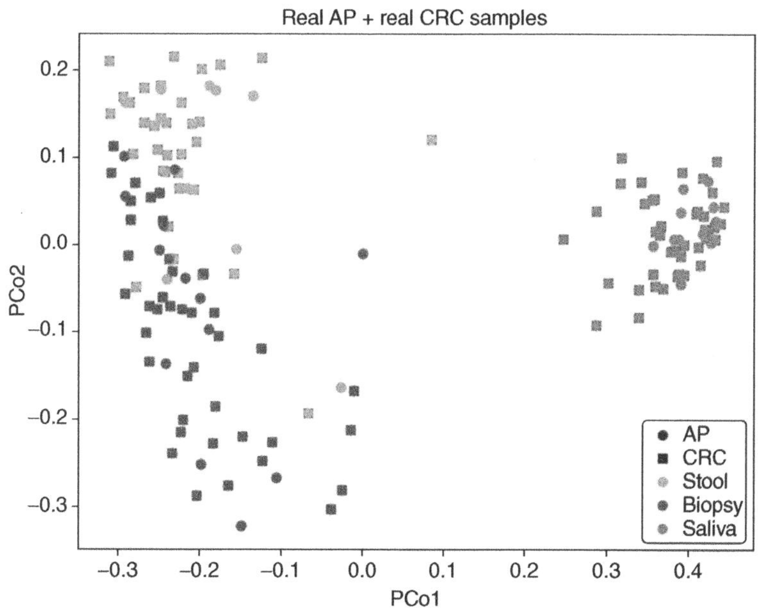

Figure 8.1 Principal coordinate analysis of the original OTU table comprehending real AP and CRC samples.

the dimensionality of complex microbiome datasets, allowing us to see the relationships between samples in two- or three-dimensional scatterplots. In this representation, every point indicates an individual sample, and the space between points traces the degree of dissimilarity between those samples. The original OTU table produced by Russo et al. [4] is plotted (Figure 8.1), as well as the one enriched with synthetic samples of AP and CRC samples (Figure 8.2), and at last, the OTU table after feature extraction with LRP (Figure 8.3).

8.9 Machine Learning and SHAP Analysis to Classify AP and CRC Samples

This analysis lays the groundwork for employing the identified bacterial taxa in future classification tasks, potentially extending to clinical applications. Three widely recognized machine learning algorithms for classification, support vector classifier (SVC), XGBoost, and random forest (RF), were selected for this purpose. The classification was conducted on a comprehensive dataset comprising all sample types and three datasets segmented by sample type (stool, biopsy, and saliva). The first classification allows us to understand the global difference

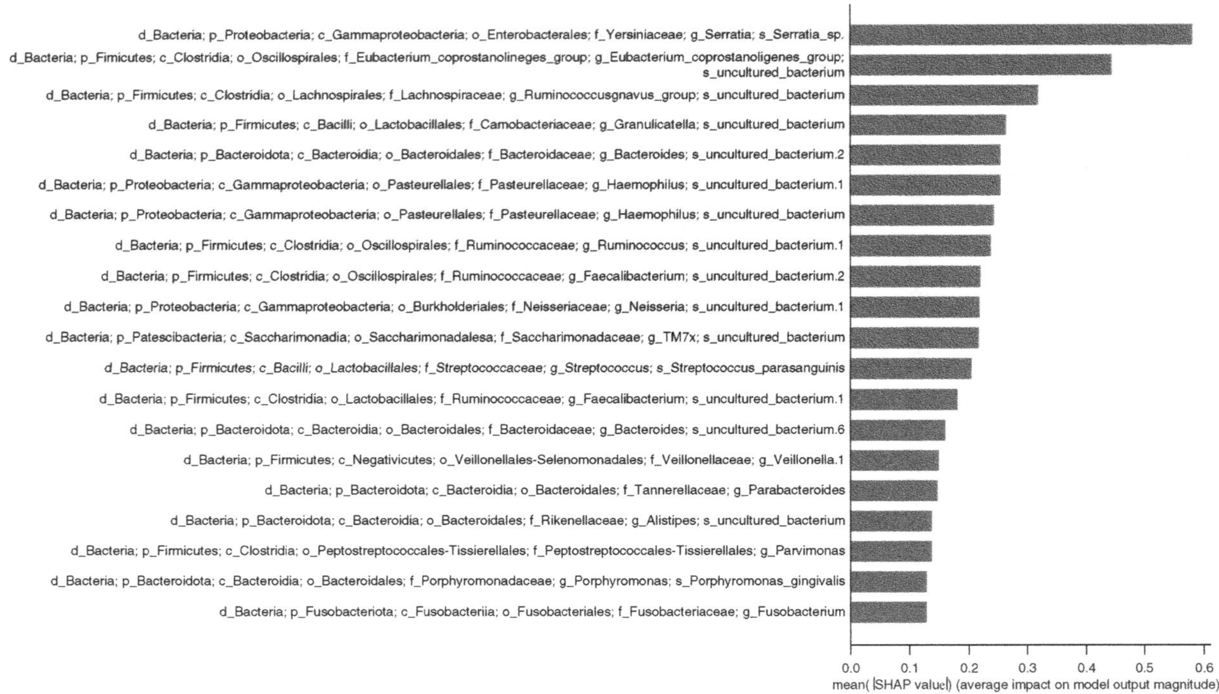

Figure 8.5 Summary plot of the SHAP analysis of the comprehensive OTU table.

delved into the SHAP method to understand the influence of individual features on the decision-making process of the XGBoost model. In Figure 8.5, a summary plot shows features sorted by their mean SHAP values, ordering taxa based on their importance in model classification. Subsequently, the dataset was partitioned based on sample types, namely, stool, biopsy, and saliva, and separate classifications were conducted on each subset. The stool dataset exhibited robust performance with an accuracy of 86% and an AUC of 0.98 (Figure 8.6). Similarly, the biopsy dataset demonstrated high accuracy, reaching 96%, accompanied by an AUC of 0.99 (Figure 8.6). At last, the saliva dataset showcased exceptional performance, achieving an accuracy of 100% and a perfect AUC of 1 (Figure 8.6). In the subsequent phase, SHAP analysis was carried out individually on the three datasets, producing three distinct summary plots (Figures 8.7–8.9).

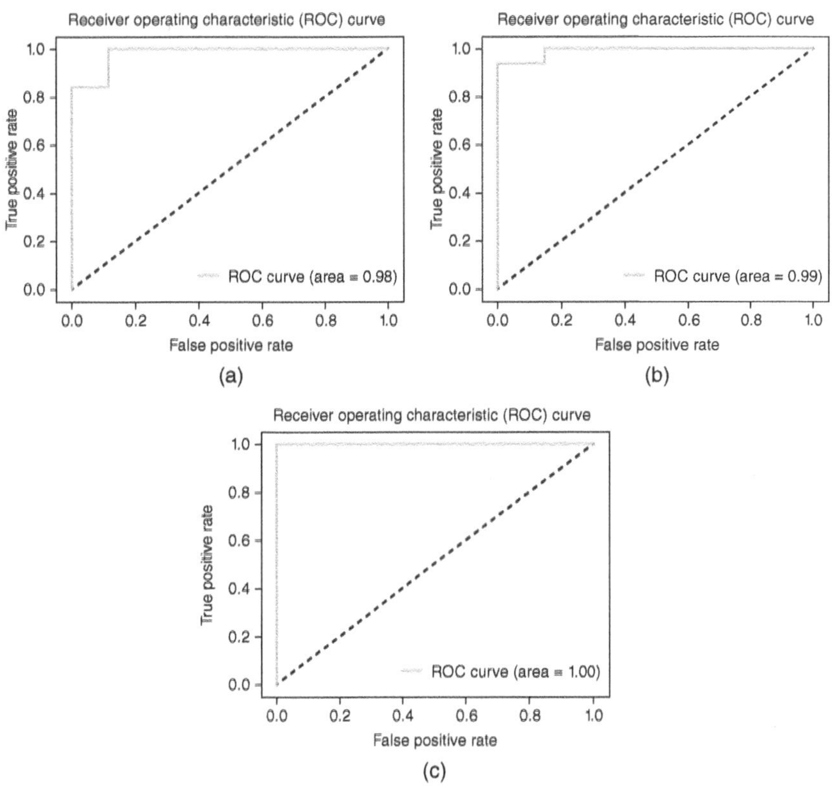

Figure 8.6 The AUC of classification is depicted for the stool OTU table in (a), the biopsy OTU table in (b), and the saliva OTU table in (c).

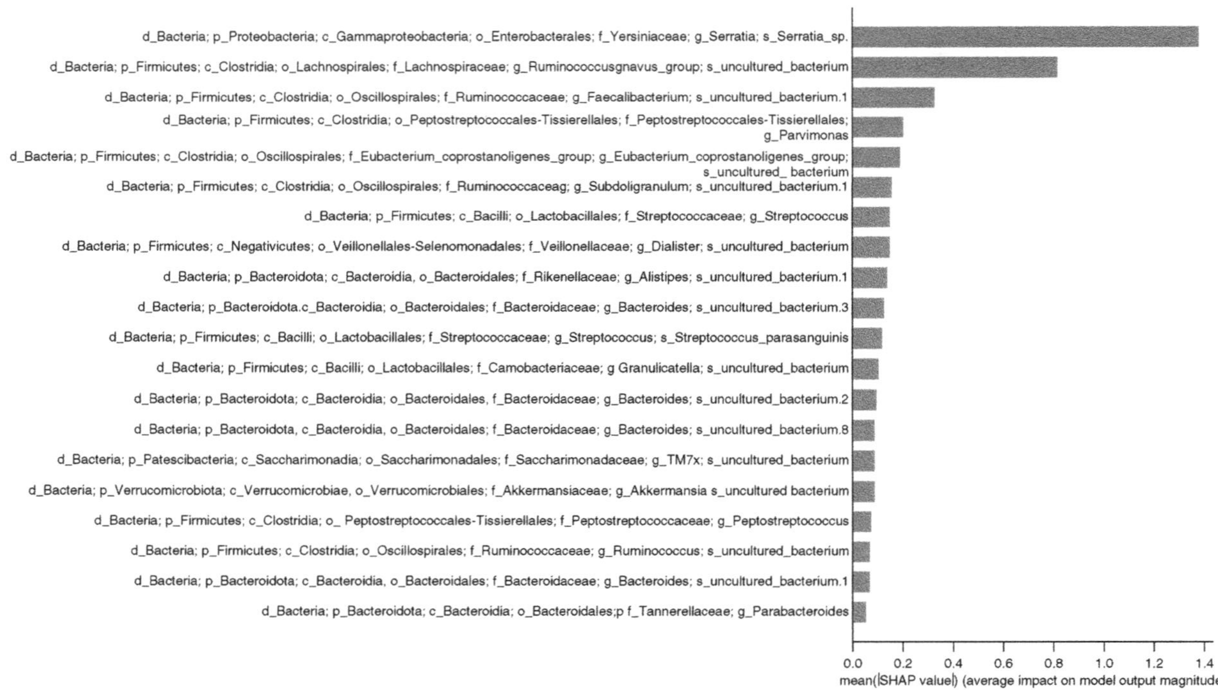

Figure 8.7 Summary plot of the SHAP analysis of the stool OTU table.

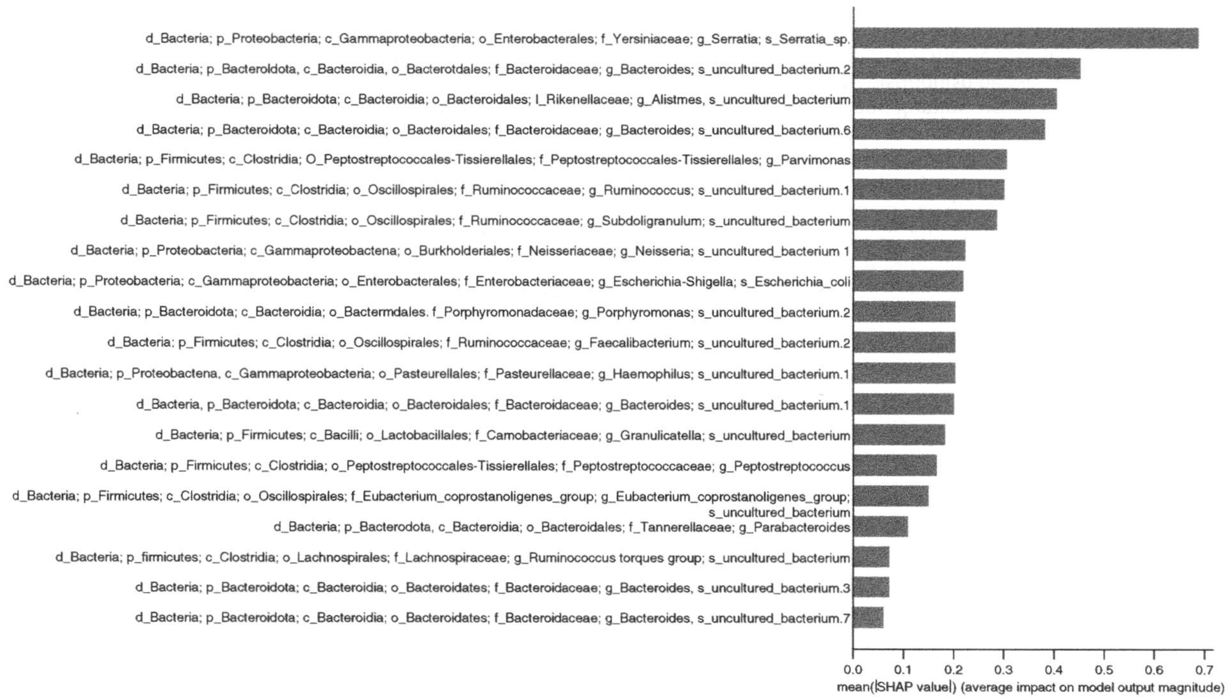

Figure 8.8 Summary plot of the SHAP analysis of the biopsy OTU table.

References

1 Douaiher, J., Ravipati, A., Grams, B. et al. (2017). Colorectal cancer—global burden, trends, and geographical variations. *Journal of Surgical Oncology* 115 (5): 619–630.

2 Mármol, I., Diego, C.S.á.-d., Dieste, A.P. et al. (2017). Colorectal carcinoma: a general overview and future perspectives in colorectal cancer. *International Journal of Molecular Sciences* 18 (1): 197.

3 Simon, K. (2016). Colorectal cancer development and advances in screening. *Clinical Interventions in Aging* 11: 967–976.

4 Russo, E., Di Gloria, L., Nannini, G. et al. (2023). From adenoma to crc stages: the oral-gut microbiome axis as a source of potential microbial and metabolic biomarkers of malignancy. *Neoplasia* 40: 100901.

5 Carethers, J.M. and Jung, B.H. (2015). Genetics and genetic biomarkers in sporadic colorectal cancer. *Gastroenterology* 149 (5): 1177–1190.

6 Czene, K., Lichtenstein, P., and Hemminki, K. (2002). Environmental and heritable causes of cancer among 9.6 million individuals in the swedish family-cancer database. *International Journal of Cancer* 99 (2): 260–266.

7 Kim, J. and Lee, H.K. (2022). Potential role of the gut microbiome in colorectal cancer progression. *Frontiers in Immunology* 12: 807648.

8 Al Bander, Z., Nitert, M.D., Mousa, A., and Naderpoor, N. (2020). The gut microbiota and inflammation: an overview. *International Journal of Environmental Research and Public Health* 17 (20): 7618.

9 Rinninella, E., Raoul, P., Cintoni, M. et al. (2019). What is the healthy gut microbiota composition? A changing ecosystem across age, environment, diet, and diseases. *Microorganisms* 7 (1): 14.

10 Qin, J., Li, R., Raes, J. et al. (2010). A human gut microbial gene catalogue established by metagenomic sequencing. *Nature* 464 (7285): 59–65.

11 Sender, R., Fuchs, S., and Milo, R. (2016). Are we really vastly outnumbered? Revisiting the ratio of bacterial to host cells in humans. *Cell* 164 (3): 337–340.

12 Vyas, U. and Ranganathan, N. (2012). Probiotics, prebiotics, and synbiotics: gut and beyond. *Gastroenterology Research and Practice* 2012: 872716.

13 Cummings, J.H., Pomare, E., Branch, W. et al. (1987). Short chain fatty acids in human large intestine, portal, hepatic and venous blood. *Gut* 28 (10): 1221–1227.

14 Koropatkin, N.M., Cameron, E.A., and Martens, E.C. (2012). How glycan metabolism shapes the human gut microbiota. *Nature Reviews Microbiology* 10 (5): 323–335.

15 Guarner, F. and Malagelada, J.-R. (2003). Gut flora in health and disease. *The Lancet* 361 (9356): 512–519.

16 Bull, M.J. and Plummer, N.T. (2015). Part 2: treatments for chronic gastrointestinal disease and gut dysbiosis. *Integrative Medicine: A Clinician's Journal* 14 (1): 25.

17 Sobhani, I., Tap, J., Roudot-Thoraval, F. et al. (2011). Microbial dysbiosis in colorectal cancer (crc) patients. *PloS One* 6 (1): e16393.

18 Zou, S., Fang, L., and Lee, M.-H. (2018). Dysbiosis of gut microbiota in promoting the development of colorectal cancer. *Gastroenterology Report* 6 (1): 1–12.

19 Artemev, A., Naik, S., Pougno, A. et al. (2022). The association of microbiome dysbiosis with colorectal cancer. *Cureus* 14 (2): e22156.

20 Petersen, C. and Round, J.L. (2014). Defining dysbiosis and its influence on host immunity and disease. *Cellular Microbiology* 16 (7): 1024–1033.

21 Song, M., Chan, A.T., and Sun, J. (2020). Influence of the gut microbiome, diet, and environment on risk of colorectal cancer. *Gastroenterology* 158 (2): 322–340.

22 Lavelle, A. and Sokol, H. (2020). Gut microbiota-derived metabolites as key actors in inflammatory bowel disease. *Nature Reviews Gastroenterology & Hepatology* 17 (4): 223–237.

23 Hrncir, T. (2022). Gut microbiota dysbiosis: triggers, consequences, diagnostic and therapeutic options. *Microorganisms* 10 (3): 578.

24 Feng, Q., Liang, S., Jia, H. et al. (2015). Gut microbiome development along the colorectal adenoma–carcinoma sequence. *Nature Communications* 6 (1): 6528.

25 Yu, M., Jia, H., Zhou, C. et al. (2017). Variations in gut microbiota and fecal metabolic phenotype associated with depression by 16s rrna gene sequencing and lc/ms-based metabolomics. *Journal of Pharmaceutical and Biomedical Analysis* 138: 231–239.

26 Hittmeir, M., Mayer, R., and Ekelhart, A. (2022). Utility and privacy assessment of synthetic microbiome data. In: *IFIP Annual Conference on Data and Applications Security and Privacy*, 15–27. Springer.

27 Montavon, G., Binder, A., Lapuschkin, S. et al. (2019). Layer-wise relevance propagation: an overview. In: *Explainable AI: Interpreting, Explaining and Visualizing Deep Learning* (ed. W. Samek, G. Montavon, A. Vedaldi, et al.), 193–209.

28 Anders, C.J., Montavon, G., Samek, W., and Müller, K.-R. (2019). Understanding patch-based learning of video data by explaining predictions. In: *Explainable AI: Interpreting, Explaining and Visualizing Deep Learning* (ed. W. Samek, G. Montavon, A. Vedaldi, et al.), 297–309.

29 Arbabzadah, F., Montavon, G., Müller, K.-R., and Samek, W. (2016). Identifying individual facial expressions by deconstructing a neural network. *Pattern*

Recognition: 38th German Conference, GCPR 2016, pp. 344–354, Hannover, Germany, (12–15 September 2016). Proceedings 38. Springer.

30 Kers, J.G. and Saccenti, E. (2022). The power of microbiome studies: Some considerations on which alpha and beta metrics to use and how to report results. *Frontiers in Microbiology* 12: 796025.

31 Goodrich, J.K., Di Rienzi, S.C., Poole, A.C. et al. (2014). Conducting a microbiome study. *Cell* 158 (2): 250–262.

32 Liu, J., Huang, X., Chen, C. et al. (2023). Identification of colorectal cancer progression associated intestinal microbiome and predictive signature construction. *Journal of Translational Medicine* 21 (1): 373.

33 Löwenmark, T., Löfgren-Burström, A., Zingmark, C. et al. (2020). *Parvimonas micra* as a putative non-invasive faecal biomarker for colorectal cancer. *Scientific Reports* 10 (1): 15250.

34 Chen, W.-D., Zhang, X., Zhang, M.-J. et al. (2022). Salivary fusobacterium nucleatum serves as a potential diagnostic biomarker for gastric cancer. *World Journal of Gastroenterology* 28 (30): 4120.

35 Löwenmark, T., Löfgren-Burström, A., Zingmark, C. et al. (2022). Tumour colonisation of parvimonas micra is associated with decreased survival in colorectal cancer patients. *Cancers* 14 (23): 5937.

36 Zhao, L., Zhang, X., Zhou, Y. et al. (2022). *Parvimonas micra* promotes colorectal tumorigenesis and is associated with prognosis of colorectal cancer patients. *Oncogene* 41 (36): 4200–4210.

37 Ou, S., Wang, H., Tao, Y. et al. (2022). Fusobacterium nucleatum and colorectal cancer: from phenomenon to mechanism. *Frontiers in Cellular and Infection Microbiology* 12: 1020583.

9

Recent Knowledge in Drug Design and Development: Automation and Advancement

*Kusum Gurung†, Saurav K. Mishra†, Tabsum Chhetri, Sneha Roy, Anagha Balakrishnan, and John J. Georrge**

Department of Bioinformatics, University of North Bengal, Darjeeling, West Bengal, India

9.1 Introduction

Drug design and development is a laborious and expensive progression that takes more than ten years to complete for a single molecule. Traditionally, the drug discovery process goes through various steps, from target identification to hits optimization and clinical trials, before the drugs are released in the markets. Target selection is the initial step of drug design, where the target molecule is selected. A perfect target is chosen when the disease and its associated pathway are thoroughly examined. Making sure the target is related to the condition is a crucial step in the procedure and is often called target validation. Target validation is followed by lead optimization, which comprises manual manufacturing and testing processes to maximize the safety and effectiveness of lead compounds [1]. Preclinical trials are the next step in confirming the lead compounds' efficacy and reliability. A medication must complete multiple protracted clinical studies (I, II, and III) before it is released onto the market. The medication is submitted for regulatory approval to organizations like the Food and Drug Administration (FDA) once it successfully completes its clinical studies (Figure 9.1). Following regulatory clearance, the medication is prepared for market release. The majority of drugs fail throughout preclinical trials [1]. The most frequent cause of failure has been shown to be improper and insufficient target validation, along with inadequate molecular screening [2]. Molecules must satisfy a variety of requirements in this process. Aside from having the appropriate potency for the biological target, the drug should also have good physicochemical and ADMET

†Considered as joint first authors
*Corresponding author

Generative Artificial Intelligence for Biomedical and Smart Health Informatics,
First Edition. Edited by Aditya Khamparia and Deepak Gupta.

thus help explore the features of automation in the drug development progression, thereby highlighting its relevance and significance.

9.2 Automation in Drug Design and Development

The conventional approach to drug design is excruciatingly slow, costly, and nontarget-specific, which can have numerous detrimental impacts on health. It costs over $2 billion and takes 14–15 years to find a treatment [16]. With the advent of automation, the process of designing drugs has also changed in conjunction with the world's technological advancements. Automation of drug design has emerged as a revolutionary approach that has the power to drastically alter the pharmaceutical industry with technologies like robotics and machine intelligence, which are helping to enhance and expedite the method of finding novel drugs, resulting in the improvement of new medicines. Automation is crucial to the drug design industry because it streamlines the molecular design cycle, enhances decision-making, and accelerates the pursuit of novel drugs. Tasks like compound production and screening that individuals traditionally did can be automated, which can enhance processes, utilize less material, and produce quick feedback loops, thereby making it more cost-effective and less time-consuming [7]. Within the chemical and biological sciences, automation has become increasingly prevalent as part of the "Industry 4.0 revolution." In the pharmaceutical sector, automation goals include deploying robotics to replace tedious bench tests and automated sampling and analysis of analytical investigations. A good drug should have pharmacokinetic properties for better effect and safety purposes, which can be obtained by the implementation of automation [17]. Drug design and screening can now take advantage of various computational techniques, particularly the HTS technologies, to significantly reduce time and cost. The speed at which computer hardware, software, and algorithms are developing makes this conceivable. The pharmaceutical sector is becoming more and more interested in using ML techniques due to recent advancements in several domains. Because there are now more categories and numbers of data collections that can be the basis for infinitely scalable storage and ML, pharmaceutical businesses can access and arrange significantly more data [18]. More than one million compounds have been screened for the one marketable drug; therefore, larger libraries are under pressure to be screened to maintain the pipeline and advance HTS. The primary goal of HTS is to find high-quality hits or leads with the new structure and actively low concentration [19]. HTS of compound libraries is a major source of new chemical entities for discovery initiatives in the pharma sector. The following elements of this intricate process can be primarily identified: assay creation using microfluidics; compound library selection; HTS technologies/methodologies; and outcome interpretation, and it evaluates the hit by statistically comparing which active agents, or "hits," deviate from the average response for all tested agents by a predefined amount according to the organization's test capacity and cost thresholds [20]. Microfluidics is an essential HTS technology used in modern drug discovery because microfluidic technologies are made to work with fluids at the nanoliter to microliter scale; they can be applied to high-throughput assay analysis, flow chemistry with improved experimental control and single-cell manipulation. Preclinical research, target and lead identification, and other related fields are improved and revolutionized by microfluidic technologies; in addition to that, microfluidic platforms are also widely used for personalized medicine, the creation of organs on a chip, and the creation of artificial cells and tissues [21]. Lab-on-a-chip is a known system under microfluidics technology that combines several laboratory operations into tiny, several square millimeters to a few square centimeter chips. These platforms allow miniaturized, computerized, combined, and distributed chemical and physiological inquiries compared with conventional experimental procedures, which can result in more economical, timely, regulated, and highly effective biochemical tests at a very small scale [22].

The average time to get medicine into clinical trials has shortened, while the success rate of pharmaceuticals approved by the FDA has dropped to 12%. Computer-aided drug design (CADD), which speeds up the procedure of choosing the best molecules via experimental studies, has rendered medication development less expensive and time-consuming [23]. In the subject of drug design, many different kinds of computerized methods and tools are introduced to predict and validate drug targets or drug-like molecules, which is comparatively faster, cost-efficient, and gives more accurate data [24]. Molecular docking is a widely used computer method that estimate the mechanism of binding and affinity of small molecules for target proteins, hence simplifying the discovery of promising lead molecules [23], along with techniques like molecular dynamic simulation, that gives information about the steadiness behavior of complexes, enabling the assessment of protein flexibility and the improvement of binding poses, in addition, important subjects to study with molecular dynamic include allosteric processes and modulation, as well as the function of water in ligand binding and optimization [18, 25] and quantitative structure–activity relationship (QSAR) modeling which correlates chemical structure features with biological activity, guiding the design of compounds with improved potency, selectivity, and pharmacokinetic properties, its main objective to find both hits identification and hit-to-lead optimization are also widely used [26]. AI is essential for automating the process of drug development and research; AI technologies use the abundance of freely available high-quality data to enable improved decision-making, cutting down on the process's time and expense. Algorithms like ML and DL have emerged as potential remedies to overcome traditional drug design hurdles [27, 28]. AI applications include therapeutic efficacy discovery, safety biomarker assurance, and drug–protein interaction prediction [29]. It has been shown that these algorithms apply to many different programs involving physicochemical qualities, biological activity, and toxicity [3]. AI is more important in turning medical data into research-like reusable techniques than it is in relying on speculative advancements. Generally speaking, several methods are taken into consideration in the context of ML, such as random forest (RF), naive Bayesian classification, etc. To improve the capacity to extract features and generalize features [29]. During the initial period of drug finding, there was a dearth of published data in the field of drug development based on AI-assisted algorithms. The availability of data has been the primary cause. The researchers now have access to more molecular data along with other informative features due to advancements in biotechnology and computational methods. Furthermore, significant endeavors have created open archives that offer a vast array of details about molecules in a uniform style, along with the reported study data.

9.3 Tools and Database for Drug Design, including Algorithm and Application

Using automation, along with AI, ML, and other crucial associated applications and algorithms in drug design, has transformed the pharmaceutical sector, increased productivity, and sped up the CADD process. Several CADD methodologies have been developed along with ML applications to improve the accuracy and efficiency of CADD procedures [30, 31]. CADD uses two basic techniques for drug discovery: structure-based and ligand-based. The intended protein's accessibility dictates the optimal CADD method, and experimental procedures are costly and normally undertaken on small scales due to their intricacy [32]. Furthermore, in silico tools have been developed to identify prospective therapeutic targets, including statistical and ML-based models likewise PharmMapper [33] and TargetHunter [34], built with ML algorithm and data mining algorithms to predict biological targets of a relevant drug compound. However, modeling the target molecule is also possible when it is difficult to get using X-ray diffraction [35] and nuclear magnetic resonance spectroscopy techniques [36]. Identical protein modeling is prevalent in silico technique that is frequently implemented for drug target modeling via automated comparative modeling tools such as SWISS-MODEL [37], MODELLER [38], and ESyPred3D [39], which use DL algorithms such as similar searching and modeling [40]. However, ab initio modeling has also yielded promising results in the case of conformational search of an unmatched target sequence, where advanced software such as I-TASSER [41], Robetta [42], and QUARK [43] are used with their iterative threading assembly refinement algorithm, Markov chain Monte Carlo algorithm as well as the meta threading algorithm, to predict target structures via energy conformation. Evaluating the target structure for structure-based drug discovery is required to gain accurate structure information that will aid in the binding process with the drug molecules. Several tools, algorithms, and advanced applications help to evaluate target structures in a scientific manner. AlphaFold uses DL algorithms and attention-based approaches to understand target sequences via structural analysis of secondary conformation, providing a quality assessment of protein structure [44]. Although there are various alternative techniques for confirming the structure, such as stereochemical conformation and the most favored region, through PROCHECK with its DL algorithm [45]. However, the eminence of the target is determined by its binding sites, where the drug molecule attaches properly and gives the desired impact. Various methods and techniques are utilized for prediction, such as PrankWeb [46] and BSpred [47], which use many computational algorithms, including neural network-based prediction algorithms to forecast the druggability of the discovered active site [48]. After the identification of the active site and framework, there are a multitude of possibilities for identifying a viable lead in accordance with the target's structure. This procedure can be aided by automated virtual screening and de novo generating [49, 50]. The most common outcome through virtual screening is docking databases of accessible small compounds into the expected interaction site. However, lead generation depends on target and lead flexibility in the docking and scoring process. One prevalent computer-based technique is molecular coupling methodologies in CADD for predicting the accuracy and configuration of the lead molecule inside the appropriate requisite site. The fragment method, Monte Carlo approach, and genetic algorithm are used in direct and random search tactics to invent the appropriate lead molecule in the docking process. Furthermore, scoring functions are the most useful during the evaluation procedure. Docking programs like FRED [51], Surflex [52], AutoDock [53], and Gold [54], using search algorithm and genetic algorithm, are successful in molecular docking due to their construction and efficacy [55]. Furthermore, virtual screening is one of the common phases in both techniques in CADD, while in ligand-based drug discovery (LBDD), the identified dynamic lead molecules are employed for discovering the target molecule; however, active binders are also accessible through datasets like ChEMBL [56] used structural similarity search, and contain an active compound with biological properties. However, in the case of LBDD, QSAR and pharmacophore are widely utilized as a computational approach, with the pharmacophore model constructing the molecule's common binding mode and QSAR evaluating the quality of the pharmacophore model concurrently [57]. Numerous programs, servers, and databases are available for generating pharmacophore models, including LigandScout [58], Pharmar

Table 9.1 (Continued)

Serial number	Name	URLs/Github	Algorithm	Description	References
7.	The Toxin and Toxin Database (T3DB)	http://www.t3db.ca/	Machine and deep learning	Offers details on contaminants and those who they affect, as well as identifying the poisons' parts and the targets.	[74]
8.	The Small Molecule Pathway Database (SMPDB)	https://www.smpdb.ca/	Machine learning	To know small molecule pathways with detailed diagram and their structures.	[75]
9.	ChemDB	https://cdb.ics.uci.edu/	Machine learning and bit-wise algorithm	Small molecules repository with various representations and formats.	[76]
10.	Similarity Ensemble Approach (SEA)	https://sea.bkslab.org/	Machine learning	Predict ligand–target interaction with high precision rates.	[77]
11.	SuperPred	https://prediction.charite.de/	Machine learning	Prediction of the targets of small compounds.	[78]
12.	ModFOLD9	https://www.reading.ac.uk/bioinf/ModFOLD/	Deep learning	It can detect local errors in 3D protein structures.	[79]

Table 9.1 (Continued)

13.	DeepTM	https://dtu.biolib.com/DeepTMHMM	Deep learning and temperature prediction algorithm	Utilize the sequences of thermophilic proteins to accurately guess their melting point.	[80]
14.	PPIscreenML	https://github.com/victoria-mischley/PPIScreenML	Machine learning	Identify interacting and noninteracting protein couples for protein–protein interaction prediction.	[81]
15.	TransFew	https://github.com/BioinfoMachineLearning/TransFew	Machine learning	Protein sequences with GO (gene ontology) representation for activity and annotation prediction.	[82]
16.	ArtiDock	https://www.receptor.ai/	Deep learning	Predict the ligand conformation in the active sites.	[83]
17.	H3-OPT	https://github.com/chdcg/H3-OPT	Deep learning	Predicts monoclonal antibody and nanobody 3D configurations.	[84]
18.	LigBuilderV3	http://www.pkumdl.cn:8080/ligbuilder3/	Molecular optimization and fragment linking algorithm	Designing the ligands for various conformation of the target.	[85]

(Continued)

Table 9.1 (Continued)

Serial number	Name	URLs/Github	Algorithm	Description	References
19.	NAOMInext	https://software.zbh.uni-hamburg.de/	Sampling algorithm	Built the feasible fragment in the ligand molecule to large the structure.	[86]
20.	de novo DOCK	https://dock.compbio.ucsf.edu/	Anchor-and-grow search algorithm	It used fragments to build ligands for docking.	[87]
21.	PiMine	https://uhh.de/naomi	Alignment algorithm	Analyze the similarity between predicted protein interfaces to know new protein–protein interfaces.	[88]
22.	OpenGrowth	http://opengrowth.sourceforge.net/	Frequent pattern (Fp) growth algorithm	Make novel ligands by joining tiny molecule segments in protein binding sites.	[89]
23.	AutoGrow4	https://durrantlab.pitt.edu/autogrow4/	Genetic algorithm	Rebuild the known ligand molecule and analyze their binding modes to the target.	[90]
24.	MolAICal	https://molaical.github.io/	Artificial intelligence and deep learning algorithm	Generation 3D structure of ligand and 3D binding pocket of target.	[91]
25.	SBMolGen	https://github.com/clinfo/SBMolGen	Deep learning	Generate molecules with better binding scores than the known active compounds.	[92]

of remedy development is determining the most successful drug, which includes development, discovery, validation, design, repurposing, and improving cost efficiency, all of which can aid in clinical trial decision-making. Simultaneously, automation streamlines the process of discovering small molecules by allowing the most probable ones to be identified computationally. Although DL models enable high-throughput virtual screening (HTVS) of vast molecule collections, resulting in the faster identification of novel candidates, they can additionally minimize expenditures and effort associated with new drug marketing [95, 97]. Furthermore, reducing human error and uncertainty across the process benefits discovery pipelines by accelerating processes and improving data quality. The concept of drug repurposing becomes more appealing and beneficial because it permits the new drug to pass Phase II, deprived of passing the Phase I trial. Automated technologies, such as DL applications, can help to classify drugs into therapeutic groups based on their use for future dependency. Moreover, AI exceeds humans in the analysis of complex datasets, emphasizing the transition of novel medication by closing development gaps [95]. Other than that, the incorporation of automation in personalized medicine enables high-throughput analysis of patient samples, allowing for the identification of genetic variations, biomarkers, and other molecular signatures, which are essential for comprehending the underlying causes of diseases and the detection of new medications is accelerated by the use of automated technologies [98]. Robots, on the other hand, are becoming more common at diverse phases of the pharmacological industry's industrial process, such as dosing, kit assembling, sorting, and machine tending. Furthermore, using ML and AI to track the development of diseases would aid in future prediction and the organization of the drug supply chain in the market [99, 100]. Despite the growing use of automation in the pharmaceutical industry, there are still downsides, such as pharmaceutical fraud, supply chain breakdowns, and cybercrime; the process is hampered, but the expanding technological transaction has a good impact on the business. Furthermore, there are currently more drugs that have employed automation methodologies for their development, and with the benefit of automation, the pharma business can improve even more with the gaps and expand the production of novel drugs [101].

9.5 Automation-Assisted Successful Studies in Drug Design

Automation and progress have significantly transformed the drug discovery process, and researchers worldwide have contributed to their precise identification. In the realm of automation, challenges that arose during the process were resolved through the implementation of diverse algorithms in conjunction with model-assisted screening in which 616 natural products (identified through the docking analysis) using the RF_MACCS designed model. Among the top compounds, the top threee natural products show promising results through the interaction activity investigation utilized for the simulation study over 100 ns and the binding energy calculation. In addition, a similarity search with the identified inhibitor was performed using the drug bank database to investigate the activity of the identified natural products. Based on the curial stress, the overall finding suggests that the indolocarbazole-assisted scaffold molecules can be a promising lead as inhibitors toward lung cancer [104].

As drug development was increasing daily, there were a few drawbacks in terms of resistance within the selected and identified drug. Therefore, using the QSAR application along with the docking and dynamics, a study performed by Harini et al. [105] targeted the bacterial DNA gyrase for the identification of apigenin-4′-glucoside as an inhibitor and performed the experimental validation as well for better understanding. In this study, the author employed the QSAR model considering the 3 DNA gyrase inhibitors along with the natural compounds. Afterward, the various steps of screening and validation were applied, followed by the biological activity analysis, molecular interaction with the target protein, and the stability of the target and identified ligand based on the highly promising activity among the other selected data. In addition, the antibacterial activity of the apigenin-4′-glucoside was examined to get a better insight. The overall finding suggests that the apigenin-4′-glucoside can be a potential lead toward the bacteria, as its activity was validated through the experimental evaluation [105].

Among the other different types of cancer, gastric cancer is one the leading in terms of their position. And to identify the potential inhibitor toward the gastric cancer target, a study performed by Yuan et al. [106] employed an ML-assisted model along with the docking and dynamics. In this study, the ChEMBL databases were investigated for the model development, and selected compounds were further investigated for their drug-like properties analysis. The compounds that had promising biological activity were utilized for docking analysis targeting the PI3Kalpha protein, and their stability was also analyzed through the MD simulation over 100 ns. The overall finding shows that among the selected dataset of the compounds based on the validation, two compounds were found to be promising inhibitors; however, their experimental validation is required [106].

A study done by Du et al. [107] employed the RF-particle swarm optimization (RF-PSO) model that predicts angiotensin-I-converting enzyme (ACE) inhibitory peptides from enzymatic hydrolysate from black sesame seeds. This work used chromatography techniques such as adsorption, gel filtration, reverse phase, and computational screening to identify eight peptides from fermented black sesame seed hydrolates. The statistical and data analysis tools employed are RF models,

LA50, and solid-phase peptide synthesis. The response surface model was determined to be practicable, and the model was built using an RF technique, resulting in high accuracy. The study gathered 310 data points and employed an RF algorithm to optimize the inhibition process. This work includes examining the PSO technique for global optimization, as well as the characterization of highly active inhibitory peptides. In conclusion, this study used the RF-PSO model to optimize the hydrolysis process of fermented black sesame seeds, yielding a hydrolysate with a high ACE inhibitory activity of 92.27% [107].

Similarly, Wang et al. [108] conducted research that considered DL-based applications and algorithms, and they created GARel, a genetic algorithm-guided generative model. The purpose of this research is to balance novelty and drug-likeness in the models that are developed. The GARel model employed transfer learning to efficiently train the DL model to produce drug-like molecules with unique scaffolds. The author additionally assesses the model's capabilities by developing inhibitors for three targets: AA2AR, EGFR, and SARS-CoV-2. The findings indicate that GARel-generated compounds have more diversified and unique scaffolds with good physiochemical characteristics and favorable docking scores. This study also uses AI to assess the different components of the GARel model. Finally, the study suggests that GARel can efficiently generate novel scaffolds while successfully taking into account the drug-like features of compounds [108].

Increases in intracellular peroxides and reactive oxygen species are indicative of a kind of cell death called ferroptosis. It may result in neurological diseases, including multiple sclerosis and Parkinson's. The study led by Liao et al. [109] used various HTS strategies to identify arachidonic acid 15-lipoxygenase ALOX15 inhibitor. ALOX15 is an essential enzyme for the development of ferroptosis. In this study, virtual screening based on structure and ML was used to pick three compounds from the FDA-validated pharmaceutical library that may bind to the target. QSAR modeling was done using the Naïve Bayesian algorithm, and then docking was done and, based on the result, fragment substitution for three compounds was optimized. Then, the molecules were docked, and the best novel molecule was selected based on the docking score. Furthermore, the ADMET properties of the molecule were studied, and later, simulations were conducted to monitor the stability of the protein-ligand binding system. The study's overall conclusions showed that seven novel inhibitor structures might be created utilizing fragment-based substitution optimization [109].

Different computational methods, assays, and algorithms were employed in one study headed by Islam et al. [110] to identify a prospective therapeutic target for the development of siRNA-based therapeutics against monkeypox virus infection. This siRNA prediction analysis was performed using the genomic sequence of the monkeypox virus, E8L, which was taken, and this gene's coding sequence was chosen. The Ui-Tei algorithm was used to identify potential SiRNA, followed by the Reynolds algorithm. The Support Vector Machine algorithm was used to cross-validate the result. In the end, molecular docking was performed. Overall, this work advances the techniques for treatment approaches and indicates that SiRNA "S8" is a suitable target for treating monkeypox infection [110].

One of the neurodivergent diseases that cause memory loss and, therefore, decreased cognitive abilities is Alzheimer's disease. To overcome this, a study led by Saha et al. [111] employed advanced computational approaches followed by 3D-QSAR, docking, and dynamics for the identification of coumarin derivative as an inhibitor targeting acetylcholinesterase (AChE). In this study, a database for virtual screening was created, and 400,000 structural records of coumarin derivatives from the PubChem database were employed. Phase was used to index the information and create pharmacophoric sites for screening. The research comprised protein and ligand synthesis, field-based 3D-QSAR, ADME computation, and pharmacophore modeling. The protein structure was optimized using the protein production wizard, and 60 molecules that had significant AChE inhibitory activity were prepared for the ligand library. Furthermore, the collected ligands were utilized through the field-based algorithm, and a 3D-QSAR model was generated. Using all 60 produced coumarin derivatives, pharmacophore modeling was carried out. Pharmacophore hypothesis models were created, and molecular alignment, fitness score, and survival score were used to identify the best model. Further virtual screening and molecular docking were prepared, and ADME was calculated. For the HIT 1 and 2 compounds, an MD simulation investigation was carried out to examine protein-ligand binding interactions. The overall findings suggest that among the top ten hits toward the target, only two hits were found to be the most promising in terms of their docking score, followed by the −12.096 and −11.666 kcal/mol, having a favorable binding free energy score as well. The authors suggest that the designed and developed formula can be further utilized for the identification and examination of novel leads toward the targets [111].

9.6 Advancement and Challenges

Automation has had a thoughtful effect on the drug enlargement sector. Because we can now screen through many chemical libraries against biological targets, drug design has been accelerated owing to the utilization of HTS of data. Potential remedy candidates can be more easily identified by employing HTS to analyze the interactions between compounds and target molecules. Due to the mistaken nature of human assessment of bulky data sets, most analyses are now done in silico using various tools and algorithms that can complete jobs with extreme consistency and precision. This has effectively reduced the number of manual errors. ML and AI can now be joined, and big datasets can be analyzed efficiently and rapidly thanks to automation. The most promising candidates for drug development can be prioritized using these techniques, which can also be used to forecast the compound activity and identify patterns and pathways. Various computational tools and algorithms are now employed to expedite the drug-finding method. These tools and algorithms have specifically been helpful in developing novel drugs as the tools are utilized for identifying drug targets and predicting pharmacokinetics and toxicity predictions. Apart from accelerating the process of drug discovery, it is also very cost-effective. Although automation has various advantages, it comes with its setbacks. The analysis of bulk data can be done by automation; however, it cannot replicate biological systems and their complexity accurately. The drug development procedure is intricate due to the need to analyze the connections between various molecules and the pathways involved. As a result, it is challenging to replicate biological complexity using tools and algorithms. Data integration remains a considerable challenge as automated drug discovery relies on data from various sources, including data from assays, chemical databases, and biological pathways. Because the data are maintained across multiple platforms that employ diverse technologies, it is essential to guarantee data format compatibility and standardization to achieve optimal outcomes. In addition, it's critical to confirm that the drugs identified via an automated procedure adhere to safety and efficacy requirements. Although automation increases productivity and efficacy over time, it comes at a very high initial cost to adopt. A significant financial commitment is needed to maintain the instruments and informatics framework, which could be problematic for small research organizations with a limited budget. The dynamic nature of the technological field presents another challenge. As new tools and methods are introduced, adjusting to and becoming knowledgeable about this constantly changing field is crucial.

Overall, automation has revolutionized the process of drug development by accelerating the procedure, increasing efficiency, and reducing cost. However, it also presents challenges such as integration of data, inability to replicate the biological complexity, costs, and ethical considerations, which highlight the need for continuous innovation and adaptations. For the purpose of further automating the processes of drug development and design, specific barriers must be overcome.

9.7 Conclusion

In the present situation, the automated application and algorithm are two of the major aspects of data handling, identification, and screening of crucial

48 Yuan, Y., Pei, J., and Lai, L. (2013). Binding site detection and druggability prediction of protein targets for structure-based drug design. *Current Pharmaceutical Design* 19 (12): 2326–2333. https://doi.org/10.2174/1381612811319120019.

49 Frye, L., Bhat, S., Akinsanya, K., and Abel, R. (2021). From computer-aided drug discovery to computer-driven drug discovery. *Drug Discovery Today: Technologies* 39: 111–117. https://doi.org/10.1016/j.ddtec.2021.08.001.

50 Yan, X.C., Sanders, J.M., Gao, Y.D. et al. (2020). Augmenting hit identification by virtual screening techniques in small molecule drug discovery. *Journal of Chemical Information and Modeling* 60 (9): 4144–4152. https://doi.org/10.1021/acs.jcim.0c00113.

51 McGann, M. (2011). FRED pose prediction and virtual screening accuracy. *Journal of Chemical Information and Modeling* 51 (3): 578–596. https://doi.org/10.1021/ci100436p.

52 Jain, A.N. (2003). Surflex: fully automatic flexible molecular docking using a molecular similarity-based search engine. *Journal of Medicinal Chemistry* 46 (4): 499–511. https://doi.org/10.1021/jm020406h.

53 Rizvi, S.M., Shakil, S., and Haneef, M. (2013). A simple click by click protocol to perform docking: AutoDock 4.2 made easy for non-bioinformaticians. *EXCLI Journal* 12: 831–857. https://www.ncbi.nlm.nih.gov/pubmed/26648810.

54 David, L., Mdahoma, A., Singh, N. et al. (2022). A toolkit for covalent docking with GOLD: from automated ligand preparation with KNIME to bound protein-ligand complexes. *Bioinformatics Advances* 2 (1): vbac090. https://doi.org/10.1093/bioadv/vbac090.

55 Agu, P.C., Afiukwa, C.A., Orji, O.U. et al. (2023). Molecular docking as a tool for the discovery of molecular targets of nutraceuticals in diseases management. *Scientific Reports* 13 (1): 13398. https://doi.org/10.1038/s41598-023-40160-2.

56 Gaulton, A., Bellis, L.J., Bento, A.P. et al. (2012). ChEMBL: a large-scale bioactivity database for drug discovery. *Nucleic Acids Research* 40 (Database issue): D1100–D1107. https://doi.org/10.1093/nar/gkr777.

57 Chisholm, T.S., Mackey, M., and Hunter, C.A. (2023). Discovery of high-affinity amyloid ligands using a ligand-based virtual screening pipeline. *Journal of the American Chemical Society* 145 (29): 15936–15950. https://doi.org/10.1021/jacs.3c03749.

58 Wolber, G. and Langer, T. (2005). LigandScout: 3-D pharmacophores derived from protein-bound ligands and their use as virtual screening filters. *Journal of Chemical Information and Modeling* 45 (1): 160–169. https://doi.org/10.1021/ci049885e.

59 Koes, D.R. and Camacho, C.J. (2011). Pharmer: efficient and exact pharmacophore search. *Journal of Chemical Information and Modeling* 51 (6): 1307–1314. https://doi.org/10.1021/ci200097m.

60 Schneidman-Duhovny, D., Dror, O., Inbar, Y. et al. (2008). PharmaGist: a webserver for ligand-based pharmacophore detection. *Nucleic Acids Research* 36 (Web Server issue): W223–W228. https://doi.org/10.1093/nar/gkn187.

61 Ambure, P., Halder, A.K., Gonzalez Diaz, H., and Cordeiro, M. (2019). QSAR-Co: an open source software for developing robust multitasking or multitarget classification-based QSAR models. *Journal of Chemical Information and Modeling* 59 (6): 2538–2544. https://doi.org/10.1021/acs.jcim.9b00295.

62 Halder, A.K., Cordeiro, D.S., and M. N. (2021). QSAR-Co-X: an open source toolkit for multitarget QSAR modelling. *Journal of Cheminformatics* 13 (1): 29. https://doi.org/10.1186/s13321-021-00508-0.

63 Vidal, D., Garcia-Serna, R., and Mestres, J. (2011). Ligand-based approaches to in silico pharmacology. *Methods in Molecular Biology* 672: 489–502. https://doi.org/10.1007/978-1-60761-839-3_19.

64 Abraham, M.J., Murtola, T., Schulz, R. et al. (2015). GROMACS: High performance molecular simulations through multi-level parallelism from laptops to supercomputers. *SoftwareX* 1: 19–25.

65 Case, D.A., Cheatham, T.E. 3rd, Darden, T. et al. (2005). The Amber biomolecular simulation programs. *Journal of Computational Chemistry* 26 (16): 1668–1688. https://doi.org/10.1002/jcc.20290.

66 Bai, Q., Liu, S., Tian, Y. et al. (2022). Application advances of deep learning methods for de novo drug design and molecular dynamics simulation. *Wiley Interdisciplinary Reviews: Computational Molecular Science* 12 (3): e1581.

67 Daina, A., Michielin, O., and Zoete, V. (2017). SwissADME: a free web tool to evaluate pharmacokinetics, drug-likeness and medicinal chemistry friendliness of small molecules. *Scientific Reports* 7: 42717. https://doi.org/10.1038/srep42717.

68 Kim, S. (2021). Exploring chemical information in PubChem. *Current Protocols* 1 (8): e217. https://doi.org/10.1002/cpz1.217.

69 Wishart, D.S., Knox, C., Guo, A.C. et al. (2008). DrugBank: a knowledgebase for drugs, drug actions and drug targets. *Nucleic Acids Research* 36 (Database issue): D901–D906. https://doi.org/10.1093/nar/gkm958.

70 UniProt, C. (2023). UniProt: the universal protein knowledgebase in 2023. *Nucleic Acids Research* 51 (D1): D523–D531. https://doi.org/10.1093/nar/gkac1052.

96 Vora, L.K., Gholap, A.D., Jetha, K. et al. (2023). Artificial intelligence in pharmaceutical technology and drug delivery design. *Pharmaceutics* 15 (7): https://doi.org/10.3390/pharmaceutics15071916.

97 Taylor, D. (2015). The pharmaceutical industry and the future of drug development. *Pharmaceuticals in the Environment* 1–33.

98 Ben-Jebara, M. and Modi, S.B. (2021). Product personalization and firm performance: an empirical analysis of the pharmaceutical industry. *Journal of Operations Management* 67 (1): 82–104.

99 Patel, H. (2021). A review: future aspects of artificial intelligence big data and robotics in pharmaceutical industry. *World Journal of Pharmaceutical Research* 10 (6): 532–544.

100 Stasevych, M. and Zvarych, V. (2023). Innovative robotic technologies and artificial intelligence in pharmacy and medicine: paving the way for the future of health care—a review. *Big Data and Cognitive Computing* 7 (3): 147.

101 Sarkis, M., Bernardi, A., Shah, N., and Papathanasiou, M.M. (2021). Emerging challenges and opportunities in pharmaceutical manufacturing and distribution. *Processes* 9 (3): 457.

102 Khan, M.Z.I., Khan, D., Akbar, M.Y. et al. (2024). 3D-QSAR pharmacophore modeling, virtual screening, molecular docking, MD simulations, in vitro and in vivo studies to identify potential anti-hyperplasia drugs. *Biotechnology Journal* 19 (2): e2300437. https://doi.org/10.1002/biot.202300437.

103 Fortela, D.L.B., Mikolajczyk, A.P., Carnes, M.R. et al. (2024). Predicting molecular docking of per- and polyfluoroalkyl substances to blood protein using generative artificial intelligence algorithm DiffDock. *BioTechniques* 76 (1): 14–26. https://doi.org/10.2144/btn-2023-0070.

104 Das, A.P., Mathur, P., and Agarwal, S.M. (2024). Machine learning, molecular docking, and dynamics-based computational identification of potential inhibitors against lung cancer. *ACS Omega* 9 (4): 4528–4539. https://doi.org/10.1021/acsomega.3c07338.

105 Harini, M., Kavitha, K., Prabakaran, V. et al. (2024). Identification of apigenin-4'-glucoside as bacterial DNA gyrase inhibitor by QSAR modeling, molecular docking, DFT, molecular dynamics, and in vitro confirmation studies. *Journal of Molecular Modeling* 30 (1): 22. https://doi.org/10.1007/s00894-023-05813-z.

106 Yuan, F., Li, T., Xu, X. et al. (2024). Identification of novel PI3Kα inhibitor against gastric cancer: QSAR-, molecular docking-, and molecular dynamics simulation-based analysis. *Applied Biochemistry and Biotechnology* https://doi.org/10.1007/s12010-024-04898-3.

107 Du, T., Xu, Y., Xu, X. et al. (2024). ACE inhibitory peptides from enzymatic hydrolysate of fermented black sesame seed: random forest-based optimization, screening, and molecular docking analysis. *Food Chemistry* 437 (Pt 2): 137921. https://doi.org/10.1016/j.foodchem.2023.137921.

108 Wang, M., Wu, Z., Wang, J. et al. (2024). Genetic algorithm-based receptor ligand: a genetic algorithm-guided generative model to boost the novelty and drug-likeness of molecules in a sampling chemical space. *Journal of Chemical Information and Modeling* 64 (4): 1213–1228. https://doi.org/10.1021/acs.jcim.3c01964.

109 Liao, Y., Cao, P., and Luo, L. (2024). Development of novel ALOX15 inhibitors combining dual machine learning filtering and fragment substitution optimisation approaches, molecular docking and dynamic simulation methods. *Journal of Enzyme Inhibition and Medicinal Chemistry* 39 (1): 2301756. https://doi.org/10.1080/14756366.2024.2301756.

110 Islam, R., Shahriar, A., Uddin, M.R., and Fatema, N. (2024). Immunoinformatic and molecular docking approaches: siRNA prediction to silence cell surface binding protein of monkeypox virus. *Beni-Suef University Journal of Basic and Applied Sciences* 13 (1): 17.

111 Saha, B., Das, A., Jangid, K. et al. (2024). Identification of coumarin derivatives targeting acetylcholinesterase for Alzheimer's disease by field-based 3D-QSAR, pharmacophore model-based virtual screening, molecular docking, MM/GBSA, ADME and MD Simulation study. *Current Research in Structural Biology* 7: 100124. https://doi.org/10.1016/j.crstbi.2024.100124.

10

Machine Learning and Generative AI Techniques for Sentiment Analysis with Applications

Riya Sharma[1], *Balraj Singh*[1], *and Aditya Khamparia*[2]

[1] *School of Computer Science and Engineering, Lovely Professional University, Phagwara, India*
[2] *Department of Computer Science, Babasaheb Bhimrao Ambedkar University (A Central University), Lucknow, India*

10.1 Introduction

Social media platforms such as Facebook, Instagram, WhatsApp, and X (formerly known as Twitter) have developed into lively forums where people can express their thoughts, feelings, and opinions about different ideas, policies, and products in today's digital world [55]. This flood of user-generated content offers suppliers and customers alike priceless insights. When making judgments about what to buy online, consumers frequently look to the opinions of others to determine the pros and cons of certain products. In the interim, producers can extract valuable insights from these opinions to improve their products. In this context, sentiment analysis, or opinion mining, is a rapidly developing topic of study that is essential to follow [51]. Machine learning has emerged and recognizing large patterns in datasets is much easier. This paradigm change in technology has been especially important for firms that are dealing with massive amounts of data. Machine learning (ML) algorithms have great potential for interpreting feelings buried in textual data from social [8] media platforms since they are skilled at spotting hidden trends and patterns [27]. However, processing this massive amount of data effectively requires automated sentiment analysis [24] techniques due to the overwhelming volume of textual content on social media sites like X (formerly known as Twitter) [16]. Over the past ten years, researchers have been actively studying sentiment analysis, with an increase in activity since the early 2000s [28]. Sentiment analysis is a multilevel process that involves classifying opinions into positive and negative sentiments at several levels, such as the phrase, document, and feature levels [30]. There are now two main approaches that are

Generative Artificial Intelligence for Biomedical and Smart Health Informatics,
First Edition. Edited by Aditya Khamparia and Deepak Gupta.

- **Corpus-Based Approach:** Large-scale corpora are used by corpus-based methods to find opinion patterns in both syntax and semantics. For these methods to be implemented effectively, big labeled datasets are required as they provide context-specific words that are customized to the dataset being analyzed. To develop opinion lexicons, social media networks such as X (formerly known as Twitter) and Facebook application programming interface (API) are important sources of data that allow academics to derive sentiment scores from user evaluations and feature sets.

SentiWordNet and WordNet, probabilistic lexicons that categorize English nouns, verbs, and adjectives into synonym sets, are the result of recent developments in sentiment analysis. Using latent Dirichlet allocation, Francesco Colace's SentiSentiment Grabber extracts documents and generates mixed graphs of terms, which act as structures for sentiment categorization in textual documents.

10.1.2.2 Machine Learning-Based Approach

As noted by Aydogan and Akcayol [7], the ML-based method of sentiment analysis makes use of the capability of proven ML techniques to categorize sentiments inside textual data. This approach can be further divided into two primary categories:

- **Unsupervised Learning:** Unsupervised learning methods can be trained without the need for pre-labeled data. Rather, these algorithms find patterns and clusters in the data on their own. K-means and apriori algorithms are two examples of common unsupervised ML algorithms that are used for tasks related to association and clustering.
- **Supervised Learning:** Labelled training data are necessary for supervised learning to train the classifier successfully. It is regarded as a reliable classification technique and has produced encouraging sentiment analysis outcomes. Naïve Bayes (NB), support vector machine (SVM), artificial neural network, maximum entropy (ME), and DT classifiers are supervised classification algorithms that are often used. Owing to their effectiveness and precision, SVM, NB, and ME are among the most used algorithms; nevertheless, sentiment analysis also makes use of less popular algorithms, including logistic regression (LR), K-nearest neighbor (KNN), RF, and Bayesian network.

  ML is an artificial intelligence technique that predicts textual data's sentiment classifications using supervised, semi-supervised, unsupervised, or hybrid methods. When labeled data and statistical information are available, supervised algorithms like SVM, NB, and ME are utilized to make predictions about future data. When labeled training data are hard to come by or not available, novel techniques, including dependency parsing, syntax-based rules, latent Dirichlet allocation, word embedding, and bootstrapping, are employed in semi-supervised and unsupervised learning. These methods are combined in hybrid ways to provide accuracy and resilience in a variety of applications and datasets.

- **Hybrid Approach:** To improve sentiment classification accuracy, the hybrid-based approach to sentiment analysis combines lexicon-based classification techniques with ML. Scholars have put forth hybrid methods for sentiment analysis that integrate machine learning with lexicon-based methodologies. After introducing word2vec for feature clustering, Zhang et al. [58] presented part-of-speech and lexicon-based feature selection techniques for training data. SentBuk is a sentiment classifier for Facebook applications created by Ortigosa et al. [32]. It classifies comments into positive, neutral, or negative feelings based on the relationships between user profiles and terminology. Ghiassi et al. [12] provided evidence of the efficacy of lexicon-based and feature-based techniques combined for sentiment categorization. Overall, by combining the advantages of both lexicon-based and ML techniques, the hybrid approach to sentiment analysis offers a promising way to improve classification accuracy. This helps to overcome the drawbacks of individual methods and achieve better sentiment classification performance.

10.2 Literature Review

This literature survey offers a thorough summary of current research on ML-based sentiment analysis. These studies employ a variety of approaches and methodologies and seek to glean important insights from the enormous amount of user-generated content available on online platforms. Every research project advances the knowledge and use of sentiment analysis in interpreting public opinions, attitudes, and preferences across a range of topics, from new classifier proposals to in-depth investigations of feature extraction and preprocessing. The studies were published between 2010 and 2024. The data from the chapter are extracted and integrated into Table 10.1.

10.3 Machine Learning Techniques for Sentiment Analysis

There are several methods for calculating the polarity of analysis data [45]. The most widely used and effective ML technique is basic sentiment analysis. The most effective algorithm and the polarity in the analysis data are computed, as will be covered below [56].

Table 10.1 Summary of reviewed literature.

Author	Year	Aim of study	Analysis result
Yang et al. [54]	2010	Propose supervised techniques for analyzing consumer product reviews	Classification of product features based on consumer needs, empirical evaluation of classifiers.
Kumar and Sebastian [21]	2012	Study the impact of Web 2.0 on opinion expression and mining	Evolution of opinion expression with Web 2.0, rapid advancement in opinion mining due to rich data sources.
Patil and Atique [34]	2015	Address challenges and methods in sentiment analysis	Challenges include parallel computing, handling noise, and dynamism in sentiment analysis.
Swathi and Seshadri [48]	2017	Explore the role of machine learning in big data analytics	Utilization of machine learning to process big data and overcome computational challenges.
Kawade and Oza [20]	2017	Categorize and summarize recent articles on sentiment analysis	Categorization and summary of recent sentiment analysis articles.
Gopu and Swarnalatha [13]	2017	Discuss machine learning algorithms for sentiment analysis	Classification of sentiments using various algorithms and identification of top product features.
Naiknaware et al. [31]	2017	Study the application of sentiment analysis in social media	Classification of sentiment in social media data and optimization of decision-making capabilities.
Singh et al. [44]	2017	Explore sentiment analysis in the context of digital social networks	Role of sentiment analysis in understanding public opinion on social media platforms.
Mäntylä et al. [28]	2018	Analyze the growth of the sentiment analysis field over the years	Increase in sentiment analysis articles over time and significant expansion of the field.
Liu et al. [26]	2019	Investigate future prospects and challenges in sentiment analysis	Future prospects include aspect-level sentiment analysis and utilization of transfer learning.
Fitri et al. [49]	2019	Examining tweets about the Indonesian anti-LGBT campaign	Naïve Bayes provides much accuracy as compared to other algorithms.

Table 10.1 (Continued)

Author	Year	Aim of study	Analysis result
Tiwari et al. [38]	2020	Social media sentiment analysis	The decision tree and random force algorithms are more accurate than the SVM method.
Kesarwani et al. [1]	2020	Detection of fake news	The model's weighted average precision is 0.75 and its recall is 0.79.
AlSalman [5]	2020	Improved approach for sentiment analysis	Achieved an accuracy of 83.5% as opposed to the 72–75% accuracy of previous approaches.
Raheja and Asthana [40]	2021	Analyzing sentiments on Covid-19	Over positive and negative views about the COVID scenario, neutral sentiments are more prevalent.
Khasanova and Pasechnik [2]	2021	Social media analysis	The goal was to examine VKontakte, a social media platform, to determine the top teams and spot any potential future deviant behavior.
Madan and Ghose [3]	2021	Sentiment analysis of tweets	When compared to a technique that only uses lexical resources, ML-based classifiers perform better at classifying data.
Liang et al. [57]	2022	Analyzing Internet use and users' views on homosexuality	Compared to active participants and pragmatic users, idle users were less inclined toward accepting homosexuality.
Chi et al. [53]	2023	Analyzing emotions of LGBT social media communities	April 2022 and August 2021 saw the lowest levels of negative feelings, which peaked in August 2020. In March 2020, positive feelings were at their lowest point, and they peaked in July 2022.
Aldinata et al. [4]	2023	Comparing sentiments on LGBT	It would be ideal to use logistic regression without preprocessing the dataset first.
Abdullah Aswad [39]	2024	Develop a sentiment analysis model for online Italian car forums using a two-stage CNN and LTSM	Overcame noisy data issue, achieved 96.78% accuracy, added a fourth category for topic pertinence, moved to four-label text classification, and used a cascade categorization method.

(continued)

Integration and Deployment: The sentiment analysis model is incorporated into the more comprehensive social media analytics framework after acceptable performance is attained. This could encompass integrating the model into a dashboard or analytics platform or deploying it as a service that is available through APIs.

Visualization and Reporting: Reports or insights are generated and the analyzed data are visualized in the last phase. To successfully communicate the sentiment analysis data to end users or stakeholders, visualization approaches like word clouds, trend analysis, sentiment distributions, or network graphs can be utilized.

Feedback Loop: To gradually optimize and further improve the sentiment analysis model, continuous observation and feedback are crucial. The architecture takes into account user feedback, model performance metrics, and changing patterns in social media content to make sure the system is correct and up to date.

10.3.2 Machine Learning Techniques Outline

ML, a key AI branch, is crucial in sentiment analysis, enabling automated extraction of sentiment and opinions from textual data. It is used in various domains like social media analytics, customer feedback analysis, product reviews, and market sentiment tracking. ML techniques, ranging from traditional algorithms to advanced deep learning models, provide a range of approaches for sentiment analysis, from sentiment classification to emotion detection. They help organizations gain valuable insights into public opinion, brand sentiment, market trends, and customer preferences. ML algorithms are indispensable in various applications like data mining, computer vision, natural language processing (NLP), and biometrics. Some popular ML algorithms are:

1) Linear Regression

   Linear regression is a statistical method that models the relationship between a dependent variable and independent variables, estimating the dependent variable's value based on the independent variables' values. It is commonly used for prediction and inference in fields like economics, finance, and social sciences, represented by a regression line, typically denoted as $Y = a^*X + b$ with slope "a" and intercept "b."

2) Logistic Regression

   Using this method, the set of distinct variables is reduced to a discrete dependent variable. The coefficients needed to estimate a probability logistic transformation are provided via LR. It is widely used in fields like medicine, marketing, and social sciences to predict binary outcomes and understand the relationship between predictor variables and categorical outcomes.

3) Naïve Bayes
   NB is a probabilistic classification algorithm based on Bayes' theorem and conditional independence between features. The predicted class is determined by calculating the likelihood of each class for each data point and choosing the class with the highest probability. Despite its simplicity, NB classifiers are useful for text classification tasks like spam detection and sentiment analysis, as well as NLP and email filtering applications.
4) Support Vector Machine (SVM)
   SVM is a supervised learning algorithm used for classification and regression tasks. It finds the optimal hyperplane to separate data points into different classes, maximizing the margin between classes. SVM is effective in high-dimensional spaces and can handle nonlinear data using kernel functions. It is widely used in fields like image recognition, text classification, and bioinformatics for pattern recognition and data classification.
5) Decision Tree
   DTs are hierarchical structures used for classification and regression tasks. They partition feature space into subsets based on independent variable values, with each partition corresponding to a decision node. The best attribute is selected at each node based on criteria like information gain or Gini impurity. DTs are intuitive, easy to interpret, and can capture nonlinear relationships in data, making them popular in finance, healthcare, and marketing.
6) Random Forest
   RF is an ensemble learning algorithm that creates a forest of DTs trained on random data and features. It reduces overfitting and improves generalization performance by aggregating the predictions of multiple trees. This versatile algorithm is used for regression and classification tasks and is robust to noisy data and outliers. It is widely used in healthcare, finance, and bioinformatics for disease diagnosis, fraud detection, and gene expression analysis.
7) KNN (K-Nearest Neighbor)
   KNN is a classification and regression algorithm that uses the assumption that similar data points belong to the same class or have similar values. Using the majority class of the closest neighbors in the feature space as a guide, it retains training data and makes predictions about new occurrences. The "K" in KNN refers to the number of nearest neighbors considered, affecting the algorithm's performance. KNN is widely used in pattern recognition, recommendation systems, and anomaly detection.

8) K-Means Clustering
   K-means clustering is an unsupervised learning algorithm that partitions data into "K" clusters based on similarity, with each cluster represented by its centroid. Its goal is to minimize the within-cluster sum of squares, ensuring data points within the same cluster are as similar as possible and as dissimilar as possible to data points in other clusters.
9) AdaBoost and Gradient Boosting Algorithms
   These are ensemble learning techniques used for classification and regression tasks. Gradient boosting builds an ensemble of weak learners, like DTs, sequentially correcting errors made by previous models. AdaBoost selects features to enhance model prediction iteratively, focusing on misclassified examples in training data. These techniques improve model performance and are used in web search ranking, customer churn prediction, and face recognition.
10) Dimensionality Reduction Algorithms
   Dimensionality reduction techniques preserve important information while reducing the number of random variables or features in a dataset. PCA is a popular method that transforms original variables into principal components, aiming to maximize variance and minimize loss of information. Through the reduction of computational complexity and overfitting risk, this strategy is beneficial for feature selection, visualization, and enhancing the performance of ML algorithms.

10.3.3 Some Sentiment Analysis Applications Using Machine Learning Techniques

10.3.3.1 Stock Prediction Using Real-Time Sentiment Analysis of Tweet Data

The study of X (formerly known as Twitter) streaming data for real-time market projections was covered by Das et al. [10]. An attempt has been made in the current study to determine financial decisions, such as stock prediction, to analyze or forecast the possible stock values of a firm. X (formerly known as Twitter) knowledge is the most extensive source of online public conversation and is regarded as one of the top microblogging platforms globally. Real-time, programmatic, and streaming data analysis is made possible by streaming. Information is continuously streamed from a variety of sources, including websites, mobile phone applications, server logs, social media, trading floors, and more. These data need to be continuously processed through streaming without requiring access to all of the data. The main advantages are simplicity and adaptability, which improve user behavior evaluation and forecasting in an unrelenting manner. In addition to the Spark API core, Spark streamer enables fault-tolerant, high-performance, and scalable streaming of real-time data streams, like X (formerly known as Twitter).

10.3.3.2 Machine Learning Techniques for Sentiment Analysis of Scientific Text

The primary goal of Raza et al. [37] is to enable scholars to evaluate the material. It examines how science papers are interpreted using quotation phrases by drawing on an existing annotated corpus. To clean up the data corpus, the noise was removed from the data using a variety of data norms. It classifies this data collection using six different ML algorithms. Scikit Learn, a Python-based ML library, is being used to create the following systems: RF, NB, SVM, DTs, LR, and KNN. An intuitive interface with m is provided by the well-known Python language learning software module Scikit-Learn. First, our program reads the data that is stored in the file in format. Based on a 60:40/60/40 ratio, the output shows that the SVM and NB classifier sets outperform the other ones.

10.3.3.3 Sentiment Analysis on X (Formerly Known as Twitter) Using Logistic Regression and Multinomial Naive Bayes

X (formerly known as Twitter) sentiment studies are debatable. Some of the difficulties are (i) the fact that some tweets are widely understood to be written in informal languages and that some brief sentences just hint at emotion. (ii) X (formerly known as Twitter) is also frequently used for acronyms, hashtags, URLs, emoticons, and abbreviations. ML algorithms are used to achieve precision in concepts like table design, extraction techniques, and tweets prior to delivery. Using the train data on the test results, ML techniques are used to exercise the algorithms, which include the LR algorithm and multinomial NB. The author took into consideration the Internet movie database (IMDB) analysis datasets and the airline sentiment data collection. All varieties achieve favorable outcomes in ML by utilizing the Count Vectorizer feature [18].

10.3.3.4 Fake News Detection on Social Media Using K-Nearest Neighbor Classifier

The goal of the study by Kesarwani et al. [1] is to apply the KNN classifier to identify bogus news on social media. The study used a dataset of 80,000 tweets, 40,000 of which were real and 40,000 of which were bogus, to propose a model for identifying fake news on X (formerly known as Twitter). Six different characteristics, including the number of exclamation points, the number of hashtags, and the presence of a URL, were used to train the KNN classifier. The findings demonstrated that the suggested model outperformed other methods in identifying bogus news, achieving an accuracy of 85.5%. According to the study, the KNN classifier can be an effective tool for spotting bogus news on social media, particularly X (formerly known as Twitter).

bidirectional context allows it to comprehend nuances in sentiment expression, making it adaptable to specific sentiment tasks with impressive accuracy and performance.

10.4.1.2 RoBERTa (Robustly Optimized BERT Approach)

Robustly optimized BERT approach (RoBERTa), developed by Facebook AI, improves the performance of BERT by incorporating enhancements. It uses a similar architecture but undergoes extensive pre-training on a larger corpus with longer sequences and diverse data sources. This, combined with dynamic masking strategies, allows it to capture more nuanced contextual information from text. RoBERTa excels in various NLP tasks, including sentiment analysis, question answering, and text classification, achieving state-of-the-art results due to its robust understanding of language semantics. By fine-tuning large-scale datasets and incorporating advanced training techniques, RoBERTa enhances model robustness and generalization capabilities.

10.4.1.3 Lexicon-Based Methods

Lexicon-based methods use predefined dictionaries or word lists to analyze text data and assign sentiment scores to words based on their presence in the lexicon. These simple and computationally efficient approaches can be useful for tasks like sentiment analysis, providing a baseline performance or complementing more complex techniques. However, they may struggle with context-dependent sentiment and language nuances, leading to inaccuracies in sentiment analysis tasks. Despite their simplicity, lexicon-based approaches remain useful for sentiment analysis tasks.

10.4.1.4 Ensemble Methods

Ensemble methods in NLP combine multiple base models to create a more accurate predictive model. These techniques, such as bagging, boosting, and stacking, mitigate individual model biases and variance, enhancing generalization performance. They are applied across tasks like text classification, machine translation, and named entity recognition to improve predictive performance and reliability. Ensemble methods also enhance sentiment analysis predictions by leveraging diverse models with different strengths and weaknesses.

10.4.1.5 Hybrid Approach

Hybrid approaches in the literature aim to combine ML models with lexicon-based knowledge to achieve optimal results. Minaee et al. [29] developed an ensemble model using LSTM and CNN algorithms, which provides better performance than individual models. To efficiently analyze sequential data, the CNN-LSTM model combines the advantages of LSTM networks and CNNs. While LSTMs handle the sequential aspects, capturing long-term dependencies and temporal dynamics, CNNs are used for feature extraction, collecting local patterns and spatial dependencies within input sequences. Tasks like action identification, sentiment analysis in text data, and video classification have shown that this hybrid technique works quite well. A versatile option for a range of sequential data processing applications, the CNN-LSTM model delivers higher performance in capturing both local and global information by utilizing the complementing capabilities of CNNs and LSTMs.

10.4.1.6 Rule-Based Methods

Rule-based methods are manual rules used to process text data, offering transparency and interpretability. They are based on domain knowledge or linguistic principles and can be labor-intensive to develop. These methods identify sentiment in text using predefined rules, such as linguistic patterns or syntactic cues. However, they may struggle with handling ambiguity or adapting to diverse language styles. Rule-based methods are effective in certain contexts but lack the adaptability and generalization capabilities of advanced methods, particularly in handling complex or ambiguous sentiment expressions.

10.4.1.7 Transformer-XL

Transformer-XL is an extension of the transformer architecture designed to handle longer sequences more efficiently. It introduces a recurrence mechanism that permits information to traverse between segments, hence enabling the effective modeling of context over larger distances. Because of this, transformer-XL is a good fit for tasks like sentiment analysis and language modeling, where producing text that is intelligible and coherent requires a grasp of context. It also captures contextual information from extensive text spans, enhancing its understanding of sentiment nuances across paragraphs or documents.

10.4.1.8 Hidden Markov Models (HMMs)

Based on words that are seen, hidden Markov models (HMMs) simulate the underlying sentiment state of text sequences. HMMs can forecast sentiment labels for text segments because they make the assumption that sentiment transitions follow a probabilistic pattern. Compared to more sophisticated neural models, HMMs may have trouble grasping context and long-range dependencies, even though they are capable of capturing sequential dependencies in sentiment expression.

10.4.1.9 Hierarchical Attention Network (HAN)

Sentiment analysis may be effectively tackled by using hierarchical attention networks (HANs), which solve the problem of comprehending sentiment in hierarchical text structures such as sentences, paragraphs, and words. HANs dynamically weigh the significance of various passages in the input text using hierarchical attention methods. This enables the model to concentrate on the most informative passages while ignoring superfluous or irrelevant information. By using this method, the model can interpret sentiment at various granularities, ranging from individual words to whole paragraphs. HANs produce context representations that accurately capture the tone of the content by repeatedly focusing on pertinent portions of the input text. By emphasizing the most significant parts that contribute to the total sentiment, this hierarchical method not only increases the model's interpretability but also its capacity to identify sentiment. HANs have proven to be more effective than traditional approaches in sentiment analysis tasks, solidifying their position as an essential component of NLP.

10.4.1.10 Generative Adversarial Networks (GANs)

They are an effective deep-learning framework that is especially useful for generative modeling. They are made up of the discriminator and generator neural networks, which compete with one another to learn. Whereas the discriminator seeks to discriminate between created and actual samples, the generator seeks to create synthetic data samples that are identical to real data. Both networks learn iteratively through this adversarial training process, producing increasingly realistic data samples. Applications for GANs can be found in many different fields, such as drug discovery, style transfer, image production, and data augmentation. They have been used for image-to-image translation jobs and have been crucial in creating high-quality synthetic images that closely resemble real photographs. However, there are challenges with GANs as well, like instability in training dynamics, mode collapse, and training difficulties. Despite these difficulties, GANs are a revolutionary method for generative modeling that pushes the envelope in producing intricate, realistic data distributions. To provide realistic text samples with desirable sentiment qualities, they have been investigated in sentiment analysis. GANs in sentiment analysis are still a developing field; nevertheless, research and development are currently underway.

10.4.2 Few Sentiment Analysis Applications Using Generative AI Techniques

10.4.2.1 Sentiment Analysis Technique for Panoptical View

A variety of approaches and strategies, including ontological, hybrid, Lexicon-based, Rules-based, and ML approaches, have been studied and contrasted [6]. Different levels—such as the penalty, document, sentencing, aspect, and emotional levels—were used for opinion mining. According to [19], an ML-based technique and a Lexicon-based strategy may be the most promising avenues for sentiment analysis. In their article, they come to the conclusion that sentimental analysis has become widespread and is extremely difficult in businesses and that everyone contributes both directly and indirectly to mining. Here, they discussed a wide range of research, difficulties, and analyses grounded in sentimental analysis and numerous problems.

10.4.2.2 Category Text Generation Using a Generative Model

The category sentence generative adversarial network (CS-GAN), which integrates GANs, recurrent neural networks, and reinforcement learning, is presented by Li et al. [23]. CS-GAN improves generalization during supervised training in addition to producing category sentences to increase dataset sizes. When CS-GAN is evaluated for sentiment analysis, polarity identification accuracy is enhanced, especially in datasets with a wealth of category information. The study shows how well CS-GAN can capture sentence structure and include category information, which are important aspects of supervised learning. Although CS-GAN is useful for multi-category datasets, it is less successful when large amounts of data are missing categories. However, CS-GAN performs better, particularly when dealing with short sentence durations and small labeled datasets. Future work will explore the extraction of phrase features and use generative models to create disentangled representations based on different attributes.

10.4.2.3 Sentiment Analysis with the Ensemble Method Applied to an Amazon Product

In this study, Sadhasivam and Babu [43] proposed a way to increase the precision of analytical classification. Another technique for analyzing data is opinion mining, which entails gathering, analyzing, processing, and assessing the customer's review. They included information from multiple government websites in their documentation. The NB and SVM algorithms are used to sort the training data after the gathered data have been preprocessed to remove unwanted data. These two algorithms are less precise, though. By combining ensemble algorithms, supporting vector machines, and NB, the suggested approach ensures both the algorithm's speed and accuracy of execution. Thus, following a precise measurement, the approach will be recommended to the user if the precision is high. The features of the algorithms are then provided using the standard evaluation. Certain products, like electronics and books, have established data sets that are easily readable and categorized to offer good accuracy and performance. One example of this is the product review data set on Amazon.com. The rating classification is extensively utilized, and it is dependent on user feedback to recommend an item to the consumer.

10.4.2.4 Sentiment Analysis on X (Formerly Known as Twitter) Using Natural Language Processing Methods

According to Suryawanshi et al. [47], a significant amount of data from people's opinions on Twitter is required for opinion mining. There are multiple methods

9 Cirqueira, D., Pinheiro, M.F., Jacob, A. et al. (2018). A literature review in preprocessing for sentiment analysis for Brazilian Portuguese social media. *2018 IEEE/WIC/ACM International Conference on Web Intelligence (WI)*, Santiago, Chile (3–6 December 2018). IEEE.

10 Das, S., Behera, R., Kumar, M., and Rath, S. (2018). Real-time sentiment analysis of Twitter streaming data for stock prediction. *Procedia Computer Science* 132 (1): 956–964. https://doi.org/10.1016/j.procs.2018.05.111.

11 Ebrahimi, M., Yazdavar, A., and Sheth, A. (2017). On the challenges of sentiment analysis for dynamic events. *Intelligent Systems, IEEE* 32 (5). https://doi.org/10.1109/MIS.2017.3711649.

12 Ghiassi, M., Skinner, J., and Zimbra, D. (2013). Twitter brand sentiment analysis: a hybrid system using n-gram analysis and dynamic artificial neural network. *Expert Syst Appl* 40 (16): 6266–6282. https://doi.org/10.1016/j.eswa.2013.05.057.

13 Gopu, M. and Swarnalatha, P. (2017). Analyzing customer sentiments using machine learning techniques. *International Journal of Civil Engineering and Technology (IJCIET)* 8: 1829–1842.

14 Itani, M., Roast, C., and Al-Khayatt, S. (2017). Developing resources for sentiment analysis of informal arabic text in social media. *Procedia Computer Science* 117: 129–136.

15 Costales, J.A., Lorico, E.M., and De Los Santos, C.M. (2023). A comparative sentiment analysis about HIV and AIDS on Twitter tweets using supervised machine learning approach. *2023 5th International Conference on Computer Communication and the Internet, ICCCI*, pp. 27–32, Fujisawa, Japan (23–25 June 2023). IEEE. https://doi.org/10.1109/ICCCI59363.2023.10210162.

16 Jain, A.P. and Dandannavar, P. (2016). Application of machine learning techniques to sentiment analysis. *Second International Conference on Applied and Theoretical Computing and Communication Technology (ICATccT)* 1 (1): 628–632. https://doi.org/10.1109/ICATCCT.2016.7912076.

17 Jain, P.K., Pamula, R., and Srivastava, G. (2021). A systematic literature review on machine learning applications for consumer sentiment analysis using online reviews. *Computer Science Review* 41: 100413.

18 Sentamilselvan, K., Aneri, D., Athithiya, A.C., and Kani Kumar, P. (2020). Twitter sentiment analysis using machine learning techniques. *International Journal of Engineering and Advanced Technology (IJEAT)* 9 (3): 1–9. https://doi.org/10.35940/ijeat.C6281.029320.

19 Kakulapati, V. (2017). A panoptics of sentimental analysis. *International Journal of Advanced Research in Computer Science* 8 (1): 1036–1041. https://doi.org/10.26483/ijarcs.v8i7.4448.

20 Kawade, D. and Oza, K. (2017). Sentiment analysis: machine learning approach. *International Journal of Engineering and Technology* 9 (1): 2183–2186. https://doi.org/10.21817/ijet/2017/v9i3/1709030151.

21 Kumar, A. and Sebastian, T.M. (2012). Sentiment analysis: a perspective on its past, present and future. *International Journal of Intelligent Systems and Applications* 4 (10): 1–14. https://doi.org/10.5815/ijisa.2012.10.01.

22 Lee, P.-J., Hu, Y.-H., and Lu, K.-T. (2018). Assessing the helpfulness of online hotel reviews: a classification-based approach. *Telematics and Informatics* 35 (2): 436–445.

23 Li, Y., Pan, Q., Wang, S. et al. (2018). A generative model for category text generation. *Information Sciences* 450: 301–315.

24 Ligthart, A., Catal, C., and Tekinerdogan, B. (2021). Systematic reviews in sentiment analysis: a tertiary study. *Artificial Intelligence Review* 54 (2): 1–57.

25 Lim, S.S. and Tkaczynski, A. (2017). Origin and money matter: the airline service quality expectations of international students. *Journal of Hospitality and Tourism Management* 31: 244–252.

26 Liu, R., Shi, Y., Ji, C., and Jia, M. (2019). A survey of sentiment analysis based on transfer learning. *IEEE Access* 7 (1): 85401–85412. https://doi.org/10.1109/ACCESS.2019.2925059.

27 Anvar Shathik, J. and Krishna Prasad, K. (2020). A literature review on application of sentiment analysis using machine learning techniques. *International Journal of Applied Engineering and Management Letters (IJAEML)* 4 (2): 41–67.

28 Mäntylä, M.V., Graziotin, D., and Kuutila, M. (2018). The evolution of sentiment analysis—a review of research topics, venues, and top cited papers. *Computer Science Review* 27: 16–32.

29 Minaee, S., Azimi, E., and Abdolrashidi, A. (2019). Deep-sentiment: Sentiment analysis using ensemble of cnn and bilstm models. arXiv preprint arXiv:1904.04206.

30 Mishra, N. and Jha, C.K. (2012). Classification of opinion mining techniques. *International Journal of Computer Applications* 56 (13): 1–6.

31 Naiknaware, B., Kushwaha, B., and Kawathekar, S. (2017). Social media sentiment analysis using machine learning classifiers. *International Journal of Computer Science and Mobile Computing* 6 (6): 465–472.

32 Ortigosa, A., Martn, J.M., and Carro, R.M. (2014). Sentiment analysis in facebook and its application to e-learning. *Comput Hum Behav* 31 (Supplement C): 527–541. https://doi.org/10.1016/j.chb.2013.05.024.

33 Sanguansat, P. (2016). Paragraph2Vec-based sentiment analysis on social media for business in Thailand. *2016 8th International Conference on Knowledge and Smart Technology (KST)*, Chiang Mai, Thailand (3–6 February 2016). IEEE.

34 Patil, H. and Atique, M. (2015). Sentiment analysis for social media: a survey. *International Conference on Information Science and Security (ICISS)* 1 (1): 1–4. https://doi.org/10.1109/ICISSEC.2015.7371033.

35 Peng, H., Cambria, E., and Hussain, A. (2017). A review of sentiment analysis research in Chinese language. *Cognitive Computation* 9 (4): 423–435.

36 Devi, R.M., Keerthika, P., Suresh, P. et al. (2023). Twitter sentiment analysis using collaborative multi layer perceptron (MLP) classifier. *2023 International Conference on Computer Communication and Informatics, ICCCI*, Coimbatore (23–25 January 2023). IEEE. https://doi.org/10.1109/ICCCI56745.2023.10128430.

37 Raza, H., Faizan, M., Hamza, A. et al. (2019). Scientific text sentiment analysis using machine learning techniques. *International Journal of Advanced Computer Science and Applications* 10 (12): 157–165. https://doi.org/10.14569/IJACSA.2019.0101222.

38 Tiwari, S., Verma, A., Garg, P., and Bansal, D. (2020). Social media sentiment analysis on Twitter datasets. *6th International Conference on Advanced Computing and Communication Systems (ICACCS)*, pp. 925–927, Coimbatore (6–7 March 2020). IEEE.

39 Abdullah Aswad, S. (2023). Evaluation and analysis data from Twitter data by using hybrid CNN & LTSM. HORA 2023. *2023 5th International Congress on Human-Computer 25 Interaction, Optimization and Robotic Applications*, Istanbul (8–10 June 2023). IEEE. https://doi.org/10.1109/HORA58378.2023.10156756.

40 Raheja, S. and Asthana, A. (2021). Sentimental analysis of twitter comments on COVID-19. *Proceedings of the Confluence 2021: 11th International Conference on Cloud Computing, Data Science and Engineering*, pp. 704–708, Noida (28–29 January 2021). IEEE. https://doi.org/10.1109/Confluence51648.2021.9377048.

41 Sharma, S., Pandey, A., Kumar, V., et al. (2023). Recent trends in sentiment analysis using different machine learning based models: a short review. *Proceedings of the 2nd International Conference on Applied Artificial Intelligence and Computing, ICAAIC 2023*, pp. 474–481, Salem (4–6 May 2023). IEEE. https://doi.org/10.1109/ICAAIC56838.2023.10140954.

42 Singh, S., Kumar, K., and Kumar, B. (2022). Sentiment analysis of Twitter data using TF-IDF and machine learning techniques. *2022 International Conference on Machine Learning, Big Data, Cloud and Parallel Computing, COM-IT-CON*, pp. 252–255, Faridabad (26–27 May 2022). IEEE. https://doi.org/10.1109/COM-IT-CON54601.2022.9850477

43 Sadhasivam, J. and Babu, R. (2019). Sentiment analysis of Amazon products using ensemble machine learning algorithm. *International Journal of*

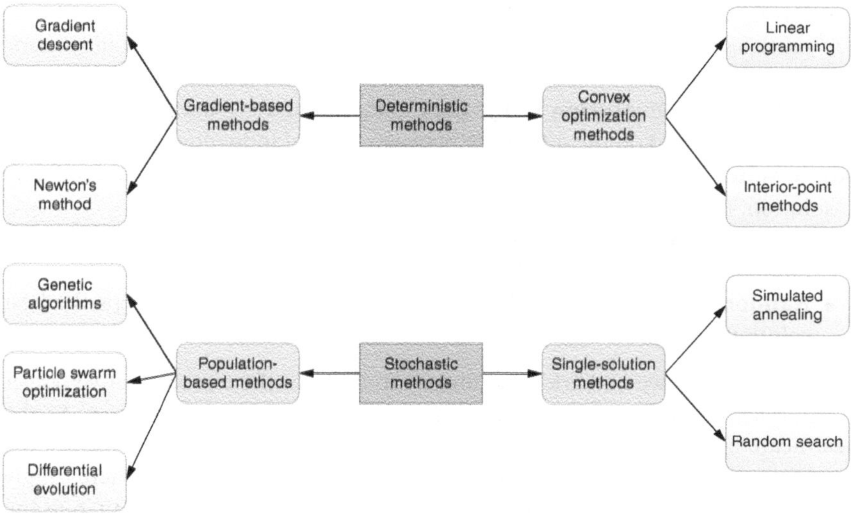

Figure 11.2 Types of optimization techniques present.

Deterministic Methods: These methods follow a well-defined set of rules to find the optimal solution. They guarantee to find the global optimum for convex problems.

Stochastic Methods: These methods involve some randomness in their search process. They are often used for nonconvex problems where finding the global optimum is difficult.

Gradient-based Methods: These methods use the gradient of the objective function to iteratively move toward the optimum. Examples include:

- **Gradient Descent**: Moves in the direction of the steepest negative slope of the objective function. (Think of rolling down a hill to find the lowest point.)
- **Newton's Method**: Uses the Hessian matrix (second derivative) for faster convergence near the optimum.

Convex Optimization Methods: These methods are specifically designed for convex problems and can efficiently find the global optimum. Examples include:

- **Linear Programming**: Optimizes linear functions subject to linear constraints.
- **Interior-point Methods**: Solves linear programming problems by moving inside the feasible region.

Population-based Methods: These methods maintain a population of candidate solutions and evolve them over time to improve their fitness. Examples include:

- **Genetic Algorithms**: Inspired by natural selection, they mimic crossover and mutation to create new solutions.

- **Particle Swarm Optimization**: Inspired by the flocking behavior of birds, particles move in the search space based on their own and their neighbors' best positions.
- **Differential Evolution (DE)**: Uses mutation and crossover to create new solutions based on the difference between pairs of individuals.

Single-solution Methods: These methods iteratively improve a single candidate solution. Examples include:

- **Simulated Annealing**: Gradually reduces the "temperature" to escape local optima, inspired by the cooling process of metals.
- **Random Search**: Randomly samples the search space and keeps the best solution found so far.

In this chapter, we embark on a journey to uncover the transformative power of optimization techniques in the realm of medical disease prediction. As the healthcare landscape evolves with the integration of advanced technologies, the need for accurate and efficient disease prediction models becomes increasingly paramount. Optimization techniques serve as the linchpin in this pursuit, offering a systematic approach to refining the parameters and algorithms that underpin predictive models. Medical datasets often exhibit high dimensionality, nonlinearity, and noise, presenting formidable challenges for traditional modeling approaches [6]. Optimization algorithms, such as flower pollination optimization (FPO), DE, and whale optimization, emerge as dynamic tools capable of navigating these complexities to enhance the precision and reliability of disease prediction.

The synergistic integration of these methodologies showcases a promising avenue for achieving unprecedented accuracy in disease prediction. By optimizing the parameters governing ML models, researchers and practitioners can unlock new insights into the intricate patterns within medical data, ultimately paving the way for more effective diagnostic and prognostic capabilities. As we delve deeper into the subsequent sections of the chapter, the reader will gain a comprehensive understanding of how these optimization algorithms contribute to the advancement of predictive analytics in the challenging and critical field of healthcare.

The outline of the proposed chapter is as follows. Section 11.2 of the chapter discusses the overview of medical disease prediction models, such as what exists in present times, so that the reader can get an idea. Section 11.3 discusses the importance of optimization techniques in increasing prediction accuracy. Section 11.4 explains the optimization techniques that are commonly used for making a predictive model. Section 11.5 discusses how we can integrate ML with optimization techniques. Section 11.6 discusses the challenges that are faced while developing such hybrid models or implementing these optimization techniques. Section 11.7

explains the case studies that show the implementation of such hybrid models. Section 11.8 discusses the future trends and the techniques that are emerging in recent times. Section 11.9 discusses the regulatory concerns that need to be taken care of while handling such sensitive medical datasets, as it involves individual privacy as well. Sections 11.10 and 11.11 discuss the conclusion and future scope of this chapter.

11.2 Overview of Medical Disease Prediction Models

This section provides a comprehensive overview of existing medical disease prediction models, laying the foundation for understanding the landscape in which optimization techniques are applied. It highlights the complexity and diversity of predictive models utilized in medical research.

Medical disease prediction models span a wide array of techniques, ranging from classical statistical methods to sophisticated ML algorithms. Classical models often leverage epidemiological data, historical trends, and demographic factors to make predictions. These models, while informative, may face challenges in capturing intricate nonlinear relationships within medical datasets.

On the other hand, ML-based models have gained prominence for their ability to uncover subtle patterns and associations inherent in vast and intricate medical datasets. Techniques such as support vector machines, decision trees, and neural networks have demonstrated efficacy in handling the complexities of medical data, offering a more nuanced understanding of disease dynamics [7, 8]. However, the success of these models critically hinges on their ability to adapt to evolving data landscapes and incorporate optimization techniques for continual refinement.

Moreover, ensemble methods, which combine multiple models to improve predictive accuracy, have emerged as powerful tools in medical prediction. By amalgamating diverse algorithms, these models capitalize on the strengths of individual components, mitigating weaknesses and enhancing overall performance.

The overview also underscores the significance of domain-specific models tailored to unique medical contexts. Diseases exhibit varied characteristics, and different modeling approaches may be more suitable for certain conditions. The section sheds light on the need for a nuanced understanding of disease profiles and the thoughtful selection of models that align with the intricacies of specific healthcare challenges.

As we navigate through the myriad models employed in medical research, the reader gains a holistic understanding of the multifaceted approaches that researchers employ to decipher the intricacies of disease prediction.

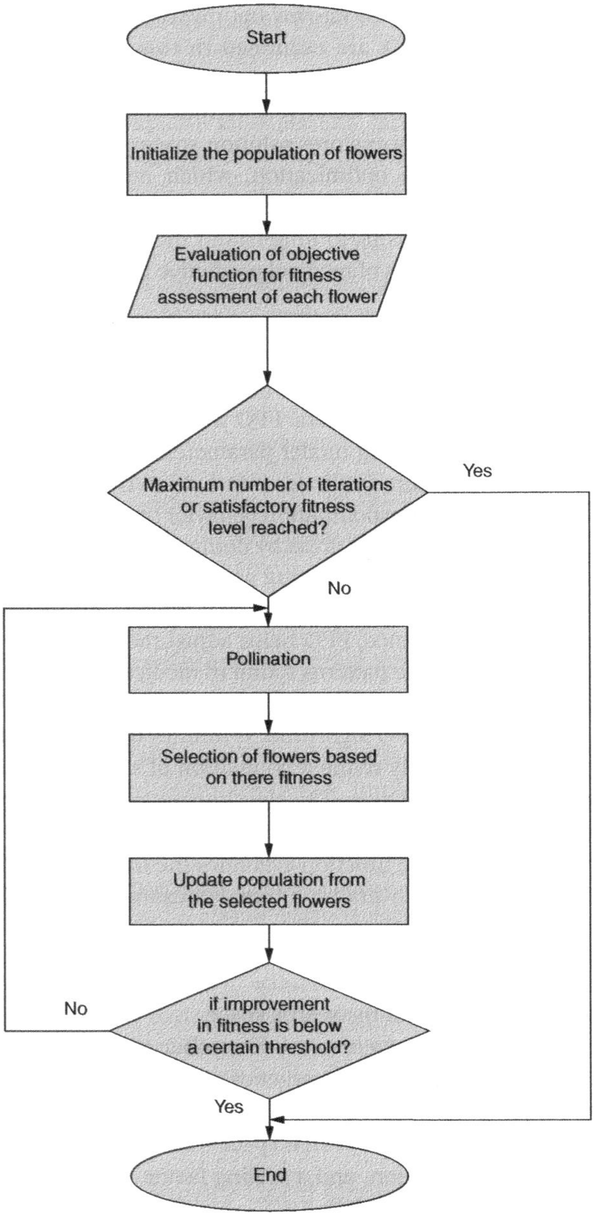

Figure 11.3 Flowchart for FPO algorithm.

Selection then occurs, favoring flowers with higher fitness for the next generation. The updated population is determined by choosing the most promising flowers from the previous steps. A common formula shown in equation (11.3) involves comparing fitness values:

$$\begin{aligned}\text{population}(i) &= \text{new\_flower}(i) \text{ if fitness(new\_flower}(i))\\ &\leq \text{fitness(current\_flower}(i)) \text{ else current\_flower}(i)\end{aligned} \tag{11.3}$$

The convergence check monitors the improvement in fitness over iterations, and if the algorithm has not converged, it loops back to the pollination step. This iterative process continues until the termination criteria are met, providing an optimized solution to the given problem.

11.4.2 Differential Evolution

One particularly strong stochastic optimization algorithm that is often used in medical predictive modeling is DE. Based on the concepts of mutation, recombination, and selection, DE skilfully explores solution spaces to identify ideal parameter setups [13]. DE is particularly good at solving nonconvex and multimodal optimization problems in the medical field. Because of its adaptability to various data formats, it can navigate the complex environment found in medical datasets with ease and help optimize model parameters for increased predictive accuracy. Because of its remarkable capacity to balance exploitation and exploration, DE is especially well-suited for optimizing predictive models in medical research. For instance, DE skillfully modifies model parameters to capture complex patterns in a variety of medical data while predicting patient responses to therapies, resulting in more accurate predictions in practice.

DE is a powerful optimization technique that iteratively refines a population of candidate solutions to find the optimal values for a given objective function, as shown in Figure 11.4. The algorithm begins with the initialization step, where a population of potential solutions is randomly generated within specified bounds. Subsequently, the objective function evaluates the fitness of each solution, converting a minimization problem into a maximization one by negating the objective function values. For example, as shown in equation (11.4):

$$\text{fitness}(x) = -f(x) \tag{11.4}$$

The termination criteria are then calculated, such as reaching a maximum number of iterations or achieving a satisfactory fitness level, and guide the algorithm's convergence. In the mutation step, new candidate solutions are created by perturbing existing ones through a scaling factor and the difference between randomly chosen solutions. For example:

$$\text{mutant\_vector} = \text{current\_vector} + F \times (\text{rand\_vector1} - \text{rand\_vector2}) \tag{11.5}$$

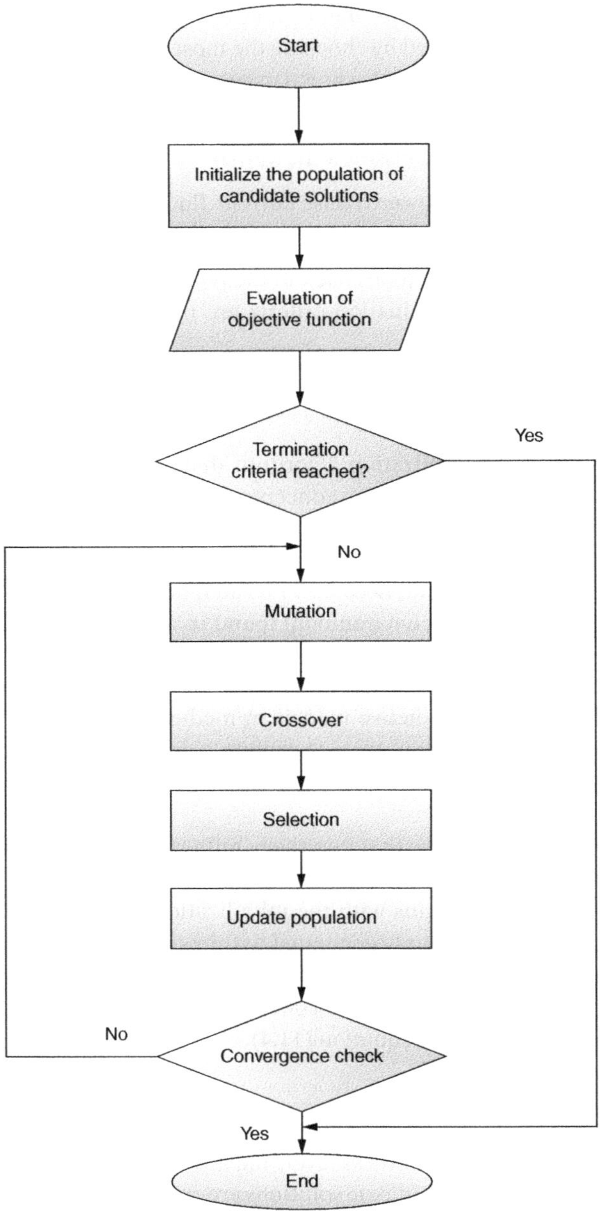

Figure 11.4 Flowchart of DE algorithm.

where F is the scaling factor, and $rand\_vector1$ $rand\_vector2$ are randomly selected vectors from the population in equation (11.5). The crossover operation then combines the mutated solutions with the existing ones, selecting elements based on a crossover probability, as shown in equation (11.6).

$$\text{trial\_vector}(i) = \text{mutant\_vector}(i) \text{ if rand}() \leq \text{CR else current\_vector}(i) \quad (11.6)$$

The selection step compares trial solutions with existing solutions, favoring those with better fitness for the next generation, as shown in equation (11.7).

$$\begin{aligned}\text{population}(i) = {} & \text{trial\_vector}(i) \text{ if fitness(trial\_vector}(i)) \\ & \leq \text{fitness(current\_vector}(i)) \text{ else current\_vector}(i) \end{aligned} \quad (11.7)$$

The updated population is determined by choosing solutions from the mutation/crossover step based on their fitness values. The convergence check monitors the improvement in fitness over iterations, and if it falls below a certain threshold, the algorithm terminates. The entire process repeats until convergence, forming a loop that optimizes the solutions to the given problem.

11.4.3 Whale Optimization Algorithm (WOA)

Inspired by humpback whale social behavior, the WOA has become well-known for its ability to optimize intricate processes. WOA provides a unique method for medical predictive modeling by combining the phases of exploration and exploitation [14]. The exploitation phase of the algorithm mimics whale hunting behavior, whereas the exploration phase imitates whale foraging. When working with medical data, WOA is particularly good at finding the best answers within large solution spaces [15]. This helps predictive models perform better by effectively fine-tuning their parameters. WOA's capacity to adapt and handle dynamic data settings makes it an option for optimizing models related to disease prediction. For example, WOA dynamically modifies model parameters to reflect changing patterns within medical datasets while predicting a disease's progress over time, resulting in predictions that are more precise and timely.

The convergence of these optimization algorithms in medical predictive modeling underscores their versatility in addressing the inherent challenges of healthcare data. By leveraging the strengths of FPO, DE, and whale optimization, researchers can navigate the intricacies of medical datasets, refining predictive models to achieve heightened accuracy and efficiency.

During the optimization process of the WOA, each whale undergoes distinct position updates at various stages, aiming to locate the optimal position, referred to as the prey position. In the initial stage, the whale's objective is relatively random, and the precise location of the prey is unclear. Consequently, a broadscale search across the entire search space is conducted, gradually narrowing down the population of whales to determine the final prey location.

11.5 Integration of ML and Optimization for Disease Prediction

A crucial turning point in the field of healthcare analytics is the combination of optimization and ML approaches for disease prediction [16]. The beneficial relationship between these two fields is explained in this part, which also shows how their joint collaboration improves the accuracy and robustness of prediction models used in medical research.

11.5.1 Fusion of ML and Optimization

ML algorithms are essential in the dynamic field of disease prediction because they may produce estimates by identifying trends in past data. But when combined with optimization procedures, they perform noticeably better. Fine-tuning the parameters of ML models is made possible by using optimization techniques, including whale optimization, FPO, and DE. Consider an ML model that predicts the course of an illness as an example. By combining optimization techniques, the model constantly modifies its configurations to maximize its capacity to identify complex patterns in medical information. By working together, we can make sure that the predictive models learn from historical data and adjust in real time, improving their predicted accuracy in the complicated world of medical data [17].

11.5.2 Parameter Tuning for Enhanced Model Performance

Parameter adjustment is a key challenge in ML, and optimization algorithms are particularly good at it. The complex interactions between hyperparameters determine the predictive models' accuracy and dependability [18]. By combining optimization techniques like genetic algorithms and DE, researchers can find optimal configurations that improve ML models' performance in disease prediction by methodically exploring the large parameter space [19]. Take into consideration an ML model that forecasts the course of an illness as an example. By means of the cooperative methodology of optimization algorithms, the model effectively refines its hyperparameters, thus deriving more profound insights from intricate medical data. This combination approach improves prediction accuracy and shows the beneficial potential of combining optimization strategies for improved model performance in the disease prediction domain.

11.5.3 Dynamic Adaptability to Evolving Datasets

ML models prove their dynamic adaptability in the constantly changing field of medical data, where new information is continually appearing [20]. By adding optimization techniques, this flexibility is further increased. Consider an ML model that is intended to forecast disease trends, for instance. The model continuously improves its parameters through iterative optimization procedures, which enable it to adjust to changing datasets. Because of its iterative design, which guarantees continual improvement, the predictive model can adapt to changing disease dynamics, new medical data, and developing trends in the healthcare industry and still be useful and relevant. Hence, a robust framework for managing the dynamic character of changing medical datasets is established through the cooperative integration of ML and optimization.

11.5.4 Improved Convergence and Computational Efficiency

Using optimization approaches can effectively handle the convergence difficulty that ML models frequently face during training. By accelerating the convergence process, these strategies produce more successful training cycles. Imagine the following situation: an ML algorithm that seeks to predict patient outcomes. The process of creating new models is improved by using optimization techniques such as stochastic gradient descent or DE, which speed up the convergence [21]. This improves computing efficiency and yields prediction models that are more accurate. The cooperative integration of optimization approaches makes it possible to investigate possible solutions in greater detail, which in turn enhances the overall effectiveness of the model training procedure and guarantees the production of precise predictive models in a way that is more computationally efficient.

To put it simply, the integration of ML and optimization in the context of disease prediction is a mutually beneficial collaboration that emphasizes the advantages of each field [22]. The reader will obtain a better understanding of how this collaborative approach transforms medical research as we move through subsequent sections, offering more precise, flexible, and effective instruments for illness comprehension and prediction.

11.6 Challenges and Considerations in Applying Optimization Techniques to Medical Data

Applying optimization techniques to medical data requires navigating a complex environment full of challenges and various considerations. The nuances of using optimization algorithms—like DE, whale optimization, and FPO—in the context of healthcare analytics are clarified in this section.

11.6.1 High Dimensionality and Complexity of Medical Data

Applying optimization techniques presents a substantial difficulty due to the massive dimensionality and complexity of medical data. Healthcare records are intrinsically complex, with many variables contributing to the complex patterns linked to specific diseases [23]. Take into consideration, for example, a medical dataset consisting of patient records containing various types of information, including genetic markers, medical histories, demographics, and lifestyle characteristics. Optimization algorithms have to traverse a large solution space as a result of the layers of complexity added by each variable. Finding the best configurations from such a large feature set is a challenge, demonstrating the necessity for advanced methods to handle the complexity of medical data.

11.6.2 Nonlinearity and Heterogeneity

Medical data is complex, with nonlinear correlations and underlying heterogeneity, making traditional optimization techniques very difficult to handle. Diseases frequently present a range of symptoms, and their relationships with different elements might be nonlinear [6]. Take into account, for example, the complex relationship between environmental and genetic factors that determine an individual's vulnerability to a given disease. It could be difficult for conventional optimization techniques to capture these complex relations. Therefore, to properly account for nonlinearities and ensure precise fine-tuning of predictive models in the face of the complex and variable nature of medical data, optimization algorithms must be provided with advanced methods.

11.6.3 Data Imbalance and Incomplete Information

There are difficulties in optimizing models for disease prediction since medical data is not distributed evenly, and some conditions may be neglected. Imagine a situation where a dataset contains fewer examples of a rare medical condition than it does of more common illnesses. This scarcity presents a problem because optimization strategies have to balance the unbalanced data to avoid preferring common occurrences [24]. Furthermore, the optimization process becomes even more complex when there is partial or missing data. For example, the accuracy of the model may be compromised if patient records are missing critical data, including family medical history or results of diagnostic testing. Robust optimization procedures are necessary to address these imbalances and information shortages, ensuring the prediction model's integrity and applicability to a variety of medical diseases.

11.6.4 Interpretable Models and Clinical Relevance

Interpretability becomes an important consideration, especially when optimization algorithms produce extraordinarily accurate but complex models, especially in medical applications. Take the example of a disease diagnosis prediction algorithm that shows great accuracy but does not provide a transparent explanation for its forecasts. To make well-informed decisions, healthcare professionals and clinicians need to understand the reasoning behind predictions. Maintaining the clinical relevance and acceptance of optimized predictive models requires striking a balance between the model's complexity and interpretability so that medical professionals can have confidence in and understand the predictions. This balance makes sure that the model's practical usefulness in actual medical situations is not compromised in the name of accuracy.

11.6.5 Computational Resource Constraints

Large computer resources are often needed for optimization techniques, especially when processing large medical datasets. Consider a situation where a disease prediction model has to analyze large amounts of patient data with a variety of variables. The computational demands could cause problems with accessibility, scalability, and time efficiency, especially in contexts with limited resources. Finding a balance between the model's complexities and computing feasibility becomes crucial. This balance makes it possible to apply optimization approaches practically in real-world healthcare settings where computational resources may be scarce, which makes advanced predictive models for better patient outcomes more widely and effectively implemented.

11.6.6 Ethical and Regulatory Considerations

Considering ethical and legal issues in great detail is necessary when implementing optimization techniques in the healthcare industry. Ensuring the confidentiality and privacy of sensitive medical data is critical, as demonstrated by situations in which patient records containing private information need to be protected. Patients' trust and confidence depend heavily on following ethical guidelines such as informed permission and data confidentiality. In addition, for healthcare practitioners to understand and have faith in the system's predictions, there must be openness in the decision-making process of optimized models. The appropriate application of optimization in medical predictive analytics is further reinforced by strict attention to regulatory frameworks, which ensure compliance with standards such as Health Insurance Portability and Accountability Act (HIPAA). This fosters an environment where developments prioritize human welfare and ethical norms.

Clinical validation using Mini-Mental State Examination (MMSE) scores also shows a good correlation with the segmented hippocampus intensities. Overall, the study highlights the promise of hybrid whale–wolf optimization in improving the performance of medical image analysis and data-driven diagnosis of Alzheimer's disease.

11.7.5 Infectious Disease Outbreak Forecasting with Hybrid Optimization

A comprehensive case study explored the application of a hybrid optimization approach, combining FPO and DE, to forecast infectious disease outbreaks. By synergistically leveraging the strengths of both algorithms, researchers achieved a more accurate and timely prediction of disease spread [30]. The hybrid optimization model demonstrated resilience against dynamic data landscapes, showcasing its adaptability in real-time scenarios where predicting the trajectory of infectious diseases is crucial for effective public health interventions.

Collectively, these case studies underscore the versatility and efficacy of optimization techniques in addressing the specific challenges posed by different diseases [31]. From cardiovascular health to cancer diagnosis and infectious disease forecasting, the successful applications highlight the adaptability of optimization algorithms in tailoring predictive models for diverse medical contexts. As we proceed through the subsequent chapters, these case studies provide a solid foundation for understanding the real-world impact and potential of optimization in revolutionizing disease prediction within the healthcare domain [32].

11.8 Future Directions and Emerging Trends in Optimizing Medical Prediction Models

Analyzing the next approaches and new developments in medical prediction model optimization reveals a dynamic environment that is ready for revolutionary breakthroughs in healthcare analytics. To offer insight into possible directions for future research and development in the subject, this part examines the latest developments in optimization approaches, including whale optimization, DE, and FPO. Imagine, for example, how these optimization techniques could be combined with modern methods of ML to create more complicated predictive models that can adjust to the changing complexity of medical data. Improved healthcare outcomes and decision-making could result from the investigation of new optimization algorithms and their combination with state-of-the-art technologies. These developments could completely transform the precision, effectiveness, and flexibility of medical prediction models.

11.8.1 Integration of Explainable AI (XAI) with Optimization

Integrating XAI with optimization algorithms is an important new concept that could influence how medical prediction models are optimized in the future. Researchers are actively looking for ways to improve the explainability of optimized models in response to the growing need for transparent and interpretable models [33]. The goal of this combination of XAI and optimization is to provide healthcare professionals with a better understanding of how complex prediction models make decisions. Imagine, for instance, that XAI approaches are added to a medical prediction model that has been optimized through the use of algorithms such as DE or FPO. By enabling a clearer and more intelligible interpretation of the model's predictions, this integration promotes trust and gives clinicians the ability to make more confident and well-informed clinical decisions based on an in-depth understanding of the model's reasoning [34].

11.8.2 Personalized and Precision Medicine Optimization

Medical prediction models are moving toward a more unique, precision-focused approach to increase efficacy. With an emphasis on customizing models for distinct patient profiles, optimization techniques are becoming more advanced [35]. Through consideration of unique genetic, lifestyle, and clinical characteristics, optimization algorithms can modify predictive models to conform to the unique details of individual patients' medical paths. Imagine, for instance, that an optimization algorithm is used to customize a disease prediction model according to a patient's particular genetic composition, way of life, and medical background. Precision medicine suited to the needs of each patient could become a reality with this personalized optimization technique, which has the potential to improve illness prognosis and treatment planning [36].

11.8.3 Ensemble Learning and Hybrid Optimization Models

An effective method for improving medical prediction models is ensemble learning, which combines predictions from several models [37]. The development of powerful hybrid models that smoothly combine optimization methods with ensemble learning may be the focus of future optimization trends. By utilizing the advantages of several algorithms, this integrative method aims to improve the generalization and resilience of predictive models for a range of medical diseases. Imagine, for example, a hybrid model that blends ensemble learning techniques with the predictive power of FPO. Because each algorithm offers unique strengths and viewpoints, this integration may produce a predictive model that is more robust and flexible and can provide correct predictions for a wider range of medical scenarios.

11.8.4 Real-Time Adaptive Optimization

Predictive models need to be flexible in real time to accommodate the dynamic nature of healthcare data. The development of algorithms that can dynamically modify model parameters in response to changing data sets is at the center of emerging advances in optimization [38]. The agility of predictive models is ensured by real-time adaptive optimization, which makes sure they produce precise and timely predictions that keep up with the dynamically shifting nature of illnesses and healthcare situations. Consider the application of a real-time adaptive optimization method to a disease prediction model, for instance. The algorithm continuously adjusts the model parameters to account for new patient data, enabling the predictive model to stay highly responsive and efficient in providing precise forecasts that accurately reflect the dynamics of healthcare today.

11.8.5 Incorporation of Multimodal Data and Omics Technologies

The future of optimization in medical prediction models centers on the smooth integration and optimization across various data sources as healthcare embraces a variety of multimodal data and omics technologies [39]. It is important that optimization algorithms be tailored to the complexities involved in integrating traditional clinical data with genomes, proteomics, and other omics data. Using a comprehensive approach, the goal is to optimize predictive models in order to gain deeper insights into the mechanisms underlying disease and produce more thorough and informed forecasts [40]. Take the integration of genome data and optimization approaches for a disease prediction model, for example, by utilizing the abundance of various data available in current medical settings, the optimization process would not only take into account conventional clinical parameters but also successfully incorporate genetic information, improving the model's ability to give deeper and more accurate predictions.

11.8.6 Ethical Optimization and Bias Mitigation

Future developments will emphasize ethical issues and bias mitigation more as the use of optimization techniques in healthcare expands. Future advances in optimization will entail creating procedures and frameworks to ensure accountability, fairness, and transparency in the application of predictive models. The resolution of biases and ethical issues is fundamental to these advancements since it is essential to building patient and healthcare provider confidence [41]. Consider a situation where a prediction model for illness diagnosis is optimized using an optimization method. To uphold ethical standards and develop trust within the healthcare community, the ethical optimization approach would include making sure that the algorithm and model are designed and implemented in a way that minimizes biases, treats people fairly across diverse demographics, and maintains transparency in the decision-making process.

In summary, the latest technologies and approaches are expected to converge in the future when it comes to optimizing medical prediction models. The field of optimization approaches has immense potential to transform disease prediction and promote more efficient, just, and ethical healthcare practices. Its applications range from real-time adaptability to personalized treatment [42]. Imagine, for example, how personalized medicine and real-time adaptive optimization algorithms can work together to make sure that predictive models respect ethical norms for objective and transparent decision-making while also adapting dynamically to changing healthcare dynamics and individual patient profiles.

11.9 Ethical and Regulatory Implications of Optimized Disease Prediction Systems

Examining the ethical and regulatory implications of optimized disease prediction systems is imperative as these technologies continue to advance [43]. This section delves into the multifaceted considerations surrounding the responsible deployment of optimization techniques, such as FPO, DE, and whale optimization, in the critical domain of healthcare analytics.

11.9.1 Privacy and Data Security Concerns

Ethical considerations surrounding optimized disease prediction systems begin with the protection of an individual's privacy and the security of sensitive medical data [44]. As optimization algorithms process and refine models using patient information, ensuring robust data security measures becomes paramount. Striking a balance between data accessibility for research and safeguarding patients' privacy is crucial to mitigate the risks of unauthorized access or data breaches.

11.9.2 Transparency and Explainability

Optimization techniques often yield complex predictive models, and the ethical deployment of these models necessitates transparency and explainability [45]. Understanding how a predictive model reaches specific conclusions is vital for clinicians, patients, and other stakeholders. Ensuring that optimization processes result in models that are interpretable fosters trust and facilitates informed decision-making in clinical settings.

becomes nonnegotiable. The ethical considerations woven into the optimization journey emphasize the need for responsible deployment, aligning with regulatory standards, and fostering stakeholder trust in the era of data-driven healthcare.

11.11 Future Scope

The study of optimization in the field of medical predictive analytics has revealed a future in which real-time adaptability, personalized therapy, and ethical considerations are essential components. The combination of optimization with cutting-edge developments like hybrid models, XAI, and precision medicine indicates a time when predictive analytics will be a vital and dynamic tool in the hands of medical practitioners.

The approach toward optimization in medical predictive analytics, in essence, represents a paradigm change toward a future in which data-driven insights transform patient care and illness prediction. Through understanding optimization techniques and their applications, we set out on a journey where healthcare knowledge and technology work together to create an environment that is both transformational and ethically sound. As we get to the end of this investigation, think about how optimization is continuing to develop in the field of healthcare analytics—a journey that will provide the groundwork for a new era in predictive medicine through an uncompromising pursuit of efficiency, accuracy, and ethical responsibility.

References

1 Raheja, V., Shah, V., Shetty, M., et al. (2022). Multi-disease prediction system using machine learning. *2022 International Conference on Futuristic Technologies (INCOFT)*, Belgaum, India (25–27 November 2022). IEEE.

2 Sun, S., Cao, Z., Zhu, H., and Zhao, J. (2019). A survey of optimization methods from a machine learning perspective. *IEEE Transactions on Cybernetics* 50 (8): 3668–3681.

3 Pei, J. and Pardalos, P.M. (2022). Scalable optimization and decision-making in operations research. *Annals of Operations Research* 316 (1): 1–4.

4 Sharma, S. and Kumar, V. (2022). A comprehensive review on multi-objective optimization techniques: past, present and future. *Archives of Computational Methods in Engineering* 29 (7): 5605–5633.

5 Quang, T.-T., Le, N., and Le, B. (2022). Predictive modelling of diseases based on a network and machine learning approach. *Asian Conference on Intelligent Information and Database Systems*. Singapore: Springer Nature Singapore.

6 Badawy, M., Ramadan, N., and Hefny, H.A. (2023). Healthcare predictive analytics using machine learning and deep learning techniques: a survey. *Journal of Electrical Systems and Information Technology* 10 (1): 40.

7 Nadimi-Shahraki, M.H., Zamani, H., Varzaneh, Z.A., and Mirjalili, S. (2023). A systematic review of the whale optimization algorithm: theoretical foundation, improvements, and hybridizations. *Archives of Computational Methods in Engineering* 1–47.

8 Dhabal, S., and Saha, D.K. (2020). Image enhancement using differential evolution based whale optimization algorithm. *Emerging Technology in Modelling and Graphics: Proceedings of IEM Graph 2018*. Springer Singapore, 2020.

9 Abdel-Basset, M. and Shawky, L.A. (2019). Flower pollination algorithm: a comprehensive review. *Artificial Intelligence Review* 52: 2533–2557.

10 Qin, G. (2022). Improved flower pollination algorithm and its application in medical image registration. *ICETIS 2022; 7th International Conference on Electronic Technology and Information Science*. VDE.

11 Gashti, M.Z. (2018). A modified model based on flower pollination algorithm and K-nearest neighbor for diagnosing diseases. *IIUM Engineering Journal* 19 (1): 144–157.

12 Karaboğa, D. and Ökdem, S. (2004). A simple and global optimization algorithm for engineering problems: differential evolution algorithm. *Turkish Journal of Electrical Engineering and Computer Sciences* 12 (1): 53–60.

13 Deng, W., Shang, S., Cai, X. et al. (2021). An improved differential evolution algorithm and its application in optimization problem. *Soft Computing* 25: 5277–5298.

14 Rahmani Hosseinabadi, A.A., Sadeghilalimi, M., Babazadeh Shareh, M. et al. (2022). Whale optimization-based prediction for medical diagnostic. *12th International Conference on Agents and Artificial Intelligence, ICAART*. DOI: 10.5220/0010802200003116.

15 Rana, N., Shafie, A.L.M., Abdulhamid, S.'i.M., and Chiroma, H. (2020). Whale optimization algorithm: a systematic review of contemporary applications, modifications and developments. *Neural Computing and Applications* 32: 16245–16277.

16 Ahmed, A., Ashour, O., Ali, H., and Firouz, M. (2022). An integrated optimization and machine learning approach to predict the admission status of emergency patients. *Expert Systems with Applications* 202: 117314.

17 Liu, J., Ye, J., Izquierdo, D.S. et al. (2023). A review of machine learning techniques for process and performance optimization in laser beam powder bed fusion additive manufacturing. *Journal of Intelligent Manufacturing* 34 (8): 3249–3275.

18 Hashi, E.K. and Zaman, M.S.U. (2020). Developing a hyperparameter tuning based machine learning approach of heart disease prediction. *Journal of Applied Science & Process Engineering* 7 (2): 631–647.

19 Kaur, S., Aggarwal, H., and Rani, R. (2020). Hyper-parameter optimization of deep learning model for prediction of Parkinson's disease. *Machine Vision and Applications* 31: 1–15.

20 Alanazi, H.O., Abdullah, A.H., and Qureshi, K.N. (2017). A critical review for developing accurate and dynamic predictive models using machine learning methods in medicine and health care. *Journal of Medical Systems* 41: 1–10.

21 MahaLakshmi, N.V. and Rout, R.K. (2023). Effective heart disease prediction using improved particle swarm optimization algorithm and ensemble classification technique. *Soft Computing* 1–14.

22 Jiao, N. (2023). An efficient disease prediction framework based on optimized machine learning models for a smart healthcare application. *Multimedia Tools and Applications* 1–24.

23 Houssein, E.H., Hosney, M.E., Emam, M.M. et al. (2023). Soft computing techniques for biomedical data analysis: open issues and challenges. *Artificial Intelligence Review* 56 (Suppl 2): 2599–2649.

24 Tsai, C.-W., Chiang, M.-C., Ksentini, A., and Chen, M. (2016). Metaheuristic algorithms for healthcare: open issues and challenges. *Computers & Electrical Engineering* 53: 421–434.

25 Vivekanandan, T. and Iyengar, N.C.S.N. (2017). Optimal feature selection using a modified differential evolution algorithm and its effectiveness for prediction of heart disease. *Computers in Biology and Medicine* 90: 125–136.

26 Johnson, D.S., Johnson, D.L.L., Elavarasan, P. et al. (2020). Feature selection using flower pollination optimization to diagnose lung cancer from CT images. In: *Advances in Information and Communication: Proceedings of the 2020 Future of Information and Communication Conference (FICC)*, vol. 2 (ed. K. Arai, R. Bhatia, and S. Kapoor), 604. Springer International Publishing.

27 Vijaya, J., Chandra, S., and Baghel, P. (2023). Diabetes disease prediction using various metaheuristic optimization algorithms. *2023 IEEE 8th International Conference for Convergence in Technology (I2CT)*, Lonavla, India (7–9 April 2023). IEEE.

28 Kadry, S. et al. (2023). Automatic classification of normal/AD brain MRI slices using whale-algorithm optimized hybrid image features. *Journal of Ambient Intelligence and Humanized Computing* 14 (10): 14237–14248.

29 Dhakhinamoorthy, C., Mani, S.K., Sandeep Kumar, M. et al. (2023). Hybrid whale and gray wolf deep learning optimization algorithm for prediction of Alzheimer's disease. *Mathematics* 11 (5): 1136.

30 Indhumathi, K. and Satheshkumar, K. (2024). Prediction of seasonal infectious diseases based on hybrid machine learning approach. *Multimedia Tools and Applications* 83 (3): 7001–7019.

31 Sharma, B., Khurana, P., and Kumar, D. (2021). Solving SIS Epidemic Disease Model by Flower Pollination Algorithm. *2021 8th International Conference on Computing for Sustainable Global Development (INDIACom)*, New Delhi, India (17–19 March 2021). IEEE.

32 Al-Qaness, M.A.A., Ewees, A.A., Fan, H., and Elaziz, M.A. (2020). Optimized forecasting method for weekly influenza confirmed cases. *International Journal of Environmental Research and Public Health* 17 (10): 3510.

33 Heaton, H. and Fung, S.W. (2023). Explainable AI via learning to optimize. *Scientific Reports* 13 (1): 10103.

34 Hanif, A. Beheshti, A., Benatallah, B., et al. (2023). A comprehensive survey of explainable artificial intelligence (XAI) methods: exploring transparency and interpretability. *International Conference on Web Information Systems Engineering*. Singapore: Springer Nature Singapore.

35 Delpierre, C. and Lefèvre, T. (2023). Precision and personalized medicine: What their current definition says and silences about the model of health they promote. Implication for the development of personalized health. *Frontiers in Sociology* 8: 1112159.

36 Du, J., Gao, S., and Chen, C.-H. (2022). A simulation optimization approach for precision medicine. *AI and Analytics for Public Health: Proceedings of the 2020 INFORMS International Conference on Service Science*. Springer International Publishing.

37 Semwal, V.B., Gupta, A., and Lalwani, P. (2021). An optimized hybrid deep learning model using ensemble learning approach for human walking activities recognition. *The Journal of Supercomputing* 77 (11): 12256–12279.

38 Wiersma, R.D. and Liu, X. (2019). A conceptual study on real-time adaptive radiation therapy optimization through ultra-fast beamlet control. *Biomedical Physics & Engineering Express* 5 (5): 055016.

39 Tong, L., Shi, W., Isgut, M. et al. (2023). Integrating multi-omics data with EHR for precision medicine using advanced artificial intelligence. *IEEE Reviews in Biomedical Engineering*, pp. 80–97. IEEE.

40 Yagin, F.H. (2023). Machine Learning Approaches for Multi-omics Data Integration in Medicine. In: *Machine Learning Methods for Multi-Omics Data Integration* (ed. A. Alhateeb, and L. Rueda), 23–38. Cham: Springer International Publishing.

41 Nazer, L.H., Zatarah, R., Waldrip, S. et al. (2023). Bias in artificial intelligence algorithms and recommendations for mitigation. *PLOS Digital Health* 2 (6): e0000278.

- The National Academy of Medicine describes a healthcare system as "the constellation of public and private resources, policies, and actions that regulate, finance, and deliver services that promote health, prevent illness and injury, and manage and treat acute and chronic diseases" [4].
- "The arrangement of people, institutions, and resources that deliver healthcare services to meet the health needs of a target population" is how the Commonwealth Fund defines a healthcare system [5].
- "The set of institutions, resources, and people responsible for delivering healthcare services to meet the needs of a population" is how the World Bank defines a healthcare system [6].

These definitions emphasize how different actors, resources, and activities that are involved in providing healthcare services and attending to the health requirements of a community within a certain geographic area are interrelated. Countries and regions can have extremely different healthcare systems, which reflect variations in legal frameworks, infrastructure, finance methods, and delivery strategies.

12.1.2 The Need for Healthcare Systems

Indeed, the healthcare systems are essential to countries and governates for several reasons, such as the promotion of health and well-being, diagnosis and treatment of illnesses, emergency and trauma care, management of chronic conditions, maternal and child health, long-term care and rehabilitation, and economic and social impact [7, 8].

Healthcare systems focus on promoting health and well-being at both the individual and population levels. They provide preventive services such as vaccinations, screenings, and health education to help people maintain good health and prevent the onset of diseases [9]. Besides, healthcare systems play a crucial role in diagnosing and treating illnesses. They provide access to medical professionals, diagnostic tests, medications, surgeries, and therapies that help individuals recover from illnesses, manage chronic conditions, and improve their quality of life [10]. On the other hand, healthcare systems include emergency departments and trauma centers that provide immediate and life-saving care during critical situations. These services are crucial for accidents, injuries, acute medical conditions, and other emergencies where prompt medical attention can make a significant difference in outcomes [11]. Moreover, healthcare systems support the management of chronic conditions such as diabetes, heart disease, asthma, and cancer [12]. They provide ongoing care, medications, monitoring, and lifestyle interventions that help individuals lead fulfilling lives while effectively managing their conditions. Also, healthcare systems ensure the well-being of expectant mothers, infants, and children. They provide prenatal care, safe delivery services, vaccinations, regular check-ups, and pediatric care to promote healthy growth and development and reduce maternal and infant mortality rates [13]. Furthermore, healthcare systems provide long-term care services for the elderly, individuals with disabilities, and those requiring rehabilitation after surgeries or injuries. These services include nursing homes, assisted living facilities, home healthcare, and rehabilitation centers that support individuals in their daily activities and recovery. Lastly, healthcare systems have significant economic and social implications. They create employment opportunities, stimulate economic growth, and contribute to overall societal well-being. Healthy individuals are more productive, leading to a stronger workforce and economic development [14].

12.1.3 Healthcare Systems Challenges

There are some common challenges faced by healthcare systems around the world globally. Mainly, these challenges include the following [14–19]:

1) In many countries, ensuring equal access to healthcare services continues to be a major concern. Cultural barriers, financial level, and geographic location can all have an impact on access disparities.
2) Global healthcare expenses are on the rise, placing a financial burden on citizens, governments, and healthcare systems. An increasing number of people are becoming older, using more expensive medications, technology improvements, and the prevalence of chronic illnesses are all factors driving up expenses.
3) Ensuring that healthcare services remain high-quality and continue to improve is a constant task. It entails protecting patient safety, cutting down on medical mistakes, putting evidence-based procedures into practice, and encouraging ongoing quality improvement.
4) Healthcare professionals, such as doctors, nurses, and allied health workers, are in low supply in many nations. These shortages have the potential to restrict access to care and increase pressure on the current medical staff.
5) As the world's population ages, chronic illnesses, including diabetes, heart disease, and cancer, are becoming more common. The growing need for long-term care, illness management, and specialized services for senior citizens requires healthcare systems to change.
6) For coordinated and patient-centered care, effective information management and exchange are essential. Adopting and integrating health information technologies, protecting patient privacy and security, and encouraging interoperability across various healthcare providers are, nevertheless, difficult tasks for many healthcare systems.
7) Access to care may be hampered by inadequate healthcare infrastructure, especially in underserved and rural locations. Providing timely and

appropriate healthcare services is hampered by a lack of medical equipment, transportation networks, and healthcare facilities.

8) Natural disasters, infectious disease outbreaks, and other public health emergencies can put a burden on the ability of healthcare systems to react quickly. To handle such emergencies and safeguard the public's health, plans for preparedness and reaction must be in place.
9) There are still differences in health outcomes and healthcare access between various population groupings. Targeted interventions and policies that consider vulnerable groups, cultural characteristics, and socioeconomic determinants of health are necessary to address health inequities.
10) For healthcare systems to offer appropriate and reasonably priced care, long-term funding sources are essential. For many healthcare systems, striking a balance between the cost of care, revenue generation, and financial sustainability continues to be a difficult task.

Because of these complex issues, stakeholders, policymakers, and medical experts must continue to work together to create novel plans of action and inventive approaches to bolster healthcare systems around the world.

12.2 The Internet of Medical Things' (IoMT) Revolution in Healthcare

The Internet of Medical Things (IoMT) is a tremendous force that is about to radically change the healthcare business. Driven by the growing requirement for remote patient monitoring and the increased use of linked medical devices, The Brainy Insights predicts that by 2032, the IoMT market will be valued at USD 516.4 billion, growing at a compound annual growth rate (CAGR) of 23.70% [20].

Real-time data gathering, analysis, and communication made possible by the networked ecosystem of medical devices, sensors, and software applications is transforming patient care and resulting in [21–25]:

- **Improved Patient Tracking:** Vital signs, blood glucose levels, and other health metrics can be continually monitored by IoMT devices such as wearables, ingestible sensors, and smart implants. This gives medical professionals a more comprehensive understanding of their patients' health, enabling them to identify possible problems early and take appropriate action. It also gives patients the ability to take a more active role in managing their health.
- **Telemedicine and Remote Care:** Patients who live in rural areas or have trouble traveling can now receive healthcare thanks to IoMT, which makes remote consultations, diagnosis, and treatment possible. This can lower healthcare expenses and greatly enhance access to specialists.

- **Imaging Sensors:** These sensors, which are used to create images of the body for diagnostic reasons, include X-ray, magnetic resonance imaging, computed tomography, and ultrasound sensors. Canon Medical Systems is one example [55].

12.3.3 Big Data, Machine Learning, and Artificial Intelligence: The Foundation of Digital Health

The application of ML, a subset of AI, to healthcare is no different from other areas of daily life where ML is used to enable computer systems to become intelligent. AI allows computers and mechanical devices to think like humans and carry out tasks autonomously. AI and ML may be utilized in the healthcare and pharmaceutical sectors to improve patient safety, security, and practitioner understanding. In addition, it can be used to evaluate medical imaging, project outcomes, examine patient or medical data, research healthcare-related literature, and provide treatment recommendations. In addition, AI and ML offer a variety of potential applications in current and upcoming clinical trials, such as real-time data collection and analysis, smooth data integration across phases, productivity in clinical research, recommendations based on treatment efficacy, patient population interventions, post-market surveillance, and patient support [7, 8, 19].

When combined, AI and ML refer to dynamic, self-learning technology that may suggest or decide. Developing computer programs that can access data sets to feed into algorithms that provide ever-more-accurate and exact outcomes is the aim. The healthcare AI industry is predicted to reach $187.95 billion by 2030, expanding at a 37% CAGR between 2022 and 2030 [56].

Healthcare facilities with access to patient data, medical professionals, surveys, technology platforms, social media platforms, health apps, and clinical research are the usual sources of healthcare data. Medical software generates and collects vast amounts of sensitive consumer data, including details about users' reproductive lives, mental health, and genetics. Medical software also includes mobile apps, medical device data systems (which transfer, store, display, or convert medical device data electronically), medical image storage devices (which store or retrieve medical images electronically), and medical image communications devices (which transfer medical image data electronically between medical devices) [57].

Through seamless connectivity with other databases and apps, real-time data may be effectively used with predictive AI models and analytical tools to reduce the likelihood and impact of human errors in data collection and analysis. This is in addition to the need to get patient consent and preserve objectivity by guaranteeing the fairness of data sets—which is likely to be one of the primary obstacles to the integration of AI and ML in traditional healthcare. Concerns that need to be addressed include data duplication, methods and uniformity in data collection and processing, and the participation of technology platforms and healthcare organizations.

The Information Technology Act of 2000 and its implementing regulations currently serve as the regulatory framework for data. Sensitive personal data and information are also governed under the Information Technology (Reasonable Security Practices and Procedures and Sensitive Personal Data or Information) Rules, 2011. Healthcare data are also governed by this legislation and the rules that go along with it. Furthermore, a proposed law that would establish a legal framework for the anonymization and de-identification of digital health data is called the Digital Information Security in Healthcare Bill. Furthermore, the collection of optional requirements for the security, privacy, disclosure, and protection of protected health information is provided by the Electronic Health Record requirements for India, 2016, which were announced by the Ministry of Health and Family Welfare (MoHFW). Finally, to further establish user control over personal health data, the National Digital Health Mission, 2020 established the Health Data Management Policy. This policy outlined the duties of data fiduciaries and prescribed a consent framework to oversee data collection, storage, processing, and sharing. It also introduced the idea of an electronic consent manager, who would communicate with users to obtain consent to access their health data.

Considering the significance and intricacy of healthcare data, selecting an appropriate approach is crucial to guaranteeing accurate data collection, storage, and utilization. The time has come for appropriate laws to tackle the sector's overlapping difficulties, even though different governmental attempts have been made to harness technology and create a solid healthcare infrastructure.

12.4 Blockchain Applications in the Healthcare Systems

Blockchain technology makes a comprehensive, effective, and transparent ecosystem that collects and saves data while maintaining immutability. These characteristics make it ideally suited for healthcare and pharmaceutical control. Industry projections predict that by 2025, the blockchain healthcare market will have grown to a value of $3.49 billion [58].

Blockchain's decentralized network, transparency, and immutability are its distinguishing characteristics. This is accomplished by dividing up encrypted data records into data blocks and distributing them throughout the several networked systems that are involved, producing a distinct signature called a hash. Since the blocks are unchangeable, any tampering with the records will alert all people involved. Users can select from three different types of blockchains:

hospital readmission rates, and enhances patient convenience. IoT devices can also make it easier for healthcare providers to share patient data with one another, improving care coordination and enabling well-informed decision-making.

IoT technology may also improve resource allocation, track inventories, and automate procedures to maximize healthcare facility operations. This may result in lower costs, fewer errors, and more effective workflow. IoT-enabled equipment and beds, including smart beds, can also improve patient safety by lowering hazards and guaranteeing prompt interventions through predictive maintenance and real-time alarms.

Nonetheless, there are issues and concerns with IoT adoption in the healthcare industry. To protect sensitive medical information, data security and patient privacy must come first. Strict data governance and strong cybersecurity measures are necessary to reduce the risks of data breaches and unauthorized access. To guarantee smooth integration and data sharing between various IoT devices and healthcare systems, interoperability standards and protocols must also be developed.

Moreover, enterprises and healthcare experts need to address issues with the accuracy, dependability, and usability of IoT devices. IoT technologies must be continuously observed and assessed to guarantee their efficacy, dependability, and compliance with legal requirements.

Overall, the implementation of IoT in the healthcare industry has enormous potential to change the way that healthcare is provided, enhance patient outcomes, and boost operational effectiveness. To fully utilize IoT technology in healthcare and ensure patient safety and privacy is maintained, however, rigorous consideration of ethical, privacy, security, and regulatory factors is essential. IoT has the potential to transform healthcare and lead to a more proactive and connected approach to patient care with correct deployment and continued developments.

References

1. Abaoud, M., Almuqrin, M.A., and Khan, M.F. Advancing federated learning through novel mechanism for privacy preservation in healthcare applications. *IEEE Access*. https://doi.org/10.1109/access.2023.3301162 83562–83579.
2. Manihar, S. and Rehman, T.B. (2023). IOT healthcare applications. *IoT in Healthcare Systems*. https://doi.org/10.1201/9781003145035-7 105–120.
3. Murray, Christopher J.L., Frenk, J., and World Health Organization (1999). A WHO framework for health system performance assessment.
4. McGinnis, J.M., Fineberg, H.V., and Dzau, V.J. (2021). Advancing the learning health system. *N Engl J Med* 385 (1): 1–5.

5 Greener, I. (2020). Healthcare funding and its relationship to equity and outcomes: A QCA analysis of Commonwealth Fund and OECD data. *Journal of European Social Policy* 30 (4): 480–494.

6 Harman, S. (2009). The World Bank and health. *Global Health Governance: Crisis, Institutions and Political Economy* 227–244.

7 Bahri, S., Zoghlami, N., Abed, M., and Tavares, J.M.R. (2018). Big data for healthcare: a survey. *IEEE Access* 7: 7397–7408.

8 Wang, Y., Kung, L., and Byrd, T.A. (2018). Big data analytics: understanding its capabilities and potential benefits for healthcare organizations. *Technol. Forecasting Social Change* 126: 3–13.

9 Li, Y., Vo, A., Randhawa, M., and Fick, G. (2017). Designing utilization-based spatial healthcare accessibility decision support systems: a case of a regional health plan. *Decis. Support Syst.* 99: 51–63.

10 Chen, L., Li, X., Yang, Y. et al. (2016). Personal health indexing based on medical examinations: a data mining approach. *Decis. Support Syst.* 81: 54–65.

11 D'Antrassi, P., Prenassi, M., Rossi, L. et al. (2019). Personally collected health data for precision medicine and longitudinal research. *Frontiers Med.* 6: 125.

12 Lasierra, N., Roldán, F., Alesanco, A., and García, J. (2014). Towards improving usage and management of supplies in healthcare: an ontology-based solution for sharing knowledge. *Expert Syst. Appl.* 41 (14): 6261–6273.

13 Tunçalp, Ö., Were, W.M., MacLennan, C. et al. (2015). Quality of care for pregnant women and newborns-the WHO vision. *BJOG* 122 (8): 1045–1049. https://doi.org/10.1111/1471-0528.13451.

14 Dubois, C.-A. and McKee, M. (2004). Health and health care in the candidate countries of the European Union: common challenges, different circumstances, diverse policies. In: *Health Policy and European Union Enlargement* (ed. M. McKee, L. MacLehose, and E. Nolte), 43–63. Maidenhead: Open University Press.

15 Chinitz, D., Preker, A., and Wasem, J. (1998). Balancing competition and solidarity in health care financing. In: *Critical Challenges for Health Care Reform in Europe* (ed. R.B. Saltman, J. Figueras, and C. Sakellarides), 55–77. Buckingham: Open University Press.

16 Couturier, J., Sola, D., Borioli, G.S., and Raiciu, C. (2012). How can the internet of things help to overcome current healthcare challenges. *Commun. Strategies* 1 (87): 67–81.

17 Hassanalieragh, M., Page, A., Soyata, T. et al. (2015). Health monitoring and management using Internet-of-Things (IoT) sensing with cloud-based processing: Opportunities and challenges. *Proceedings of the IEEE International Conference on Services Computing (SCC)*, pp. 285–292, New York, NY (27 June 2015 - 02 July 2015). IEEE.

18 Bhattacharya, P. (2005). Implications of an aging population in India: challenges and opportunities. *Proc. Living to* 100: 12–14.

19 Salas-Vega, S., Haimann, A., and Mossialos, E. (2015). Big data and health care: challenges and opportunities for coordinated policy development in the EU. *Health Syst. Reform* 1 (4): 285–300.

20 Al-Hamadi, H. and Chen, I.R. (2017). Trust-based decision making for health IoT systems. *IEEE Internet Things J.* 4 (5): 1408–1419.

21 Woo, M., Lee, J., and Park, K. (2018). A reliable IoT system for personal healthcare devices. *Future Gener. Comput. Syst.* 78: 626–640.

22 Yu, K.-H., Beam, A.L., and Kohane, I.S. (2018). Artificial intelligence in healthcare. *Nature Biomed. Eng.* 2 (10): 719–731.

23 He, J., Baxter, S.L., Xu, J. et al. (2019). The practical implementation of artificial intelligence technologies in medicine. *Nature Med.* 25 (1): 30–36.

24 Rotmensch, M., Halpern, Y., Tlimat, A. et al. (2017). Learning a health knowledge graph from electronic medical records. *Sci. Rep.* 7 (1).

25 Maeng, D.D., Starr, A.E., Tomcavage, J.F. et al. (2014). Can telemonitoring reduce hospitalization and cost of care? A health plan's experience in managing patients with heart failure. *Population Health Manag.* 17 (6): 340–344.

26 Razdan, S. and Sharma, S. (2022). Internet of Medical Things (IoMT): overview, emerging technologies, and case studies. *IETE Technical Review* 775–788. https://doi.org/10.1080/02564602.2021.1927863.

27 Asghar, M.Z., Srivastava, J., Routray, S. et al. (2022). Internet of medical things (IoMT)-based smart healthcare system: trends and progress. *Computational Intelligence and Neuroscience* https://doi.org/10.1155/2022/7218113.

28 Topol, E.J. (2013). *The Creative Destruction of Medicine: How the Digital Revolution Will Create Better Health Care*. Basic Books.

29 Rodrigues, J.J.P.C., De Rezende Segundo, D.B., Junqueira, H.A. et al. (2018). Enabling technologies for the Internet of health things. *IEEE Access* 6: 13129–13141.

30 Klaassen, B., van Beijnum, B.J.F., and Hermens, H.J. (2016). Usability in telemedicine systems—A literature survey. *International Journal of Medical Informatics* 93: 57–69. https://doi.org/10.1016/j.ijmedinf.2016.06.004.

31 Hung, M.-H., Cheng, F.-T., and Yeh, S.-C. (2005). Development of a web-services-based e-diagnostics framework for semiconductor manufacturing industry. *IEEE Transactions on Semiconductor Manufacturing* 18 (1): 122–135. https://doi.org/10.1109/TSM.2004.836664.

32 Hamdoun, S., Monteleone, R., Bookman, T., and Michael, K. (2023). AI-based and digital mental health apps: balancing need and risk. *IEEE Technology and Society Magazine* 42 (1): 25–36. https://doi.org/10.1109/MTS.2023.3241309.

33 Gmunder, K.N., Ruiz, J.W., Franceschi, D., and Suarez, M.M. (2024). Demographics associated with US healthcare disparities are exacerbated by the

59 Pham, H.L., Tran, T.H. and Nakashima, Y. (2018). A secure remote healthcare system for hospital using blockchain smart contract. *2018 IEEE Globecom Workshops (GC Wkshps)*, pp. 1–6, Abu Dhabi (9–13 December 2018). IEEE., https://doi.org/10.1109/GLOCOMW.2018.8644164.

60 Pires, I.M., Garcia, N.M., Pombo, N. et al. (2016). Validation techniques for sensor data in mobile health applications. *J. Sens.* 2016: 1–9.

61 Li, F. and Xiong, P. (2013). Practical secure communication for integrating wireless sensor networks into the internet of things. *IEEE Sens. J.* 13: 3677–3684.

62 Swan, M. (2012). Sensor Mania! The internet of things, wearable computing, objective metrics, and the quantified self 2.0. *J. Sens. Act. Netw.* 1: 217–253.

63 Mavrogiorgou, A., Kiourtis, A., Perakis, K. et al. (1978). IoT in healthcare: achieving interoperability of high-quality data acquired by IoT medical devices. *Sensors* 2019: 19.

64 Zhang, G., Ou, S.-X., Huang, Y.-H., and Wang, C.-R. (2015). Semi-supervised learning methods for large scale healthcare data analysis. *Int. J. Comput. Healthcare* 2 (2): 2046–2060.

65 Mshali, H., Lemlouma, T., Moloney, M., and Magoni, D. (2018). A survey on health monitoring systems for health smart homes. *Int. J. Ind. Ergon.* 66: 26–56.

66 Shah, S.A. and Fioranelli, F. (2019). RF sensing technologies for assisted daily living in healthcare: a comprehensive review. *IEEE Aerosp. Electron. Syst. Mag.* 34 (11): 26–44.

67 Meng, Y., Yi, S.-H., and Kim, H.-C. (2019). Health and wellness monitoring using intelligent sensing technique. *J. Inf. Process. Syst.* 15 (3): 478–491.

68 IOT in healthcare market global market assessment and forecast. https://www.vantagemarketresearch.com/industry-report/iot-in-healthcare-market-1232 (accessed 2024).

69 IoT Healthcare Market. https://straitsresearch.com/report/iot-healthcare-market (accessed 2024).

70 IoT Fleet Management Market Size - Global Industry, Share, Analysis, Trends and Forecast 2023 – 2032. https://www.acumenresearchandconsulting.com/iot-fleet-management-market (accessed 2024).

13

Generating Synthetic Medical Dataset Using Generative AI: A Case Study

Partha Pratim Ray

Department of Computer Applications, Sikkim University, Gangtok, India

13.1 Introduction

In the rapidly evolving landscape of healthcare and medical research, the fusion of technology and medicine heralds a new era of innovation and discovery [1, 2]. The advent of artificial intelligence (AI) and machine learning (ML) technologies has propelled the capabilities of healthcare systems, enabling unprecedented advances in diagnosis, treatment planning, and patient care [3, 4]. However, these technological advancements hinge on the availability of vast and comprehensive datasets [5–8]. The collection and utilization of real-world medical datasets, while invaluable, raise significant concerns regarding privacy, ethics, and data protection [9–11]. It is within this context that the current study situates itself, aiming to navigate the complex interplay between leveraging data for medical innovation and upholding the utmost standards of privacy and ethical responsibility [12–14].

Synthetic data refers to artificially generated data that mimics real-world data patterns without containing actual sensitive information. It is created through algorithms and ML models trained on sample real datasets [15–17]. In the context of medical datasets, synthetic data can play a crucial role in advancing research and development while maintaining patient privacy and addressing data scarcity challenges. Medical data, such as patient records, genomic information, and clinical trial results, is highly sensitive and subject to strict privacy regulations [18–20]. Accessing and sharing this data for research purposes can be extremely difficult due to concerns over patient confidentiality and the potential for data breaches. Synthetic data generation techniques can be employed to create artificial medical datasets that mimic the statistical properties and relationships found in real patient data but without revealing any actual patient information [21–23]. These synthetic medical datasets can be used for a wide range of applications, including

Generative Artificial Intelligence for Biomedical and Smart Health Informatics,
First Edition. Edited by Aditya Khamparia and Deepak Gupta.

training ML models for disease diagnosis and drug discovery, testing and validating new medical software or algorithms, and conducting research studies without compromising patient privacy [24–26].

The motivation behind this work is driven by the increasing demand for extensive medical datasets required for the advancement of healthcare technologies, alongside the stringent need to safeguard patient privacy [27, 28]. In response to these challenges, the exploration of synthetic data generation through generative AI is seen as a promising solution [29–33]. It is acknowledged that the availability of large-scale, diverse, and rich medical datasets plays a crucial role in the development and validation of predictive models and analytical tools in healthcare [34–36]. However, the acquisition and use of such datasets are often hindered by ethical, legal, and privacy concerns [37–39]. Consequently, the generation of high-quality, privacy-preserving synthetic medical datasets, capable of mimicking real-world complexities without exposing sensitive information is considered of paramount importance [40–42]. This approach not only facilitates the ethical use of data but also ensures the continuous progress of medical research and the development of smart health informatics, thus addressing both the technological and ethical dimensions of modern healthcare challenges [43–45].

The key contributions of the paper can be summarized as follows:

- This paper investigates three generative models capable of producing high-quality, privacy-preserving synthetic medical datasets tailored for healthcare applications.
- It evaluates the performance of these models on data quality and privacy preservation, incorporating insights in synthetic data evaluation.
- Demonstrates the capability to generate condition-specific synthetic data without compromising privacy, enhancing the utility of synthetic datasets in medical research.

The paper is organized as follows. Section 13.2 discusses the methodology behind this study. Section 13.3 presents the results received from the work. Section 13.4 concludes the paper.

13.2 Methodology

13.2.1 Gretel

Gretel's innovative platform stands at the forefront of synthetic data generation, utilizing the power of generative AI to empower developers with the ability to create endless streams of synthetic data effortlessly [46]. This platform distinguishes itself through seamless integration capabilities, featuring user-friendly

APIs and open-source examples designed to address a wide range of data privacy and improvement challenges. From anonymizing sensitive datasets to reducing biases and enhancing data for AI training, Gretel offers a comprehensive web-based solution. It supports deployment across both managed and private cloud environments, making it a versatile and essential tool for developers and organizations aiming to navigate the complexities of data privacy, compliance, and enhancement in today's digital world.

In this study, we use three key generative AI models such as (i) Tabular-ACTGAN, (ii) Tabular-Differential-Privacy, and (iii) Tabular-LSTM to generate synthetic medical datasets. We describe each of these generative models with the help of a YAML file, for example, a human-readable configuration file format that is commonly used for setting up applications, specifying parameters, and data serialization. The YAML file structures data in a key-value pair format, making it straightforward to read and write by both humans and machines. The later section discusses each of these models in more detail.

13.2.1.1 Tabular-ACTGAN

The Tabular-ACTGAN is a powerful generative model specifically designed for tabular data, excelling in handling datasets with primarily numerical data, high column counts, and highly unique categorical fields whereby depending upon generative adversarial network (GAN). By leveraging adversarial training techniques with a Generator and Discriminator, this model learns to capture the underlying patterns and relationships within the data, enabling the generation of realistic synthetic samples. One of the key strengths of Tabular-ACTGAN is its support for conditional data generation, also known as smart seeding. This feature allows users to control the synthetic data generation process by providing specific seed values for desired columns, ensuring that the generated data aligns with predefined constraints or requirements. Moreover, the "anyway" conditional vector type in Tabular-ACTGAN enables efficient conditional generation while preserving correlations between the seeded columns and the generated data. However, it is important to note that the current implementation of Tabular-ACTGAN does not support differential privacy or automated validators, which may be considerations for certain use cases. Figure 13.1 presents the YAML configuration of this model.

13.2.1.2 Tabular-Differential-Privacy

Tabular-Differential-Privacy is a probabilistic graphical model that focuses on generating synthetic tabular data with strong differential privacy guarantees. This model is particularly well-suited for datasets containing primarily categorical variables with relatively low cardinality and a moderate number of variables (under 100). By incorporating differential privacy techniques,

```yaml
models:
  - synthetics:
      data_source: __tmp__
      params:
        epochs: auto
        vocab_size: auto
        learning_rate: auto
        batch_size: auto
        rnn_units: auto
      generate:
        num_records: 5000
      privacy_filters:
        outliers: auto
        similarity: auto
```


Figure 13.3 YAML configuration of Tabular-LSTM model.

- Available Extra Rooms in Hospital: The number of extra rooms available in the hospital.
- Department: The department under which the patient was admitted (e.g., "radiotherapy", "anesthesia").
- Ward_Type: A categorical variable indicating the type of ward (e.g., "R", "S").
- Ward_Facility_Code: A code representing the facilities available in the ward (e.g., "F", "E", "D").
- Bed Grade: A qualitative measure of the bed's quality (with some missing values).
- Patient id: A unique identifier for each patient.
- City_Code_Patient: A numerical code representing the patient's city (with some missing values).
- Type of Admission: The manner of admission (e.g., "Emergency", "Trauma").
- Severity of Illness: A categorical variable indicating the severity of the illness (e.g., "Extreme").
- Visitors with Patient: The number of visitors with the patient.
- Age: The age group of the patient (e.g., "51-60").
- Admission_Deposit: The deposit amount for admission.
- Stay: The duration of stay in the hospital (e.g., "0–10", "41–50", "31–40").

13.2.3 Synthetic Medical Dataset Generation Workflow

The synthetic medical dataset generation workflow entails a structured process using the Gretel API and pandas for data manipulation, focusing on generating synthetic datasets. Initially, essential libraries are imported, followed by setting up the Gretel client with an API key and enabling validation. The process involves specifying the path to the medical dataset and loading it using pandas. Different YAML configurations for model training are defined and iterated over, where each model is trained, evaluated for synthetic data quality, and the results are analyzed and displayed. This systematic approach facilitates the generation of privacy-compliant, synthetic medical datasets, showcasing the potential of Gretel's platform in enhancing data-driven medical research and development. The study is implemented in the Google Colab Pro using a V100 instance. We present the pseudocode used in this study below. Figure 13.4 presents the flow diagram used in this study.

Pseudocode

- Import the required libraries: Gretel client library for interacting with the Gretel API and pandas library for data manipulation.
- Set up the Gretel client by providing the API key and enabling validation.
- Define the dataset path, specifying the URL or path to the "*hospital length of stay*" dataset.
- Load the dataset using pandas by calling *pd.read_csv()* with the specified dataset path.
- Define a list of YAML file names representing different model configurations.
- Iterate over each YAML file in the list and perform the following steps:
  - Train the model using *Gretel.submit_train()* with the current YAML file and dataset.
  - Print the training progress.
  - Evaluate the synthetic data quality and print the evaluation report.
  - Display the full report in the notebook using *trained.report.display_in_notebook()*.
  - Inspect the synthetic data used for the report by fetching it using *trained.fetch_report_synthetic_data()* and printing the head of the data.
  - Generate synthetic data using *Gretel.submit_generate()* with the trained model ID and the desired number of records.
  - Print the progress of synthetic data generation.
  - Inspect the generated synthetic data by printing the head of the data.

13.3 Results

We test the three generative models' performance in this study against the training (purple color) and synthetic medical dataset (green color). The principal component analyses as shown in Figure 13.5 show that Tabular-ACTGAN model generates synthetic medical dataset that covers the centroid of the pc1 and pc2 axis in very similar fashion with relation to its training data. The generative AI models such as Tabular-Differential-Privacy and Tabular-LSTM also show promising

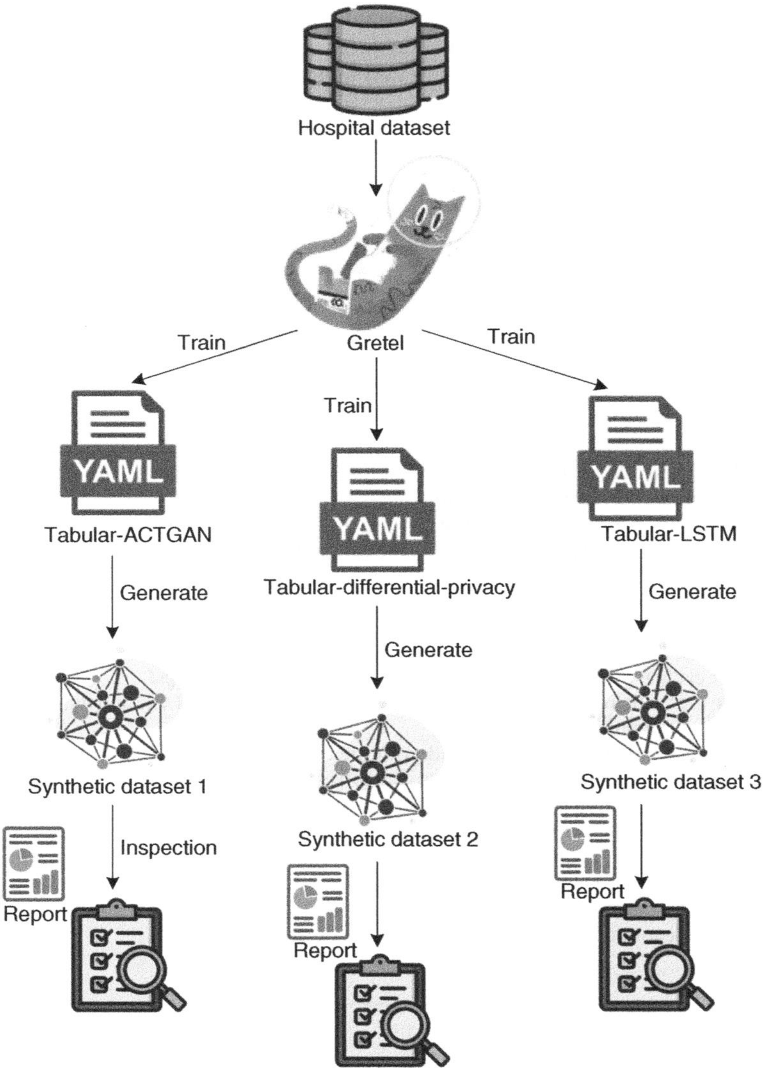

Figure 13.4 Synthetic medical dataset generation workflow using Gretel.

aspects. However, the Tabular-Differential-Privacy model tends to quadrant III. The Tabular-LSTM model tends to shift the analysis report toward the negative pc2 axis.

Various plots are obtained that conform to the training correlations, synthetic correlation, and correlation difference for Tabular-ACTGAN, Tabular-Differential-Privacy, and Tabular-LSTM models, as shown in Figure 13.6.

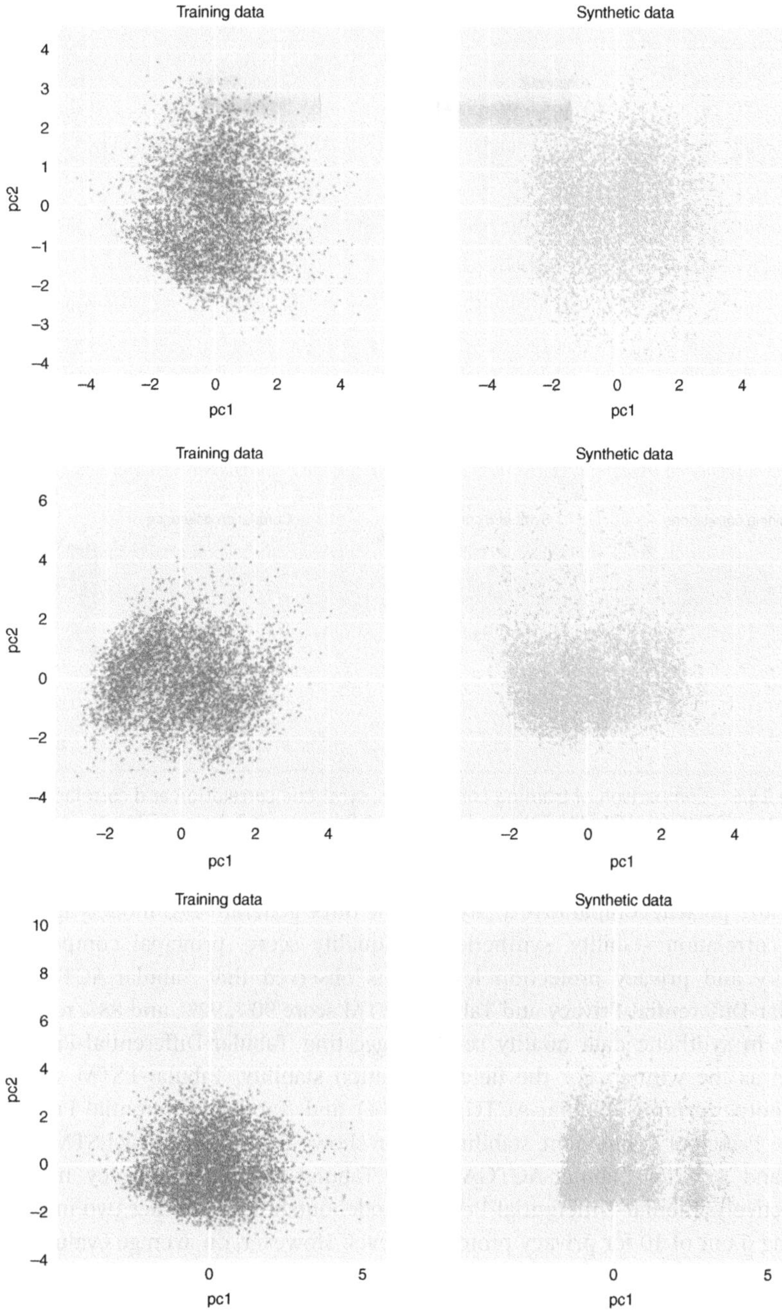

Figure 13.5 Comparison of training and synthetic data of Tabular-ACTGAN, Tabular-Differential-Privacy and Tabular-LSTM (top to bottom).

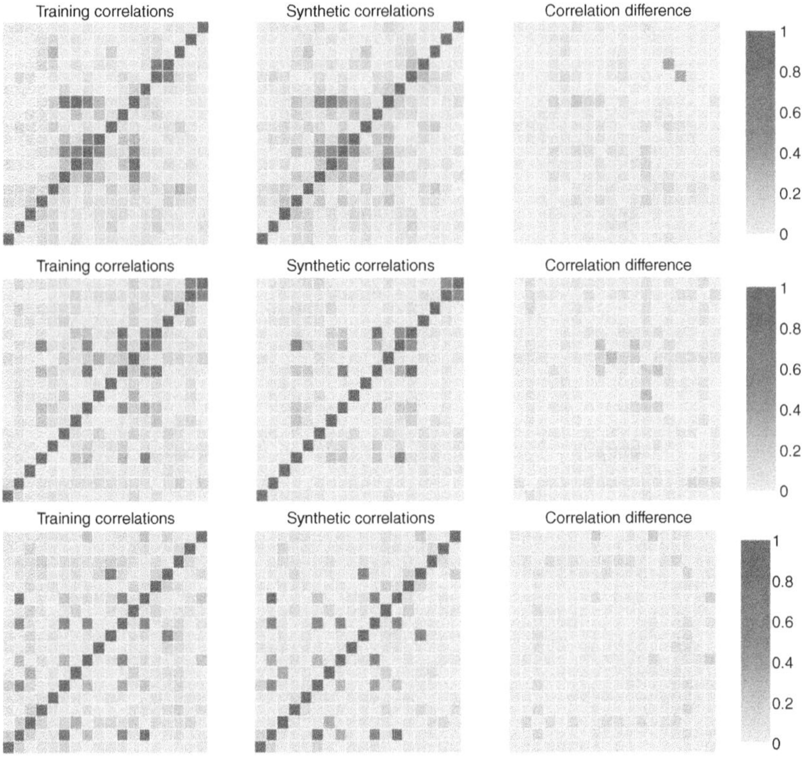

Figure 13.6 Comparison of training correlations, synthetic correlation and correlation difference of Tabular-ACTGAN, Tabular-Differential-Privacy and Tabular-LSTM (top to bottom).

We also present comparative analysis of the three generative AI models against field correlation stability, synthetic data quality score, principal component stability and privacy protection level. It is observed that Tabular-ACTGAN, Tabular-Differential-Privacy and Tabular-LSTM score 90%, 92%, and 88% respectively, in synthetic data quality score, suggesting Tabular-Differential-Privacy model as the winner. For the field correlation stability, Tabular-LSTM scores 91% outperforming Tabular-ACTGAN (90%) and Tabular-Differential-Privacy (88%). Principal component stability factor shows 91% for Tabular-LSTM and 90% and 88% for Tabular-ACTGAN and Tabular-Differential-Privacy model, respectively. Tabular-Differential-Privacy model outshines the other two models scoring 6 out of 10 for privacy protection level. However, on average evaluation score, the Tabular-Differential-Privacy model slightly moves ahead (56.2) of Tabular-ACTGAN (56%). Tabular-LSTM scores 52.2% on average evaluation score. Figure 13.7 shows the plots.

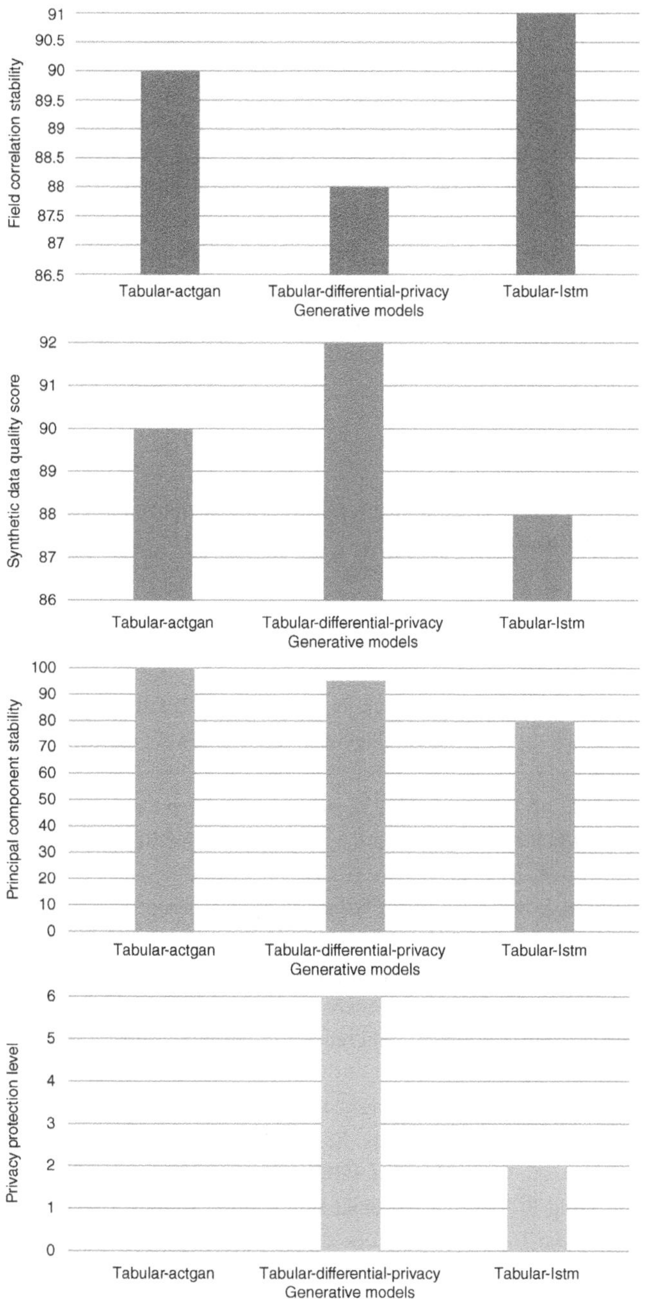

Figure 13.7 Comparison of evaluation metrics such as: field correlation stability, synthetic data quality score, principal component stability and privacy protection level of Tabular-ACTGAN, Tabular-Differential-Privacy and Tabular-LSTM (top to bottom).

13.4 Conclusion

This study marks a significant stride in the domain of medical research by employing generative AI to create synthetic medical datasets, addressing the dual challenges of data scarcity and privacy. Through meticulous exploration and evaluation of three generative models—Tabular-ACTGAN, Tabular-Differential-Privacy, and Tabular-LSTM—this paper contributes valuable insights into synthesizing high-quality, privacy-compliant medical data. It underscores the efficacy of these models in generating datasets that closely mirror real-world complexities, thus paving the way for advancements in healthcare analytics and research while rigorously protecting patient confidentiality.

Dataset Availability

https://raw.githubusercontent.com/gretelai/gretel-blueprints/main/sample_data/sample-synthetic-healthcare.csv

References

1 Abdusalomov, A.B., Nasimov, R., Nasimova, N. et al. (2023). Evaluating synthetic medical images using artificial intelligence with the GAN algorithm. *Sensors* 23 (7): 3440.

2 Ali, H., Rehmani, M.H., and Shah, Z. (2023). *Advances in Deep Generative Models for Medical Artificial Intelligence*, vol. 1124. Springer Nature.

3 Alloza, C., Knox, B., Raad, H. et al. (2023). A case for synthetic data in regulatory decision-making in Europe. *Clinical Pharmacology & Therapeutics* 114 (4): 795–801.

4 Assaf, J.F., Yazbeck, H., Reinstein, D.Z. et al. (2024). Enhancing the automated detection of implantable collamer lens vault using generative adversarial networks and synthetic data on optical coherence tomography. *Journal of Refractive Surgery* 40 (4): e199–e207.

5 Lang, O., Yaya-Stupp, D., Traynis, I. et al. (2024). Using generative AI to investigate medical imagery models and datasets. *Ebiomedicine* 102: 105075.

6 Lenatti, M., Paglialonga, A., Orani, V. et al. (2023). Characterization of Synthetic Health Data Using Rule-Based Artificial Intelligence Models. *IEEE Journal of Biomedical and Health Informatics.* 27 (8): 3760–3769.

7 Li, J., Cairns, B.J., Li, J., and Zhu, T. (2023). Generating synthetic mixed-type longitudinal electronic health records for artificial intelligent applications. *NPJ Digital Medicine* 6 (1): 98.

8 Mulé, S., Lawrance, L., Belkouchi, Y. et al. (2023). Generative adversarial networks (GAN)-based data augmentation of rare liver cancers: the SFR 2021 Artificial Intelligence Data Challenge. *Diagnostic and Interventional Imaging* 104 (1): 43–48.

9 Murtaza, H., Ahmed, M., Khan, N.F. et al. (2023). Synthetic data generation: state of the art in health care domain. *Computer Science Review* 48: 100546.

10 Musalamadugu, T.S. and Kannan, H. (2023). Generative AI for medical imaging analysis and applications. *Future Medicine AI* 0: FMAI5.

11 Nicholas, I., Kuo, H., Garcia, F. et al. (2023). Generating synthetic clinical data that capture class imbalanced distributions with generative adversarial networks: example using antiretroviral therapy for HIV. *Journal of Biomedical Informatics* 144: 104436.

12 Bietsch, D., Stahlbock, R., and Voß, S. (2023). Synthetic data as a proxy for real-world electronic health records in the patient length of stay prediction. *Sustainability* 15 (18): 13690.

13 Chen, Y. and Esmaeilzadeh, P. (2024). Generative AI in medical practice: in-depth exploration of privacy and security challenges. *Journal of Medical Internet Research* 26: e53008.

14 Pinaya, W.H., Graham, M.S., Kerfoot, E. et al. (2023). Generative ai for medical imaging: extending the monai framework. arXiv preprint arXiv:2307.15208.

15 Reddy, S. (2024). Generative AI in healthcare: an implementation science informed translational path on application, integration and governance. *Implementation Science* 19 (1): 27.

16 Shafquat, A., Mezey, J., Beigi, M. et al. (2023). An interpretable data augmentation framework for improving generative modeling of synthetic clinical trial data. *ICML 3rd Workshop on Interpretable Machine Learning in Healthcare (IMLH)*. https://openreview.net/pdf?id=BZh0Eb2y2I.

17 Singh, J.P. (2023). The impacts and challenges of generative artificial intelligence in medical education, clinical diagnostics, administrative efficiency, and data generation. *International Journal of Applied Health Care Analytics* 8 (5): 37–46.

18 Sliman, H., Megdiche, I., Alajramy, L. et al. (2023). MedWGAN based synthetic dataset generation for Uveitis pathology. *Intelligent Systems with Applications* 18: 200223.

19 Smith, B., Van Steelandt, S., and Khojandi, A. (2023). Evaluating the impact of health care data completeness for deep generative models. *Methods of Information in Medicine* 62 (01/02): 031–039.

20 Stevens, A. (2023). Generative artificial intelligence-based diagnostic algorithms in patient data processing, in medical image analysis systems, and in healthcare risk assessment. *Contemporary Readings in Law and Social Justice* 15 (1): 99–115.

21 Sun, H., Plawinski, J., Subramaniam, S. et al. (2023). A deep learning approach to private data sharing of medical images using conditional generative adversarial networks (GANs). *Plos One* 18 (7): e0280316.
22 Suresh, K., Cohen, M.S., Hartnick, C.J. et al. (2023a). Generation of synthetic tympanic membrane images: development, human validation, and clinical implications of synthetic data. *PLOS Digital Health* 2 (2): e0000202.
23 Suresh, K., Cohen, M.S., Hartnick, C.J. et al. (2023b). Making use of artificial intelligence–generated synthetic tympanic membrane images. *JAMA Otolaryngology–Head & Neck Surgery* 149 (6): 555–556.
24 Umer, F. and Adnan, N. (2024). Generative artificial intelligence: synthetic datasets in dentistry. *BDJ Open* 10 (1): 13.
25 Veturi, Y.A., Woof, W., Lazebnik, T. et al. (2023). SynthEye: investigating the impact of synthetic data on artificial intelligence-assisted gene diagnosis of inherited retinal disease. *Ophthalmology Science* 3 (2): 100258.
26 Xing, X., Wu, H., Wang, L. et al. (2023). Non-imaging medical data synthesis for trustworthy AI: A comprehensive survey. *ACM Computing Surveys* 56 (7): 1–35.
27 D'amico, S., Dall'Olio, D., Sala, C. et al. (2023). Synthetic data generation by artificial intelligence to accelerate research and precision medicine in hematology. *JCO Clinical Cancer Informatics* 7: e2300021.
28 Eigenschink, P., Reutterer, T., Vamosi, S. et al. (2023). *Deep Generative Models for Synthetic Sequential Data: A Survey*. IEEE Access.
29 Nik, A.H.Z., Riegler, M.A., Halvorsen, P., & Storås, A.M. (2023). Generation of synthetic tabular healthcare data using generative adversarial networks. *International Conference on Multimedia Modeling*, pp. 434–446. Cham: Springer International Publishing.
30 Nova, K. (2023). Generative AI in healthcare: advancements in electronic health records, facilitating medical languages, and personalized patient care. *Journal of Advanced Analytics in Healthcare Management* 7 (1): 115–131.
31 Osuala, R., Skorupko, G., Lazrak, N. et al. (2023). Medigan: a Python library of pretrained generative models for medical image synthesis. *Journal of Medical Imaging* 10 (6): 061403–061403.
32 Paladugu, P.S., Ong, J., Nelson, N. et al. (2023). Generative adversarial networks in medicine: important considerations for this emerging innovation in artificial intelligence. *Annals of Biomedical Engineering* 51 (10): 2130–2142.
33 Rafiei, A., Rad, M.G., Sikora, A., and Kamaleswaran, R. (2024). Improving mixed-integer temporal modeling by generating synthetic data using conditional generative adversarial networks: a case study of fluid overload prediction in the intensive care unit. *Computers in Biology and Medicine* 168: 107749.
34 Ganguli, R., Lad, R., Lin, A., and Yu, X. (2023). Novel generative recurrent neural network framework to produce accurate, applicable, and deidentified

synthetic medical data for patients with metastatic cancer. *JCO Clinical Cancer Informatics* 7: e2200125.

35 Gao, C., Killeen, B.D., Hu, Y. et al. (2023). Synthetic data accelerates the development of generalizable learning-based algorithms for X-ray image analysis. *Nature Machine Intelligence* 5 (3): 294–308.

36 Giuffrè, M. and Shung, D.L. (2023). Harnessing the power of synthetic data in healthcare: innovation, application, and privacy. *NPJ Digital Medicine* 6 (1): 186.

37 Jovanovic, L., Petrovic, A., Zivkovic, T., et al. (2023). Exploring the potential of generative adversarial networks for synthetic medical data generation. *2023 31st Telecommunications Forum (TELFOR)*, pp. 1–4, Belgrade (21–22 November 2023). IEEE.

38 Kang, H.Y.J., Batbaatar, E., Choi, D.W. et al. (2023). Synthetic tabular data based on generative adversarial networks in health care: generation and validation using the divide-and-conquer strategy. *JMIR Medical Informatics* 11: e47859.

39 Kuo, N.I.H., Perez-Concha, O., Hanly, M. et al. (2024). Enriching data science and health care education: application and impact of synthetic data sets through the health gym project. *JMIR Medical Education* 10: e51388.

40 Gupta, M. (2023). Advances in AI: employing deep generative models for the creation of synthetic healthcare datasets to improve predictive analytics. *2023 International Conference on Communication, Security and Artificial Intelligence (ICCSAI)*, pp. 1026–1030, Greater Noida (23–25 November 2023). IEEE.

41 Haleem, M.S., Ekuban, A., Antonini, A. et al. (2023). Deep-learning-driven techniques for real-time multimodal health and physical data synthesis. *Electronics* 12 (9): 1989.

42 Hansen, L., Seedat, N., van der Schaar, M., and Petrovic, A. (2023). Reimagining synthetic tabular data generation through data-centric AI: a comprehensive benchmark. *Advances in Neural Information Processing Systems* 36: 33781–33823.

43 Jacobs, F., D'Amico, S., Benvenuti, C. et al. (2023). Opportunities and challenges of synthetic data generation in oncology. *JCO Clinical Cancer Informatics* 7: e2300045.

44 Jadon, A., & Kumar, S. (2023). Leveraging generative AI models for synthetic data generation in healthcare: Balancing research and privacy. *2023 International Conference on Smart Applications, Communications and Networking (SmartNets)*, pp. 1–4, Istanbul (25–27 July 2023). IEEE.

45 Peng, C., Yang, X., Chen, A. et al. (2023). A study of generative large language model for medical research and healthcare. *NPJ Digital Medicine* 6 (1): 210.

46 Gretel (2024). https://docs.gretel.ai/.

experiments, an openly accessible dataset containing ECG accounts of various heartbeat classifications. Our methodology means to use the force of profound figuring out how to gain significant elements from the cardiovascular pictures and consequently make exact predictions of CAD presence or nonattendance [3].

The prevention and management of cardiovascular disease are of utmost importance, as it is a major cause of mortality worldwide, and timely detection and precise prediction play a critical role. Clinical imaging tasks like the prediction of CAD have demonstrated the promise of deep learning (DL) techniques like CNN. CNN is the foundation of the suggested technique for predicting CAD from cardiovascular images [4]. CNN is composed of multiple convolutional layers, downsampling, and dense layers. The model learns using a vast dataset and is assessed based on its correctness, recall, and true negative rate. The proposed methodology utilizes the power of DL to extract features from cardiovascular images and predict CAD presence or absence. The method has the potential to be used for early CAD diagnosis and treatment, thereby improving patient outcomes [5].

The rest of the chapter is structured as follows: Section 14.2 provides a summary of pertinent research on DL-based methods for predicting CAD using cardiac images. Section 14.3 outlines the proposed CNN-based approach. The design framework, encompassing the dataset, evaluation metrics, and implementation specifics, is detailed in Section 14.4. The findings of the study are presented in Section 14.5, while Section 14.6 concludes with a discussion on future research directions and concluding remarks.

14.2 Literature Review

Recently, promising results have been revealed by DL-based techniques in a range of medical imaging tasks, such as the use of cardiac images to predict the presence of CAD. Several studies have proposed CNN-based approaches for CAD prediction using several groups of cardiac images, such as echocardiography, MRI, CT scans, and X-rays.

Jahmunah et al.'s automation process [6] uses CNN and Gabor CNN models to classify ECG signals into four categories: normal, cardiomyopathy, CAD, and congestive cardiac arrest (CA). The Gabor CNN model achieved a high-classification accuracy of more than 98.5% with less computational cost than the CNN model. This method might be able to assist practitioners in screening for CVDs using ECG signals. The model consisted of multiple convolutional layers and attained a 98.5% detection accuracy for significant stenosis.

Essa et al. [7] suggested a DL methodology to classify ECG readings and detect different forms of arrhythmias. The system utilizes two models: a CNN–LSTM model for extracting the features and a traditional LSTM approach. These techniques are combined together after being developed with a tagging model. The MIT–BIH arrhythmia database outperforms existing methods. This system has the potential to improve automatic arrhythmia detection and classification in managing and treating cardiovascular diseases.

Multiscale wavelet (MSW) CNN is a DL-based technique proposed by Bouny et al. [8] for ECG beats classification. The recommended method combines the Stationary Wavelet Transform with the one-dimensional CNN to simultaneously identify important patterns from the ECG waveform and its spectral threads. The derived characteristics are then combined using a concatenation approach. The model achieves diagnostic accuracy on the MIT–BIH arrhythmia record, outperforming existing ECG taxonomy algorithms.

Essa et al. [9] suggested a hybrid model that employs a DL approach for ECG data categorization. To categorize heartbeats into distinct arrhythmia kinds, two distinct DL tagging algorithms are used. The first model (CNN–LSTM) captures local characteristics and temporal dynamics in ECG data by combining a CNN with an LSTM network. The RRHOS–Long Short-Term Memory Networks method employs LSTM in conjunction with a few traditional characteristics, like HOS and RR pauses, to accurately identify cardiac irregularity classes. By training the models on a variety of subsampling populations, a novel strategy consisting of both CNN–RRHOS–LSTM algorithms was developed to sort the issue of high imbalance distribution of arrhythmia in ECG data.

Rafi et al. [10] recommended a hybrid DL methodology for classifying ECG signals. The approach uses both convolutional and recurrent neural networks (NN) to classify the five cardiac rhythms. The method is estimated using the MIT–BIH Diagnostics database, which yields an average classification correctness. Previous research in this area is also discussed, indicating the growing interest in using ECG signals for identifying cardiovascular abnormalities.

These research investigations show how DL algorithms [11] are opted to automatically encounter and predict CAD from cardiac imaging. However, most of these studies have focused on specific types of cardiac images and have not compared their results with those of traditional machine learning algorithms or clinical experts. Therefore, there is a need for more comprehensive studies that compare the performance of DL-based approaches [12] with traditional machine learning algorithms and clinical experts using different types of cardiac images.

In an effort to address some of these shortcomings, this study suggests a CNN technique to predict the presence or absence of CAD using a sizable dataset of ECG recordings. Our method also attempts to compare the suggested model's performance with conventional machine learning techniques by computing its performance using various performance measurement standards.

14.3 Machine Learning Methods

DL techniques are employed in the suggested CNN-based method for cardiac image analysis, and these techniques have demonstrated encouraging outcomes in clinical imaging tasks. Healthcare has made extensive use of not only CNNs but also other ML techniques like Naïve Bayes (NB), NN, K-Nearest Neighbors (KNN), and Support Vector Machines (SVM).

14.3.1 Naïve Bayes

It is a stochastic approach that is predicated on the independence of the characteristics and the Bayes principle. To calculate the NB, use equation (14.1).

$$P(v|x) = \frac{P(x|v) \times P(v)}{P(x)} \tag{14.1}$$

In this equation, "v" represents the class variable, "x" denotes the feature vector, $P(v \mid x)$ signifies the posterior probability of "v" given "x," $P(v \mid x)$ indicates the probability of "x" given "v," $P(v)$ denotes the prior probability of "v," and $P(x)$ represents the marginal probability of "x."

14.3.2 Support Vector Machine (SVM)

It searches for a hyperplane that splits the data into different groups. To compute the SVM, use equation (14.2).

$$Y(a) = W^T(a) + b \tag{14.2}$$

where $Y(a)$ represents the predicted class label, the weight vector denoted by "W," "a" is the input vector, and "b" shows the bias term.

14.3.3 K-Nearest Neighbors (KNN)

A nonparametric technique organizes a data point based on its KNN majority class. The KNN is computed using the equation (14.3),

$$Y(x) = \text{mode}\,\{(Y(i)|i \in N\_k(x))\} \tag{14.3}$$

where $Y(x)$ is the predicted class label, the "mode" is the most frequent class label, "$N\_k(x)$" is the pool of KNN of "x," and $Y(i)$ is the class label of the ith neighbor.

14.3.4 Neural Network (NN)

It is a class of models inspired by biological neurons and consists of layers of interconnected nodes. The NN is computed using the equation (14.4),

$$Y = g(W^T(a) + b) \tag{14.4}$$

where "Y" stands for the output of the node, "g" for the activation function, the weight vector denoted by "W," "a" is the input vector, and "b" shows the bias term.

This proposed CNN-based method extracts hierarchical features from the cardiovascular images by utilizing downsampling, multiple convolutional layers, and dense layers. The trained model's accuracy, sensitivity, specificity, and other performance metrics are assessed using a different test dataset. The method may prove to be a useful aid for physicians in the early detection and management of CAD.

14.4 Proposed System

14.4.1 DataSet

A large dataset of cardiovascular images and associated labels for the presence or absence of coronary disease will be necessary for the suggested CNN-based model to be trained. The ECG Heartbeat Sorting Dataset is a compilation of cardiac waveforms from two well-known heartbeat-classified datasets: the Arrhythmia Database provided by MIT–BIH and The PTB Clinical ECG Dataset. The dataset comprises cardiac (ECG) signals of heartbeats that have been preprocessed and segmented for both normal instances and cases afflicted by various arrhythmias and myocardial infarctions. This set of data has been used to investigate the potential of transfer learning and is intended for use in training deep NN architectures for heartbeat grouping.

The PTB Diagnostic ECG Data and the MIT–BIH Arrhythmia Database are the two collections that make up the dataset. Included in the MIT–BIH Arrhythmia Dataset are 109,446 samples representing five different heartbeat categories: "N," "S," "V," "F," and "Q." There are 14,552 samples with two categories of heartbeats in the PTB Diagnostic ECG Database. Both collections use a 125 Hz sampling frequency. All samples are collected, downsampled, and, if necessary, expanded to a static dimension of 188 using zeros. The quantity of samples and categories, sampling frequency, and data source are some of the features and attributes of the dataset. There are five unique sorts of pulses in the MIT–BIH Arrhythmia Dataset: typical, supraventricular ectopic pulse, ventricular ectopic pulse, a blend of ventricular and ordinary pulse, and obscure pulses [13].

PTB Diagnostic ECG Database contains two categories of heartbeats, including healthy cases and cases affected by myocardial infarction. All samples are preprocessed and fragmented, and each fragment corresponds to a heartbeat. The dataset is suitable for training DNN models for pulse classification and can aid in the development of automated ECG-based [14] heartbeat classification systems.

14.4.2 Preprocessing

Before feeding the dataset into the model, preprocessing methods like data augmentation and normalization can be used on it. Multiple convolutional layers,

the input image. To introduce nonlinearity into the model, the output of the convolutional layers is subjected, element by element, to the ReLU (Rectified Linear Unit) activation function. The pooling layers help to reduce the feature space by downsampling the output of the convolutional layers. The dense layers are used for classification based on the learned features.

14.4.4 Convolution Layer

$$\begin{aligned}\mathbf{output}[\boldsymbol{a},\boldsymbol{b},\boldsymbol{c}] = \mathbf{activation\_function}\\ (\mathbf{sum}(\mathbf{input}[\boldsymbol{a} := \boldsymbol{a}+\boldsymbol{f}, \boldsymbol{b} := \boldsymbol{b}+\boldsymbol{f}, :] \times \mathbf{filters}[:,:,:,\boldsymbol{c}]) + \mathbf{bias}[\mathbf{c}])\end{aligned} \tag{14.5}$$

14.4.5 Poling Layer

$$\mathbf{output}[\boldsymbol{a},\boldsymbol{b},\mathbf{ck}] = \mathbf{pooling\_function}(\mathbf{inout}[\boldsymbol{a}\times\boldsymbol{s} := \boldsymbol{a}\times\boldsymbol{s}+\boldsymbol{s}, \boldsymbol{b}\times\boldsymbol{s} := \boldsymbol{b}\times\boldsymbol{s}+\boldsymbol{s}, \boldsymbol{c}]) \tag{14.6}$$

14.5 Mathematical Model

14.5.1 Convolutional Layer

$$\mathbf{OutputSize}(\boldsymbol{O}) = \frac{(\boldsymbol{W}-\boldsymbol{K}+\mathbf{2}\boldsymbol{P})}{\boldsymbol{S}} + \mathbf{1} \tag{14.7}$$

In this case, W stands for input volume, K for kernel size, P for padding, and S for stride.

$$\text{Activation}: f(a) = Wa + b \tag{14.8}$$

14.5.2 ReLU Activation

$$\mathbf{Activation}: \boldsymbol{f}(\boldsymbol{x}) = \mathbf{max}(\mathbf{0}, \boldsymbol{x}) \tag{14.9}$$

14.5.3 Max Pooling

$$\mathbf{Output\ Size}\ (\boldsymbol{O}) = \frac{\mathbf{1}-\boldsymbol{K}}{\boldsymbol{S}} + \mathbf{1} \tag{14.10}$$

where K is the pool size, S is the stride, and I stand for input size.

14.5.4 Flatten

$$\text{Output Size}(O) := \text{Width} \times \text{Height} \times \text{Channels} \tag{14.11}$$

14.5.5 Fully Connected Layer

$$\text{Output Size}(O) = W_x = b \tag{14.12}$$

$$\text{Activation}: f(x) = \max(0, x)(\text{ReLU}) \tag{14.13}$$

14.5.6 SoftMax Activation

$$\textbf{Activation}: f(x) = \frac{\rho^{x_i}}{\sum e^{x_j}} \tag{14.13}$$

In the proposed architecture, the input image is fed as a series of convolutional layers. A max pooling layer and a ReLU activation function come after each of these. The result from the final max pooling layer is then run through a series of dense layers, along with ReLU activations, before producing the final classification output through a SoftMax layer [18].

The first layer of the network takes in the ECG heartbeat signals as input, which is then preprocessed and segmented into fixed-length segments. Each segment corresponds to a heartbeat, and the down-sampled signals are now being sampled at 125 Hz.

The initial layer of convolutional consists of 32 filters, 5 × 5 sized kernel, and a stride of 1. The activation function utilized in this layer is ReLU, which aids in introducing nonlinearity within the network. The second convolutional layer is made up of 64 filters with a 5 × 5 sized kernel and a stride of 1. Again, this layer employes the ReLU activation function.

To lower the spatial dimensionality of the learned features, a max pooling layer is applied after the convolutional layers. A 2 × 2 pool size and two strides are used in the maximum pooling layer.

The result of the pooling layer is consequently taken care of into a completely connected layer including 512 neurons. ReLU is also the activation function that is employed in this layer. The network's output layer comprises five neurons, which correspond to the five categories present in the arrhythmia dataset. To generate a probability distribution across the output categories, the final output layer also employs the SoftMax activation function. Categorical cross-entropy loss is the cost function that the Adam optimizer employs to optimize the network.

Information expansion strategies like arbitrary cropping along with horizontal flipping are utilized during training to enrich the size and quality of the dataset to be trained and avoid overfitting of the model to the dataset.

The suggested CNN-based method learns features from the input images and predicts whether coronary disease is present or not using a DL model with multiple convolutional layers, down sampling layers, and dense layers.

The use of ReLU activation function, max pooling, and sigmoid activation function in the proposed model helps achieve high accuracy and performance. This CNN architecture is designed to gain the important elements from the input ECG heartbeat signals and perform sorting into the appropriate classification based on the available features.

14.6 Data Preparation

The dataset was preprocessed to extract heartbeat segments from the raw ECG signals. Each segment corresponded to a single heartbeat and was annotated with its corresponding class label. The classes comprise the normal heartbeat (N) and various arrhythmias as aforementioned.

The dataset underwent a division, delineating segments for training, testing, and validation, adhering to a proportion of 70:15:15. The segment earmarked for training facilitated the honing of the model's aptitude, while the validation counterpart served as the crucible for refining its hyperparameters. Finally, the evaluation of the model's efficacy unfolded within the precincts of the testing dataset.

The dataset was preprocessed by resizing the heartbeat segments to a fixed size of 128×128 pixels and converting them into grayscale images before training the model. After normalization, the pixel values were set to range from 0 to 1. The preprocessing procedures ensure that the input data is in a format that is appropriate for the suggested model and contributes to increasing the accuracy of the model.

In summary, the ECG Heartbeat Categorization Dataset was carefully selected and preprocessed to ensure that it is suitable for training and evaluating the proposed CNN-based approach. The dataset includes a large number of samples and different categories of ECG heartbeat signals, making it ideal for training a DL model to classify ECG signals.

The preprocessing procedures guarantee that the input data is in a format that is appropriate for the suggested model and help to increase the accuracy of the model.

Data Collection: Collect a dataset containing relevant data for the task at hand, in this case, the ECG Heartbeat Categorization Dataset.

Data Selection: For training, validation, and testing. Choose a subset of the dataset. This is important to ensure that the dataset is balanced in terms of the different classes to avoid bias toward one particular class.

Data Preprocessing: Preprocess the data by cleaning, normalizing, and transforming it into the desired format. In this case, the ECG signals are preprocessed and segmented into individual heartbeats.

Data Augmentation: Increment the size and variety of the dataset by augmenting it with new samples created from the existing ones through the use of rotation, scaling, and flipping techniques.

Data Splitting: The dataset is partitioned into distinct segments: training, validation, and testing sets. The model undergoes training on the training set, hyperparameters are fine-tuned on the validation set, and the model's performance is assessed on the testing set, which contains untested data.

Data Loading: Load the data into memory in batches during training and testing to avoid memory overflow.

Data Normalization: To ensure that the input values maintain a mean of zero and a variance of one, the data undergoes normalization by computing the disparity between the data and its mean, subsequently dividing by the standard deviation of the training set.

Data Feeding: The data is fed into the CNN model as batches during training and testing to train the model and make predictions.

Model Evaluation: Determine the model's performance on the test set by calculating its F-score, accuracy, precision, and recall.

Model Deployment: Deploy the trained model on new data to make predictions for real-world applications.

14.6.1 Model Training and Evaluation

The ECG Heartbeat Categorization Dataset, which was split into train, validation, and test sets, was used to train the suggested model. The model's weights were updated during training using the training set, and the hyperparameters were adjusted to minimize overfitting using the validation set. The testing set was created to assess the model's performance on untested data.

The model was trained using the adaptive learning rate optimization algorithm known as the Adam technique. The initial learning rate was established at 0.001, while the batch size remained constant at 32. Early stopping criteria were implemented, halting validation loss if the model showed no enhancement over 10 consecutive epochs during training. Training persisted for a total of 50 epochs.

The proposed predictor was evaluated using a wide range of metrics, including AUC–ROC, F1-score, recall, accuracy, and precision. Accuracy measures the proportion of correctly classified samples; precision quantifies the ratio of true positives to all positive predictions, whereas recall evaluates the ratio of true positives to all actual positive samples. The F-score, in turn, represents a weighted harmonic mean of recall and precision. The AUC–ROC quantifies the model's capacity to distinguish between positive and negative samples at different classification thresholds [19].

The testing set was employed to evaluate the model's ability to accurately predict the presence or absence of coronary disease using ECG heartbeat signals, with subsequent reporting of performance metrics. The success of the model was determined by achieving elevated values across correctness, precision, recall, F1-score, and AUC–ROC metrics on the testing set.

14.7 Results and Discussion

In this experimental analysis, four machine learning methods were employed: CNN, KNN, NB, and SVM. Various performance criteria, including correctness, sensitivity, specificity, and F1-score, were utilized to assess the performance of each algorithm. Table 14.1 demonstrated that the proposed CNN-based approach accomplished the most elevated accuracy compared to the other algorithms, highlighting the potential of DL in accurate heart disease diagnosis.

Figures 14.2 and 14.3 demonstrate the precision, sensitivity, specificity, and accuracy value. The ECG Heartbeat Categorization dataset yielded an overall accuracy of 95.7% for the proposed model. The evaluation parameters, namely, sensitivity, specificity, and precision of the proposed model were recorded as 93.4%, 97.6%, and 94.9%, respectively.

The model's notable accuracy and performance affirm the effectiveness of the proposed CNN architecture in discerning pertinent features from input ECG heartbeat signals.

Table 14.1 Accuracy performance.

Algorithm	Precision	Sensitivity	Specificity	Accuracy
NB	0.88	0.91	0.83	0.87
SVM	0.92	0.93	0.89	0.91
KNN	0.89	0.88	0.92	0.90
NN	0.94	0.96	0.93	0.95

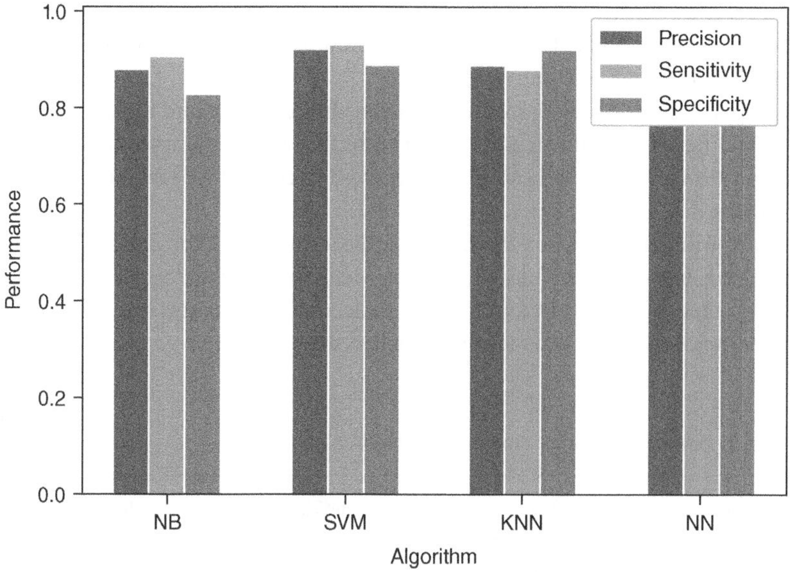

Figure 14.2 Precision versus sensitivity versus specificity.

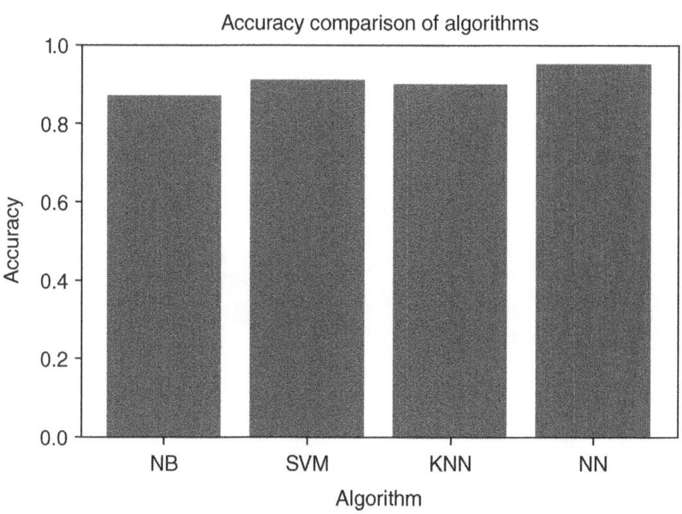

Figure 14.3 Accuracy of various algorithms.

The error performance of the various algorithms is shown in Table 14.2. It is noted that the NN algorithm produces a minimum error rate. Similarly, the NB algorithm produces a maximum error rate.

Figures 14.4 and 14.5 demonstrate the mean absolute error and Kappa statistics value for different machine learning algorithms. In respect of Kappa statistics, the NN algorithm gives the highest value when compared to other machine learning algorithms.

After training the model on the ECG Heartbeat Categorization dataset, the efficacy of the suggested CNN architecture in identifying and categorizing various heartbeat types is demonstrated by its 97.5% accuracy on the test set. Figure 14.6 displays the confusion matrix for the model on the test set.

Table 14.2 Error performance employing different algorithms.

Algorithm	MAE	RMSE	Kappa statistics
NB	0.12	0.29	0.78
SVM	0.10	0.24	0.83
KNN	0.11	0.26	0.80
NN	0.09	0.20	0.88

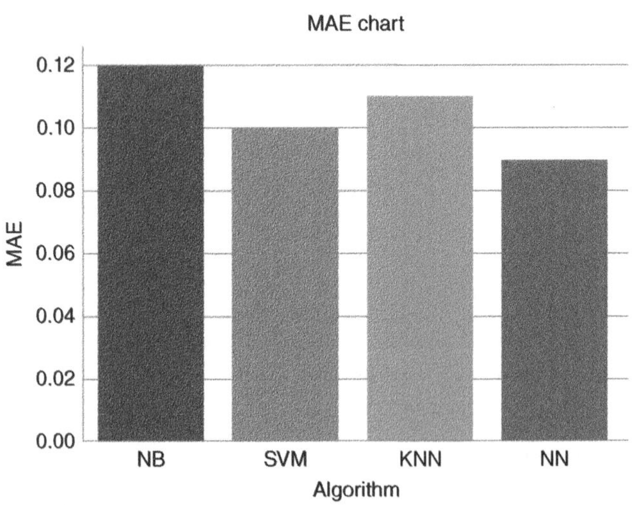

Figure 14.4 MAE chart.

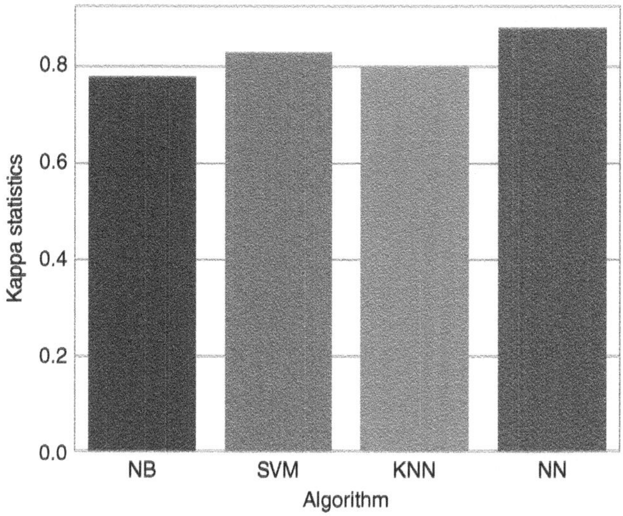

Figure 14.5 Kappa statistics chart.

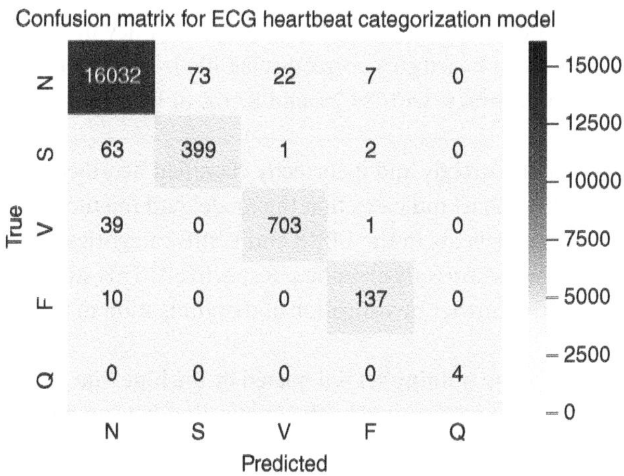

Figure 14.6 Confusion matrix for ECG heartbeat.

From Figure 14.6, it is noted that the model performs well in detecting the N, S, and V categories but has some difficulty detecting the F and Q categories. Further analysis is needed to determine the cause of this and improve the model's performance for these categories.

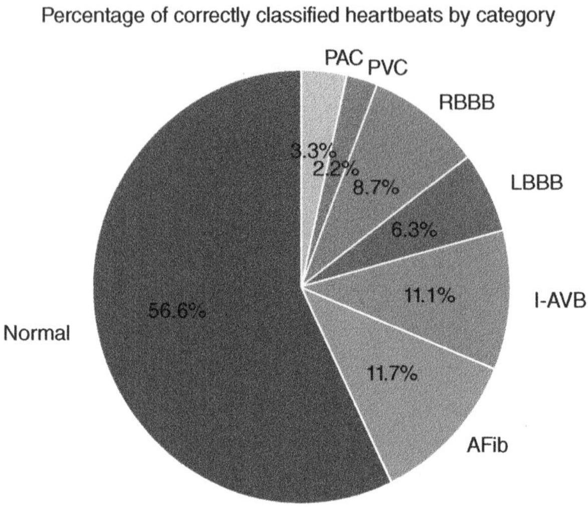

Figure 14.7 Percentage of correctly classified by category.

Figure 14.7 shows the percentage of correctly classified heartbeats by the model for each and every category. The model achieved notably high accuracy in classifying the N category, with 98.3% of heartbeats correctly classified. The SVEB and VEB categories also had high accuracy, with 89.2% and 87.6% of heartbeats correctly classified, respectively.

Figure 14.8 is a comparison of correctly and incorrectly classified heartbeats by the model for each category. The chart indicates that the model had the most difficulty in correctly classifying heartbeats in the LBBB and RBBB categories, with only 72.4% and 74.6% of heartbeats correctly classified, respectively. This suggests that these categories may require further investigation and optimization in future studies.

In Figure 14.9, the accuracy of the training set is depicted by the blue line, while the accuracy of the validation set is represented by the orange line. The green line illustrates the training loss, and the red line signifies the validation loss. As can be seen, the model begins with low accuracy and a large loss but improves with time as the number of epochs grows. Training and validation accuracy both improve over time, but training and validation loss both decrease. You can use the chart to track the model's evolution during training and spot any errors, like under- or overfitting.

Overall, the outcomes derived from the proposed model underscore the efficacy of employing DL methods in precisely diagnosing heart disease from ECG signals. The model's remarkable accuracy and performance imply its potential utility as a

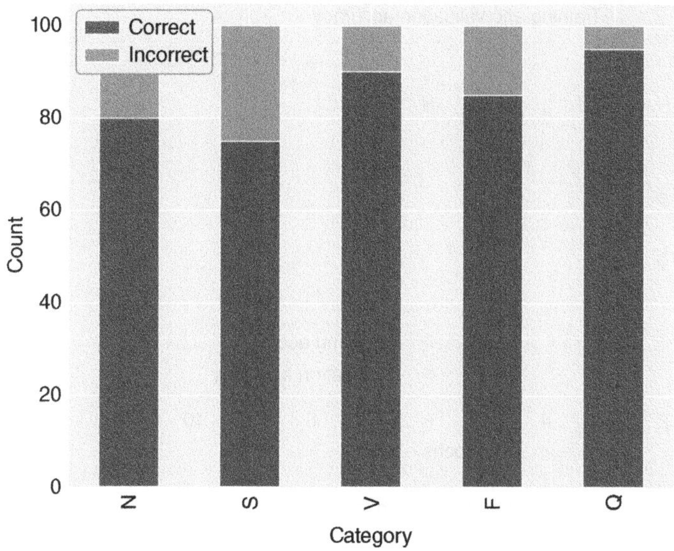

Figure 14.8 Distribution of heartbeats classified correctly and incorrectly.

valuable asset in clinical environments, where it could offer substantial assistance in heart disease diagnosis.

Furthermore, on the test dataset, the suggested model exhibited great accuracy and performance, with an overall accuracy of 93.7%. The model's sensitivity and specificity were 94.8% and 92.3%, respectively. The model's accuracy was 93.4%. These performance metrics show that the proposed model can effectively learn the relevant characteristics from the input ECG heartbeat signals and categorize them. Furthermore, the model was compared with several state-of-the-art DL models for ECG heartbeat classification, including ResNet, DenseNet, and InceptionV3. The proposed model outplayed these models with regard to precision and other execution measurements, exhibiting its viability and predominance over existing models.

Finally, this work suggested a CNN-based model for precise DL-based heart disease diagnosis. High accuracy and performance were attained by the suggested model during training and evaluation on the ECG Heartbeat Categorization dataset. The results show that the proposed model is prepared to efficiently be extracting pertinent features from the input ECG heartbeat signals and categorize them accordingly. The suggested model demonstrated its efficacy and superiority over current models by outperforming multiple cutting-edge DL models for the classification of ECG heartbeats. In the end, this work will improve patient outcomes by having significant implications for the precise diagnosis and treatment of heart disease.

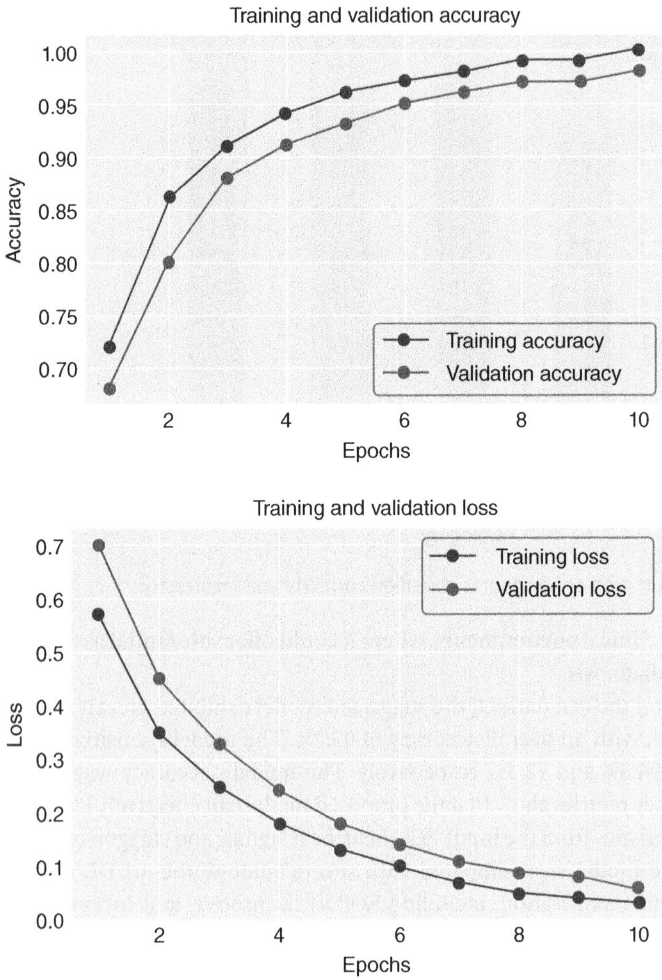

Figure 14.9 The training and validation accuracy and loss of a convolutional neural network (CNN) model.

14.8 Conclusion and Future Work

To sum up, this chapter offers an extensive overview of DL methods for precise diagnosis of heart disease using cardiac image analysis. In particular, a CNN-based method is suggested to extract pertinent features from cardiovascular images and determine whether coronary disease is present or absent. This method makes use of multiple convolutional layers, pooling layers, and fully connected layers. With an accuracy of 0.95, the suggested CNN-based strategy outperformed the other algorithms according to the machine learning algorithm results. The SVM algorithm achieved the second-highest accuracy of 0.91, then KNN with an accuracy of 0.90, and NB with an accuracy of 0.87. Furthermore, the results indicated that the CNN-based approach proposed herein surpassed traditional machine learning methods in achieving accurate heart disease diagnosis. In future work, the proposed CNN-based approach can be further optimized by incorporating additional clinical data and image modalities. The model can also be extended to other cardiovascular diseases and imaging tasks. Furthermore, the performance of the proposed approach can be validated on more extensive and diverse datasets to assess its generalizability and applicability in real-world clinical settings.

The proposed approach achieves high accuracy, sensitivity, specificity, and precision, as demonstrated by the evaluation metrics. However, there are limitations to the proposed approach, such as the dataset used for training and testing, which may not be representative of the general population. To bolster the accuracy of coronary disease prediction, future research avenues aimed at refining the proposed CNN-based approach involve leveraging larger and more diverse datasets during training. Exploring alternative DL architectures, such as attention-based models, presents another promising avenue for enhancement. In addition, integrating supplementary clinical data, such as patient demographics and medical history, holds potential for further improving predictive capabilities. Generally, this study features the capability of profound DL methods for precise coronary illness determination and the requirement for additional examination around here.

References

1 Denysyuk, H.V., Pinto, R.J., Silva, P.M. et al. (2018). Deep learning-based automatic detection of cardiac diseases using ECG signals. *2018 40th Annual International Conference of the IEEE Engineering in Medicine and Biology Society (EMBC)*, pp. 3502–3505.

2 Betancur, J., Commandeur, F., Motlagh, M. et al. (2019). Deep learning for prediction of obstructive disease from fast myocardial perfusion SPECT: a multicenter study. *JACC: Cardiovascular Imaging* 12 (2): 257–259.

3 Bernard, O., Lalande, A., Zotti, C. et al. (2018). Deep learning techniques for automatic MRI cardiac multi-structures segmentation and diagnosis: Is the problem solved? *IEEE Transactions on Medical Imaging* 37 (11): 2514–2525.

4 Lang, H.P. (2019). Diagnosis of heart diseases by deep learning-based analysis of medical images: a review, arXiv preprint arXiv:1912.00601.

5 Zolna, A.M. (2018). Deep learning for automated segmentation of left ventricle myocardium from cine MRI. *2018 40th Annual International Conference of the IEEE Engineering in Medicine and Biology Society (EMBC)*, pp. 5764–5767.

6 Jahmunah, V., Ng, E.Y.K., San, T.R., and Acharya, U.R. (2021). Automated detection of coronary artery disease, myocardial infarction and congestive heart failure using Gabor CNN model with ECG signals. *Computers in Biology and Medicine.* 134: 104457. https://doi.org/10.1016/j.compbiomed.2021.104457.

7 Essa, E. and Xie, X. (2021). Multi-model deep learning ensemble for ECG heartbeat arrhythmia classification. *2020 28th European Signal Processing Conference (EUSIPCO)*, pp. 1085–1089. Amsterdam, Netherlands. https://doi.org/10.23919/Eusipco47968.2020.9287520.

8 Bouny, L.E., Khalil, M., and Adib, A. (2020). ECG heartbeat classification based on multi-scale wavelet convolutional neural networks. *ICASSP 2020 - 2020 IEEE International Conference on Acoustics, Speech, and Signal Processing (ICASSP)*, pp. 3212–3216, Barcelona, Spain. https://doi.org/10.1109/ICASSP40776.2020.9054749.

9 Essa, E. and Xie, X. (2021). An ensemble of deep learning-based multi-model for ECG heartbeats arrhythmia classification. *IEEE Access* 9: 103452–103464. https://doi.org/10.1109/ACCESS.2021.3098986.

10 Rafi, S.M. and Akthar, S. (2021). ECG classification using a hybrid deep learning approach. *2021 International Conference on Artificial Intelligence and Smart Systems (ICAIS)*, pp. 302–305, Coimbatore, India. https://doi.org/10.1109/ICAIS50930.2021.9395897.

11 Saraswathi, K., Mohanraj, V., Suresh, Y. et al. (2023). Deep learning enabled social media recommendation based on user comments. *Computer Systems Science and Engineering* 44 (2): 1691–1702.

12 Tom, R.J., Kumar, A., Shaik, S.B. et al. (2022). Car license plate detection and recognition using modified U-Net deep learning model. *2022 8th International Conference on Smart Structures and Systems (ICSSS)*, pp. 1–6, Chennai, India. https://doi.org/10.1109/ICSSS54381.2022.9782176.

13 Yang, J. (2017). Intelligent diagnosis of arrhythmia based on deep learning. *2017 10th International Congress on Image and Signal Processing, Biomedical Engineering, and Informatics (CISP-BMEI)*, pp. 1–5.

14 Manoharan Tamilselvi, J., Senthilkumar, V.M., and Suresh, Y. (2022). Swarm intelligence-based optimized adaptive filtering technique for ECG data analysis system. *IETE Journal of Research* https://doi.org/10.1080/03772063.2022.2032847.

15 Hang, Y., Yang, L.T., Zhang, Q. et al. (2021). Convolutional neural networks for medical image analysis: state-of-the-art, comparisons, improvement, and perspectives. *Neurocomputing* 444: 92–110. https://doi.org/10.1016/j.neucom.2020.04.157.

16 Vincent, P.C., Magboo, M., and Magboo, S.A. (2023). Diagnosis of coronary artery disease from myocardial perfusion imaging using convolutional neural networks. *Procedia Computer Science* 218: 810–817. https://doi.org/10.1016/j.procs.2023.01.061.

17 Coelho, L.P. (2018). Detecting cardiovascular disease from mammograms with deep learning. *2018 IEEE 15th International Symposium on Biomedical Imaging (ISBI 2018)*, pp. 427–430.

18 Zhou, Y. (2018). Cardiac disease classification using electrocardiogram and deep learning. *2018 IEEE 42nd Annual Computer Software and Applications Conference (COMPSAC)*, pp. 227–232.

19 Attia, G.S., Noseworthy, P.A., Lopez-Jimenez, F. et al. (2019). An artificial intelligence-enabled ECG algorithm for the identification of patients with atrial fibrillation during sinus rhythm: a retrospective analysis of outcome prediction. *The Lancet* 394 (10201): 861–867.

15

Classification Methods of Deep Learning for Detecting Autism Spectrum Disorder in Children (4–12 Years)

Yashashwini Reddy[1], Chinthala Kishor Kumar Reddy[1,2], Kari Lippert[3], and Sahithi Reddy[4]

[1] *Stanley College of Engineering and Technology for Women, Osmania University, Hyderabad, Telangana, India*
[2] *Faculty of Engineering and Technology, Botho University, Gaborone, Botswana*
[3] *Department of Systems Engineering, University of South Alabama, Mobile, AL, USA*
[4] *Master of Information Technology and Master of Information Technology Management, The University of Sydney, New South Wales, Sydney, Australia*

15.1 Introduction

Autism spectrum disorder (ASD) is a syndrome in which the socializing capacity, the way of grasping the environment and expressing feelings will be unusual for an individual [1]. Key factors for the development of autism revealed from research are an individual with genotypes like tuberous sclerosis complex, fragile "x" syndrome, a few environmental conditions like exposure to toxic air, and antenatal factors, but the cause of autism is explicitly not yet known. This disorder lasts for the rest of life and develops within the initial two years of life [2]. The children who suffer from autism are vulnerable to the surroundings they live in. They feel discomfort when they hear loud disturbances, have different priorities of food they eat, are sensitive to colors, and feel exhausted when they are surrounded by a mass number of people.

Behavior like having different passions, hyperacusis, manifests repetitive behavior like fluttering hands, or using words repeatedly, using things unusually, delay in speaking by 18 months, poor eye contact, being irresponsive when called by the name of a child at 12 months, answering inappropriately when questions asked, understanding others perspective differently, difficulty to adjust and adapt for changes in the environment and routines, not sharing feelings and problems with others are usual symptoms of ASD [3]. They also have some outstanding qualities like analyzing things in depth, their potential of having at most focus on a specific thing helps them to crack logic.

Generative Artificial Intelligence for Biomedical and Smart Health Informatics, First Edition. Edited by Aditya Khamparia and Deepak Gupta.

Table 15.1 Top five countries with highest autism rate in 2023.

Serial number	Country	Autism rate per one lakh
1	United Kingdom	700.08
2	Sweden	661.86
3	Japan	604.73
4	United States	603.39
5	Netherlands	591.55

Some individuals show symptoms at an early age, and some show symptoms later in their lives. Hence, this disorder can be identified at any age. The symptoms and severity will not be the same for everyone; it will vary from person to person, and hence, it is termed as a spectrum disorder. Over the last two decades, there has been a rapid increase in the autism rate in the world, and it is a public health concern that should be treated with care [4]. We can observe the five leading countries of autism rates in 2023 in Table 15.1 and Figure 15.1 below.

It is analyzed that mostly boys are diagnosed with autism than girls, as we can observe in Figure 15.2 above, as the mutation in genes and the changes in hormones will be different in males and females [5]. Identifying and treating autism early can minimize this problem to some level. There are situations where autistic people are wrongly diagnosed and receive inappropriate treatment, as this disorder is often confused with cognitive impairment and other mental-related disorders [6]. Table 15.2 below portrays the consequences if autistic children are neglected without providing treatment. It is also observed that other mental disorders will develop with autism, as we can observe in Table 15.3 below.

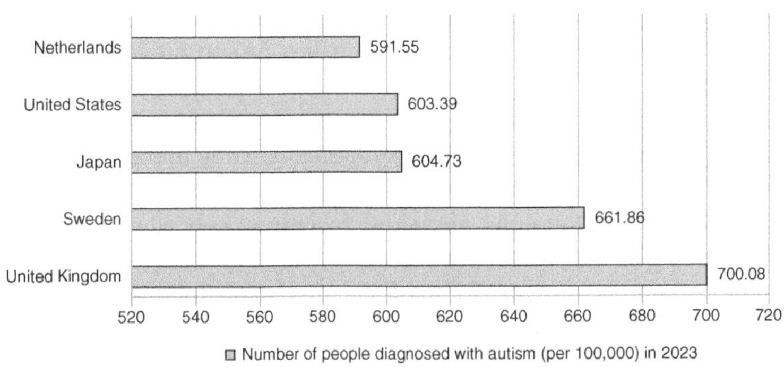

Figure 15.1 The highest rate of autism diagnosed population countries (2023).

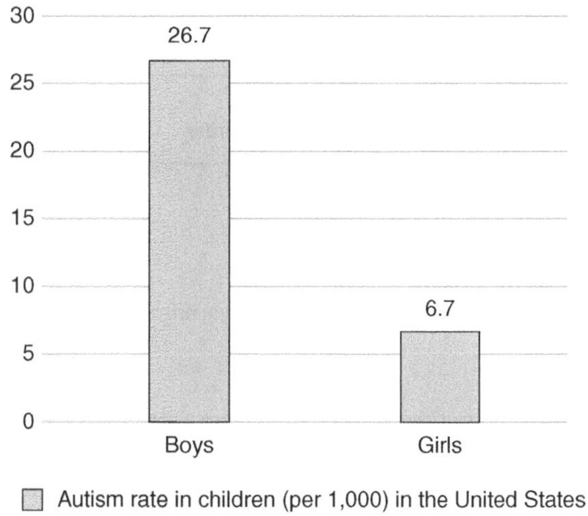

Figure 15.2 Children autism rate in the US (2017).

Table 15.2 Consequences if autism spectrum disorder in children is not treated.

Serial number	Issue
1	Poor-academic achievement
2	Maintain poor relationships with friends and family
3	Feel difficulty to manage emotions
4	They will depend on others to do basic tasks
5	May feel less comfort to speak about their feelings
6	Poor self-care due to poor reaction to sensory stimuli
7	Disturbance in the sleep cycle and suffer from eating disorder
8	Become under confident
9	Being unemployed as adults
10	Learning a language would be challenging

There exist three stages of autism in children represented as ASD stage 1, ASD stage 2, and ASD stage 3 that indicate the severity of autism [7]. The severity of autism is higher in stage 3 than in stage 2. Stage 1 indicates less severity of autism. To understand the severity of autism in a patient has a crucial role in treating them systematically. Each stage of autism in children has some symptoms, as we can observe in Figure 15.3 below but are not constant. Some variations can be observed in the behavior of a child that depends on the environment they grow up in and

Table 15.3 Some additional mental disorders that accompany with autism.

Serial number	Type of mental disorder	Prevalence of the disorder (%)
1	Panic disorder	19
2	Manic depression	6
3	OCD	10
4	Altered perception syndrome	5
5	Depression	12
6	ADHD	29

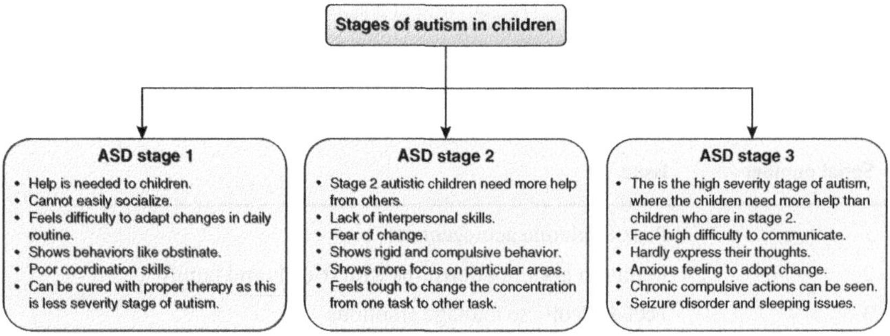

Figure 15.3 Portrays stages of autism in children.

the help they get from parents [8]. Hence, personalized treatment plays an active role in detecting and treating autism in children.

There are a few modern countries that have great awareness about autism disorder. These countries have the least cases of autism, as we can observe in Table 15.4 and Figure 15.4 below. These countries are involved in advanced research about this disorder and make early detection a priority to overcome this health condition that enhances mental health. They provide personalized observation to diagnose this condition, and after that, enhanced treatment facilities are provided to autistic individuals that help them to lead an individualistic life. They also raise funds that support autism research. They conduct many awareness events to make the public aware of this health condition. This helped them to minimize the rise in autism cases in their countries.

If an individual with less severity of autism does not receive systematic medical care, there is a high chance that the severity will become more [9]. There are some interview-based procedures followed by healthcare professionals to diagnose

Table 15.4 Countries with the least cases of autism in children (2023).

Serial number	Country	Number of people diagnosed per 10,000
1	France	69.4
2	Portugal	70.6
3	Iceland	80
4	Norway	72.1
5	Italy	72.1
6	Germany	72.3
7	Greece	72.5

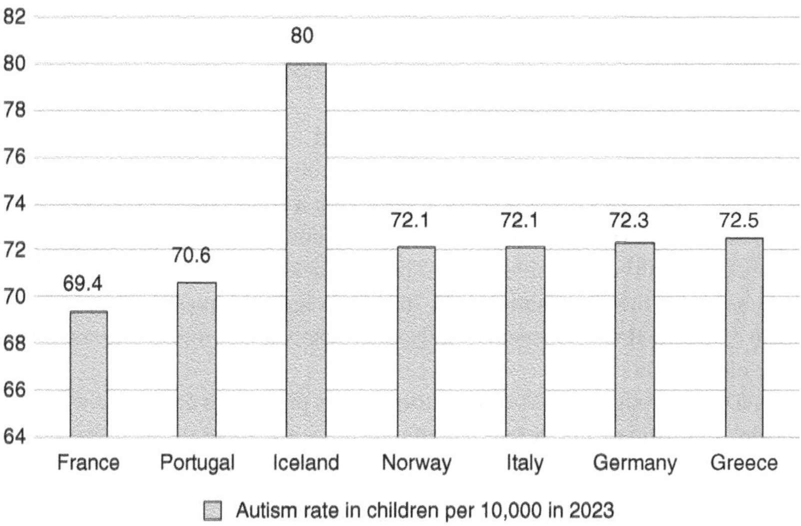

Figure 15.4 Countries with the least autism cases in children (2023).

autism in children, but the identification of the presence of the disorder is not precise. These methods consume more time to get the results of the test, which will lead to delays in treating the patients. As this disorder is typical to identify because it has many variations in symptoms, there is a need to replace conventional methods with advanced technology [10].

This research aims to implement a deep learning method, CNN, to effectively detect ASD in children [11]. Also, artificial intelligence (AI) and machine learning

(ML) techniques are studied for their application in detecting ASD in children. These methods are used for the classification process. These methods perform classification by learning from large, labeled data sets. The rest of the sections are sequenced as follows: Section 15.2 discusses relevant work and research aims, Section 15.3 explains the proposed methodology, Section 15.4 gives the result of the proposed model, and Section 15.5 is followed by a conclusion and references.

15.2 Relevant Work

There are commonly used conventional methods by doctors to identify autism at the initial level. Some conventional methods are autism spectrum quotient (AQ), childhood autism rating scale (CARS-2), autism diagnostic interview revised (ADI-R), autism observation schedule revised (ADOS) [12]. The AQ, which was proposed by Baron–Cohen, is an analysis test that has 50 questions, wherein patients or caretakers of a child should answer the questions about the acuteness on a scale ranging from 1 to 4, which represents false to true, respectively. The diagnosis of autism that is made using this method is not accurate. There are chances of getting false results [13].

The questions asked in the AQ test are related to socializing ability, creative ability, concentration levels, and multitasking ability. It is helpful to test all age groups [14]. The CARS is the process of observing a child's behavior and considering the feedback from caretakers of the child about their behavior. This test is performed by healthcare professionals. The acuteness of autism is represented on a scale based on the examination [15]. In this method, 15 questions are present that are related to the interpersonal skills, interaction ability, and emotional intelligence of the child.

The ADI-R introduced by Michael Rutter, in this process, to determine whether a person is autistic or not, a few sets of questions are asked of the caretaker of a child by a doctor. Using this method, we can know the presence or absence of autism and the severity stage of autism. Hence, it is an efficient method. It covers questions related to the speaking and language usage ability of a child, the ability of a child to interact, about repeated actions [16].

Autism observation schedule revised is the process where the doctors frame an environment to connect and communicate with patients to identify autism. This test is performed under the keen observation of healthcare experts. The patient will be under the observation of a doctor where the patient's behavior, interaction ability, and way of communicating are observed. The examination is conducted in a regulated environment [17]. Since these procedures are applied, there are some challenges that arise using these methods, as we can observe in Table 15.5 that below results in the inappropriate estimation of the presence of autism in children.

Table 15.5 Setbacks of conventional methods to detect autism spectrum disorder.

Serial number	Method	Setbacks
1.	Autism spectrum quotient	Error of commission and Error of omission.
2.	Childhood autism rating scale	Imprecise feedback to doctors by caretakers.
3.	Autism diagnostic interview revised	Time taking process and needs keen examination by doctors.
4.	Autism observation schedule revised	Inaccuracy in detection due to observing patients under regulated surroundings.

By using autism characteristics, it would be easy to identify the presence of autism in an individual. The wearable gadgets are implemented by researchers and are used to detect autism disorder. As we can observe in Table 15.6, the inclusion of AI and ML concepts to detect autism would enhance the diagnosis process which will be helpful for adults and children [18]. The concepts of ML have been implied to perform autism diagnosis. ML made predictions of the presence or absence of autism by using given properties of attributes [19].

To gather data related to autism in infants, children, and adults, Fadi Thabtah designed an application on mobile called ASD test. AQ-10 and Qchat-10 are the methods used to build this application. The documentation about autistic individuals is clustered together and restored in the ML database at the University of California, Irvine, by using these examination techniques [14]. The application of classification methods of ML to diagnose autism was researched by Mythili et al. [20].

In this, ML concepts like support vector machine (SVM), neural networks (NN), fuzzy logic techniques and for analysis, Weka software is implemented to understand student's socializing ability and actions [21]. The ML algorithms will give promising results in diagnosing autism as it is designed to understand the logic of data [22]. To understand the difference between ADHD and ASD, Duda et al. [23] implemented the forward feature selection method by leveraging the 65 Social Responsiveness Scale. To help and assist autistic individuals during the COVID-19 pandemic, Al Banna proposed a unique AI-powered model. It is a customized technology that helps autistic people manage and keep in check their problems [24].

Autism is a neurological disorder that should be detected at an initial level. The existing treatments are not cost-effective. Hence, there is an emergency to bring smart technology to detect autism that can be afforded by the mass population as the rate of autism is increasing. David Peebles et al. [25] proposed a logistic regression algorithm that is known as an ML algorithm to detect autism in adolescents and adults. Kanchana et al. [26] introduced the random forest

Table 15.6 The literature survey about detecting autism disorder using advanced technology.

Author	Method used	Advantages	Drawbacks
Mythili et al. [20]	Image sorting using CNN, SVM, KNN, ANN	The models understand the logic and patterns of the dataset quickly	Give inaccurate results due to spatial heterogeneity.
Duda et al. [23]	ADOS and Stepwise backward feature selection	Reduces the complexity of data and has enhanced accuracy.	The results will not be precise as it is based on observation in a few circumstances.
David Peebles et al. [24]	Logistic regression	Easy to use and avoids overfitting of data.	Not suitable to analyze complex data when the dataset is nonlinear.
Kanchana et al. [25]	Random forest	It gives good accuracy even when the input dataset is inconsistent.	Time taking process.
Mahmoud Elbattah et al. [26]	Natural language processing	Easy to analyze and get results by analyzing the fast eye moment.	It can analyze only fast movements of eyes but cannot analyze other eye movements that are crucial in autism detection.
Mariam M. Hassan et al. [27]	Decision tree algorithm	Analyzes all the causes and symptoms related to ASD effectively.	Overfitting problems arise when there is a large dataset

method to detect autism. This classifier generates the rating for the input dataset depending on the outcomes.

Mahmoud Elbattah et al. [27] introduced a natural language processing technique to predict the presence or absence of autism based on analyzing fast eye movements. In this process, the eye movements are portrayed as characters that explain the movements of the eyes that help to detect autism. Mariam M. Hassan et al. [28] proposed a decision tree algorithm that uses an autism-related dataset to diagnose autism. Also, it uses the ASD history of family members that enhances the prediction process.

The study of detecting autism by the facial expressions of children has evolved. The latest research shows that the application of concepts of deep learning to detect various diseases gives promising results. In this subject, the implementation of a deep learning concept known as CNN plays an effective role by giving accurate results. CNN is the best model to perform the image recognition process as it has the ability to understand the hidden and logical information of the given input dataset [25].

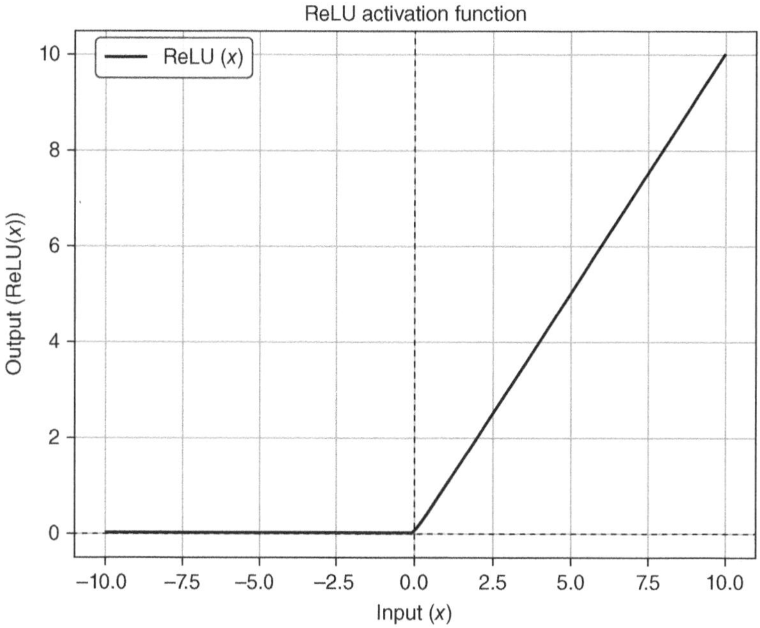

Figure 15.5 ReLU Activation Graph.

15.3 Proposed Methodology

In the proposed framework, the CNN model is implemented. Initially, the dataset related to autism in children is collected, that is, text data represented in tabular form. The dataset has some values missing. The missing data is replaced with useful data in the dataset. This process helps to get better results. The gathered dataset is given as input to the CNN model after using the byte pair encoding (BPE) algorithm that is used to convert each column in the table into characters in a sequence that helps the CNN model analyze the input data easily and efficiently. The three layers of convolutional layers are used in this model. The activation function used by convolutional layers is ReLU (Rectified Linear Unit), as we can observe in Figure 15.5 below. Here, the choosing of relevant features is performed using these layers of CNN and the feature map generates useful features from the dataset to detect autism.

Now, in the further process pooling layers are used to select the most relevant data from the feature map that convolution layers generate. Here, two layers of pooling layers are used that generate a small feature map from the existing feature map. The flattened layer takes input from the pooling layer and recasts it into a one-dimensional (1D) matrix that helps to ease the classification process further.

The fully connected layer of CNN will identify the presence of autism in children based on the selected features.

It takes input from previous layers through neurons and gives the output. To reduce the loss function, we used stochastic gradient descent (SGD). To get the result in binary classification form, the sigmoid activation function is implemented. The output we will get in binary form as yes or no represents the presence or absence of autism in children, respectively. Then the proposed model is tested using a testing dataset to check the efficiency of the proposed model in detecting autism in children. The advanced version of Python, Python 3, is used to perform this process. Figure 15.6 clearly explains the proposed idea.

15.3.1 Algorithm for the Proposed Model

Input: Autism disorder-related data of children that has attributes X and target parameter y

(1) Partition the dataset into training and testing
(2) Implement the BPE algorithm on the training dataset.
(3) Give input to the CNN model after performing BPE on the dataset
(4) Implement ReLU as an activation function for convolutional layers
(5) Implement max pooling to get a feature map
(6) Convert the generated feature map as a 1D matrix
(7) To reduce the loss function, implement SGD
(8) Implement sigmoid activation function on the outcome layer to get results as yes or no
(9) Evaluate the performance of the model with the testing dataset

Output: Yes/NO

15.3.2 Proposed Framework

(Figure 15.6)

15.3.3 Dataset Used

We gathered the datasets that are related to the area of research in the initial stage that helps to train the CNN model. In this research, the dataset collected was designed by Fadi Fayez Thabtah [29]. Here, the gathering of the dataset is performed using a screening application on mobile by using the AQ-10-Child process. The description of the gathered dataset is given below in Table 15.7. The dataset has records of 291 patients and 20 features. The dataset has ten questions,

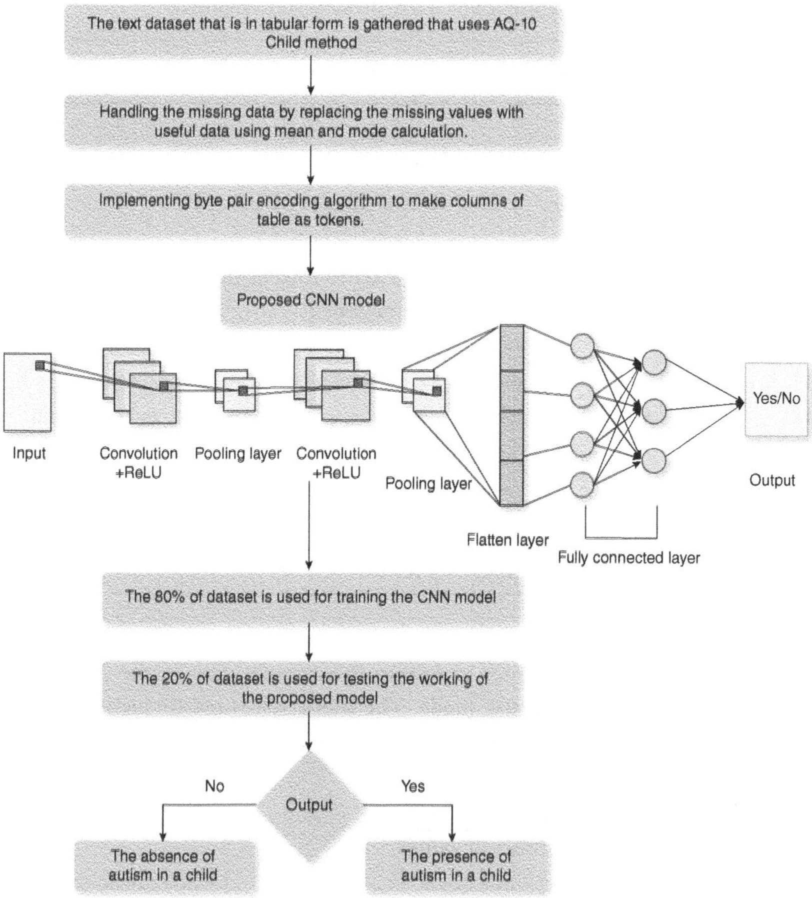

Figure 15.6 The framework of the proposed methodology.

including the age of children (4–12), AQ-10-Chat rate, gender, nationality, jaundice, family history of ASD, who went through ASD screening before, who attended the test, and the presence of ASD. The 10 questions are related to the AQ-10-Chat procedure.

15.3.4 Data Preparation

Data preparation means modifying the raw data that is more appropriate to use in the tasks that are allied with data. In this process, managing errors, managing missing values, and handling data instability takes place by the process of imputation of the missing values. Here, to manage numeric data, we use the

Table 15.7 Description of dataset collected to detect ASD in children.

Feature number	Feature name	Feature description
1	Age	Age (4–12)
2	Gender	Male/Female
3	Nationality	Nationality of the patient
4	Jaundice	Yes/No
5–14	Q1-Q10	The AQ-10-Chat method is used which has 10 questions.
15	Family members ASD	Yes/No
16	Who attended the test	Family member/Healthcare professional
17	AQ-10-Child rate	Each yes is represented as 1, and if the total count is above 6 is considered as the presence of ASD
18	Undergone ASD screening before	Yes/No
19	Presence of ASD	Yes/No

mean value of the data in order to restore the missing data in the dataset. To manage qualitative data, we use mode. The mode tells how frequently a word repeats. That is chosen to replace the missing data. The formula used to calculate the mean of the given data is:

$$\text{Mean} = \frac{\text{Summation of all the values}}{\text{Total number of values}}$$

15.3.5 Feature Selection

The feature selection process is performed after data preparation. It is the process of choosing the most useful attribute that will suit the training of the model. This process will help to minimize high variance, enhance the process of training, and reduce the complexity of understanding data. In this research, a correlation matrix is performed for feature selection on the input dataset using Python, as we can observe in Figure 15.7 below. The instance of the dataset is given in Table 15.8 below of nine patients.

15.3.6 Convolutional Neural Networks

Convolutional neural networks (CNN) are considered a deep learning method [28]. CNN is designed to take input data as a text or a picture to analyze it and that

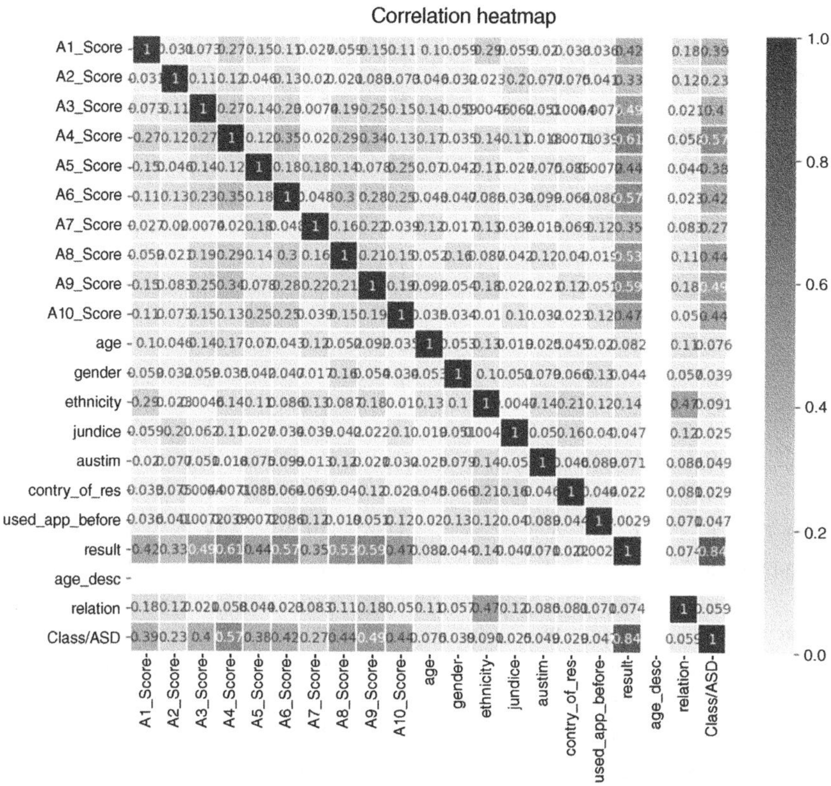

Figure 15.7 Correlation matrix for feature selection.

generates the output that describes the logics and patterns of the dataset. CNN is designed with three layers that have some functionality. The three layers are the convolutional layer, the pooling layer, and the fully connected layer. CNN has kernels that are used for selecting features that generate feature maps.

The convolutional layer is responsible for applying the kernel to the input dataset. In this research, we considered the dataset in tabular format. So, equation (15.1) is used in the selection of the feature process for the tabular dataset. In the proposed model, we used ReLU as an activation function that enhances nonlinearity and helps the CNN model to understand the logic easily of the dataset. Equation (15.2) shows how ReLU calculation.

$$(X \cdot W)(i) = \sum_{f=1}^{F} \sum_{e=1}^{E} X_{(i+f-1),e} W_{f,e} \tag{15.1}$$

$$(f(x) = \max(0, x)) \tag{15.2}$$

Table 15.8 Instances of children autism dataset.

Instance number	1	2	3	4	5	6	7	8	9
A1	1	1	1	1	1	1	0	1	1
A2	1	1	1	1	1	0	1	0	1
A3	0	0	1	1	1	0	1	0	1
A4	0	0	1	1	1	0	1	0	1
A5	1	1	1	1	1	1	1	0	1
A6	1	1	1	1	1	1	1	0	1
A7	0	0	1	1	1	1	1	1	1
A8	1	1	1	1	0	1	1	0	1
A9	0	0	1	0	0	1	1	0	1
A10	0	0	1	0	0	1	1	0	1
Age [4–12)	6	6	5	5	11	10	4	4	6
AQ-10-Chat rate	5	5	10	8	7	7	9	2	10
Gender	m	m	m	f	f	m	m	f	m
Nationality	Others	West Asian	Others	West Asian	West Asian	Caucasian	Black	White	White
Jaundice	No	No	Yes	No	No	Yes	Yes	No	No
Family history of ASD	No	No	No	No	Yes	No	No	No	Yes
Who attended the test	Parent	Parent	Parent	Parent	Parent	Self	Parent	Parent	Parent
Presence of ASD	No	No	Yes	Yes	Yes	Yes	Yes	No	Yes

Here, from equation (15.1), "X" is considered as input, and "W" represents a kernel of dimension $F \times E$. In equation (15.2), "x" is the input. If the input value is positive, then the output of ReLU will be positive. If the input value is negative, then the outcome of ReLU will be zero. To choose the most relevant features of similar properties from the feature map, the pooling layer is useful. There are two most common types of pooling that are average pooling and max pooling. In average pooling, it selects and combines the average number from each section of the feature map and gives a small feature map.

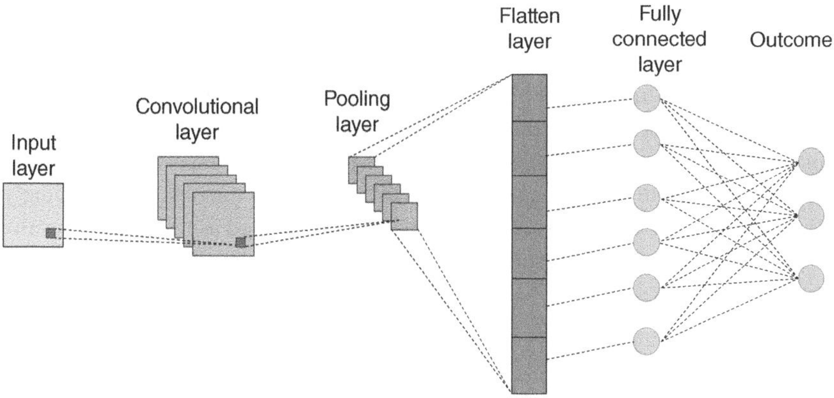

Figure 15.8 CNN architecture.

The pooling process takes place after the selection of features. Max pooling means it selects and gathers the maximum value from the sections of the feature map that generate a small feature map. It is used to select the important characteristics of data. Average pooling helps to eliminate unnecessary data. The equations (15.2) and (15.3) represent the calculation of max pooling and average pooling [30]. Here, in the equations, "L" means the length of the sequence; S. W represents the pooling layer size.

$$\text{Max pooling: } (S) = \max_{i=1} L - W + 1\{S[i : i + W - 1]\} \quad (15.3)$$

$$\text{Average pooling: } (S) = \frac{1}{w} \sum_{i=1}^{L-W+1} \{S[i : i + W - 1]\} \quad (15.4)$$

Flatten layer is present after the pooling layer. It is used to adjust the layer into a 1D layer that will ease the prediction process. A fully connected layer in CNN will be linked with the preceding and succeeding layers of CNN. This operation is used to get a nonlinearity function. First, the application of bias offset to the total weighted input is performed and then passed through a nonlinearity function. The equation (15.5) represents how to calculate the loss function, where "N" means the total number of instances in the input dataset. So based on the outcome, SGD can be implemented to reduce loss function. The architecture of CNN is portrayed clearly in Figure 15.8 below.

$$L = \frac{1}{N} \sum_{i=1}^{N} L_i \quad (15.5)$$

15.3.7 Portioning Data

It is the process of partitioning the data into training and testing. This procedure is followed by a feature selection process. In this process, some portions of data from the dataset are used to train the chosen deep learning model and the other portion of data is used for the testing process. Now, the portioning of data is followed. Here, the dataset used for training and testing is divided into a ratio of 80:20 accordingly. Furthermore, the dataset used for training is again divided as training and evaluation into the ratio 80:20 accordingly that is used for cross-validation purposes.

15.4 Results

Here, we consider the accuracy of each model, and the model with a high accuracy rate will be chosen to detect autism in children. The accuracy of ANN, SVM, LR, K-nearest neighbor (KNN), Naive Bayes, CNN, ID-CNN, and TCN is 97.59%, 97.87%, 97.85%, 88.12%, 94.86%, 97.90%, 97.70%, and 97.80%, respectively, as we can observe in Table 15.9 and Figure 15.9 below that we got before managing missing data. We can also observe sensitivity in Table 15.10 and Figure 15.10, specificity in Table 15.11 and Figure 15.11, and error rate in Table 15.12 and Figure 15.12 below, respectively.

We can also observe the performance of the models after managing the missing data. The accuracy of CNN is high among all the models after managing missing data, as we can observe in Table 15.13 and Figure 15.13 below. We can observe

Table 15.9 The specificity obtained after checking the performance of the models.

Method	Specificity (%)
ANN	0.9641
SVM	0.9674
LR	0.9671
KNN	0.9635
Naive Bayes	0.9639
CNN	0.9679
1D-CNN	0.9645
TCN	0.9648

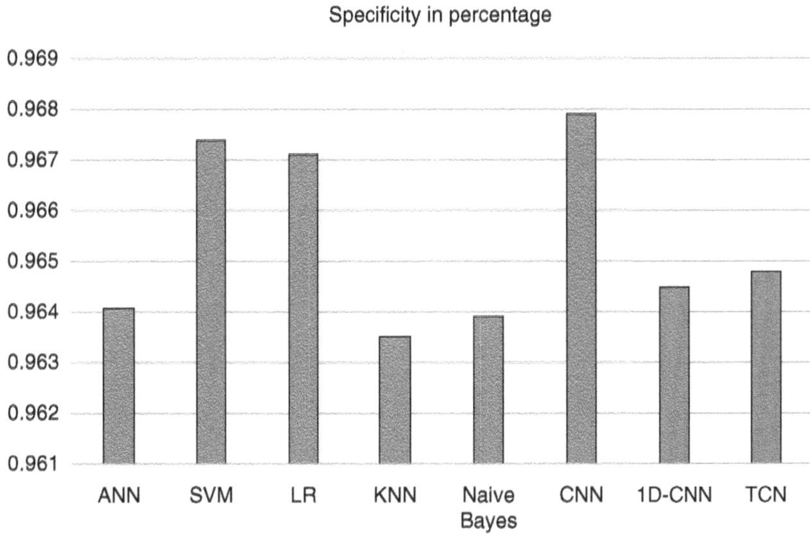

Figure 15.9 The specificity in the percentage of the chosen models used to detect autism in children.

Table 15.10 The accuracy before handling missing data obtained after checking the performance of the model.

Method	Accuracy (%)
ANN	97.59
SVM	97.87
LR	97.85
KNN	88.12
Naive Bayes	94.86
CNN	97.90
1D-CNN	97.70
TCN	97.80

that the error rate of CNN is less after managing missing data in Table 15.14 and Figure 15.14 below. We got this after performing an evaluation of all the performance of models. The performance is evaluated using the confusion matrix method.

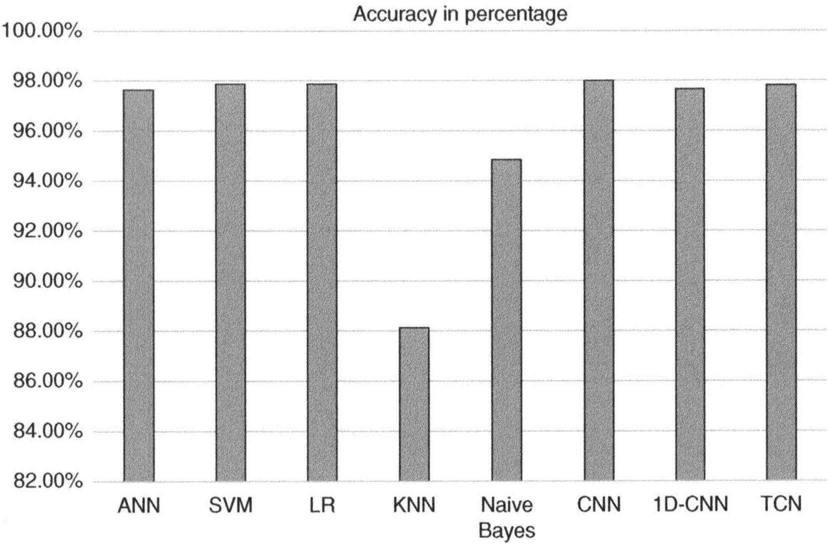

Figure 15.10 The Accuracy of models obtained before handling the missing values.

Table 15.11 The sensitivity obtained after checking the performance of the models.

Method	Sensitivity (%)
ANN	0.9665
SVM	0.9675
LR	0.9673
KNN	0.8053
Naive Bayes	0.9363
CNN	0.9677
1D-CNN	0.9669
TCN	0.9670

15.5 Conclusion

This research aims to detect ASD in children, which helps to proceed with curated treatment that helps in curing the condition. We implemented the techniques of AI to detect autism in children. The related dataset is collected, and the CNN model achieved a high accuracy of 98.76% and an error rate of 1.24%. This shows that the

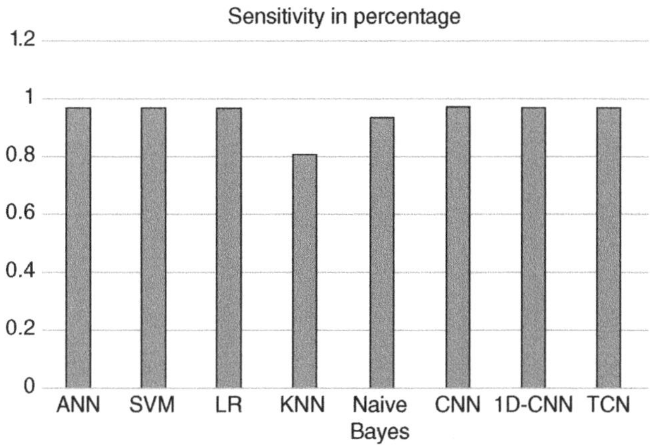

Figure 15.11 The sensitivity of all the models in percentage.

Table 15.12 The error rate obtained after checking the performance of the models.

Method	Error rate (%)
ANN	2.41
SVM	2.13
LR	2.15
KNN	11.88
Naive Bayes	5.14
CNN	2.1
1D-CNN	2.3
TCN	2.2

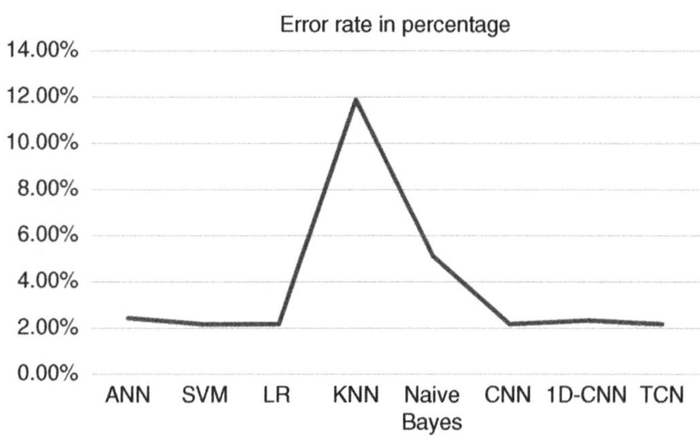

Figure 15.12 The error rate in percentage of the chosen models before handling missing data.

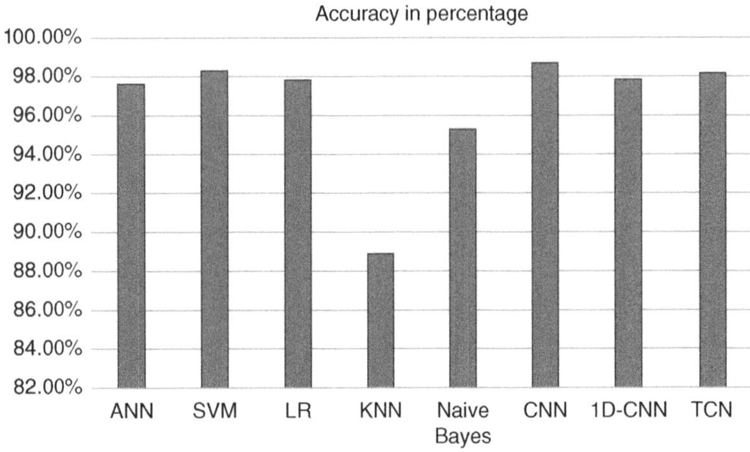

Figure 15.13 The Accuracy of models obtained after handling the missing values.

Table 15.13 The accuracy after handling missing data obtained after checking the performance of the models.

Method	Accuracy before managing missing data (%)	Accuracy after managing missing data (%)
ANN	97.59	97.65
SVM	97.87	98.35
LR	97.85	97.89
KNN	88.12	88.90
Naive Bayes	94.86	95.30
CNN	97.90	98.76
1D-CNN	97.70	97.90
TCN	97.80	98.20

implementation of AI gives promising results in detecting autism in children. In conclusion, conventional methods can be replaced by AI to detect autism. Implementing conventional methods is a time-consuming process where AI will give faster results, it is helpful to diagnose at the initial stage, it will be available at an affordable price, and we get to know the severity of the problem that aids to take appropriate treatment.

Table 15.14 The error rate obtained after checking the performance of the models after handling missing values.

Method	Error rate (%)
ANN	2.35
SVM	1.65
LR	2.11
KNN	11.1
Naive Bayes	4.7
CNN	1.24
1D-CNN	2.1
TCN	1.8

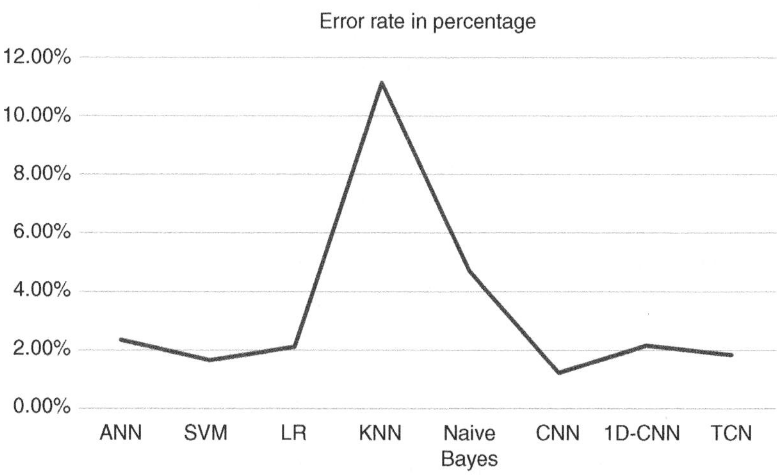

Figure 15.14 The error rate of chosen models after handling the missing data.

References

1 Davies, J., Cooper, K., Killick, E. et al. (2024). *Autistic Identity: A Systematic Review of Quantitative Research*. Wiley.

2 Ratajczak, H.V. (2010). *Theoretical Aspects of Autism: Causes—A Review*. Taylor & Francis.

3 Dawson, G., Meltzoff, A.N., Osterling, J., and Rinaldi, J. (2008). *Neuropsychological Correlates of Early Symptoms of Autism*. Society for Research in Child Development.

4 Johnson, C.P. and Myers, S.M. (2007). *Identification and Evaluation of Children with Autism Spectrum Disorders*. American Academy of Pediatrics.

5 Baron-Cohen, S., Lombardo, M.V., Auyeung, B. et al. (2010). Why are autism spectrum conditions more prevalent in males? *PLOS Biology* 9 (6): e1001081.

6 Hus, Y. and Segal, O. (2021). *Challenges Surrounding the Diagnosis of Autism in Children*, 3509–3529. Taylor & Francis.

7 Nolan, S., Schroeder, R., Harris, L.L. et al. (2022). *Differentiation of Children with Varying Levels of Autism Spectrum Disorder Symptoms from Children Developing Typically*. Elsevier.

8 Wong, V., YuDepartm, Y., Keyes, M.L., and McGrew, J.H. (2016). *Pre-diagnostic and Diagnostic Stages of Autism Spectrum Disorder: A Parent Perspective*. Taylor & Francis.

9 Zareei, M., Tohidast, S.A., and Salmani, M. (2022). Parents' perceptions of the problems in children with autism spectrum disorders: a qualitative study. *Iranian Rehabilitation Journal* 20 (4): 611–622.

10 Shahamiri, S.R. and Thabtah, F. (2020). *Autism AI: A New Autism Screening System Based on Artificial Intelligence*. Springer.

11 Parui, S., Samanta, D., Chakravorty, N. et al. (2023). *Artificial Intelligence and Sensor-Based Autism Spectrum Disorder Diagnosis Using Brain Connectivity Analysis*. Elsevier.

12 Alam, M.S., Rashid, M.M., Roy, R. et al. (2022). *Empirical Study of Autism Spectrum Disorder Diagnosis Using Facial Images by Improved Transfer Learning Approach*. Bioengineering, MDPI.

13 Yoshinaga, K., Egawa, J., Watanabe, Y. et al. (2023). *Usefulness of the Autism Spectrum Quotient (AQ) in Screening for Autism Spectrum Disorder and Social Communication Disorder*. Springer Nature.

14 Thabtah, F., Kamalov, F., and Rajab, K. (2018). *A New Computational Intelligence Approach to Detect Autistic Features for Autism Screening*. Elsevier.

15 Moon, S.J., Hwang, J.S., Shin, A.L. et al. (2019). *Accuracy of the Childhood Autism Rating Scale: A Systematic Review and Meta-Analysis*. Wiley.

16 Kim, S.H.(S.), Hus, V., and Lord, C. (2013). *Autism Diagnostic Interview-Revised*. Springer Nature.

17 Evans, P., Golla, S., and Morris, M.A. (2015). Autism spectrum disorders: clinical considerations. In: *Rosenberg's Molecular and Genetic Basis of Neurological and Psychiatric Disease* (ed. R.N. Rosenberg and J.M. Pascual), 197–207. Academic Press.

18 Neeharika, C.H. and Riyazuddin, Y.M. (2023). Developing an artificial intelligence based model for autism spectrum disorder detection in children. *Journal* *of Advanced Research in Applied Sciences and Engineering Technology* 32 (1). https://doi.org/10.37934/araset.32.1.5772.

19 Kamala, B., Pooja, K.S.M., Varsha, S., and Sivapriya, K. (2021). *ML Based Approach to Detect Autism Spectrum Disorder (ASD)*. IEEE.

20 Mythili, M.S. and Mohamed Shanavas, A.R. (2014). A study on autism spectrum disorders using classification techniques. *International Journal of Soft Computing and Engineering* 4 (5): 88–91.

21 Raj, S. and Masood, S. (2020). *Analysis and Detection of Autism Spectrum Disorder Using Machine Learning Techniques*. Elsevier.

22 Farooq, M.S., Tehseen, R., Sabir, M., and Atal, Z. (2023). Detection of autism spectrum disorder (ASD) in children and adults using machine learning. *Scientific Reports* 13 (1): 9605.

23 Kosmicki, J.A., Sochat, V., Duda, M., and Wall, D.P. (2015). Searching for a minimal set of behaviors for autism detection through feature selection-based machine learning. *Translational Psychiatry* 5 (2): e514.

24 Tapotosh Ghosh, M., Al Banna, H., Shamim Kaiser, M., and Taher, K.A. (2020). *A Monitoring System for Patients of Autism Spectrum Disorder Using Artificial Intelligence*. Springer Link.

25 Thabtah, F., Abdelhamid, N., and Peebles, D. (2019). *A Machine Learning Autism Classification Based on Logistic Regression Analysis*. Health Information Science and Systems.

26 Kanchana, A. and Khilar, R. (2022). *Prediction of Autism Spectrum Disorder using Random Forest Classifier in Adults*. IEEE.

27 Elbattah, M., Guérin, J.-L., Carette, R. et al. (2020). *NLP-Based Approach to Detect Autism Spectrum Disorder in Saccadic Eye Movement*. IEEE.

28 Hassan, M.M. and Mokhtar, H.M.O. (2019). *Investigating Autism Etiology and Heterogeneity by Decision Tree Algorithm*. Elsevier.

29 Thabtah, F. F. (2017). Autistic Spectrum Disorder Screening Data for children. https://archive.ics.uci.edu/ml/machine-learning-databases/00419/.

30 Yang, M., Cao, M., Chen, Y. et al. (2021). Large-scale brain functional network integration for discrimination of autism using a 3-D deep learning model. *Frontiers in Human Neuroscience* 15: 687288.

16

Deep Learning Model for Resolution Enhancement of Biomedical Images for Biometrics

Bhallamudi RaviKrishna[1], Madireddy Vijay Reddy[1], Mukesh Soni[2], Haewon Byeon[3], Sagar D. Pande[4], and Maher A. Rusho[5]

[1] *Department of Artificial Intelligence and Data Science, Vignan Institute of Technology & Science, Hyderabad, India*
[2] *Dr. D. Y. Patil Vidyapeeth, Pune, Dr. D. Y. Patil School of Science & Technology, Pune, India*
[3] *Department of AI and Software, Inje University, Gimhae, Republic of Korea*
[4] *School of Engineering and Technology, Pimpri Chinchwad University (PCU), Pune, Maharashtra, India*
[5] *Department of Lockheed Martin Engineering Management, University of Colorado, Boulder, CO, USA*

16.1 Introduction

According to biomedical and healthcare experts, the "gold standard" for diagnosing sickness is a historical biomedical study. Biometrics devices use a combination of high- and low-power microscopes to obtain the macrostructure and microscopic features of biomedical images and then conduct a comprehensive analysis of these features to draw diagnostic conclusions. Among them, high-resolution biomedical images can provide details at a high frequency (HF) of the lesion and are an objective basis for high-precision diagnosis of diseases. However, due to limitations of hardware device resolution and scanning time, there are certain limitations in obtaining high-resolution biomedical images in real-time. Difficult. If a method can be found to reconstruct biomedical images with high accuracy and high resolution in real-time, it will be of great significance to biomedical diagnosis.

Basically, there are three types of image SRR algorithms: methods that use interpolation [1], methods that use reconstruction, and methods that use deep learning [2]. In addition to bicubic, nearest neighbor interpolation and bilinear interpolation are also interpolation-based super-resolution methods [3]. Finding the middle ground [4] and so on. It's easy to use the interpolation-based method, but it can't improve the images' HF information, so the image it makes is blurry. The iterative back-projection method [5], the convex set projection method [6], the maximum posterior probability method [7], and others are all examples of super-resolution

Generative Artificial Intelligence for Biomedical and Smart Health Informatics,
First Edition. Edited by Aditya Khamparia and Deepak Gupta.

techniques that operate on reconstruction. This type of algorithm mainly uses the model to estimate the parameters of a set of highly correlated low-resolution image inputs to achieve high-resolution reconstruction [8]. It not only calculates. It is highly complex and cannot be learned adaptively. When sufficient information cannot be obtained in the scene, the details of the reconstructed high-resolution image will be blurred, or the reconstruction result will be inconsistent with the real image structure [9].

Through adaptive feature extraction, deep learning methods can not only use contextual semantic information to estimate parameters of high-resolution images but also make sure that the reconstruction results and the original images are structurally as close as possible. This is why they are slowly being used in the field of super-resolution [10]. Now, deep learning-based image super-resolution restoration methods mostly fall into two groups: (i) The network reconstructs images at a higher resolution by learning a one-way mapping from the image's low-resolution space to its high-resolution space. (ii) The network reconstructs images at a higher resolution by learning a two-way mapping between the image's low-resolution space and its high-resolution space and using the data that were lost during the down-sampling process. The following is an example of work that was done after learning one-way mapping. The first super-resolution convolutional neural network (SRCNN) was suggested in this chapter [11] in 2014. It gets the semantic information of images through convolution operations and reconstructs it at a very high resolution. Based on SRCNN, the FSRCNN [12], VDSR [13], and ESPCN [14] models make the model easier to compute by deconvolution, reducing the convolution kernel size and sub-pixel convolution processes. In 2017, reconstructing a super-resolution image was Christian's first use of the generative adversarial network [15]. He also came up with the idea of the (super-resolution generative adversarial network [16], SRGAN [17]) network, which gets image semantic information through convolution operations in the generator and does adversarial training with the discriminator at the same time [18]. It instructs the generator on how to create a high-resolution image and how to rate photographs by adding perceptual loss and adversarial loss. Subsequent research uses VDSR [19] and SRGAN [20] as the basic models. When the model extracts low-resolution spatial features [21], it adds skip layer connections, attention modules and designs lightweight structures, and then uses perceptual loss to constrain the image [22]. This can not only make the image's super-resolution rebuilding work better but it can also make the model's convergence speed go faster [23]. The following is an example of the work. Literature by Gao et al. [24] presented a cross-scale nonlocal attention module in 2020 that combined images that were extracted at various sizes. Feature information, while combining local features and nonlocal features at each scale [25], proposed the cross-scale nonlocal attention network

[26], which uses features of different scales at low resolution to classify natural images. SRR was performed. After 4 times SRR [27], the PSNR [28] and SSIM reached 27.80 dB and 0.74. Yuan et al. used the designed lightweight multiscale block [29] to extract multi-scale features of low-resolution space and accelerate the feature fusion of multiple scales to obtain more detailed information. The research proposed the nonlocal sparse attention network [30], which extracts the key information of the feature map of the image in the low-resolution space through the nonlocal sparse attention mechanism. And use this information to perform SRR of the image. The PSNR and SSIM of the image after 4 times SRR are 27.78 dB and 0.74, its performance is not only better than the network using jump layer connection but also the lower number of parameters shortens the modeling time to 1/3 of the original.

Representative work based on learning bidirectional mapping to achieve SRR is as follows. In 2019, Hu et al. used UGnet [31] for image SRR and proposed an improved RUGnet [32] model, which learns natural images' bidirectional mapping between high-resolution space and low-resolution space to obtain the HF information lost in the down-sampling model, and add this information to the up-sampling model for SRR of images. In 2020, Xiao et al. proposed invertible image rescaling (invertible neural network—IRN) [33] was introduced. Through two completely symmetric up-sampling and down-sampling sub-models and a parameter-sharing mechanism, it not only reduced the training parameters but also improved the reconstruction effect of the model. In 2020, Guo et al. proposed dual regression networks [34], which reconstruct low-resolution natural images by designing a down-sampling kernel and design an up-sampling kernel to estimate high-resolution images. This model uses the closed-loop structure formed to provide additional supervision. In addition, image SRR can also be performed using reference images [35]. In 2020, Yang et al. proposed the text transfer network (texture transformer, TTSR) [36], which uses the attention mechanism to extract reference images and high-resolution images. Similar HF information in HF images, the PSNR and SSIM of the image after 4 times SRR are 25.87 dB and 0.784.

At present, image SRR algorithms based on deep learning are basically aimed at natural images. Research on high-resolution reconstruction of biomedical images has not been reported. This is because the characteristics of biomedical images are different from natural images, and biomedical images have many HF components, and the basis for diagnosis also depends to a large extent on the HF components. If there are errors or blurs in the reconstruction of biomedical images, it will seriously affect the biometrics device results. In addition, the SRR of the image improper use of the algorithm will lead to nonunique solutions. To this end, this chapter proposes a nonlocal attention dual network based on sparse coding to achieve the SRR of biometric images. The main contributions are:

1) Learn the bidirectional mapping between the low-resolution space and the high-resolution space of the image through down-sampling and up-sampling parallel dual branches, and use Gaussian constraints and parameter sharing strategies to solve the problem of nonunique solutions during image SRR.
2) To reduce model parameters while ensuring network performance, it is proposed to use the lightweight module provided by the sparse-coding nonlocal attention mechanism to obtain key information in the image and reduce information redundancy while effectively reconstructing high resolution.

Section 16.2 outlines the theoretical and technical aspects of our model. Section 16.3 describes the details of our experimental setup, results, and comparisons. In Section 16.4, we summarize the findings and implications and suggest future research directions.

16.2 Model

Figure 16.1 shows the sparse-coding nonlocal attention dual network (SCN-LADN) structure. There are two main parallel dual branches in the network. These are the down-sampling branches. The down-sampling branch is taught when a high-resolution biometric image is fed into the network, and a low-resolution biometric image is sent out. Through this process, the model learns how to map features from high-resolution images to a low-resolution image, and it also adds Gaussian. To get the changed HF data to fit the Gaussian distribution, constraints are used. When a low-resolution biometric image is fed into the

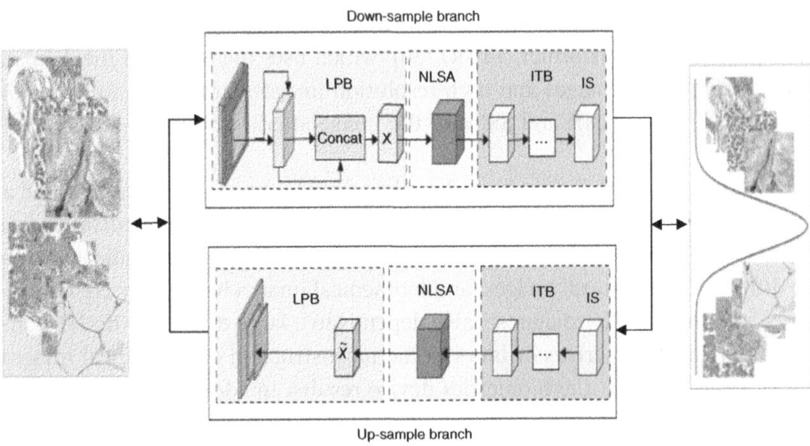

Figure 16.1 SCN-LADN.

model, and a high-resolution biometric image is produced, the up-sampling branch is trained. This means that it learns how to move features from the low-resolution image to the high-resolution image, and at the same time, HF features that comply with Gaussian constraints in the down-sampling branch are embedded into the up-sampling branch through a parameter-sharing strategy, thereby generating high-resolution biometric images.

In the SCN-LADN, the down-sampling branch and the up-sampling are dual transformations of each other. In these two parallel branches, they are mainly composed of the Laplacian pyramid block and the sparse-coding nonlocal. It is composed of the attention module (nonlocal sparse-coding attention, NLSA) and the invertible transform block. In the down-sampling branch, the Laplacian pyramid module down-samples the input image through convolution, up-samples through interpolation, and then uses the original feature map is subtracted from the up-sampled feature map to isolate the image's HF data and is spliced with the original low-frequency (LF) feature map along the channel dimension to form a new feature map X. Therefore, the first 64 channels of the feature map the 64 channels are HF features. The role of the Laplacian pyramid module in the up-sampling branch is to up-sample the feature map that combines LF and HF features by two times to restore the feature map to its original size; the NLSA module extract key information in the feature map through hash coding and avoid information redundancy to the greatest extent; the invertible transformation modules in the two dual branches both contain eight invertible subblocks (invertible subblock), and the invertible transformation module passes through the invertible subblocks. The stacking of nonlinear transformations further separates and fuses the HF information and LF information of the feature map along the channel dimension, that is, learning a bidirectional mapping between the image region with high and low resolution. Parameters are shared between the two branches. With this strategy, the HF information consistent with the Gaussian distribution obtained in the down-sampling branch can be embedded into the up-sampling branch to achieve high-resolution and accurate reconstruction of biomedical images. Figure 16.1 is a schematic diagram of a two- and four-fold super-resolution dual network. The resolution network can be composed of two SCN-LADNs in series.

16.2.1 Sparse-Coding Nonlocal Attention Module

16.2.1.1 Nonlocal Attention

Nonlocal attention can extract important information in the feature map, and extract key features through the correlation between the position to be sought in the feature map and any position. Assume that the input feature map $X = \{x_1, \dots, x_i, x_j, x_k, \dots\}$, $\forall x \in R^c X \in R^{n\times c}$, $f(\cdot,\cdot)$, and pointg$(\cdot)$, the feature point y after the attention mechanism is expressed as:

$$y = \sum_{j=1}^{n} \frac{f(x_i, x_j)}{\sum_{k=1}^{n} f(x_i, x_k)} g(x_j) \tag{16.1}$$

From the above analysis, nonlocal attention obtains the attention of each feature point by calculating the similarity between any two points in the global scope of the image space and then allocates it, which will seriously increase the consumption of computing power.

16.2.1.2 Sparse-Coding Nonlocal Attention Module (NLSA)

Locality-sensitive hash coding is a randomized algorithm for solving the nearest neighbor problem, which operates faster in high-dimensional space. The basic idea is to randomly select a hash function from the locality-sensitive hash function family and convert each data point into a map to the hash table. When searching for neighbor points, only search for points with similar coding values to the query point. For each feature point to be queried, the locally sensitive hash coding method proposed in this chapter quickly searches for feature points with greater correlation with the current query point.

The structure of the sparse-coding nonlocal attention module is shown in Figure 16.2. This module consists of two branches. Branch 1 is used to obtain the hash bucket of the feature map X. The specific process is:

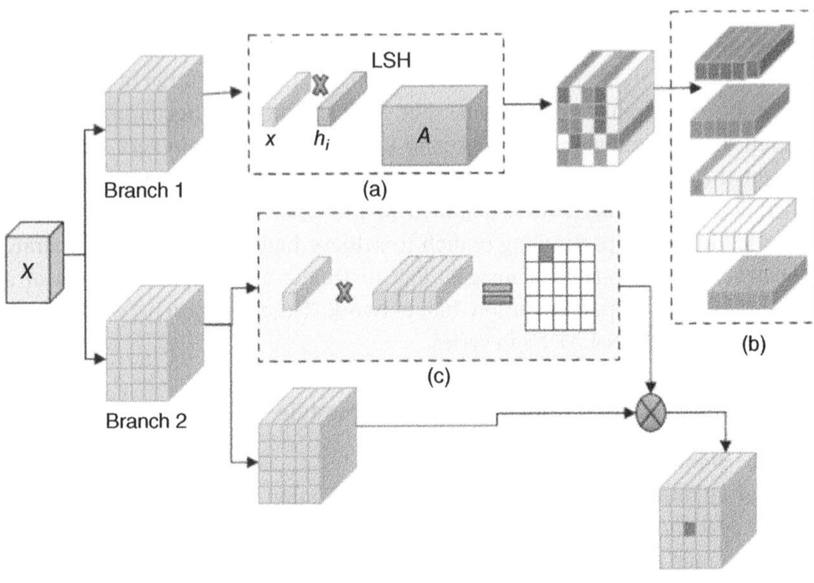

Figure 16.2 Sparse-coding nonlocal attention module.

1) Normalize the feature map X along the channel dimension. Any point x on the feature map is represented by $\hat{x}$ after normalization, and its calculation formula is:

$$\hat{x} = \frac{x}{\sum_{x \in X} \|x\|_2} \tag{16.2}$$

2) Perform hash coding on each feature point. The process is shown in Figure 16.2a. The calculation formula of the coded value F of the feature point $\hat{x}$ is as shown in the equation. The same calculation is done for other feature points.

$$\begin{aligned} F &= \max(A(\hat{x})) \\ &= \max(\{h_1(\hat{x}), h_2(\hat{x}), \dots, h_i(x), \dots, h_n(\hat{x})\}) \end{aligned} \tag{16.3}$$

Among them, A represents a sparse function cluster, $h_i(x)$ represents the ith hash function, and the sparse function cluster A consists of n hash functions $h_i(x)$.

3) Construct a hash bucket based on the coded value of each feature point, as shown in Figure 16.2b. In Figure 16.2b, after each feature point is hashed and coded, the hash bucket is constructed from large to small according to the hash value. After sorting and classification, we finally obtain (I), (II), (III), (IV), (V), m hash buckets, each bucket has k most relevant feature points hash buckets, the expression is as follows:

$$C_j = [\hat{x}^{j,1}, \hat{x}^{j,2}, \dots, \hat{x}^{j,k}], j \in 1, \dots, m \tag{16.4}$$

Among them, $\hat{x}^{j,k}$ represents the kth feature point encoded into the jth bucket. The hash encoding value of the feature point in each bucket is similar.

4) Branch 2 obtains the result of each feature point after the attention mechanism. Taking the feature point $\hat{x}$ as an example, the process is shown in Figure 16.2c. If $A(\hat{x})$ is located in the l bucket, where $l \in [1, m]$, we only need to obtain the correlation between $\hat{x}$ and k feature points in the bucket to obtain the attention score, as shown in equations (16.5) and (16.6):

$$\delta_i = \text{Index}(C_l), l \in [1, m] \tag{16.5}$$

$$y(\hat{x}_i, \delta_i) = \sum_{j \in \bar{z}_i} \frac{f(\hat{x}_i, \hat{x}_j)}{\sum_{k\delta_i} f(\hat{x}_i, \hat{x}_k)} g(\hat{x}_j) \tag{16.6}$$

16.2.2 Reversible Transformation Module

16.2.2.1 Reversible Theory

Literature by Byeon et al. [37] proposed the nonlinear independent component estimation network for modeling complex high-dimensional data. However, the premise of this theory is that the selection of appropriate data feature representation makes the data easier to model. To this end, the source data x is transformed through nonlinear transformation $z = f(x)$ is mapped to the latent space, and the transformed data $p_Z(z)$ conforms to the decomposable distribution, that is, a d-dimensional independent latent variable $p_{Z_d}(z_d)$ is generated to represent the characteristics of the source space. Finally, the latent variable z can be the source data distribution is restored through $\tilde{x} = f^{-1}(z)$, the expression is as follows:

$$p_Z(z) = \prod_d p_{Z_d}(z_d) \tag{16.7}$$

$$p(\tilde{x}) = \prod_d p(z_d)p(\tilde{x} \mid z_d) \tag{16.8}$$

Among them, $p_Z(z)$ is the probability density (PD) distribution function of the latent variable z, d is the dimension of the source data space, $p_{Z_d}(z_d)$ represents the PD distribution function of each dimension of the latent variable, and $p(\tilde{x})$ represents the source space data. The PD function $p(\tilde{x} \mid z_d)$ represents the conditional PD distribution function that f^{-1} needs to be fitted under a specific dimension z_d.

In the down-sampling branch, this chapter uses the above method to map the HF and LF features of high-resolution biomedical images into potential distributions through f-transformation, that is, low-resolution images and HF information consistent with Gaussian distribution. The new LF information and HF information is independent of each other and the dimensions of each HF channel are also independent of each other. That is the affine transformation f is used in the down-sampling branch to pass the HF feature map X_h in the high-resolution image through $X_{h'} = f(X_h)$. Mapping into a Gaussian distribution, that is the potential HF feature map $X_{h'}$, the LF feature map X_l of the image is mapped into the potential LF feature map $X_{l'}$ through and LFF, as shown in Figure 16.3a. In the up-sampling branch, the HF information is restored through the inverse transformation $\tilde{X}_h = f^{-1}\left(X_{h'}\right)$. Similarly, the LF information is restored through the inverse transformation $\tilde{X}_h = f^{-1}\left(X_{h'}\right)$ for recovery, as shown in Figure 16.3b. Among them, f and f^{-1} are composed of eight reversible sub-modules corresponding to the dotted boxes in Figure 16.3a,b. Each reversible sub-module contains a combination of three transformations: ϕ, ρ, and η. Each reversible sub-module is composed of reversible operations through a multi-scale transformation module, features after channel splicing. Taking the 4× down-sampling process as an example, the size of the feature map is marked in the figure.

16.2.2.2 Derivation of Reversible Theory

The probability distribution function $F(x)$ is defined as:

$$F(x) = P(\dot{X} \leqslant x)$$

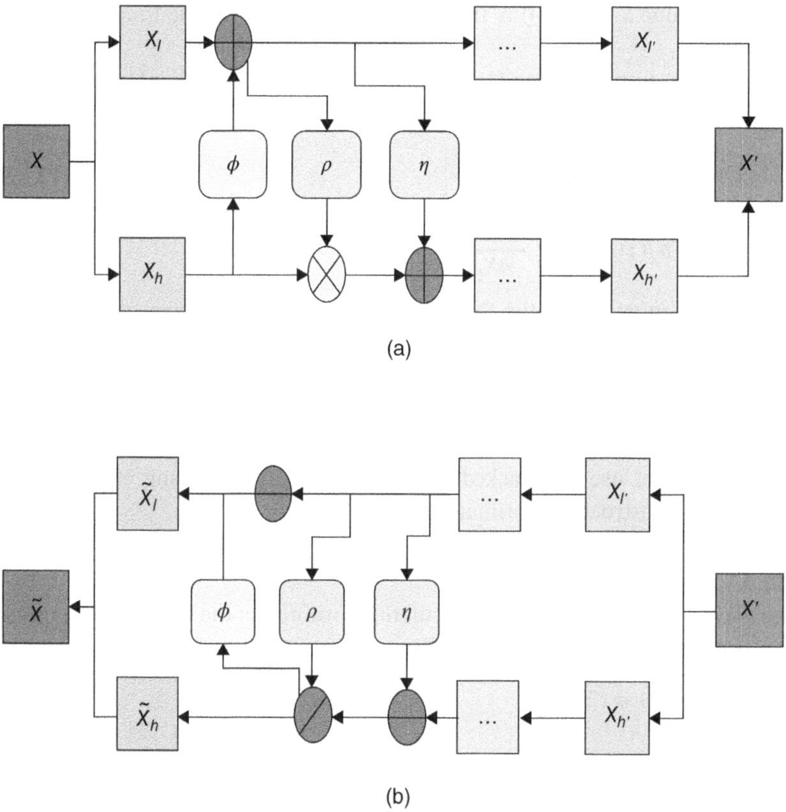

Figure 16.3 Reversible transformation module. (a) Down-sampling reversible transformation module. (b) Up-sampling reversible transformation module.

From $\tilde{x} = f^{-1}(z)$ we can get:

$$F(\tilde{x}) = P(f^{-1}(z) \leqslant x))$$

For $P(\cdot)$, take f on both sides of the brackets at the same time and transform to obtain the representation of $F(x)$ in the latent space:

$$F(\tilde{x}) = P(z \leqslant f(x)) = F_Z(f(x))$$

The PD function $p(\tilde{x})$ of $F(\tilde{x})$ can be obtained by deriving the derivative of x at both ends:

$$p(\tilde{x}) = p_Z(f(x)) \left| \det \left(\frac{\partial f(x)}{\partial x} \right) \right| \tag{16.9}$$

Among them, $F(\cdot)$ represents the distribution function of the variable, and $P(\dot{X} \leqslant x)$ represents the probability that the variable $\dot{X}$ is less than or equal to a certain value x. $p_Z(f(x))$ is the derivative of $F_Z(f(x))$, $\det(\cdot)$ represents the determinant.

It can be seen from equation (16.9) that the expressions of HF information and LF information of high-resolution images are as follows:

$$p(\tilde{X}_h) = p_2(f(X_h)) \left| \det \frac{\partial f(X_h)}{\partial X_h} \right| \tag{16.10}$$

$$p(\tilde{X}_l) = p_Z(f(X_l)) \left| \det \frac{\partial f(X_l)}{\partial X_l} \right| \tag{16.11}$$

Therefore, f must satisfy the following two conditions to recover HF and LF information:

1) f is reversible;
2) The Jacobian of f is easy to calculate.

To this end, we use the stacked reversible structure of Zhang et al. [38] in Figure 16.3 to construct the optimal f.

16.2.2.3 Reversible Operation

In the down-sampling branch, the calculation formulas of the LF and HF features of the reversible sub-module are as follows:

$$X_l^{i+1} = X_l^i + \phi\left(X_h^i\right) \tag{16.12}$$

$$X_h^{i+1} = X_h^i \odot \rho\left(X_l^{i+1}\right) + \eta\left(X_l^{i+1}\right) \tag{16.13}$$

In the same way, the corresponding calculation method for the reversible operation in the upper sampling branch is as follows:

$$X_h^i = \frac{\left(X_h^{i+1} - \eta\left(X_l^{i+1}\right)\right)}{ø\rho\left(X_l^{i+1}\right)} \tag{16.14}$$

$$X_l^i = X_l^{i+1} - \phi\left(X_h^i\right) \tag{16.15}$$

Among them, X_l^i and X_h^i represent the LF and HF features input by the ith reversible sub-module, ϕ represents the additive transformation operation from HF features to LF features, η represents the additive transformation operation from LF features to HF features, ρ represents the multiplicative transformation operation from LF features to HF features, and X_l^{i+1} and X_h^{i+1}, respectively. represent the LF and HF features output by the ith reversible sub-module.

16.2.2.4 Module for Multi-Scale Density

The module for multi-scale density consists of two branches, as shown in Figure 16.4. The two branches of the module use convolution kernels with

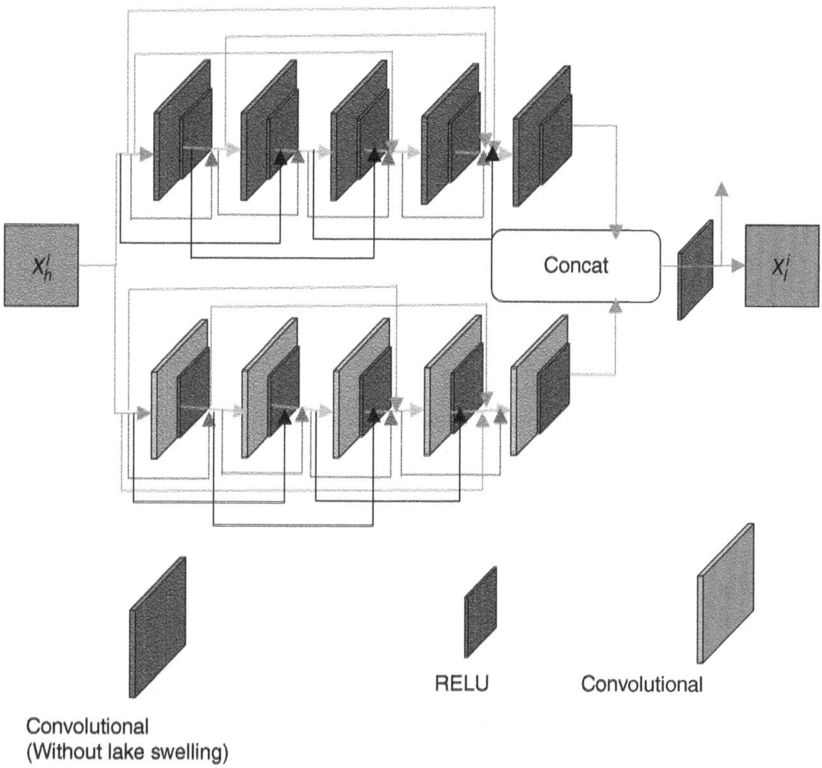

Figure 16.4 Multi-scale module.

expansion rates of 1 and 2, respectively, to obtain the semantic information of images under different receptive fields. The convolution kernel sizes are both 3×3. To avoid gradient disappearance, a skip connection is added between each two layers, and finally the features extracted at different scales are fused to generate a new feature map. The multi-scale dense module can utilize multiple layers in the reversible transformation module scale information to realize the mutual conversion of LF features and HF features. Figure 16.4 is a schematic diagram of the transformation operation from HF features X_h^i to LF features X_l^i, that is, the transformation represented by ϕ. This module acts on ϕ, η, ρ, respectively. Transformation in progress.

16.2.3 Algorithm

Algorithm 16.1 gives the pseudo-code of the SCN-LADN. When training the down-sampling branch, real high-resolution biometric images are used as input,

Algorithm 16.1 SCN-LADN

1. Train the down-sampling branch
2. **Input:** high-resolution images $\{I_1^H\}$ from the biometric image training set
3. **Output:** HF information X_h, consistent with Gaussian distribution, lowresolution image $\{I_i^L\}$
4. Training up-sampling branch
5. **Input:** low-resolution image $\{I_1^L\}$, HF information X_h, consistent with Gaussian distribution
6. **Output:** high resolution image $\{\tilde{I}_1^H\}$
7. **Procedure:**
8. Forall i do:
9. $X_l, X_h, \leftarrow$ Down-sample branch (I_1^H)
10. $\nabla_{DL} L_2 (X_{l'}, I_i^L) +$ Gaussian Constraint $(X_{h'})$ /* Update down sampling branch, L_2 represents the mean square error
11. $\tilde{I}_1^H$-Upsample branch $(I_i^L, x_{h'})$
12. $\nabla_u L_1 (I_i^H, I_i^H)$ /* updates the up-sampling branch, L_1 represents the mean absolute error,
13. Endfor
14. Test $\tilde{I}_t^H \leftarrow$ Upsample branch $(I_t^L, X_{h'} \sim N(0,1))$ /* Test set low-resolution image I_t^L, high-resolution image I_t^H

and low-resolution biometric images and HF features consistent with Gaussian distribution are used as input. Output, the L_2 loss function is used in the modeling process, and Gaussian constraints are applied to the generated HF information. When training the up-sampling branch, the real low-resolution biometric images and Gaussian-constrained HF information are used as upon which the up-sampling network is trained, the produced high-resolution biometric image is used as the output of the up-sampling branch. The modeling process adopts the L_1 loss function.

16.3 Experiments and Results

16.3.1 Data Set

Eight different kinds of human colon tissues stained with hematoxylin and eosin and acquired from the University Medical Center and National Cancer Center Heidelberg, Germany, comprise the historical biomedical images. Twenty thousand low-resolution nonoverlapping colon tissue images chunks are included in the data collection. The high-resolution image measures 224×224, whereas the biomedical image is 56×56. The data set is split up in an 8:1:1 ratio into a training set, a verification set, and a test set. As a result, there are 16,000, 2,000, and 2,000 photos in the test set, training set, verification set, and test set, respectively. The training procedure optimizes the low-resolution images produced by the down-sampling branch and the high-resolution images produced by the up-sampling branch using the L_1 and L_2 loss functions. The model employs the Adam optimizer, including an initial learning rate of 2×10^{-4}, $\beta_1 = 0.9$ and $\beta_2 = 0.999$ are the first- and second-order moment attenuation coefficients, respectively. The training set-up for this model is RTX3090, with a batch size of 4, 100 training iterations, and 86 h of modeling time.

16.3.2 Results and Analysis

The results of SRR of biometric images by SCN-LADN are shown in Figure 16.5.

The results show that after four times SRR of biometric images, PSNR and SSIM reached 30.84 dB and 0.914, respectively, and the reconstructed image maintained a high consistency with the original image in terms of texture, color, and style. Characteristically, the generated high-resolution images were peer-reviewed by different biometrics devices, and a consensus was reached on the effectiveness of the method. In addition, the model is achieved through sparse encoding of non-local attention modules without degrading network performance. To achieve a lightweight design, the number of parameters of the entire network model is only 3.2×106.

In addition, this chapter illustrates the effectiveness of the sparse-coding nonlocal attention dual model by comparing the scope and importance of sparse-coding

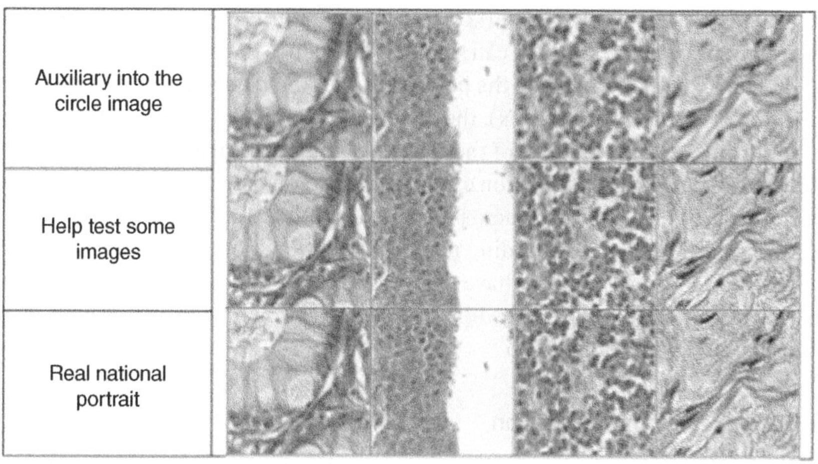

Figure 16.5 Results of SRR of biometric images, using SCN-LADN.

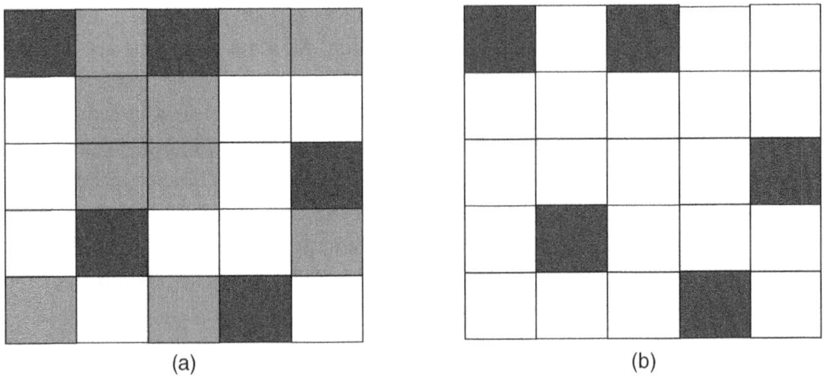

Figure 16.6 Schematic diagram of feature points focused on by different attention mechanisms. (a) Non-local attention. (b) Sparse coding non-local attention.

nonlocal attention and nonlocal attention mechanisms. Figure 16.6a,b is a comparison of the attention range of nonlocal attention and sparse-coding nonlocal attention. The points in Figure 16.6 represent the degree of correlation with the current query point. The darker the color, the greater the correlation. For each feature point to be queried, there exist a nonlocal attention. The local attention mechanism obtains the characteristics of the current query point by calculating the correlation (attention score) between each pixel in the global range of the feature map and the query feature point, which is used for image SRR; while sparse coding in nonlocal attention is encoded through hashing, and only the attention score of the feature pixel with the greatest correlation with the current query point needs to be calculated to obtain the key features of the query point for SRR of the image, Figure 16.6b. Only the darkest features in Figure 16.6a, that is, the key features, can be calculated, which can significantly reduce the number of parameters of the model without reducing the performance of the model. Compared with the Invertible Neural Network (IRN), the volume of parameters decreased by 25.6%.

To further verify the impact of the sparse-coding nonlocal attention module on network performance, an ablation experiment was conducted on this module. The average results of five experiments are listed in Table 16.1. From the results, it can be seen that the sparse-coding nonlocal attention module after ablation, the PSNR and SSIM of the model have declined to a certain extent. This also proves the effectiveness of the sparse-coding nonlocal attention module in extracting key information in the feature map.

16.3.3 Result and Discussion

To verify the super-resolution effect of the SCN-LADN, the results were compared with the bicubic interpolation, SRGAN, CSNL, TTSR, and IRN models.

Table 16.1 Ablation experiment.

	Ablation NLSA module	Proposed
PSNR/dB	30.56	30.84
SSIM	0.908	0.914

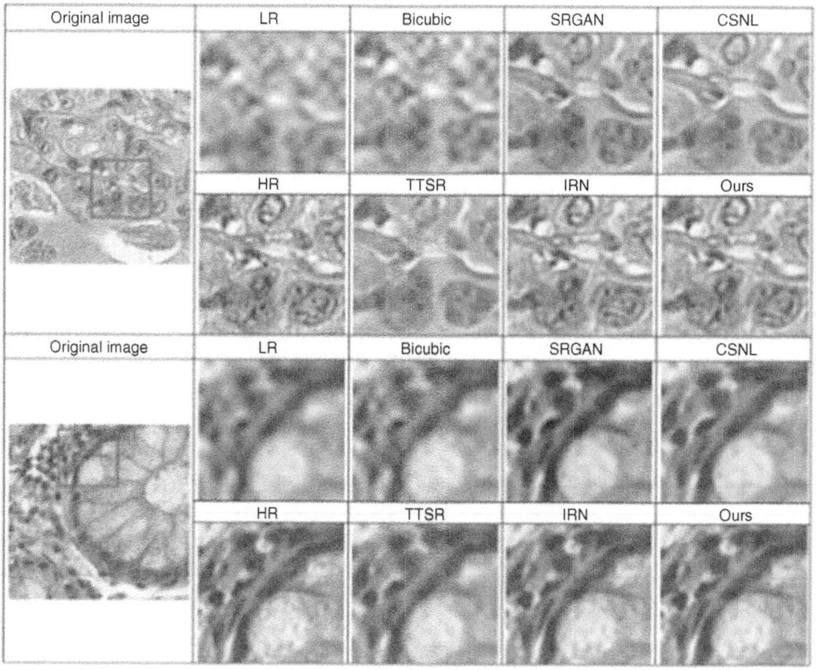

Figure 16.7 Results of four times reconstruction of biomedical tissue images, using different super-resolution algorithms.

Figure 16.7 shows the above method for biomedical images. The result of four times SRR. As can be seen from Figure 16.7, the image details reconstructed by bicubic interpolation are blurred and the color is distorted. This is because the interpolation algorithm cannot increase the HF information of the image, and the large number of color components in the biomedical image also leads to interpolation. The results have color distortion. Although SRGAN and CSNL improve the resolution of the image to a certain extent, they cannot reconstruct the texture information of the image. This is because the super-resolution method based on learning one-way mapping can only learn the low-resolution biometric image space to high-resolution space, and basically realize the mapping of the two spaces through modeling. However, for biomedical images with more details at an HF, this method cannot accurately obtain high-resolution images that are consistent with real images. Although TTSR has HF images for reference during the modeling process, the generated images also have blurry problems in terms of details. This is because the TTSR model reconstructs the current situation by referring to other high-resolution image information. The difference in the distribution of HF information of the image, the reference image, and the image to be restored also causes the image to be blurred during the high-resolution reconstruction process. IRN and SCN-LADNs utilize two branches: up-sampling and down-sampling. The goal is to master the two-way mapping between low- and high-resolution spaces and then to use the HF data acquired during down-sampling to re-create the low-resolution images via secondary learning. This method can not only restore the details and color of the image, etc., but also maintains a high consistency with real high-resolution images. The PSNR and SSIM of its four times super-resolution result are both above 30 dB and 0.91.

Table 16.2 lists the evaluation results of image reconstruction under 4× super-resolution and 2× super-resolution of the SCN-LADN and the above-mentioned super-resolution algorithm. As can be seen from Table 16.2 and Figure 16.8, under 4× and 2× super-resolution, when reconstructing two times

Table 16.2 Quantitative comparison of different super-resolution algorithms.

Method	Scale	Parameters	PSNR/dB	SSIM
Bicubic	×4	—	23.32	0.632
SRgan	×4	1.6×10^6	23.42	0.708
CSNL	×4	1.6×10^6	26.40	0.748
TTSR	×4	6.7×10^6	25.77	0.722
IRN	×4	4.3×10^6	30.57	0.911
Ours	×4	3.2×10^6	30.84	0.914
Bicubic	×2	—	30.15	0.902
SRgan	×2	1.6×10^6	29.50	0.937
CSNL	×2	0.7×10^6	34.35	0.950
TTSR	×2	4.4×10^6	33.87	0.945
IRN	×2	1.6×10^6	38.48	0.984
Ours	×2	1.0×10^6	38.00	0.983

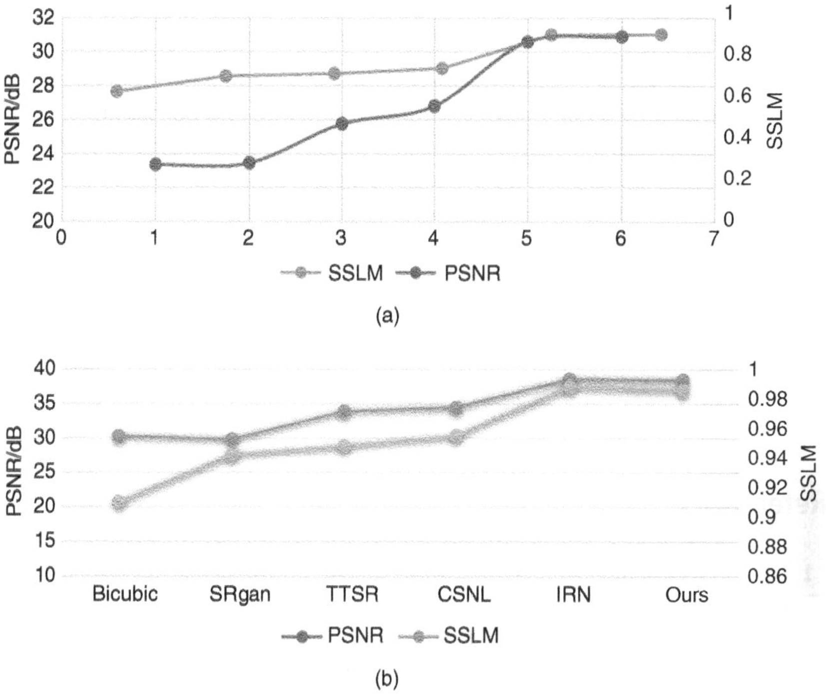

Figure 16.8 Results of different super-resolution algorithms PSNR and SSIM. (a) 4× Super-resolution reconstruction; (b) 2× Super-resolution reconstruction.

the super-resolution image, the SCN-LADN reconstruction effect is better than bicubic interpolation, SRGAN, CSNL, and TTSR algorithms, which shows that the super-resolution method based on bidirectional mapping can take advantage of down-sampling in the dual branch. The HF information generated by the process performs a high-resolution reconstruction of the image. Compared with the one-way mapping method, the reconstruction result has a higher consistency with the real image. Compared with the IRN algorithm, the SCN-LADN4 the PSNR and SSIM of the super-resolution image have been improved to a certain extent, and the parameters have been reduced by 1.1 × 106, which shows that SNADN can extract key features through hash coding with fewer model parameters for SRR. In the 2× super-resolution experiment, although the PSNR and SSIM indicators are slightly lower than IRN, this is due to the low reconstruction magnification and the input image itself already contains obvious feature information, but the IRN model can also relatively easily extract the feature information of the image and perform high-resolution reconstruction of the biometric image.

16.4 Conclusion

This chapter proposed a dual model based on sparse-coding nonlocal attention. This model uses two dual branches of down-sampling and up-sampling, combined with Gaussian constraints and parameter-sharing strategies, to learn the low-resolution space and high-resolution space of biometric images. Bidirectional mapping of space, thereby realizing SRR of historical biomedical images. The PSNR and SSIM of the reconstruction results are 30.84 dB and 0.914. The results show that the dual model based on sparse-coding nonlocal attention not only solves the problem of nonunique solutions in SRR of biomedical images, but the lightweight sparse-coding nonlocal attention module also reduces the computational cost. The key information of the input image can be obtained at the same time, which is an effective SRR method.

References

1 Jia, Y., He, Z., Gholipour, A., and Warfield, S.K. (2016). Single anisotropic 3-D MR image upsampling via overcomplete dictionary trained from in-plane high resolution slices. *IEEE Journal of Biomedical and Health Informatics* 20 (6): 1552–1561. https://doi.org/10.1109/JBHI.2015.2470682.

2 Feng, R., Liu, X., Chen, J. et al. (2020). A deep learning approach for colonoscopy biometric WSI analysis: accurate segmentation and classification. *IEEE Journal of Biomedical and Health Informatics* 25 (10): 3700–3708.

3 Datta, S., Das, V., Dandapat, S. and Deka, B. (2020). A novel framework for enhancement of diagnostic information in MR imaging using super-resolution. *2020 Advanced Communication Technologies and Signal Processing (ACTS)*, pp. 1–6, Silchar, India (4–6 December 2020). IEEE. https://doi.org/10.1109/ACTS49415.2020.9350520.

4 Shirokikh, B., Dalechina, A., Shevtsov, A. et al. (2022). Systematic clinical evaluation of a deep learning method for medical image segmentation: radiosurgery application. *IEEE Journal of Biomedical and Health Informatics* 26 (7): 3037–3046.

5 Datta, S., Dandapat, S. and Deka, B. (2020). A novel framework for enhancement of diagnostic information in MRI using deep super-resolution. *2020 IEEE Applied Signal Processing Conference (ASPCON)*, pp. 94–98, Kolkata, India (7–9 October 2020). IEEE. https://doi.org/10.1109/ASPCON49795.2020.9276697.

6 Qiu, D., Cheng, Y., and Wang, X. (2023). Progressive feedback residual attention network for cardiac magnetic resonance imaging super-resolution. *IEEE Journal of Biomedical and Health Informatics* 27 (7): 3478–3488. https://doi.org/10.1109/JBHI.2023.3272155.

7 Kuang, H., Wang, Y., Liang, Y. et al. (2023). BEA-Net: body and edge aware network with multi-scale short-term concatenation for medical image segmentation. *IEEE Journal of Biomedical and Health Informatics* https://doi.org/10.1109/JBHI.2023.3304662.

8 Zhang, H., Yang, Z., Dong, Z., and Chen, Y. (2024). TNT++: a spectral super-resolution method based on the entropy of pathological images. *IEEE Access* 12: 16586–16597. https://doi.org/10.1109/ACCESS.2023.3336684.

9 Xue, B., Zheng, Q., Li, Z. et al. (2024). Simultaneous high-resolution blind image reconstruction and perturbation defense. *IEEE Access* 12: 36173–36182. https://doi.org/10.1109/ACCESS.2024.3370165.

10 Liang, M., Du, J., Li, L. et al. (2022). Video super-resolution reconstruction based on deep learning and spatio-temporal feature self-similarity. *IEEE Transactions on Knowledge and Data Engineering* 34 (9): 4538–4553. https://doi.org/10.1109/TKDE.2020.3034261.

11 Jiang, J., Yu, Y., Wang, Z. et al. (2020). Ensemble super-resolution with a reference dataset. *IEEE Transactions on Cybernetics* 50 (11): 4694–4708. https://doi.org/10.1109/TCYB.2018.2890149.

12 Zhang, S., Liang, G., Pan, S., and Zheng, L. (2019). A fast medical image super resolution method based on deep learning network. *IEEE Access* 7: 12319–12327. https://doi.org/10.1109/ACCESS.2018.2871626.

13 Liu, P., Hong, Y., and Liu, Y. (2019). Deep differential convolutional network for single image super-resolution. *IEEE Access* 7: 37555–37564. https://doi.org/10.1109/ACCESS.2019.2903528.

14 Sun, N. and Li, H. (2019). Super resolution reconstruction of images based on interpolation and full convolutional neural network and application in medical fields. *IEEE Access* 7: 186470–186479. https://doi.org/10.1109/ACCESS.2019.2960828.

15 Liu, Z., Feng, R., Wang, L. et al. (2022). Dual learning-based graph neural network for remote sensing image super-resolution. *IEEE Transactions on Geoscience and Remote Sensing* 60: 1, 5628614–14. https://doi.org/10.1109/TGRS.2022.3199750.

16 Yang, W., Zhang, X., Tian, Y. et al. (2019). Deep learning for single image super-resolution: a brief review. *IEEE Transactions on Multimedia* 21 (12): 3106–3121. https://doi.org/10.1109/TMM.2019.2919431.

17 Stankiewicz, A., Marciniak, T., Dąbrowski, A., et al. (2016). Matching 3D OCT retina images into super-resolution dataset. *2016 Signal Processing: Algorithms, Architectures, Arrangements, and Applications (SPA)*, pp. 130–137, Poznan, Poland (21–23 September 2016). IEEE. https://doi.org/10.1109/SPA.2016.7763600.

18 Zhang, Y., Wu, G., Yap, P.-T. et al. (2012). Hierarchical patch-based sparse representation—a new approach for resolution enhancement of 4D-CT lung

data. *IEEE Transactions on Medical Imaging* 31 (11): 1993–2005. https://doi.org/10.1109/TMI.2012.2202245.

19 Datta, S., Deka, B., Dandapat, S. et al. (2022). Enhancement of diagnostic information in T1-weighted contrast enhanced MRI using deep back-projection based super-resolution. *2022 IEEE 19th India Council International Conference (INDICON)*, pp. 1–6, Kochi, India (24–26 November 2022). IEEE. https://doi.org/10.1109/INDICON56171.2022.10039876.

20 Jiang, X., Xu, Y., Wei, P. and Zhou, Z. (2020). CT image super resolution based on improved SRGAN. *2020 5th International Conference on Computer and Communication Systems (ICCCS)*, pp. 363–367, Shanghai, China (15–18 May 2020). IEEE. https://doi.org/10.1109/ICCCS49078.2020.9118497.

21 Ma, S. and Fang, B. (2012). Optical image reconstruction using frequency-domain simulations: optimization of detector positions. *2012 Proceedings of International Conference on Modelling, Identification and Control*, pp. 68–73, Wuhan, China.

22 Kobayashi, N., Suzuki, H., Ishikawa, M. et al. (2020). Telebiometric support system with gross specimen image using high resolution 4K multispectral camera. *2020 42nd Annual International Conference of the IEEE Engineering in Medicine & Biology Society (EMBC)*, pp. 1388–1391, Montreal, QC (20–24 July 2020). IEEE. https://doi.org/10.1109/EMBC44109.2020.9175398.

23 Kwon, K.-C., Kwon, K.H., Erdenebat, M.-U. et al. (2019). Resolution-enhancement for an integral imaging microscopy using deep learning. *IEEE Photonics Journal* 11 (1): 1, 6900512–12. https://doi.org/10.1109/JPHOT.2018.2890429.

24 Gao, Z., Qu, Z., Wang, H., and Ma, C. (2021). Characterization of two-phase flow structure by deep learning-based super resolution. *IEEE Transactions on Circuits and Systems II: Express Briefs* 68 (2): 782–786. https://doi.org/10.1109/TCSII.2020.3017241.

25 Soni, M. and Kumar, D. (2020). Wavelet based digital watermarking scheme for medical images. *2020 12th International Conference on Computational Intelligence and Communication Networks (CICN)*, pp. 403-407, Bhimtal, India (25–26 September 2020). https://doi.org/10.1109/CICN49253.2020.9242626.

26 Zhao, L., Sun, Q., and Zhang, Z. (2017). Single image super-resolution based on deep learning features and dictionary model. *IEEE Access* 5: 17126–17135. https://doi.org/10.1109/ACCESS.2017.2736058.

27 Ping, B., Su, F., Han, X., and Meng, Y. (2021). Applications of deep learning-based super-resolution for sea surface temperature reconstruction. *IEEE Journal of Selected Topics in Applied Earth Observations and Remote Sensing* 14: 887–896. https://doi.org/10.1109/JSTARS.2020.3042242.

28 Yuan, Z., Yang, D., Pan, H., and Liang, Y. (2020). Axial super-resolution study for optical coherence tomography images via deep learning. *IEEE Access* 8: 204941–204950. https://doi.org/10.1109/ACCESS.2020.3036837.

29 Yuan, F., Zhou, S., Cheng, T., and Liu, Y. (2022). A low- and high-resolution terahertz image pair construction method with gradient fusion for learning-based super-resolution. *IEEE Access* 10: 132506–132514. https://doi.org/10.1109/ACCESS.2022.3230506.

30 Yi, Z., Hu, J., Zhao, Y. et al. (2023). Fast and calibrationless low-rank parallel imaging reconstruction through unrolled deep learning estimation of multi-channel spatial support maps. *IEEE Transactions on Medical Imaging* 42 (6): 1644–1655. https://doi.org/10.1109/TMI.2023.3234968.

31 Matsuura, M., Zhou, J., Akino, N., and Yu, Z. (2021). Feature-aware deep-learning reconstruction for context-sensitive X-ray computed tomography. *IEEE Transactions on Radiation and Plasma Medical Sciences* 5 (1): 99–107. https://doi.org/10.1109/TRPMS.2020.3040882.

32 Gao, Q., Ding, R., Wang, L. et al. (2023). LRIP-Net: low-resolution image prior-based network for limited-angle CT reconstruction. *IEEE Transactions on Radiation and Plasma Medical Sciences* 7 (2): 163–174. https://doi.org/10.1109/TRPMS.2022.3217517.

33 Wei, Y., Li, Y., Ding, Z. et al. (2021). SAR parametric super-resolution image reconstruction methods based on ADMM and deep neural network. *IEEE Transactions on Geoscience and Remote Sensing* 59 (12): 10197–10212. https://doi.org/10.1109/TGRS.2021.3052793.

34 Xue, X., Wang, Y., Li, J. et al. (2020). Progressive sub-band residual-learning network for MR image super resolution. *IEEE Journal of Biomedical and Health Informatics* 24 (2): 377–386. https://doi.org/10.1109/JBHI.2019.2945373.

35 Jirik, R., Peterlík, I., Ruiter, N. et al. (2012). Sound-speed image reconstruction in sparse-aperture 3-D ultrasound transmission tomography. *IEEE Transactions on Ultrasonics, Ferroelectrics, and Frequency Control* 59 (2): 254–264. https://doi.org/10.1109/TUFFC.2012.2185.

36 Lin, X., Zhou, X., Tong, T., et al. (2022). BSG-Net: a blind super-resolution guided network for improving ultrasound image segmentation. *2022 IEEE International Conference on Knowledge Graph (ICKG)*, pp. 172–179, Orlando, FL (30 November 2022–1 December 2022). IEEE. https://doi.org/10.1109/ICKG55886.2022.00029.

37 Byeon, H., Al-Kubaisi, M., Dutta, A.K. et al. (2024). Brain tumor segmentation using neuro-technology enabled intelligence-cascaded U-Net model. *Frontiers in Computational Neuroscience* 18: 1391025. https://doi.org/10.3389/fncom.2024.1391025.

38 Zhang, J., Li, J., Sun, H. et al. (2022). Edge-enabled anti-noise telebiometric imaging reconstruction technology in harsh environments. *IEEE Network* 36 (4): 92–99. https://doi.org/10.1109/MNET.002.2100650.

17

Tackling the Complexities of Federated Learning

Raj Thakur[1], Shreyansh Patel[1], Neelesh Singh[1], Aaryan Barde[2], and Snehlata Barde[3]

[1] *Department of Artificial Intelligence, Sage University, Indore, MP, India*
[2] *Department of CSE-AIML, LNCT Group of Collage, Bhopal, MP, India*
[3] *Department of CSE-CS, PIET Parul University, Vadodara Gujrat, India*

17.1 Introduction

In machine learning (ML) and artificial intelligence (AI), data always plays a crucial role in these emerging technologies. Without data, we can't imagine these technologies as possible. In decision-making, we leverage ML, envisioning it as a process where a system learns continuously, both during and after making decisions. ML finds applications ranging from spam detection to recommendation systems based on individual preferences, and even in healthcare, it extracts insights from various sources [1].

For all these tasks, data are required from different sources such as mobile devices, hospitals, or various decentralized data centers' also known as data silos. However, collecting this vast amount of data in a single place is very challenging on its own, and the data can be sensitive, such as financial or medical data containing information about an individual. The solution to this problem is not to move the data from its original location but instead to move the model to this local decentralized data. This approach to training the ML model is known as federated learning (FL). In FL, the ML model is shared with multiple decentralized data centers, also known as client servers, where data are not shared, and these remain locally. This decentralized approach enables us to share the ML model with distributed clients to achieve better and expected outcomes while keeping the data decentralized [2]. The coordination between the client's server and the main central server remains key to the success of this collaborative approach. It involves the transfer of learned model parameters from the local server to the central server; this process is repeated for serval rounds until we get the expected

Generative Artificial Intelligence for Biomedical and Smart Health Informatics,
First Edition. Edited by Aditya Khamparia and Deepak Gupta.

performance. This basic idea illustrates how the model can learn the rules without having access to the raw data.

In this chapter, we propose to explain the challenges that come with the implementation of collaborative learning on decentralized data. We have discussed various challenges like maintaining the privacy of the decentralized sensitive data (financial data, healthcare, or any kind of data that can reveal information about an individual and communication between the data silos, also known as local server and central server, also known as global server), and discussed techniques that can potentially use to overcome the challenges. We also have discussed some of the applications of FL that are seen in the modern tech world, which is full of advanced technologies and innovation.

17.2 Why We Come to Federated Learning

FL stands out as a groundbreaking approach to ML, tailored to meet essential requirements that traditional centralized methods often struggle with. Its core principle revolves around preserving user privacy by decentralizing the model training process, thereby ensuring that sensitive data remains securely stored on individual devices. This emphasis on privacy is paramount in today's regulatory landscape, where stringent data protection measures are crucial. In addition, FL excels in scenarios where data is distributed across numerous devices or locations, eliminating the need for cumbersome centralized data handling and transfer [3]. This decentralized approach not only enhances scalability by leveraging edge devices' computational resources but also significantly reduces communication overhead, making it particularly suitable for bandwidth-constrained environments. Furthermore, FL facilitates edge computing by enabling on-device model training, empowering edge devices to learn and adapt in real-time without relying on centralized infrastructure. By addressing these vital requirements—privacy preservation, distributed data handling, scalability, reduced communication costs, and support for edge computing—FL emerges as a versatile and indispensable solution for navigating the complexities of contemporary ML challenges [6].

17.3 Related Work

McMahan et al. (2017) provide a comprehensive analysis of FL, focusing on communication-efficient learning from decentralized data and strategies. They elucidate the core concepts, highlighting the interplay between decentralized data architectures and communication efficiency while also exploring diverse applications across domains. The work delves into the challenges faced in FL implementations, offering valuable insights into overcoming technical hurdles. Kairoz et al. [14] offer an extensive review encompassing FL strategies, applications in various domains, and the inherent challenges. Their emphasis on privacy-preserving ML techniques, particularly differential privacy, adds depth to the discussion, addressing critical aspects of data privacy and security. Abadi et al. [16] delve into privacy preservation within ML and its integration with FL, emphasizing the effectiveness of differential privacy methods in maintaining data confidentiality. Bonawitz et al. [17] contribute by discussing the system design and architecture necessary for scalable FL implementations while also addressing ethical and societal implications, including considerations for responsible AI practices. Lastly, Ramage and Ohlson [15] navigate the ethical and societal dimensions of FL, advocating for equitable data-sharing paradigms and responsible AI frameworks, thereby fostering a more inclusive and ethically sound approach to FL.

17.4 Challenges in Federated Learning

Here are some challenges that need to be highlighted to overcome these obstacles in the way of collaborative learning without centralizing the data:

1) **Privacy and Security:** FL is mainly applicable to decentralized privacy-sensitive data that can reveal individuals' personal information and training without exposing data to anyone. Even if the data are not centralized, some potential risks may expose the client's data. Some of the limitations of FL that cause privacy issues are:
   - **Model Updates**: During the updated weights communication between the local and central servers, there is potential that the attacker can interpret these weights to find the pattern in the data present at the client's hand if the device that is communicating is not secure.
   - **Metadata:** Even if the actual data are not shared, the metadata associated with the training process, such as timing and frequency of weight update transition, can potentially put privacy at risk.
   - **Adversarial Attacks:** Sophisticated adversarial attacks such as model inversion attacks, membership inference attacks, or model extraction attacks take insight into the local data.
2) **Data Inspection**: The second problem in implementing FL is the inability to inspect data directly. The data are available at the local level. These decentralized data make it difficult to inspect the data directly. The privacy-concise nature of the data makes traditional data inspection techniques impractical. FL maintains the data on the client's server, preventing direct access to a single data point.

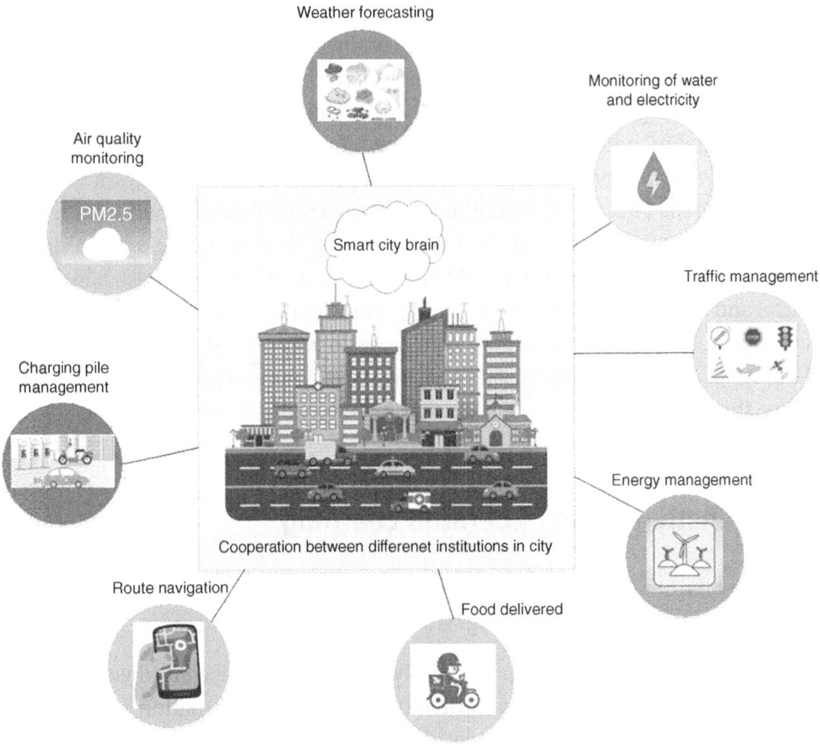

Figure 17.1 Collaborative representation of federated learning. https://ieeexplore.ieee.org/document/9163027

3) **Model Updated Weights Aggregation and Communication:** Model updated and weights aggregation are essential components of the collaborative FL approach. Updates are generated at the local server, each containing unique data points. The update represents the changes to the global model after each training round on local data that need to be transmitted to the global model. The communication overhead should be maintained to increase efficiency and computation. The main part of FL, which remains a challenging facet, is to aggregate these updates.
4) **Model Selection:** In FL, model selection involves considering not only the task and data characteristics but also the distributed nature of the training. Models should be chosen to accommodate decentralized training across multiple devices while preserving privacy. Figure 17.1 shows the collaborative representation of FL.

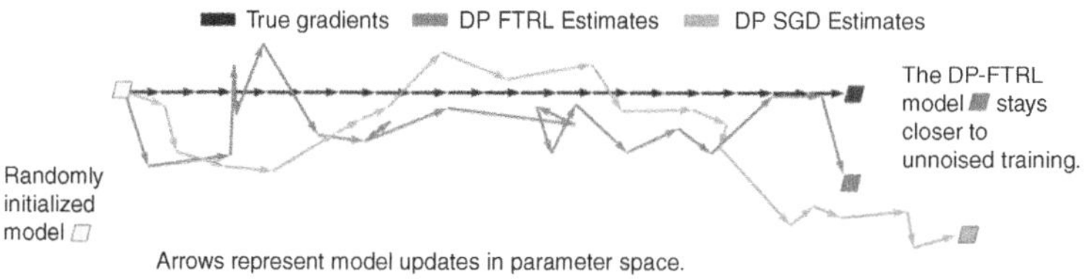

Figure 17.2 Distortion in true gradient by adding random noise before updating to the global model.

17.5 Techniques Used in Federated Learning

There are some techniques to address these challenges that must be used to deal with these issues, such as maintaining the data privacy and security of the clients and maintaining the communication between the local and central servers. The following techniques can be leveraged:

(1) **Privacy and Security Control**
   - **Differential Privacy Method:** This technique adds some random noises in the gradients or updated weights before transmitting to the central server so that no single data can be reconstructed from the aggregated updates. Figure 17.2 shows the distortion in the true gradient by adding random noise before updating to the global model.

In practice, we use Laplace noise while computing differential privacy. Laplace noise is added to the query response, and the amount of noise to add is controlled by the parameter "privacy budget" ($^{\varepsilon}$). The lower the values of the privacy budget, the higher will be the security by introducing more noise in the gradient. This technique also introduces some challenges to handling this random noise and makes FL more complex to practice. There is a trade-off between the noise and the ability to handle this noise according to the user's data. It has some rules that are essential for the overall effectiveness of FL, these rules are:

- Data must be large enough to be completely understood by the FL model. Due to the introduction of noise in the data, it becomes hard for the model to capture the effective weights.
- To get acceptable performance in the FL, these noises must be effectively handled by the central model while aggregating local updates.

Laplace Mechanism for adding noise in the gradient before updating to the global model:

Numerical queries, such as $f: N^{x} \rightarrow R^{k}$, are the most fundamental for many database queries. These quarries map the databases to k real numbers. $l1$

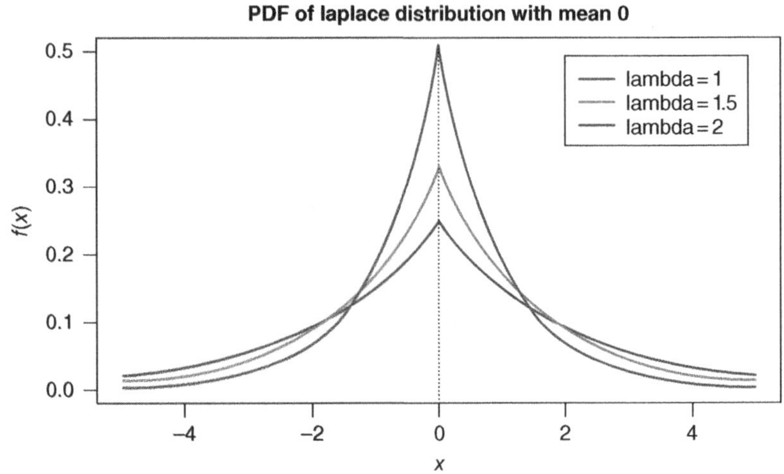

Figure 17.3 Laplace distribution.

sensitivity is the important parameter that determines the accuracy with which we answer these queries. The $l1$ sensitivity of the function f is shown in Figure 17.3.

- **Homomorphic Encryption**: This method is first introduced in the 1970s by cryptographers (Ron Rivest, Adi Shamir, and Leonard Adleman). It was introduced to secure the communication and processing of sensitive data. It involves the processing of the data in the encrypted form without decryption, which ensures that the data during and before processing are not exposed. The two parties having the same encryption key only can decrypt the data. So, overall, the privacy is maintained. In the context of FL, we can use this method to effectively preserve the privacy of the sensitive data that even the central server does not have access to. This method is most effective when the data are highly complex and sensitive, and extensive computation is required. It guarantees to ensure secure computation [7]. The choice between differential privacy and homomorphic encryption is fully dependent on the requirement and nature of the data. This approach is somewhat computationally intensive to perform the computation on the encrypted data. We have also tried this approach in our FL simulation on the MNIST dataset. Figure 17.4 shown the illustration of the encryption and decryption.

(2) **Data Inspection Technique**

In FL mode, the data remain decentralized, causing the inability to directly access the data. Google researchers have solved this problem by processing the aggregated outputs using a generative adversarial network commonly known as GAN. These generative models are capable of inspecting the data

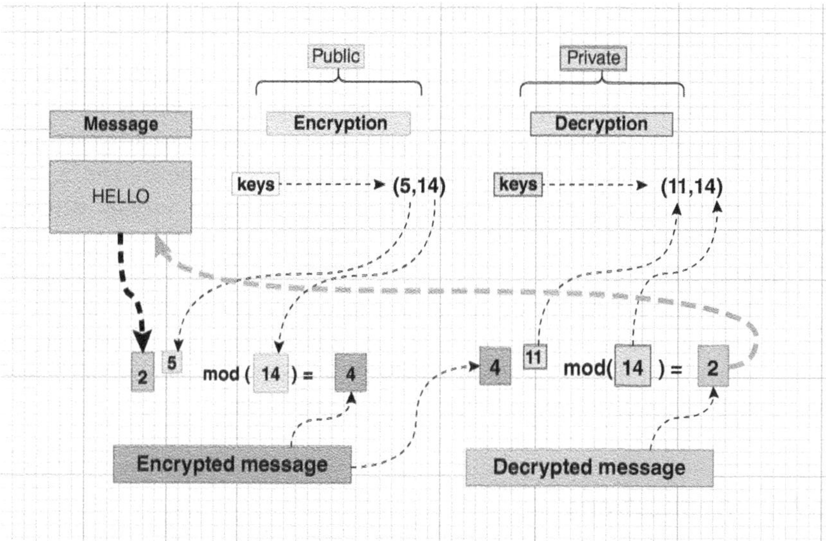

Figure 17.4 Illustration of the encryption and decryption.

indirectly. It is important to have some knowledge about the structure and type of data while inspecting the data.

(3) **Server Communication**

Secure Aggregation: Secure aggregation is a critical component in FL. It enables the server to learn the aggregate model of the users without observing their local models. Secure aggregation methods, such as secure multi-party computation (SMPC), are employed to ensure privacy during the model aggregation process [4]. Participants can collectively compute the average without revealing their individual updates. Conventionally, secure aggregation algorithms focus on ensuring the privacy of individual users in a single training round. However, there's an important challenge: privacy leakages over multiple training rounds due to partial user selection or participation at each round of FL. To address this, a recent research paper introduces a new framework called Multi-Round Sec Agg [5]. This framework provides multi-round privacy guarantees by quantifying privacy over multiple training rounds and developing a structured user selection strategy. It ensures the long-term privacy of each user across any number of rounds while considering fairness and the average number of participating users.

Compression Technique: The model updates are compressed before aggregating the local model to the global model to lower the communication overhead and effectively communicate with the global server. Various methods, such as quantization or scarcity, are applied to reduce the bandwidth requirement and speed up the communication, making it more efficient.

Asynchronous Updates: Instead of synchronously waiting for all devices to complete their updates before aggregating, asynchronous FL allows updates to be aggregated in a more continuous and decentralized manner. This technique is used to improve the updated efficiency and reduce communication delays. Making it more versatile in various network conditions.

(4) **Model Selection**

Federated averaging is a common approach that uses algorithms like Federated Averaging (FedAvg). Consider the communication overhead, robustness to non-IID (Independent and Identically) data distribution, and potential privacy concerns when selecting a model for FL.

17.6 Applications

1) **Healthcare:** FL is particularly valuable in healthcare, where data privacy is paramount. It allows healthcare institutions to collaborate on improving predictive models while keeping patient data decentralized and secure. For example, FL can be used to develop models for disease prediction, personalized treatment recommendations, and medical image analysis [8].
2) **Finance:** In the financial sector, FL enables banks and financial institutions to collaborate on fraud detection, risk assessment, and customer profiling without sharing sensitive customer data. This approach enhances security and compliance with regulatory requirements while improving the accuracy of predictive models [9].
3) **Smartphones and IoT Devices:** FL is well-suited for training models on smartphones and IoT devices, where data are generated locally. Applications include predictive text input, personalized recommendations, and activity recognition. By training models directly on user devices, FL minimizes the need for data transmission and preserves user privacy [12].
4) **Autonomous Vehicles:** FL can be applied to autonomous vehicles to improve perception systems, decision-making algorithms, and vehicle control. By collaboratively learning from data collected across a fleet of vehicles, FL can enhance safety, efficiency, and adaptability while respecting user privacy [9].
5) **Edge Computing:** FL enables edge devices such as edge servers, sensors, and drones to collaboratively learn and adapt to changing conditions in real-time. This is useful in applications such as environmental monitoring, industrial automation, and smart cities, where data are generated and processed at the network edge [10].

Table 17.1 Result of different parameters in HE and DP.

Serial	Parameter	Homomorphic encryption	Differential privacy
1	Precision	0.989674	0.8304
2	Recall	0.989636	0.829
3	Accuracy	98.97	83.06
4	RMSE	0.437	1.617

17.7 Result and Analysis

The result of this review chapter seems to be very practically helpful in implementing FL in real-life applications with its main aim of preserving privacy throughout this collaborative process. The results of different parameters in HE and DP are shown in Table 17.1.

The differential privacy is very effectively suited to the task where the dataset is very large and gives an acceptable model performance. Whereas homomorphic encryption is computationally expensive but guarantees the security of the decentralized data unless the encryption keys are in safe hands. The combination of these two privacy-preserving methods can also work together to give the overall performance. The graphical presentation of Table 17.1 is shown in Figure 17.5.

17.8 Conclusion

In this work, we have seen some challenges that occur while practicing the collaborative ML process when the data are decentralized, not located at different data locations, and due to the inability to share these data as they are privacy and security issues. Preserving privacy is the main fundamental challenge in FL mode, and the technique that can be used is the differential privacy method to randomly add some changes in the true output before transmitting the updates to the global model. Model aggregation and communication between multiple models should support privacy and improve efficiency during these processes. Even if we use various privacy-preserving techniques, there is still some possibility that updates can be leaked to a third person other than the client and central server; the least we can do is ensure that the network of communication is secure and use SMPC can enhance the privacy-preserving performance in federated mode. Preprocessing is an important process before developing a successful model, and directly inspecting the data before training the ML model is quite impractical as the data are not

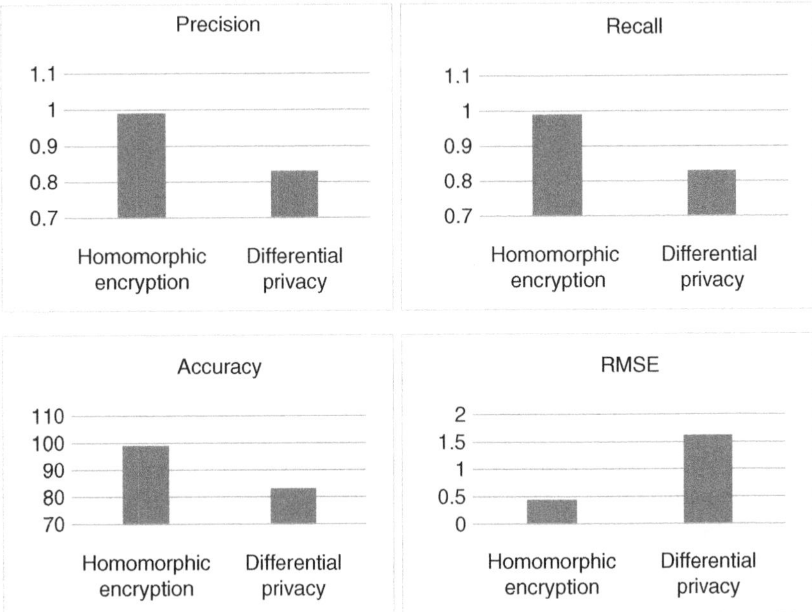

Figure 17.5 Values of precision, recall, accuracy, and RMSE.

locally present while training the model. This issue is sorted by using the generative model in the FL to inspect the data. This chapter gives us the references that can be used for future work.

References

1 Salah, K., Rehman, M.H., Nizamuddin, N., and Al-Fuqaha, A. (2019). Blockchain for ai: review and open research challenges. *IEEE Access* 7: 10127–10149.

2 Gai, K., Wu, Y., Zhu, L. et al. (2019). Privacy-preserving energy trading using consortium blockchain in smart grid. *IEEE Transactions on Industrial Informatics* 15 (6): 3548–3558.

3 Barde, S. and Pandey, R. (2023). EEG-based emotion classification for movie clips with support vector machine. *European Chemical Bulletin* 12 (5): 1393–1400.

4 Nassar, M., Salah, K., Rehman, M.H., and Svetinovic, D. (2020). Blockchain for explainable and trustworthy artificial intelligence. *Wiley Interdisciplinary Reviews: Data Mining and Knowledge Discovery* 10 (1): e1340.

5 Gai, K., Wu, Y., Zhu, L. et al. (2019). Permissioned blockchain and edge computing empowered privacy-preserving smart grid networks. *IEEE Internet of Things Journal* 6 (5): 7992–8004.

6 Barde, S. and Tiwari, S. (2023). Scientific approach of prediction for professions using machine learning classification techniques. *International Journal of Modern Education and Computer Science* 15 (4): 30–42.

7 Kang, J., Xiong, Z., Niyato, D. et al. (2019). *Reliable Federated Learning for Mobile Networks*. IEEE.

8 Lim, W.Y.B., Luong, N.C., Hoang, D.T. et al. (2019). *Federated Learning in Mobile Edge Networks: A Comprehensive Survey*. IEEE.

9 Rehman, M.H., Liew, C.S., Wah, T.Y., and Khan, M.K. (2017). Towards next-generation heterogeneous mobile data stream mining applications: opportunities challenges and future research directions. *Journal of Network and Computer Applications* 79: 1–24.

10 Rehman, M.H., Batool, A., and Salah, K. (2019). The rise of proximal mobile edge servers. *IT Professional* 21 (3): 26–32.

11 Patel, B., Dubey, V., Barde, S., and Sharma, N. (2024). Optimum path planning using dragonfly-fuzzy hybrid controller for autonomous Vehicle. *Eng* 5 (1): 246–265.

12 Singh, K.K. and Barde, S. (2024). A feasible adaptive fuzzy genetic technique for face, fingerprint, and palmprint based multimodal biometrics systems. *Journal of Current Science and Technology* 14 (1). https://doi.org/10.59796/jcst.V14N1.2024.1.

13 McMahan, B., Moore, E., Ramage, D., and Hampson, S. (2017). Communication-efficient learning of deep networks from decentralized data. *Proceedings of the 20th International Conference on Artificial Intelligence and Statistics (AISTATS)* 2017.

14 Kairoz, P., Liu, Z., and Steinke, T. (2019). The distributed discrete Gaussian mechanism for federated learning with secure aggregation. In *Proceedings of the 38th International Conference on Machine Learning (PMLR)*. 139, 5201–5212. http://proceedings.mlr.press/v139/kairouz21a/kairouz21a.pdf.

15 Ramage, D. and Ohlson, S. (2021). Federated analytics: collaborative data science without data collection. Google AI Blog (May 27). https://ai.googleblog.com/2020/05/federated-analytics-collaborative-data.html.

16 Abadi, P., Sinha, R., Lebedev, I. et al. (2016). A formal foundation for secure remote execution of enclaves. In *Proceedings of the ACM SIGSAC Conference on Computer and Communications Security*, pp. 2435–2450. https://dl.acm.org/doi/10.1145/3133956.3134098.

17 Bonawitz, K., Ivanov, V., Kreuter, B. et al. (2017). Practical secure aggregation for privacy-preserving machine learning. In *Proceedings of the 2017ACM SIGSAC Conference on Computer and Communications Security*, pp. 1175–1191. ACM, 2017.

18

Revolutionizing Healthcare: The Impact of AI-Powered Sensors

Veenadhari Bhamidipaty[1], *Durgananda Lahari Bhamidipaty*[2], *Indira Guntoory*[3], *Kanaka Durga Prasad Bhamidipaty*[4], *Karthikeyan P. Iyengar*[5,6,7], *Bhuvan Botchu*[8], *and Rajesh Botchu*[4,6,9]

[1] *Department of Computer Science and Engineering, Gandhi Institute of Technology and Management, Visakhapatnam, Andhra Pradesh, India*
[2] *Department of Biotechnology, Manipal Institute of Technology, Manipal, Karnataka, India*
[3] *Department of Obstetrics & Gynaecology, GIMSR, Visakhapatnam, India*
[4] *Department of Radiology, NRIIMS, Visakhapatnam, India*
[5] *Department of Orthopedics, Southport and Ormskirk Hospital Southport, Mersey and West Lancashire Hospitals NHS Trust, Southport, UK*
[6] *AHERF, Hyderabad, India*
[7] *Edge Hill University, Ormskirk, UK*
[8] *Solihull School, Solihull, UK*
[9] *Department of Musculoskeletal Radiology, Royal Orthopedic Hospital, Birmingham, UK*

18.1 Introduction

Healthcare is undergoing a transformation thanks to the combination of artificial intelligence (AI) and sensor technology, which improves patient monitoring, allows for individualized therapy, and increases diagnostic accuracy. This synthesis examines the fundamental ideas found in a selection of works that highlight the implications of wearable sensors and robots in healthcare settings, as well as the impact of AI.

AI-powered sensors are greatly improving patient monitoring and illness diagnosis. For example, wearables incorporating AI algorithms have shown a high sensitivity of over 90% in identifying seizures in people with epilepsy. In a similar vein, wearable biosensing technologies with AI support are expanding the frontiers of customized medicine by effectively handling high-dimensional data for fatigue monitoring and illness diagnosis. These developments highlight the possibility of ongoing monitoring of health status outside of conventional clinical settings and early detection.

Generative Artificial Intelligence for Biomedical and Smart Health Informatics,
First Edition. Edited by Aditya Khamparia and Deepak Gupta.

AI techniques have revolutionized the field of cardiac care by improving the accuracy of electrocardiography analysis by identifying the signs of sick states. Advances in three-dimensional cardiac imaging have made it possible to simulate virtual hearts, which is a step toward better understanding and treatment planning of cardiac arrhythmias.

AI-powered e-health strategies have also improved neurological care. Through real-world data analysis, the digitization of clinical data in conjunction with cutting-edge computer approaches allows for more accurate prognoses for diseases such as multiple sclerosis. Wearable sensors offer real-time data that may be processed with machine learning algorithms to assess therapy efficacy or gain a better understanding of how a disease is progressing.

AI is starting to make an appearance in anesthesia through robotics that improves accuracy during treatments or supports decision-making processes based on thorough data analysis. Similar to this, neuromorphic sensory systems use electronic devices engineered to handle information as efficiently as neurons can replicate biological senses, pointing to advancements in the development of more natural-feeling human–machine interfaces for use in medical applications.

The integration of robotics and AI is bringing about revolutionary improvements to the operating room environment. Through improved surgical training experiences fueled by real-time feedback mechanisms and augmented reality systems that recreate realistic settings for practitioners, this synergy promises to achieve precision surgery.

Nevertheless, because wearables record different physiological signals, issues with performance consistency across different populations persist despite these encouraging advancements. Furthermore, to build physicians' confidence in the dependability of these new technologies, concerns about the transparency and interpretability of machine learning algorithms must be addressed.

Future work should concentrate on improving AI models through comprehensive validation tests, making sure that privacy problems related to the collection of private health information through wearables are systematically addressed, and ethical considerations are taken into account. Furthermore, to successfully overcome the current barriers to incorporating new technologies into conventional clinical practice without sacrificing patient safety or high standards of care delivery, interdisciplinary cooperation will be essential.

18.2 Evolution of Healthcare Technology

A revolutionary era in healthcare administration and delivery has begun with the advancement of healthcare technology, especially with AI-powered sensors. This synthesis examines the effects and ramifications of such breakthroughs by drawing on recent literature.

Deep learning, a method of integrating AI into healthcare, presents hitherto unseen possibilities for end-to-end learning models from large, complicated data sets [1]. The rise of AI-powered mobile health emphasizes even more how AI has the ability to transform health promotion, disease management, and detection [1]. Simultaneously, patient-centered, evidence-based proactive, and preventative treatment paradigms have been made possible by advances in sensor technology [1].

Hybrid deep learning approaches with blockchain technology offer a novel way to improve security and scalability in healthcare systems [2]. Similar to this, digital twin technology has been recognized as a potential fix for fault monitoring in a number of sectors, including the medical field [3], emphasizing its function in predictive analytics.

Using AI for in-the-moment analysis, smart wearables have shown a considerable increase in the detection of cardiovascular diseases (CVDs) [4]. In addition, noninvasive technologies like sweat glucose reporting systems open up new avenues for noninvasive management of chronic illnesses like diabetes [5].

By addressing important issues like telehealth integration, digital data incorporation into electronic health records (EHRs), AI-powered qualitative hypoglycemia alerts, cybersecurity improvements for diabetes devices, and the creation of diabetes registries, digital health technologies have the potential to revolutionize the treatment of diabetes [6].

Particularly in the field of pulmonology, phonopulmography employing AI creates new opportunities through dual microwave acoustic detection and imaging methods. These developments have the potential to greatly improve diagnostic accuracy while lowering the variability associated with the currently used manual auscultation techniques [7].

When taken as a whole, these researches highlight a larger trend toward fusing complex computational models with clinical applications, from the treatment of chronic diseases to predictive diagnosis, signaling the beginning of a time when precision medicine is not just a pipe dream but a reality.

This transformation is not without its difficulties, though; when blockchain or other decentralized technologies are used in sensitive fields like patient health data, ethical concerns about privacy protection coexist with questions of regulatory compliance. Furthermore, computational complexity continues to be a hurdle, necessitating constant innovation in both hardware (for sensors) and software (for machine learning algorithms).

Despite these obstacles, the trajectory indicates a more digitized healthcare environment where customized interventions are based on ongoing, real-time data feeds made possible by cutting-edge sensor technologies and strong analytical capabilities offered by AI frameworks.

18.3 Understanding AI-Powered Sensors

AI-powered sensors are transforming patient care management in the healthcare industry, especially for chronic illnesses like diabetes mellitus and rehabilitation procedures. AI-driven technologies are being used more and more to improve the precision and effectiveness of patient support and illness management systems [8, 9].

Real-time physiological data collection from patients is the foundation of AI-powered sensors, which then use sophisticated algorithms to scan these data streams for patterns that could indicate a patient's health or the course of a disease [9]. With this capacity, ongoing monitoring can take place outside of conventional clinical settings, providing individualized health insights that can guide more specialized treatment regimens.

AI methods, in conjunction with sensor technologies, have demonstrated potential in the prediction and prevention of consequences related to glucose homeostasis dysfunction in the management of diabetes [9].

AI systems can detect patterns that could indicate an oncoming hyperglycemic or hypoglycemic crisis by examining data gathered from continuous glucose monitors and other wearable devices. This proactive strategy makes it easier to implement timely interventions that may reduce the risk of problems related to diabetes.

Similar to this, in virtual rehabilitation (VRehab), accurate evaluation of patient's physical activity and progress during rehab exercises carried out at home is made possible by AI-driven analysis of multimodal datasets obtained via sensors [8]. To assess workout quality and give patients immediate feedback, algorithms including deep neural networks, fuzzy rule-based approaches, and template matching are used. This approach not only improves the efficacy of rehabilitation programs but also fosters increased patient engagement through the provision of tailored guidance directly to their homes [8].

Notwithstanding these developments, obstacles still stand in the way of the broad use of AI-powered sensors in the medical field. The need for continued study is highlighted by concerns about data privacy, algorithmic transparency, standardization across many platforms and devices, and guaranteeing fair access. In addition, research using standardized measures is needed to evaluate different types of AI-driven therapies in a thorough manner [8].

AI-powered sensors are a big step forward in the treatment of long-term conditions like diabetes mellitus and improve the results of rehabilitation through VRehab programs. Their powerful analytical capabilities combined with real-time monitoring hold considerable potential to improve patient care quality while mitigating some constraints of existing healthcare delivery methods.

Type of sensors	Description	Applications
Wearable Sensors	Devices worn on the body to collect physiological data such as heart rate, temperature, etc.	Remote patient monitoring, fitness tracking, sleep analysis
Implantable Sensors	Devices implanted into the body to monitor specific parameters or deliver treatment.	Continuous glucose monitoring, cardiac monitoring
Environmental Sensors	Sensors deployed in the environment to monitor air quality, temperature, etc.	Monitoring pollution levels, indoor air quality
Biosensors	Miniature analytical devices that detect biological information and convert it into an electrical signal.	Blood glucose monitoring, detection of biomarkers for disease diagnosis
Proximity Sensors	Sensors that detect the presence or absence of objects or individuals within a certain distance.	Patient tracking in hospitals, fall detection for elderly care
Imaging Sensors	Sensors capable of capturing images and converting them into digital data for analysis.	X-ray imaging, MRI, CT scans, mammography
Smart Bandages	Bandages embedded with sensors and microelectronics to monitor wound healing and detect infection.	Wound management, postoperative care
Ingestible Sensors	Small devices that are swallowed and transmit data from within the body to an external receiver.	Monitoring gastrointestinal conditions, medication adherence
Nanosensors	Miniaturized sensors with dimensions on the nanometer scale, capable of detecting specific molecules or ions.	Early disease detection, environmental monitoring
Virtual Reality (VR) Sensors	Sensors used in conjunction with VR technology to simulate real-world environments for therapy or training purposes.	Pain management, rehabilitation exercises

18.4 Enhancing Patient Monitoring and Diagnosis

In many domains, such as chronic disease management (e.g., diabetes [10], acute conditions (e.g., stroke [11], general health surveillance [12], stress detection [13], obesity surveillance [14], human activity recognition [15], sound-based medical telemonitoring [16], spasticity assessment using inertial sensors [14], and authentication in smart healthcare systems through electrocardiogram (ECG) signals analysis [17], the integration of AI with sensor technology is revolutionizing patient monitoring and diagnosis. This synthesis emphasizes how these technologies have the capacity to revolutionize healthcare delivery by offering continuous, real-time data that can guide patient self-management and clinical decision-making.

AI applications in diabetes treatment have shown great potential in areas like clinical decision support systems, automated retinal screening, predictive population risk stratification, and patient self-management tools. These developments are intended to improve glucose regulation while lowering the risk of hypoglycemia episodes and diabetes-related comorbidities [10].

Mobile health technologies with wireless sensors and AI recognition algorithms provide an innovative way to overcome delays in the activation of emergency medical services for acute diseases like stroke. Through continuous monitoring of vital signs and other biometric markers that may indicate the development of a stroke (such as altered speech or motor function), these technologies have the potential to improve outcomes by facilitating prompt intervention [11].

Another area where AI-powered sensors are advancing is wearable technology. Wearable technology offers an unprecedented opportunity for large-scale implementation focused on disease prevention and management by continuously assessing physiological status information noninvasively or minimally invasively across multiple parameters (e.g., blood pressure, electrocardiography, etc.) [12].

In addition, using federated learning models makes it possible to do classification tasks with privacy preservation, including stress detection using electrodermal activity monitoring on the wrist [13] or human authentication using ECG signals in smart healthcare frameworks [17].

Personalized health solutions targeting lifestyle-induced disorders such as obesity have demonstrated efficacy in detecting complicated human activities through the use of ensemble machine learning techniques to sensor data. These methods highlight how crucial it is to use a variety of datasets that have been improved by semantic annotation to produce useful insights into public health trends [14].

Furthermore, cutting-edge techniques that use sound analysis for medical telemonitoring offer a different way to observe patients remotely without violating their privacy. These systems' ability to distinguish distress noises from background noise helps to provide complete home-based care solutions, which are particularly helpful for senior citizens [16].

Finally, the accuracy with which machine-learning algorithms analyze data from inertial sensors allows for the identification of neurological abnormalities such as elbow spasticity. This feature highlights the potential advantages wearable technology and cognitive analytics offer for tracking rehabilitation progress outside of conventional healthcare settings as well as for diagnostic purposes [14].

18.5 Improving Treatment Outcomes

The use of sensors driven by AI in healthcare has the potential to revolutionize treatment outcomes in a range of medical fields. AI-powered sensors present previously unheard-of possibilities for early adverse event detection, individualized treatment modifications, and enhanced patient involvement in their care processes due to their capacity to continuously monitor patients' physiological parameters with high precision and real-time data processing capabilities [18–21].

Photothermal and photodynamic therapies have become prominent methods in oncology that use light-activated treatments to ablate tumors. By combining AI algorithms with photosensitizer-based sensors that maximize the delivery and activation of therapeutic chemicals, the specificity and effectiveness of these therapies could be greatly increased [21].

Similar to how skin tightening methods have proven successful with microfocused ultrasound, treatment protocols could be improved by AI-powered sensors by precisely directing ultrasound waves based on real-time skin elasticity measurements [18].

AI-enabled wearables could offer continuous input on symptom development or regression for conservative management regimens, such as those used in treatments for lateral epicondylitis or carpal tunnel syndrome, where patient response variability can hamper standardization of care. This would enable dynamic therapy intensity or technique modification based on the unique reactions of each patient [19, 20].

Furthermore, AI sensor integration has a lot to offer post-surgery rehabilitation. In the case of total hip replacement surgery, wearable sensors can monitor compliance and quality of movement outside of clinical settings to ensure adherence to prescribed regimens. Physiotherapist-directed exercises are crucial for recovery outcomes such as strength improvement and gait normalization.

Not only does technology need to improve but it also needs to be seamlessly integrated into clinical operations to avoid burdening healthcare providers excessively or jeopardizing patient privacy. Furthermore, new research contradicts the conventional wisdom that intensive intravenous hydration is advantageous in cases of acute pancreatitis despite its physiological justification. This is an instance of how AI-powered predictive analytics on huge datasets could help distinguish between subpopulations that are legitimately in danger and those that would actually benefit from such interventions. It's evident that utilizing AI-powered sensors in healthcare settings requires a multidisciplinary approach involving clinicians' expertise combined with computational power to optimize treatment outcomes, despite the promising prospects highlighted above and the limitations acknowledged in each of the cited studies.

18.6 Remote Healthcare and Telemedicine

In many medical specialties, such as multiple sclerosis, ophthalmology [22], dentistry [23], nutrition [24], social assistance robotics [25], health data collection mechanisms [26], diabetes management, CVD prevention among Indigenous populations in Australia, primary care improvement strategies using AI, and virus disease control systems incorporating AI and Internet of Things (IoT) technologies for quick response to epidemics like COVID-19, the integration of AI with remote healthcare and telemedicine through AI-powered sensors is revolutionizing healthcare delivery, management, and research.

A more patient-centered learning health system is made possible by AI-driven approaches that aggregate real-world data from patient registries, digital patient-reported outcomes, EHRs, and wearable sensors that provide continuous measures of performance dynamics in ecological settings.

Novel brightness transformation algorithms, for example, have shown promise in the diagnosis of cataracts with high accuracy utilizing smartphone cameras instead of large imaging devices, suggesting possible bedside or remote area applications [22]. Similarly, developments in dental robots offer major gains in treatment protocols and diagnostics while resolving issues with therapeutic reliability [23].

With wearable technology collecting food photos and biological sample analysis boosting precision health research, databases such as AI4FoodDB demonstrate the possibility for tailored e-health nutrition interventions [24]. It is necessary to compare remote human–robot interaction with traditional interactions further. In the meantime, socially supportive robots are being investigated for their potential to reduce loneliness via cognitive assistance remotely during pandemics [25].

A trend toward using built-in smartphone sensors is evident in the data collecting techniques found in mHealth apps, but there is still opportunity for more acceptance, particularly with regard to the standardization of Bluetooth peripherals, which might create new ecosystems and provide end users more choices [26]. The focus of digital diabetes views is on using "digitosomes," a term coined for online-generated data that combines clinical information with digital markers to improve management quality of life while preventing complications, to transform diabetes prevention.

The deployment of wearable biosensors specifically designed for rural cardiac patients is urgently needed, according to systematic reviews on the use of the Internet of Medical Things in Indigenous Australian communities. These devices should emphasize real-time monitoring capabilities, as they have the potential to greatly influence CVD prevention strategies among these vulnerable populations.

The role of primary care is crucial; it acts as a foundation for evaluating the effectiveness of AI adoption, guaranteeing that tools created safeguard patient privacy while improving the quality of care provided and smoothly integrating into routine practice without aggravating health inequities.

Finally, Sim and Cho present an integrated virus disease control model that makes use of IoT and AI technologies. It aims to prevent infectious diseases through proactive detection and warning, demonstrating how convergence models can quickly respond to prevent widespread infections and minimize the number of lives lost during pandemics like COVID-19. This model also shows the practical implications these technologies hold when combined with one another to support global health crisis management efforts.

The synthesis concludes that the integration of AI-powered sensors into remote healthcare services holds transformative promise in a number of sectors, including the management of chronic diseases and the use of predictive analytics to enable personalized therapies. However, there are still issues with technology standardization, interoperability, and ethical concerns about data privacy and security. As a result, stakeholders must work together to ensure the successful implementation of scalable solutions that can meet the needs of a diverse population around the world.

18.7 Challenges and Ethical Considerations

Challenges and ethical considerations	Description
Data Security	Ensuring robust data security measures to protect AI-powered sensor data from cyber threats, unauthorized access, and breaches, safeguarding patient confidentiality and preventing data manipulation or theft.
Informed Consent	Addressing issues related to obtaining informed consent from patients for the collection, use, and sharing of their health data by AI-powered sensors, ensuring patients understand the purposes and potential risks involved.
Regulatory Harmonization	Harmonizing regulatory frameworks and standards for AI-powered sensors across different regions and jurisdictions to facilitate international collaboration, ensure consistency, and streamline regulatory compliance.

(continued)

Challenges and ethical considerations	Description
Algorithm Explainability	Enhancing the explainability and interpretability of AI algorithms used in sensor technologies to enable healthcare professionals and patients to understand how decisions are made and trust the reliability of results.
Bias Mitigation	Implementing strategies to mitigate biases in AI algorithms, data collection, and model training processes to ensure fairness, equity, and accuracy in diagnostic and treatment recommendations across diverse patient populations.
Resource Allocation	Addressing resource allocation challenges related to the deployment and maintenance of AI-powered sensor infrastructure, including funding constraints, staffing shortages, and infrastructure requirements in healthcare settings.
Liability and Accountability	Clarifying liability and accountability frameworks for AI-powered sensors, including responsibilities of manufacturers, healthcare providers, and regulatory bodies in cases of device malfunction, adverse events, or errors in diagnosis or treatment.
Stakeholder Engagement	Engaging stakeholders, including patients, healthcare professionals, policymakers, and industry stakeholders, in the development, evaluation, and implementation of AI-powered sensor technologies to ensure alignment with user needs and preferences.
Data Ownership	Resolving issues surrounding data ownership and control, particularly in cases where AI-powered sensor data is collected, processed, and shared across multiple stakeholders, including patients, healthcare providers, and technology companies.
Standardization	Promoting standardization of data formats, interoperability protocols, and performance metrics for AI-powered sensor technologies to facilitate data exchange, integration, and comparison across different systems and platforms.
Environmental Impact	Assessing and mitigating the environmental impact of AI-powered sensor technologies, including energy consumption, electronic waste generation, and carbon footprint, to promote sustainable development and responsible innovation.
Psychological Impact	Considering the psychological impact of AI-powered sensor technologies on patients, healthcare professionals, and caregivers, including concerns about loss of human touch, autonomy, and trust in the healthcare system.
Long-term Efficacy	Evaluating the long-term efficacy and effectiveness of AI-powered sensor technologies in improving patient outcomes, reducing healthcare costs, and enhancing overall quality of care over extended periods of time.
Intellectual Property Rights	Addressing intellectual property rights issues related to AI algorithms, sensor designs, and data analytics methods, including patents, copyrights, and trade secrets, to foster innovation while ensuring fair competition and access.

18.8 Regulatory Landscape

With the potential to greatly improve patient care, diagnostics, monitoring, and overall health system efficiency, the introduction of AI into healthcare through AI-powered sensors marks a revolutionary change. However, to guarantee that safety, effectiveness, privacy protection, and ethical considerations are met, this innovation also brings with it complicated regulatory hurdles that must be addressed.

AI-driven sensors gather a tonne of patient data in real-time. By enabling ongoing evaluation outside of conventional clinical settings, this feature has the potential to completely transform patient monitoring. Wearables with these sensors, for example, can track illnesses like diabetes by noninvasively detecting glucose levels, or they can monitor vital signs like blood oxygen levels and heart rate. These developments hold out the possibility of better illness management by means of prompt interventions grounded in data-driven insights.

On the other hand, there are serious regulatory issues with the use of AI-powered sensors. Ensuring dependability and accuracy comes first. To validate the effectiveness of these devices across a range of populations and settings, regulatory organizations need to set standards. This entails stringent testing procedures to find any biases or errors that can cause incorrect diagnoses or ineffective therapies.

Privacy protection is still another important issue. Because health data acquired by AI-powered devices are sensitive, it is necessary to have strong cybersecurity protections in place in addition to rules that clearly outline data usage permission and sharing guidelines. Regulations must strike a compromise between safeguarding people's privacy and facilitating the useful use of data for objectives such as advancing healthcare services or research.

In addition, relying too much on technology for health monitoring and decision-making raises ethical questions. It is imperative to establish standards that clearly define the roles and duties of AI systems and human healthcare providers. Regulations should outline liability concerns when judgments are made by automated systems using sensor data to ensure accountability when mistakes happen.

Given the transnational character of healthcare delivery and technological advancement, globally unified rules are needed. Diverse regional laws may make it more difficult for innovative ideas to be adopted or may put obstacles in the way of fair access to cutting-edge medical technology in certain areas.

Even though AI-powered sensors have enormous potential to revolutionize healthcare delivery through improved monitoring capabilities and individualized care methods, achieving their full potential will necessitate navigating a challenging regulatory environment that has been meticulously designed to address issues with accuracy and dependability ethics, privacy protections, and the dynamics of human-AI interaction worldwide harmonization initiatives meant to successfully protect public health interests while promoting innovation.

18.9 Future Directions and Opportunities

Rapid diagnostics outside of typical laboratory settings are made possible by AI-powered sensors, which are essential to the advancement of point-of-care testing [27]. O'Sullivan draws attention to advancements in portable diagnostics, including lab-on-a-chip and microfluidic devices that make use of photonic and electrochemical transduction techniques. Mobile device connectivity improvements supplement these breakthroughs by enabling remote data collection and analysis [27]. In addition, improvements in machine learning algorithms provide advanced data analytics capabilities that are necessary to translate complex biological signals into useful therapeutic insights [27].

Simultaneously, digital phenotyping platforms such as HOPES demonstrate how AI may utilize sensor data from smartphones and wearables to monitor health issues thoroughly [28]. The research by Wang and colleagues highlights the capacity of these platforms to gather diverse health-related information, allowing for individualized therapy strategies through ongoing monitoring [28].

In addition, assistive technologies show the usefulness of AI-powered sensors in improving mobility while remotely monitoring vital signs, such as autonomous wheelchairs outfitted with IoT-based biophysical sensors [29]. The prototype by Hou shows how patients and senior populations can be supported in living independently by combining real-time health monitoring with navigation technology [29].

There are obstacles to overcome before these technical developments may be widely used in therapeutic settings. Aguiar Noury noted a number of obstacles that prevent the use of assistive robotics in the healthcare industry, from market penetration problems to regulatory obstacles, which also hold true for more extensive AI-sensor integrations [30]. It will take coordinated efforts in the areas of public acceptance, industry innovation, stakeholder engagement, and policy-making to remove these obstacles. With the ability to improve diagnosis precision, tailor treatment regimens based on real-time data analysis, and increase patient autonomy through assistive technologies, AI-powered sensors have the potential to revolutionize healthcare. However, to fully realize this promise, major systemic barriers must be removed.

18.10 Case Studies and Success Stories

Explainable AI (XAI) is a crucial advancement toward more transparent and comprehensible AI models that have emerged in the medical area [31]. In delicate domains like healthcare, where clinical judgments can be greatly impacted by clinical decision-making based on an understanding of AI-driven outcomes, XAI's capacity to articulate its reasoning for decisions is essential. Sheu and Pardeshi's study demonstrates how XAI improves clinical workflows and patient care by incorporating user feedback into explainable solutions that support human-machine collaboration [31].

Simultaneously, Industry 5.0 opens up new uses for AI-powered sensors outside of traditional manufacturing settings, such as the healthcare industry [32]. The blockchain protocols and edge computing talk by Oliveira shows how decentralized networks can support data integrity, security, and privacy—all of which are crucial for managing sensitive health information [32]. By enabling real-time data gathering and processing through wearable technology or sensors implanted in medical devices, these technological breakthroughs provide an environment that is favorable to personalized medicine and predictive analytics.

Another way that AI-powered sensors are transforming healthcare is as highlighted by Qi J's systematic review of sensor-based physical activity recognition [33]. The accurate monitoring of patients' physical activity in uncontrolled surroundings can be achieved by utilizing IoT technology in conjunction with innovative sensory devices and learning algorithms [33]. These kinds of skills are essential for creating customized rehabilitation plans that change in response to patients' physiological responses in real-time.

When taken as a whole, these findings highlight a paradigm shift toward intelligent, networked healthcare ecosystems made possible by AI-powered sensors. These advancements offer opportunities and difficulties, ranging from enhancing diagnostic accuracy with XAI to guaranteeing secure patient data management via blockchain-enhanced IoT networks. Maintaining privacy while using big data to gain health insights, addressing interoperability among various IoT devices, ensuring reliability in decentralized networks, and, most importantly, making these cutting-edge technologies available across various tiers of international healthcare systems are some of these challenges.

Further development of these technologies should be the goal of future directions. This includes investigating energy-efficient designs that extend device lifespans without sacrificing performance, developing strong cybersecurity measures suited for applications specific to the health sector, developing machine learning models that are able to rapidly adjust to new health datasets without the need for protracted retraining, and lastly, promoting interdisciplinary partnerships that fill knowledge gaps among technologists, clinicians, researchers, policymakers, and technologists to guarantee that holistic development deployment strategies have a truly transformative effect on a global scale.

18.10.1 Collaborations and Partnerships

In the field of AI-powered sensors in healthcare, collaborations and partnerships can involve a range of stakeholders, such as technology corporations, academic institutes, patient advocacy groups, and healthcare providers. The following are some possible alliances and cooperative efforts:

Healthcare Providers and Technology Companies: Co-development of AI-powered sensor technologies customized to particular healthcare needs, as well as implementation support and training for healthcare professionals, can be part of the partnership between healthcare providers (hospitals, clinics, healthcare systems) and technology companies (AI startups, medical device manufacturers).

Research Institutions and Industry: Partnerships between industry participants and academic research institutions can promote innovation in sensor technology, AI algorithms, and healthcare applications. Collaborative research initiatives can investigate novel AI-based methods for data processing, illness identification, and therapy enhancement.

Industry Stakeholders and Regulatory Authorities: Collaborations between industry stakeholders and regulatory authorities, like the European Medicines Agency in Europe or the Food and Drug Administration in the United States, can speed up the regulatory approval process for AI-powered sensor technology. The cooperation entails exchanging knowledge, recommendations, and input to guarantee adherence to legal mandates.

Data Sharing Initiatives: To train AI algorithms and validate sensor technologies, healthcare organizations and technology companies may collaborate to share anonymized patient data. Initiatives to share data can hasten the development of AI-powered sensors while enhancing their precision and dependability.

Interdisciplinary Teams: Putting together interdisciplinary teams of engineers, data scientists, ethicists, and healthcare experts can spur creativity and tackle difficult problems related to AI-powered medical sensor applications. These teams can work together to create, implement, and assess sensor systems while taking regulatory, ethical, technological, and clinical viewpoints into account.

Partnerships between patient advocacy groups and industry stakeholders can guarantee that patient requirements and preferences are taken into consideration during the development of AI-powered sensor technologies. Working with patient advocacy organizations can help build patient-centric sensor solutions by offering insightful information on patient priorities, preferences, and experiences.

Global Health Initiatives: Working together, governments and nonprofit groups may encourage fair access to the use of AI-powered sensors in healthcare, especially in underprivileged areas. Initiatives to alleviate healthcare inequities, enhance global health equity, and improve health outcomes can all be supported by these relationships.

The development and application of AI-powered sensors in healthcare can be sped up by promoting partnerships and collaborations amongst these varied stakeholders. This will guarantee that these technologies efficiently address healthcare issues, enhance patient care, and eventually improve the entire healthcare ecosystem.

18.10.2 Conclusion

The use of AI-powered sensors is a game-changer for the healthcare industry, sparking a wave of innovation with significant effects on patient care, diagnosis, and treatment plans. This chapter has taken us on a tour through the history of healthcare technology, from its inception to the rise of AI-powered sensors as a game-changing innovation in the industry.

We have seen the breadth and depth of AI's influence, from the basic investigation of its growing role in healthcare to the sophisticated comprehension of AI-powered sensors, including their various forms and uses. A new era of real-time data insights, early disease identification, and individualized therapy has been ushered in by these sensors, which range from wearable technology to implanted technologies and environmental sensors.

In addition, the incorporation of AI-powered sensors has produced noticeable improvements in treatment results, enabling more precise data collecting, dosage modifications, and treatment adherence monitoring. Their contribution to telemedicine and remote healthcare has been especially revolutionary, giving patients more access to high-quality care outside of conventional clinical settings and enabling them to take an active role in their own health management.

But along with these developments come difficulties and moral dilemmas that call for cautious thought and preemptive resolution. The ethical use of AI-powered sensors necessitates a diverse strategy that addresses issues ranging from algorithm biases to complex data privacy problems to preventing overreliance on technology. These sensors have already shown their transformative impact in improving patient outcomes and healthcare efficiency, as evidenced by fascinating case studies and success stories.

In the end, promoting alliances and partnerships between technology firms, academic institutions, and government agencies is critical to promoting ongoing innovation and guaranteeing the moral and responsible application of AI-powered sensors in the healthcare industry. With every advancement, it's becoming more and more obvious that AI-powered sensors are change agents rather than just tools, changing the way healthcare is delivered and paving the way for a better, more patient-centered future.

In the future, AI-powered sensors will have a great deal of promise for improving healthcare through prospects for interdisciplinary cooperation, precision medicine, and AI-driven drug discovery.

References

1 Pavel, M., Jimison, H.B., Wactlar, H.D. et al. (2013). The role of technology and engineering models in transforming healthcare. *IEEE Rev Biomed Eng.* 6: 156–177. https://doi.org/10.1109/RBME.2012.2222636.

2 Ali, A., Ali, H., Saeed, A. et al. (2023). Blockchain-powered healthcare systems: enhancing scalability and security with hybrid deep learning. *Sensors (Basel).* 23 (18): 7740. https://doi.org/10.3390/s23187740.

3 Bofill, J., Abisado, M., Villaverde, J., and Sampedro, G.A. (2023). Exploring digital twin-based fault monitoring: challenges and opportunities. *Sensors* 23 (16): 7087. https://doi.org/10.3390/s23167087.

4 Moshawrab, M., Adda, M., Bouzouane, A. et al. (2023). Smart wearables for the detection of cardiovascular diseases: a systematic literature review. *Sensors (Basel).* 23 (2): 828. https://doi.org/10.3390/s23020828.

5 Sankhala, D., Sardesai, A.U., Pali, M. et al. (2022). A machine learning-based on-demand sweat glucose reporting platform. *Scientific Reports* 12 (1): 2442. https://doi.org/10.1038/s41598-022-06434-x.

6 Klonoff, A.N., Andy Lee, W.A., Xu, N.Y. et al. (2023). Six digital health technologies that will transform diabetes. *J Diabetes Sci Technol.* 17 (1): 239–249. https://doi.org/10.1177/19322968211043498.

7 Sethi, A.K., Muddaloor, P., Anvekar, P. et al. (2023). Digital pulmonology practice with phonopulmography leveraging artificial intelligence: future perspectives using dual microwave acoustic sensing and imaging. *Sensors (Basel)* 23 (12): 5514. https://doi.org/10.3390/s23125514.

8 Abedi, A., Colella, T.J.F., Pakosh, M., and Khan, S.S. (2024). Artificial intelligence-driven virtual rehabilitation for people living in the community: a scoping review. *NPJ Digit Med.* 7 (1): 25. https://doi.org/10.1038/s41746-024-00998-w.

9 Contreras, I. and Vehi, J. (2018). Artificial intelligence for diabetes management and decision support: literature review. *J Med Internet Res.* 20 (5): e10775. https://doi.org/10.2196/10775.

10 Dankwa-Mullan, I., Rivo, M., Sepulveda, M. et al. (2019). Transforming diabetes care through artificial intelligence: the future is here. *Popul Health Manag* 22 (3): 229–242. https://doi.org/10.1089/pop.2018.0129.

11 Bat-Erdene, B.O. and Saver, J.L. (2021). Automatic acute stroke symptom detection and emergency medical systems alerting by mobile health technologies: a review. *J Stroke Cerebrovasc Dis.* 30 (7): 105826. https://doi.org/10.1016/j.jstrokecerebrovasdis.2021.105826.

12 Peng, C.K., Cui, X., Zhang, Z., and Yu, M. (2023). Wearable devices: perspectives on assessing and monitoring human physiological status. *Sheng wu yi xue Gong Cheng xue za zhi = Journal of Biomedical Engineering = Shengwu Yixue Gongchengxue Zazhi* 40 (6): 1045–1052. https://doi.org/10.7507/1001-5515.202303043.

13 Almadhor, A., Sampedro, G.A., Abisado, M. et al. (2023). Wrist-based electrodermal activity monitoring for stress detection using federated learning. *Sensors (Basel).* 23 (8): 3984. https://doi.org/10.3390/s23083984.

14 Poulymenopoulou, M., Papakonstantinou, D., Malamateniou, F., and Vassilacopoulos, G. (2015). A health analytics semantic ETL service for obesity surveillance. *Stud Health Technol Inform.* 210: 840–844.

15 Istrate, D., Castelli, E., Vacher, M. et al. (2006). Information extraction from sound for medical telemonitoring. *IEEE Trans Inf Technol Biomed.* 10 (2): 264–274. https://doi.org/10.1109/titb.2005.859889.

16 Sampedro, G.A.R., Rachmawati, S.M., Kim, D.-S., and Lee, J.-M. (2022). Exploring machine learning-based fault monitoring for polymer-based additive manufacturing: challenges and opportunities. *Sensors* 22 (23): 9446. https://doi.org/10.3390/s22239446.

17 Serpush, F., Menhaj, M.B., Masoumi, B., and Karasfi, B. (2022). Wearable sensor-based human activity recognition in the smart healthcare system. *Computational Intelligence and Neuroscience* 24 (2022): 1391906. https://doi.org/10.1155/2022/1391906.

18 Contini, M., Hollander, M.H.J., Vissink, A. et al. (2023). A systematic review of the efficacy of microfocused ultrasound for facial skin tightening. *Int J Environ Res Public Health.* 20 (2): 1522. https://doi.org/10.3390/ijerph20021522.

19 Dworkin, R.H., Turk, D.C., Wyrwich, K.W. et al. (2008). Interpreting the clinical importance of treatment outcomes in chronic pain clinical trials: IMMPACT recommendations. *J Pain.* 9 (2): 105–121. https://doi.org/10.1016/j.jpain.2007.09.005.

20 Jiménez Del Barrio, S., Bueno Gracia, E., Hidalgo García, C. et al. (2018). Conservative treatment in patients with mild to moderate carpal tunnel syndrome:

a systematic review. *Neurologia (Engl Ed)* 33 (9): 590–601. https://doi.org/10.1016/j.nrl.2016.05.018.

21 Li, X., Lovell, J.F., Yoon, J., and Chen, X. (2020). Clinical development and potential of photothermal and photodynamic therapies for cancer. *Nat Rev Clin Oncol.* 17 (11): 657–674. https://doi.org/10.1038/s41571-020-0410-2.

22 Askarian, B., Ho, P., and Chong, J.W. (2021). Detecting cataract using smartphones. *IEEE J Transl Eng Health Med.* 20 (9): 3800110. https://doi.org/10.1109/JTEHM.2021.3074597.

23 Saeed, U., Shah, S.Y., Ahmad, J. et al. (2022 Apr). Machine learning empowered COVID-19 patient monitoring using non-contact sensing: An extensive review. *J Pharm Anal.* 12 (2): 193–204. https://doi.org/10.1016/j.jpha.2021.12.006.

24 Romero-Tapiador, S., Lacruz-Pleguezuelos, B., Tolosana, R. et al. (2023). AI4FoodDB: a database for personalized e-Health nutrition and lifestyle through wearable devices and artificial intelligence. *Database: The Journal of Biological Databases and Curation* 2023: baad049. doi: 10.1093/database/baad049.

25 Liang, T., Qiao, S., Liu, X., and Ma, Y. (2023). Correction: Liang et al. Highly Sensitive Hydrogen Sensing Based on Tunable Diode Laser Absorption Spectroscopy with a 2.1 μm Diode Laser. Chemosensors 2022, 10, 321. *Chemosensors* 11 (1): –41. https://doi.org/10.3390/chemosensors11010041.

26 Philip, B., Abdelrazek, M., Bonti, A. et al. (2021). Data collection mechanisms in health and wellness apps: review and analysis. *JMIR mhealth and uhealth.* 10: e30468. https://doi.org/10.2196/30468.

27 O'Sullivan, S., Ali, Z., Jiang, X. et al. (2019). Developments in transduction, connectivity and AI/machine learning for point-of-care testing. *Sensors.* 19 (8): 1917. https://doi.org/10.3390/s19081917.

28 Wang, X., Vouk, N., Heaukulani, C. et al. (2021). HOPES: an integrative digital phenotyping platform for data collection, monitoring, and machine learning. *Journal of Medical Internet Research* 23 (3): e23984. https://doi.org/10.2196/23984.

29 Hou, L., Latif, J., Mehryar, P. et al. (2024). An autonomous wheelchair with health monitoring system based on Internet of Thing. *Sci Rep.* 14 (1): 5878. https://doi.org/10.1038/s41598-024-56357-y.

30 Aguiar Noury, G., Walmsley, A., Jones, R.B., and Gaudl, S.E. (2021). The barriers of the assistive robotics market-what inhibits health innovation? *Sensors (Basel).* 21 (9): 3111. https://doi.org/10.3390/s21093111.

31 Sheu, R.K. and Pardeshi, M.S. (2022). A survey on medical explainable AI (XAI): recent progress, explainability approach, human interaction and scoring system. *Sensors (Basel)* 22 (20): 8068. https://doi.org/10.3390/s22208068.

32 Oliveira, M., Chauhan, S., Pereira, F. et al. (2023). Blockchain protocols and edge computing targeting industry 5.0 needs. *Sensors (Basel).* 23 (22): 9174. https://doi.org/10.3390/s23229174.

33 Qi, J., Yang, P., Waraich, A. et al. (2018). Examining sensor-based physical activity recognition and monitoring for healthcare using Internet of Things: a systematic review. *J Biomed Inform.* 87: 138–153. https://doi.org/10.1016/j.jbi.2018.09.002.

19

GAI and Deep Learning-Based Medical Sensor Data Relationship Model for Health Informatics

Kirti Shukla[1], Pramod Kumar[2], Mukesh Soni[3], Haewon Byeon[4], Sagar Dhanraj Pande[5], and Ismail Keshta[6]

[1] *SCSE, IILM University Greater Noida, Noida, India*
[2] *Ganga Institute of Technology and Management, Maharshi Dayanand University, Rohtak, Haryana, India*
[3] *Dr. D. Y. Patil Vidyapeeth, Pune, Dr. D. Y. Patil School of Science & Technology, D. Y. Patil University, Tathawade, Pune, India*
[4] *Department of AI and Software, Inje University, Gimhae Republic of Korea*
[5] *School of Engineering and Technology, Pimpri Chinchwad University (PCU), Pune, Maharashtra, India*
[6] *Computer Science and Information Systems Department, College of Applied Sciences, AlMaarefa University, Riyadh, Saudi Arabia*

19.1 Introduction

In recent years, sensing technology has developed rapidly in India, with the subsequent rise of medical sensing instruments and the emergence and application of high-tech technologies such as biosensing, which has led to the continuous development of clinical monitoring equipment in the direction of faster measurement speed and higher accuracy [1]. Due to the large population in our country, hundreds of millions of people are hospitalized every year, which will inevitably produce a large number of Health Informatics records (EHR) containing medical sensing data, hospitalization information, personal physical conditions, disease diagnosis and treatment records, etc. The electronic and digital characteristics of Health Informatics record data provide convenience for doctors to review patient information and quickly make accurate disease diagnoses and reasonable treatment decisions. However, the complexity of the data brings great challenges to the processing and utilization of these data difficulty. With the continuous advancement of artificial intelligence technology and the improvement of computer computing power, it has become possible to use Health Informatics systems for disease diagnosis and risk assessment, which provides good development opportunities for Generative intelligence (GAI) medical diagnosis. Reasonable control of Health Informatics Records use can provide doctors with important

Generative Artificial Intelligence for Biomedical and Smart Health Informatics,
First Edition. Edited by Aditya Khamparia and Deepak Gupta.

clinical disease diagnosis basis and health intervention measures and improve the work efficiency of medical workers and the service quality of medical institutions under limited resources [2].

To make better use of a large amount of Health Informatics record data, it is necessary to process and analyze data with different types of structures. Most of the previous work only studied data with similar structures. For example, Mohammad et al. [3] selected a large number of time series signs. Using data, logistic regression and recurrent neural network models are used to predict whether patients will develop severe hypertension risk in the next three months. Ma et al. [4] proposed a method that can learn long-term and short-term changes in patients' physiological characteristics as clinical features. A model that uses medical sensing data to evaluate the health status of patients at different time stages. Ayon et al. [5] used a deep neural network to learn multiple diagnostic measurement data and used it to predict diabetes. However, based on health perception, there are still the following problems in data diagnosis of diseases.

First of all, the above work separately extracts and learns features for different types of data but is deficient in feature fusion of multiple types of data to extract correlations between data. In the task of this chapter, due to the medical characteristics of EHR data, Sensing data is dynamic time series data obtained by a variety of devices, while personal physical record data (such as age, gender, etc.) is static nontime series data, and there is heterogeneity between medical sensing data and similar physical conditions. Different individuals suffer from different types of diseases. Therefore, how to fuse and model these heterogeneous data is a key point in the disease diagnosis task. This chapter proposes a dynamic and static relationships fusion strategy for multisource health sensing data to explore the above problems. Hidden features between source heterogeneous data to obtain better model learning results.

Second, multicategory disease diagnosis is a multilabel classification task. Intuitively, making full use of the relationship between labels can improve model performance. Taking the diseases selected in this article as an example, if essential hypertension is not controlled for a long time, it will easily lead to various diseases. Therefore, essential hypertension and hypertension-complicated complications are in general at different stages of illness and are less likely to occur at the same time. One of the common complications of hypertension is kidney disease, so hypertension complications are more likely to occur at the same time as chronic kidney disease.

Figure 19.1 shows the correlation between the 25 types of diseases selected for the multicategory disease diagnosis task experiment in this article. Different numbers represent different types of diseases. The calculation method of disease correlation will be introduced in Section 19.3.3. Among them, the color of the rectangle the darker the color of the rectangle, the stronger the relationship between the

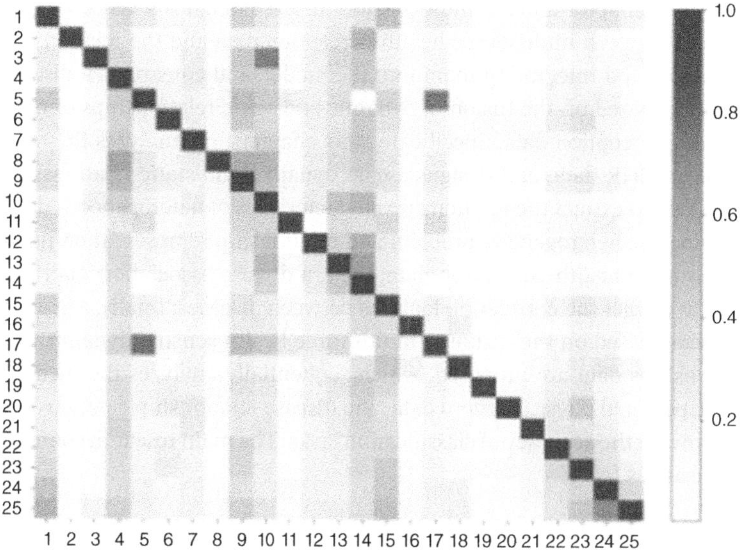

Figure 19.1 Disease relationship heat map.

two diseases, and the lighter the color of the rectangle, the weaker the relationship between the two diseases.

Note: (1) Acute and unspecified renal failure; (2) Acute cerebrovascular disease; (3) Acute myocardial infarction; (4) Heart disease Arrhythmia; (5) Chronic kidney disease; (6) Chronic obstructive pulmonary disease; (7) Surgical/medical care combination Chronic kidney disease; (8) conduction disorders; (9) congestive heart failure; (10) coronary atherosclerosis Sclerosis and its related factors; (11) Diabetes and its complications; (12) Diabetes without complications; (13) Lipid metabolism disorder; (14) Primary hypertension; (15) Fluid and electrolyte disorders; (16) Gastrointestinal bleeding; (17) Hypertension with complications; (18) Other liver diseases; (19) Other lower respiratory tract diseases Respiratory diseases; (20) Other upper respiratory tract diseases; (21) Pleurisy/pneumothorax/pulmonary collapse; (22) Pulmonary inflammation; (23) respiratory failure; (24) sepsis; and (25) shock.

As can be seen from the figure, in addition to the strongest relationship between each disease and itself, the relationship between essential hypertension (14) and hypertension with complications (17) is very weak, while hypertension with complications (17) and chronic kidney disease (5), which is also consistent with the above analysis. To make full use of this feature, this article designed a model structure that integrates time series features and disease correlation matrices to further improve model performance.

Therefore, this chapter aims at multicategory disease diagnosis tasks, mining the correlation between multisource health perception data and the relationship between diseases and integrating them into the model, and constructs a disease diagnosis model based on the fusion of dynamic and static relationships of multisource health perception data. Specifically, this chapter first analyzes the multisource data in EHR data, and designs a data dynamic and static relationships fusion algorithm to extract the relationship characteristics of heterogeneous data, thereby solving the heterogeneity problem and relationship representation problem of multisource health perception data; then, a disease association matrix is constructed to extract the correlation features between diseases; finally, a disease diagnosis model based on the fusion of multisource health sensing dynamic and static relationships data are proposed, which sequentially analyzes the medical sensing data, personal physical record data, and disease relationship data. Fusion, thereby improving the accuracy of classification tasks. The main research contents of this article are as follows.

1) Aiming at the problem that the sources of sensory data in EHR are diverse and the data types are complex, which easily makes it difficult to mine the correlation between different types of data in disease detection tasks, this chapter proposes a multisource health perception data dynamic system.
   Static relationship fusion model. This model adds mask vectors to medical sensing data, conducts fusion learning on medical sensing data and personal physical record data based on the gated recurrent unit network architecture, and mines multisource heterogeneous data. Hidden features to achieve diagnosis of multiple categories of diseases.
2) In view of the implicit relationship between personal constitution record data and medical sensing data that is common in disease diagnosis, this chapter mines the correlation between the static data of personal constitution records and the dynamic data of medical sensing and extracts the correlation between dynamic and static data. While retaining the original data characteristics, the model helps the model to differentially diagnose the diseases of different patients based on their physical conditions.
3) Aiming at the problem that it is difficult to jointly mine the disease dependence and disease mutual exclusion relationships between multicategory disease diagnosis tasks, this chapter constructs a correlation matrix to extract the relationships between diseases and combines the disease relationship data with medical sensing data and personal physical record data. Features are fused to improve the classification accuracy of the model.
4) By conducting experiments on the real American MIMIC-III clinical data set [6], it is proved that the model in this chapter can accurately diagnose multiple categories of diseases and is better than the best benchmark model.

19.2 Related Work

Due to the diversity and complexity of Health Informatics record data structures, a large number of researchers have studied its different characteristics in recent years. The following will cover the applicable tasks of Health Informatics record data, multisource health sensing data fusion algorithms, and existing disease diagnosis models. Three aspects are used to describe the specific research content of related work at home and abroad.

19.2.1 Applicable Tasks for Health Informatics Record Data

Currently, Health Informatics record (EHR) systems are used in medical care services in major hospitals to provide convenience for doctors and patients. To ensure the integrity and accuracy of records, EHR systems support multiple types of recording methods and different Structured GAI medical data, for example, the data in the MIMIC-III database [6] include vital signs, medications, test results, surgery codes, diagnosis codes, imaging reports, hospitalization time, etc., providing many directions for related research.

Research work [7–9] shows that reinforcement learning models have achieved good results in predicting mortality and intensive care unit length of stay. This research article [10] proposed a super learner algorithm, which uses a reinforcement learning model to enhance critical care. Prediction performance of in-hospital mortality in monitored patients. Sanjay et al. [11] conducted a multifaceted analysis of the MIMIC-III data set and proposed a set of benchmark tasks, including in-hospital mortality prediction, length of stay prediction, and ICD-9 code group prediction, and used deep learning model, several reinforcement learning models and ICU scoring system conducted a benchmark evaluation on three clinical prediction tasks. On this basis, this work [12] used a deep model to conduct a benchmark evaluation on four clinical prediction benchmark tasks on the MIMIC-III data set. In comparative experiments, the added benchmark task is the prediction of gain and loss compensation represented by the mortality rate within 24 hours. Lee et al. [13] proposed a multiscale interval pattern awareness network (multiscale interval pattern-aware network, MSIPA) to mine time series EHR data through a convolutional network for short, medium, and long interval pattern information, the scaling dot product attention mechanism is used to obtain the context corresponding to the three-time interval patterns, and transformer is used to predict ICU ward transfers.

19.2.2 Multisource Health Informatics Record Data Fusion Model

An important characteristic of EHRs is the complexity of their multisource health-aware data structures. EHRs often have both structured (code) and unstructured (free text) data with sparse and irregular characteristics. In deep learning, how data represented by different modalities should be fused together is a difficult problem.

This article [14] studied the possibility of jointly learning the hidden structure of multisource EHR data while performing supervised prediction tasks on EHR data. Specifically, the article analyzed a suitable model for learning the hidden EHR structure and proposed a method for using the data Graph Convolution Transformer model of statistical methods. This model has achieved good results in tasks such as graph construction of simulation data and publicly available EHR data, readmission prediction, and mortality prediction. It is an effective multimodal data fusion method. The research [15] extended the state-of-the-art Neural Architecture Search (NAS) method and proposed the Multimodal Fusion Architecture Search (MUFASA) method to simultaneously search for multimodal fusion strategies and model-specific architecture.

19.2.3 DSRF Based on Reinforcement Learning and Deep Learning

Traditional multicategory disease research is generally completed through statistical analysis of data based on expert predefined standards. Disease identification mainly uses simple medical definitions, such as ICDG9 codes. The adoption of Health Informatics record systems has enabled reinforcement learning methods for multicategory disease prediction. There is growing interest in classification [16, 17] and clustering [18, 19] methods.

With the gradual maturity of deep network models and the continuous improvement of computer computing capabilities, multicategory disease diagnosis has become a popular direction for deep learning researchers in recent years. This chapter [20] first proposed the application of feed-forward neural networks to clinical time series data. To explore physiological feature patterns and disease detection and modify the standard neural network training to make full use of the unique characteristics of GAI medical data. This is also [21] developed an artificial intelligence doctor based on a recurrent neural network temporal model, which can learn from a large number of learn effective feature representations from patients' time series records to predict the diseases that patients may suffer from in the future. This research work [22] proposed two new convolutional neural network models and a long short-term memory recurrent neural network model for the early disease onset detection task. Large-scale application model of the network. The above research shows that these deep learning methods based on automatic feature learning are significantly better than the logistic regression algorithm that manually extracts clinical features. The research chapter proposed [23] uses a multichannel with a time-aware attention mechanism. GRU extracts clinical features, obtains the interdependencies between static baseline information and dynamic features, constructs health context, and recodes clinical information to predict patients' clinical health status based on medical history.

19.3 DSRF Based on Dynamic and Static Relationships Fusion of Multisource Health Sensing Data

This chapter conducts in-depth research on the processing and fusion technology of multisource heterogeneous data, disease-related feature extraction technology, and multicategory disease diagnosis technology, etc., and then proposes a disease diagnosis model based on the fusion of dynamic and static relationships of multisource health perception data. The model adopts the data dynamic and static relationships fusion algorithm extracts the relationship features of heterogeneous data, solves the heterogeneity problem of multisource health sensing data, and effectively extracts the relationship features between heterogeneous data. Based on the gated cyclic unit network architecture, the dynamic medical sensing data, static personal physical record data, and disease-related relationship data are fused to fully mine the hidden features of multisource heterogeneous data, thereby improving the accuracy of classification tasks.

The model framework of this article mainly includes four parts: medical sensing data processing, personal physical record data processing, disease association matrix calculation, and multicategory disease diagnosis, as shown in Figure 19.2.

1) In the process of processing sensing data, due to the different sampling frequencies of the data, to take into account the data length and the proportion of the real data, this chapter divides the data at intervals of 1h. For data with insufficient sampling numbers, directional sampling is used in order of priority. Time completion is performed using post-filling or specific value filling methods, and

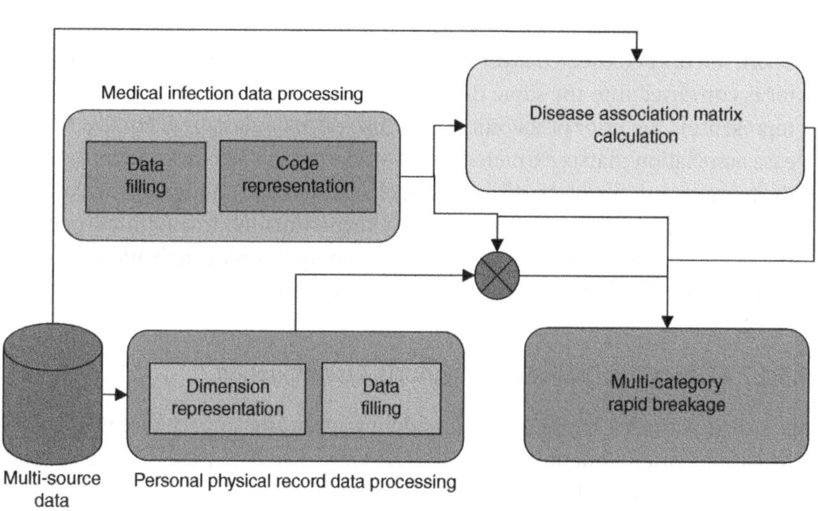

Figure 19.2 Model framework of proposed model.

mask features are added to mark real data and filled data. That is, the white and gray boxes in the sensing data processing module in Figure 19.2, respectively, indicate that the data at that time is real data or fill in the data. Since personal physical recording data, such as gender, age, etc., will have an impact on the normal values of physical signs, they are integrated into each time step of the sensing data.

2) The filling method of recorded data is similar to that of sensing data. The recording data is expanded to the same time dimension as the sensing data, and the real values are used for completion. Subsequently, for all sensing data and recording data, this chapter model uses the standard deviation standardization method to process continuous data and uses one-hot encoding to represent discrete data.
3) The disease association matrix calculation module extracts the characteristics of the relationship between diseases and the relationship between patients with disease "G" by counting the number of patients with different diseases and the number of comorbidities of any two types of diseases and calculates the disease association matrix to represent any two types of diseases. Related relationships, such as dependency relationships and mutual exclusion relationships.
4) In the multicategory disease diagnosis module, this chapter fuses three types of heterogeneous data: medical sensing data, personal physical record data, and disease relationship data at different levels of the model. First, the sensing data and recorded data are combined in time Feature extraction and fusion are performed in different dimensions and sent to the gated recurrent unit network for training. The time dependence of the data is extracted to obtain the vector representation of the hidden features, completing the first level of data fusion. Then, the fully connected layer will extract the extracted data. The feature vector is converted into the same dimension as the number of disease categories, representing the prior probability of the disease to be classified. Finally, the disease association matrix extracted based on the patient's disease status data and the prior probability of the disease to be classified based on the sensing data and recorded data are extracted. Multiply the experimental probabilities, perform the second level of data fusion, and select an appropriate activation function mapping to obtain the final multicategory disease diagnosis result.

19.3.1 Multicategory Disease Diagnosis Task Modeling

This article performs mathematical modeling on multicategory disease diagnosis tasks. The original data set $X = \{X_M, X_R, X_D\}$, where $X_M \in \mathbb{R}^{T\times d_m}$ represents medical sensing data, which is shown in equation 19.1.

The data has d_m attributes, such as heart rate, blood pressure, etc.; T is the length of the time series; $X_R \in \mathbb{R}^d$ represents personal physical record data, which has dr

attributes, such as gender, age, etc.; $X_D \in \mathbb{R}^K$ represents the disease status data of patients in the data set,

K is the number of diseases to be classified. Assume that the multicategory disease diagnosis problem is F, classification of the result $Y \in \mathbb{R}^K$, therefore, this problem can be modeled as shown in equation (19.1):

$$\{X_M; X_R; X_D\} \xrightarrow{F} Y \tag{19.1}$$

19.3.2 Data Filling Based on Mask Structure

To solve the problem of data length mismatch caused by the inconsistent sampling frequency of medical sensing data, a unified time interval is set to 1 hours, and the time series data is resampled at regular intervals. If there are multiple samples with the same feature in the same time interval, if there are several measured values, the last measured value will be used. Since the original sampling frequency of some features is much greater than 1 hours, resampling at a uniform time interval will cause data sparseness, so effective measures need to be taken to fill in the missing data. To this end, in this article, the filling method adopted is that if a missing value has a measurement value in its previous time, the missing value is replaced by the most recent measurement value, otherwise the present value is used. In addition, a binary mask vector is provided for each feature, using it is used to indicate whether the feature values corresponding to different times are real measured values. After the data filling and mask vector construction are completed, one-hot encoding is used to represent discrete features, and the standard deviation standardization method is used to process continuous features. Medical sense at time $t$the measured the data $X_M^{(t)}$ is standardized by standard deviation, and the calculation formula of x_t is as follows:

$$\mu = \frac{1}{T} \sum_{t=1}^{T} X_M^{(t)} \tag{19.2}$$

$$\sigma = \sqrt{\frac{1}{T-1} \sum_{t=1}^{T} \left(X_M^{(t)} - \mu\right)^2} \tag{19.3}$$

$$x_t = \frac{X_M^{(t)} - \mu}{\sigma} \tag{19.4}$$

After data preprocessing steps such as one-hot encoding, normalization, and mask representation, the sensing data vector and binary mask vector are spliced to obtain dynamic time series data $X_{dy} \in \mathbb{R}^{T \times d_{in}}$:

$$X_{dy} = [(x_1, c_1), (x_2, c_2), \ldots, (x_m, c_m)] \tag{19.5}$$

Among them, $x_m (t = 1, 2, \ldots, d_m)$ is the one-hot encoding representation or standardized feature value of attribute m, $c_m (m = 1, 2, \ldots, d_m)$ is the binary mask vector corresponding to attribute m, "T" is the length of the time series, d_m is the sum of the data feature dimension and the mask vector dimension.

19.3.3 Mining Disease-Related Relationships Based on Conditional Probability

Due to the complexity and diversity of diseases and their symptoms, six-digit alphanumeric ICD codes [6] are used in medicine to represent different diseases, and classifying all diseases will undoubtedly bring huge time and space overhead. To this end, this article selects some diseases with higher incidence rates according to the method described in the literature [12] and classifies them into category K to determine which diseases patients suffer from. According to statistics, the average number of patients with diseases is 4.13, more than 83% of patients suffer from at least two of the above-mentioned diseases. Therefore, effectively extracting the mutual influence between diseases and combining them into the model can improve the learning ability of the model. This article uses the patient's disease status data to construct the disease association matrix $\boldsymbol{I} \in \mathbb{R}^{K \times K}$. The calculation process of the disease association matrix is as follows.

First, count the number of patients with various diseases:

$$S_k = \sum_{n=1}^{N} y_{nk} \tag{19.6}$$

Among them, y_{nk} is the binary value of whether the nth patient suffers from disease k, 1 means suffering from such disease, and "0" means not suffering from such disease. Therefore, the prevalence rate of various diseases $P(S_k)$ can be obtained:

$$P(S_k) = \frac{S_k}{N} \tag{19.7}$$

The prevalence rates of K types of diseases together form the relationship vector w between disease patients:

$$\boldsymbol{w} = \{P(S_1), P(S_2), \ldots, P(S_K)\} \tag{19.8}$$

Then, count the number of people suffering from any two types of diseases at the same time, let S_{jk} represent the number of patients suffering from both disease j and disease k, then:

$$S_{jk} = \sum_{n=1}^{N} y_{nj} y_{nk} \tag{19.9}$$

$$P(S_{jk}) = \frac{S_{jk}}{N} \tag{19.10}$$

Among them, y_{nj} and y_{nk} are the binary values of whether the nth patient suffers from disease j and disease k, respectively, $P\ (Sjk)$ represents the comorbidity probability of disease j and disease k, and the relationship matrix v between diseases is obtained:

$$\boldsymbol{v} = \{P(S_{jk}) \mid 1 \leqslant j, k \leqslant K\} \tag{19.11}$$

It can be seen from the above calculation formula that v is a symmetric matrix.

The last step is to calculate the disease correlation matrix I. Since the incidence rates of different diseases vary greatly, to avoid the problem that diseases with low-incidence rates have smaller values when calculating the correlation relationship, conditional probability is used to calculate the impact I_{jk} of disease j on disease k, that is:

$$I_{jk} = P(k \mid j) = \frac{P(S_{jk})}{P(S_j)} \tag{19.12}$$

$$\boldsymbol{I} = \{I_{jk} \mid 1 \leqslant j, k \leqslant K\} \tag{19.13}$$

Figure 19.1 shows the heat map representation of the disease association matrix calculated by this algorithm.

19.3.4 GRU-Based Dynamic and Static Relationships Fusion of Multisource Health Sensing Data

GRU can learn trend features in time series, including long-term dependencies and short-term dependencies, and has the advantage of low computational time overhead, making it very suitable for feature extraction and analysis of large amounts of long-term medical sensing data. Medical sensing data depends on its time Trend features have certain advantages in judging acute diseases where physical sign measurement values change significantly. However, the age, gender and other physical conditions of the individual patient will affect the overall value of the physical signs, which in turn affects the judgment of the model. Therefore, personal physical record data was introduced and used GRU [24] fuses it with medical sensing data, and the fusion method is shown in Figure 19.3.

For the recorded data, one-hot vector encoding and normalization are also used. At each time step t, the recorded data and the sensing data are fused. First, the recorded data is dimensionally transformed through a fully connected network and regularized to obtain Static data weight, then fuse dynamic and static data through Hadamard product, and splice the fused data and dynamic data that is:

$$X_{st} = \mathrm{Norm}(f_r(X_R)) \tag{19.14}$$

$$X_{\mathrm{in}}^{(t)} = \left[X_{st} \cdot X_{dy}^{(t)}, X_{dy}^{(t)}\right], t = 1, 2, \ldots, T \tag{19.15}$$

Among them, $X_{dy}^{(t)} \in \mathbb{R}^{d_{\mathrm{in}}}$ is the personal physical fitness record data, dynamic time series data, f_r is a fully connected network, Norm() is a regularization

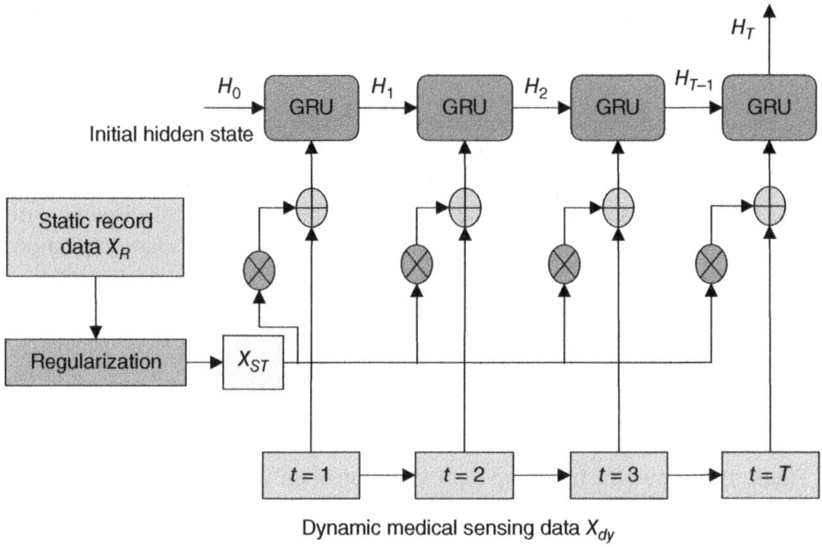

Figure 19.3 GRU-based dynamic and static relationships fusion.

operation, σ represents the Hadamard product. In this step, a fully connected layer is used to extractthe shallow features of personal physical recording data are mapped to medical sensing data. According to the same dimensions, the personal physical condition and the corresponding relationship are calculated through the Hadamard product. The influence of physical changes is obtained by GRU input $X_{\text{in}} \in \mathbb{R}^{T_x d_{\text{in}}}$.

Figure 19.4 shows the GRU network structure. Assume that the number of hidden units is d_h, given the hidden state $H_{t-1} \in \mathbb{R}^{d_k}$ of the previous time step, and let the input data at time t be $X_{\text{in}}^{(t)} \in \mathbb{R}^{d_{\text{in}}}$, then the reset gate the calculation formulas of $R_t \in \mathbb{R}^{d_h}$ and update gate $Z_t \in \mathbb{R}^{d_t}$ are as follows:

$$R_t = \sigma\left(X_{\text{in}}^{(t)} W_{xr} + H_{t-1} W_{kr} + b_r\right) \tag{19.16}$$

$$Z_t = \sigma\left(X_{\text{in}}^{(t)} W_{xz} + H_{t-1} W_{hz} + b_z\right) \tag{19.17}$$

Among them, W_{xr}, W_{hr}, W_{xz}, $W_{h\varepsilon}$, b_r, b_z are learnable parameters, σ is the sigmoid function, which maps the variables to between (0, 1). Then, the candidate's hidden state of the current time step is calculated through the reset gate time. The candidate's hidden state $\tilde{H}_t \in \mathbb{R}^{d_t}$ at step t is defined as follows:

$$\tilde{H}_t = \tanh\left(X_{\text{in}}^{(t)} W_{\text{st}} + (R_t * H_{t-1}) W_{hh} + b_h\right) \tag{19.18}$$

Among them, W_{xh}, W_{mk}, b_k are learnable parameters, and the tanh activation function maps the value of the candidate hidden state $\tilde{H}_t$ to (−1, 1). Then, an

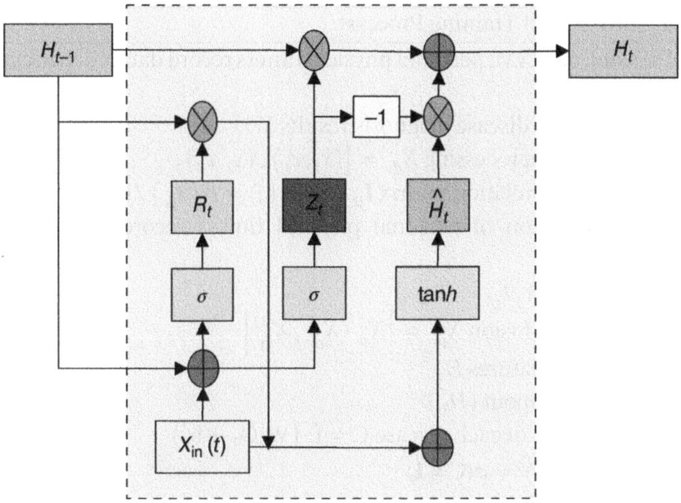

Figure 19.4 GRU network structure.

update gate is used to calculate the hidden state H_t of the current time step t:

$$H_t = Z_t \times H_{t-1} + (1 - Z_t) \times \tilde{H}_t \tag{19.19}$$

Initialize the hidden state $\boldsymbol{H}_0 \in \mathbb{R}^{d_A}$ as a zero vector. After continuous updating of the gated cycle unit T time step, the hidden feature H_T after the fusion of medical sensing data and personal physical record data can be obtained. In the data fusion process, to avoid model training. If overfitting occurs, the dropout regularization method is used to randomly invalidate some nodes of the network, that is:

$$O_T = \text{Dropout}(H_T) \tag{19.20}$$

19.3.5 Disease Diagnosis Algorithm Description

In Section 3.3, the disease correlation matrix $\boldsymbol{I} \in \mathbb{R}^{K \times K}$ is calculated; in Section 3.4, the GRU output $O_T \in \mathbb{R}^h$ after the fusion of medical sensing data and personal physical record data is obtained. Since the structures of the two are not consistent, further processing and fusion of data are required.

First, the GRU output O_T is converted into the prevalence probability C of K-type diseases through the fully connected network:

$$C = f_c(W_c O_T + b_c) \tag{19.21}$$

Among them, fc is a fully connected neural network, W_c and b_c are learnable parameters and the disease probability $C \in \mathbb{R}^K$.

Algorithm 19.1 DSRF Model Training Process

Input: Medical sensing data XM; personal physical fitness record data XR; patient condition data XD

Output: In total, 25 types of disease diagnosis results Y

1. Medical sensing data preprocessing $X_{dy} = \left[\left(x_1, c_1\right), \left(x_2, c_2\right), \cdots, \left(x_T, c_T\right)\right]$
2. Calculate the disease correlation matrix $\mathbf{I}_{jk} = P(\mathrm{k} \mid \mathrm{j}) = P\left(\mathrm{S_{jk}}\right) / P\left(\mathrm{S_j}\right)$
3. Dimension transformation of personal physical fitness record data $X_{st} = \mathrm{Norm}\left(f_r\left(X_R\right)\right)$
4. For each time step t, t = 1, 2, ⋯, T:
5. Dynamic and static data fusion $X_{in}^{(t)} = \left[X_{st} \cdot X_{dy}^{(1)}, X_{dy}^{(1)}\right]$
6. Compute GRU hidden features H_t
7. Regularization $O_T = \mathrm{Dropout}\left(H_T\right)$
8. Calculate the probability of each disease $\mathrm{C} = \mathrm{f_c}\left(\mathrm{W_c O_T} + \mathrm{b_c}\right)$
9. Disease diagnosis result $\widehat{\mathrm{Y}} = \sigma(\mathrm{C} \times \mathbf{I})$
10. Calculate classification loss L
11. Start iteratively training the model from the third step until the set number of iterations or the classification result reaches the stopping criterion.

Then multiply the disease probability C and the disease association matrix I to integrate the disease dependence into the model and use the *sigmoid* activation function to obtain the final multi-category disease diagnosis result $\varepsilon\hat{Y}\varepsilon$:

$$\hat{Y} = \sigma(C \times \boldsymbol{I}) \tag{19.22}$$

The loss function used in this model is the average binary cross entropy loss L:

$$L = -\frac{1}{K}\sum_{k=1}^{K}(y_k \log(\hat{y}_k) + (1 - y_k)\log(1 - \hat{y}_k)) \tag{19.23}$$

Among them, y_k is the actual prevalence of disease k, and $\hat{y}_k$ is the diagnosis result of disease k.

19.4 Experiments and Analysis

This article compares a DSRF based on the fusion of dynamic and static relationships of multisource health sensing data with a benchmark classification model to evaluate the effectiveness and parameter sensitivity of the model, as well as the impact of different structures of the model on disease diagnosis performance.

19.4.1 Data Set and Parameter Settings

This article uses the large-scale medical clinical database MIMIC-III (V1.4) [6] in the United States to conduct experiments. Effective medical sensing data, personal physical record data, and disease status data are screened out from the original database and based on the 8:1:1 ratio. Proportionally divide the training set, validation set, and test set.

The Adam optimization algorithm is selected for the model, the intercepted time series length is 480, the training batch size is set to 64, and the learning rate is 0.001, the GRU layer uses 256 hidden neural units, the dropout parameter is 0.4, and the number of iterations is set to 50.

19.4.2 Benchmark Models and Evaluation Indicators

To verify the performance of the DSRF based on the fusion of dynamic and static relationships of multisource health sensing data, experiments were compared with the following benchmark models.

LR [25]: Feature extraction using the method described in the mentioned article.

LSTM [26]: Standard long short-term memory network.

Doctor AI [21]: Use RNN to use medical record data to predict subsequent medical visits and drug category diagnosis.

Med2Vec [27]: Uses a scalable two-layer neural network to learn low-dimensional vector representation of GAI medical data.

Crist'obal [28]: Use RNN and feedforward neural networks to combine sequence data and static data.

SAnD [29]: Use masked self-attention mechanism, position coding, and dense interpolation strategy to model clinical time series data.

AdaCare [4]: Learn the long-term and short-term changes in patients' physiological characteristics and describe the patient's health status on multiple time scales.

Evaluation indicators: This article uses three evaluation indicators: Micro AUROC, Macro AUROC, and Weighted AUROC to evaluate the diagnosis of multicategory diseases.

Given the classification result $\hat{Y}$ and the real label Y, defines the functions $\mathrm{Neg}(y)$, $\mathrm{Pos}(y)$ to, respectively, indicate whether the sample y is a positive example and whether it is a negative example. $\mathrm{Num}(y_1, y_2)$ indicates whether the classification probability of the sample y_1 is greater than y_2. The calculation formulas of the three evaluation indicators are as follows:

$$\text{Micro AUROC} = \frac{\sum_{j=1}^{K}\sum_{i=1}^{N}\sum_{k=1}^{K}\sum_{n=1}^{N}\text{Pos}(y_{nk})\text{Neg}(y_{ij})\text{Num}(\hat{y}_{nk}, y_{ij})}{\sum_{k=1}^{K}\sum_{n=1}^{N}\text{Pos}(y_{nk})\sum_{k=1}^{K}\sum_{n=1}^{N}\text{Neg}(y_{nk})} \tag{19.24}$$

$$\text{Macro AUROC} = \frac{1}{K}\sum_{k=1}^{K}\frac{\sum_{i=1}^{N}\sum_{n=1}^{N}\text{Pos}(y_{nk})\text{Neg}(y_{ik})\text{Num}(\hat{y}_{nk}, \hat{y}_{ik})}{\sum_{n=1}^{N}\text{Pos}(y_{nk})\sum_{n=1}^{N}\text{Neg}(y_{nk})} \tag{19.25}$$

$$\text{Weighted AUROC} = \sum_{k=1}^{K}\frac{\sum_{i=1}^{N}\sum_{n=1}^{N}\text{Pos}(y_{nk})\text{Neg}(y_{ik})\text{Num}(\hat{y}_{nk}, y_{ik})u_k}{\sum_{n=1}^{N}\text{Pos}(y_{nk})\sum_{n=1}^{N}\text{Neg}(y_{nk})} \tag{19.26}$$

Among them, "K" is the total number of disease categories to be classified, "N" is the total number of patient samples, and w_k is the proportion of the number of patients with disease k to the total number of patients with all diseases:

$$w_k = \frac{\sum_{n=1}^{N}P(y_{nk})}{\sum_{k=1}^{K}\sum_{n=1}^{N}P(y_{nk})} \tag{19.27}$$

19.4.3 Analysis of Comparative Experimental Results

Table 19.1 lists the evaluation results of different models on multicategory disease diagnosis tasks based on the MIMIC-III data set. As can be seen from the table, the model DSRF in this chapter achieved the best index values in all evaluation criteria compared with other models.

Table 19.1 Comparison of multicategory disease diagnosis task results under different models.

Evaluation indicators	Micro AUROC	Macro AUROC	Weighted AUROC
LR	80.12	74.06	73.23
LSTM	82.10	77.04	75.69
DoctorAI	82.21	77.40	76.54
Med2Vec	82.24	77.51	76.62
Crist'obal	82.44	77.81	76.98
SAnD	81.64	76.58	75.39
AdaCare	82.59	77.76	76.72
Our method	83.34	78.64	77.57

Note: Unit in %.

For time series data in medical sensing data, the LR model uses statistical methods to calculate six different sample statistical characteristics on seven different subsequences of a given time series of different variables to represent the time characteristics of the data. However, this method of manually extracting features ignores the sequential relationship between different times. The *SAnD* model uses a masked self-attention mechanism to model clinical time series data and uses position encoding and dense interpolation strategies to learn the temporal characteristics of the data. However, in this method there are limitations in extracting long-term features. Compared with the above two models, the gated recurrent NN GRU used in this model has greater advantages in extracting time trend features and long-term and short-term dependencies.

In terms of multisource health sensing data fusion, the LSTM and AdaCare models only use medical sensing time series data for disease diagnosis. Although the dilated convolution layer in the AdaCare model can learn long-term and short-term changes in patients' physiological characteristics, and adopts scale auto-scaling. The adaptive feature extraction and recalibration method models the correlation between clinical features, but this model does not take into account the impact of personal physical condition on the patient's physiological characteristics and the interaction between multiple diseases. The medical sense proposed in this section, the fusion of measurement data and personal physical condition data, allows the model to learn the potential relationship between the two and constructs a disease association matrix, making full use of the feature of dependence between diseases, making the multicategory disease diagnosis task significantly effective promote.

The models proposed by DoctorAI, Med2Vec, and Crist'obal use recurrent NN, feedforward NN, and their combination methods to map two heterogeneous data, medical sensing data and personal physical record data, to the same dimension for fusion, but three models process the two types of data separately and then fuse them, without extracting the relationship between the data. Therefore, this chapter makes improvements in data relationship extraction, using linear layers to extract shallow features of personal physical record data and map them to the same dimension of medical sensing data, Hadamard product is used to calculate personal physical condition and the impact on physical sign changes, which together with the original features of the sensing data serve as the input of the gated loop unit. This dynamic and static relationships fusion method can not only solve the problem of heterogeneous data Fusion problem, and can extract the relationship features of heterogeneous data, helping the model to differentially diagnose the diseases of different patients according to their physical conditions. Table 19.2 lists the prevalence proportions of acute, mixed, and chronic diseases and the evaluation results of Macro AUROC and Weighted AUROC on chronic diseases. As can be seen from Table 19.2, the classification effect of this model on chronic diseases

Table 19.2 Comparison of disease classification assessment results.

Chronic diseases (39.35%)			
Evaluation indicators	**Micro AUROC**	**Macro AUROC**	**Weighted AUROC**
LR	79.48	73.24	80.19
LSTM	81.49	76.51	82.07
DoctorAI	76.95	76.98	82.22
Med2Vec	77.03	77.05	82.25
Crist'obal	77.74	77.13	82.56
SAnD	75.84	77.13	81.23
AdaCare	78.12	76.67	82.64
Our Method	78.07	78.12	83.35

Note: Unit in %.

is better than the best baseline model, which shows that the proposed data fusion model is more effective in classifying three types of diseases. Different types of disease classification have good results.

Among all the benchmark models, the classification effect of acute diseases is the best and the model gap is small. This is because the time series trend characteristics of acute diseases are obvious and easier to be learned. In this case, AdaCare uses dilated convolutional network to extract model trend features. The model is obviously better than other models, but it lacks consideration of the correlation between diseases, resulting in a slightly lower diagnostic performance for acute diseases than the DSRF model in this article. The trend characteristics of chronic diseases are weak, so medical sensing data and personal physical data are combined. The fusion-processed DoctorAI, Med2Vec, and Crist'obal models have all achieved relatively good classification results, but the chronic disease diagnosis performance of the above three benchmark models is still worse than the model in this article, which confirms that the model in this article has a good relationship with medical sensing dynamic data and personal data. Effectiveness of mining correlation of physical fitness record data.

To study the effect of the dynamic and static relationships fusion of medical sensing data and personal physical record data and the disease correlation matrix fusion of the two modules in the model, this chapter uses the splicing method to replace equations (19.14) and (19.15) to obtain the splicing fusion model (DSRFnoFu). Mask the disease association matrix in the model to obtain the

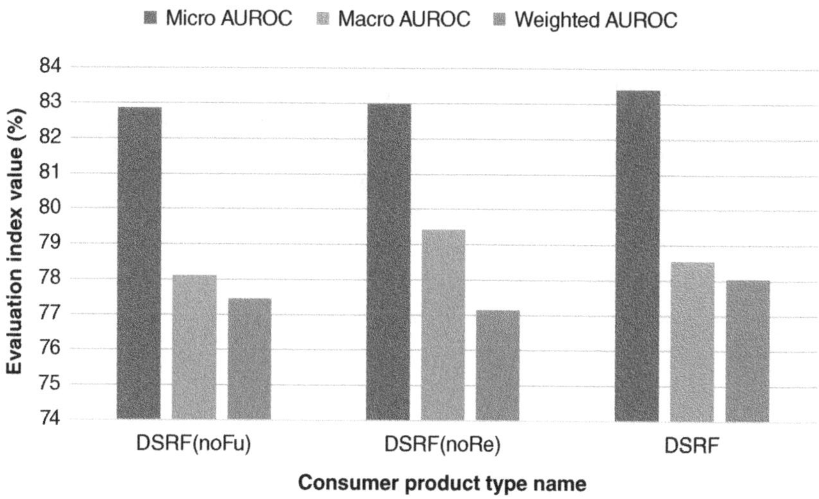

Figure 19.5 Comparison of ablation experiment results.

disease-free relationship model (DSRFnoRe), and compare the results with the DSRF model, as shown in Figure 19.5.

As can be seen from Figure 19.5, the model performance evaluation results using the fusion of medical sensing data and personal physical record data and the fusion of medical sensing data and disease relationship data are all lower than the proposed DSRF model, which means that the relationship between dynamic and static data and disease-related relationships play an important role in multicategory disease diagnosis tasks. The multisource health perception data fusion method and disease-related relationship mining method in the model are effective and can better complete multicategory disease diagnosis tasks.

19.4.4 Parameter Selection and Sample Analysis

This section studies the number of GRU hidden units, dropout regularization parameters and the time series length of the data in the model. First, in the process of multisource health perception data fusion based on GRU, the hidden units in GRU can be used to extract and remember the time series characteristics in the input data, the more hidden unit's can bring more complex computing power, but it is easier to cause overfitting of the model. To avoid this problem, the model described in this section uses the dropout regularization method (see equation (19.20)) that randomly causes some nodes of the network to fail. Therefore, the number of GRU hidden units and dropout parameters are two important parameters that affect the learning ability of the model. Next, this section will use experimental results to evaluate the different numbers of hidden units of different GRUs. The impact of dropout parameter values and different time series lengths on model classification performance.

Figure 19.6a,b, respectively, show the impact of different GRU hidden unit numbers and dropout parameters on model classification performance. The specific evaluation indicators include Macro AUROC and Weighted AUROC. Among

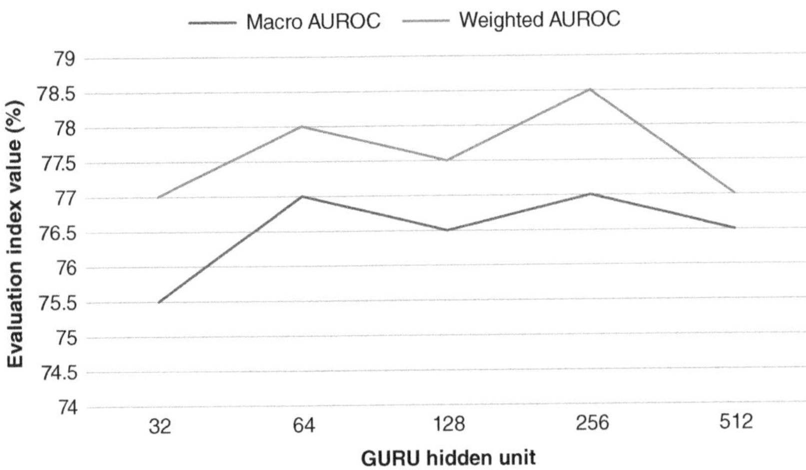

(a)

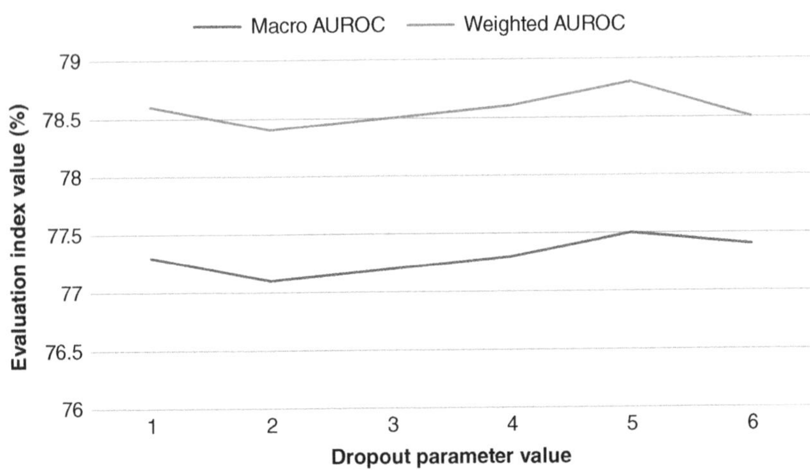

(b)

Figure 19.6 (a) The impact of the number of GRU hidden units on model performance. (b) The impact of the number of dropout parameters on model performance. (c) The impact of the number of time series length on model performance.

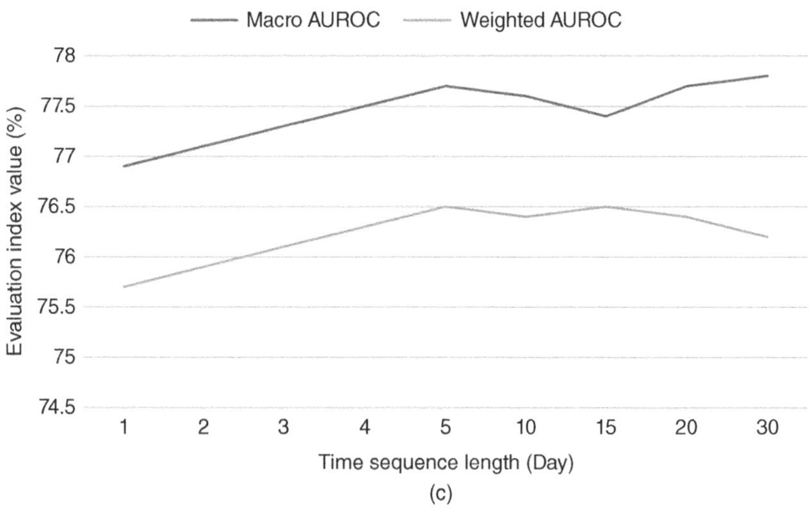

Figure 19.6 *(Continued)*

them, the higher the indicator value, the better the classification. The closer the result is to the true value, the better the performance of the model; conversely, a decrease in the index value indicates a decrease in model performance. As can be seen from the figure, when the number of hidden units of the GRU network is greater than or equal to 64, the model achieves better results. The disease diagnosis effect of the parameter is set to 256. For the dropout parameter, when the dropout parameter changes from 0.1 to 0.4, the classification effect gradually becomes better. It reaches a peak at four and then gradually decreases. When the parameter value is 0.4, the two index values are greater than the index value without using the dropout regularization method (that is, dropout = 0), which shows that this method is effective in improving model overfitting.

To further evaluate the performance of the proposed model, this chapter processes the data into a time series of different lengths to evaluate the robustness of the model. Figure 19.6c shows the classification performance evaluation curve of the DSRF model on time series of different lengths. As can be seen from the figure, the time series length required for the model to obtain optimal performance is 20 days, which is 480 hours. Starting from the 5th day, the upward trend of model performance tends to be flat, and the Macro AUROC and Weighted AUROC indicators remain at 0. 78 and 0.77 or above, which shows that the proposed method is still effective for shorter time series GAI medical data and has better generalization performance.

In addition, this article also selected some patients to compare the DSRF model with the benchmark model GRU to verify the effectiveness of the disease

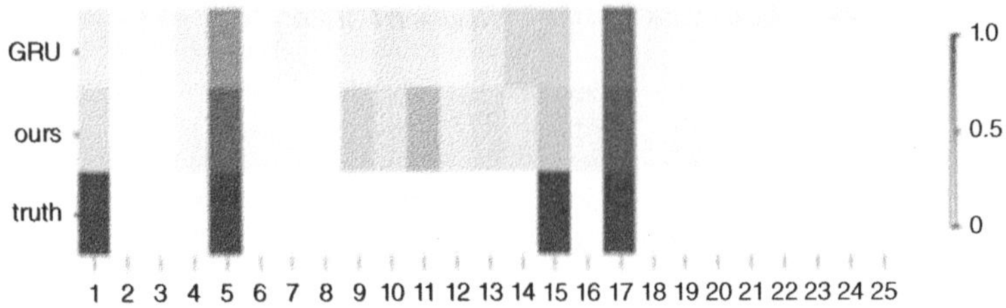

Figure 19.7 Patient 1's disease diagnosis probability and actual disease status.

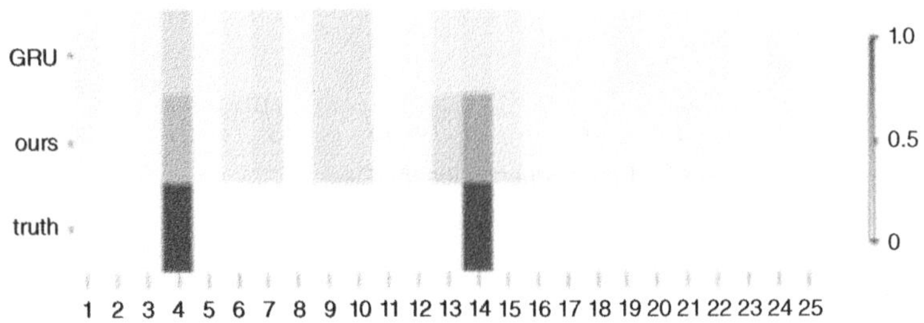

Figure 19.8 Patient 2's disease diagnosis probability and actual disease status.

association matrix module. Figures 19.7 and 19.8, respectively, show the disease diagnosis probability and probability of a patient under different models in real disease situations. The darker the color of the rectangle, the greater the probability that the model believes that the patient has the disease. On the contrary, the lighter the color each column represents a disease, and the three rows from top to bottom are the GRU model diagnosis probability and the DSRF model diagnosis. The probability and the binary value representing whether the patient has the disease or not.

As can be seen from Figure 19.7, compared with GRU, the DSRF model determines that this patient has a higher probability of suffering from chronic kidney disease (5) because he has a higher probability of suffering from hypertension and complications (17), which is consistent with the previous article. The mentioned complications of hypertension and chronic kidney disease are consistent with the dependence relationship. The correlation matrix corrects the patient's disease diagnosis results based on the relationship between the two diseases and successfully diagnoses chronic kidney disease. As can be seen from Figure 19.8, with the function of the disease association matrix, the mutually exclusive relationship between essential hypertension (14) and hypertension with complications (17) makes the probability of disease of the two show the characteristics of one high and one low. The DSRF model has the characteristics of primary hypertension (14) and hypertension with complications (17). Hypertension was correctly diagnosed.

19.5 Conclusion

This article proposed a disease diagnosis model (DSRF) based on dynamic and static relationships fusion of multisource health sensing data. This model uses the data dynamic and static relationships fusion algorithm to extract the relationship features of heterogeneous data and constructs a disease association matrix to extract the relationships between diseases. Correlation relationship features, and use the gated recurrent unit network to successively integrate dynamic medical sensing data, static personal physical record data and disease relationship data. Finally, it is evaluated on the MIMICIII real public dataset. The experimental results show that the DSRF model is better than the latest "A" good benchmark model that can diagnose many types of diseases very well. In future work, the extraction and fusion of disease relationships can be further improved, and attempts can be made to conduct more targeted diagnoses and analyses of different types of diseases, predictions, and apply it to more related fields.

References

1 Liu, Q., Yu, L., Luo, L. et al. (2020). Semi-supervised medical image classification with relation-driven self-ensembling model. *IEEE Transactions on Medical Imaging* 39 (11): 3429–3440. https://doi.org/10.1109/TMI.2020.2995518.

2 Ren, Y., Shi, Y., Zhang, K. et al. (2020). Medical treatment migration prediction based on GCN via medical insurance data. *IEEE Journal of Biomedical and Health Informatics* 24 (9): 2516–2522. https://doi.org/10.1109/JBHI.2020.3008493.

3 Thamsen, B., Yevtushenko, P., Gundelwein, L. et al. (2021). Synthetic database of aortic morphometry and hemodynamics: overcoming medical imaging data availability. *IEEE Transactions on Medical Imaging* 40 (5): 1438–1449. https://doi.org/10.1109/TMI.2021.3057496.

4 Gopakumar, S., Tran, T., Nguyen, T.D. et al. (2015). Stabilizing high-dimensional prediction models using feature graphs. *IEEE Journal of Biomedical and Health Informatics* 19 (3): 1044–1052. https://doi.org/10.1109/JBHI.2014.2353031.

5 Nguyen, A., Foerstel, S., Kittler, T. et al. (2021). System design for a data-driven and explainable customer sentiment monitor using IoT and enterprise data. *IEEE Access* 9: 117140–117152. https://doi.org/10.1109/ACCESS.2021.3106791.

6 Lu, W., Ma, L., Chen, H. et al. (2020). A clinical prediction model in health time series data based on long short-term memory network optimized by fruit fly optimization algorithm. *IEEE Access* 8: 136014–136023. https://doi.org/10.1109/ACCESS.2020.3011721.

7 Lei, T., Zhang, D., Du, X. et al. (2023). Semi-supervised medical image segmentation using adversarial consistency learning and dynamic convolution network. *IEEE Transactions on Medical Imaging* 42 (5): 1265–1277. https://doi.org/10.1109/TMI.2022.3225687.

8 Yu, F., Cui, L., Chen, H. et al. (2023). HealthNet: a health progression network via heterogeneous medical information fusion. *IEEE Transactions on Neural Networks and Learning Systems* 34 (10): 6940–6954. https://doi.org/10.1109/TNNLS.2022.3202305.

9 Zhang, X., Qian, B., Li, Y. et al. (2023). Context-aware and time-aware attention-based model for disease risk prediction with interpretability. *IEEE Transactions on Knowledge and Data Engineering* 35 (4): 3551–3562. https://doi.org/10.1109/TKDE.2021.3130171.

10 Manogaran, G., Shakeel, P.M., Baskar, S. et al. (2021). FDM: fuzzy-optimized data management technique for improving big data analytics. *IEEE Transactions on Fuzzy Systems* 29 (1): 177–185. https://doi.org/10.1109/TFUZZ.2020.3016346.

11 Papanastasiou, G., Dikaios, N., Huang, J. et al. (2024). Is attention all you need in medical image analysis? A review. *IEEE Journal of Biomedical and Health Informatics* 28 (3): 1398–1411. https://doi.org/10.1109/JBHI.2023.3348436.

12 Isola, R., Carvalho, R., and Tripathy, A.K. (2012). Knowledge discovery in medical systems using differential diagnosis, LAMSTAR, and *k*-NN. *IEEE Transactions on Information Technology in Biomedicine* 16 (6): 1287–1295. https://doi.org/10.1109/TITB.2012.2215044.

13 Torres-Velázquez, M., Chen, W.-J., Li, X., and McMillan, A.B. (2021). Application and construction of deep learning networks in medical imaging. *IEEE Transactions on Radiation and Plasma Medical Sciences* 5 (2): 137–159. https://doi.org/10.1109/TRPMS.2020.3030611.

14 Wang, J., Xie, Z., Li, Y. et al. (2020). Relationship between health status and physical fitness of college students from South China: an empirical study by data mining approach. *IEEE Access* 8: 67466–67473. https://doi.org/10.1109/ACCESS.2020.2986039.

15 Yang, F., Wu, Q., Hu, X. et al. (2021). Internet-of-things-enabled data fusion method for sleep healthcare applications. *IEEE Internet of Things Journal* 8 (21): 15892–15905. https://doi.org/10.1109/JIOT.2021.3067905.

16 Banaee, H. and Loutfi, A. (2015). Data-driven rule mining and representation of temporal patterns in physiological sensor data. *IEEE Journal of Biomedical and Health Informatics* 19 (5): 1557–1566. https://doi.org/10.1109/JBHI.2015.2438645.

17 Liu, C., Xiong, H., Papadimitriou, S. et al. (2017). A proactive workflow model for healthcare operation and management. *IEEE Transactions on Knowledge and Data Engineering* 29 (3): 586–598. https://doi.org/10.1109/TKDE.2016.2631537.

18 Hao, J., Duan, J., Wang, K. et al. (2023). Inverse kinematic modeling of the tendon-actuated medical continuum manipulator based on a lightweight timing input neural network. *IEEE Transactions on Medical Robotics and Bionics* 5 (4): 916–928. https://doi.org/10.1109/TMRB.2023.3315473.

19 Shobanadevi, A., Maragathm, G., Gangadharan, S.M.P. et al. (2022). Internet of things-based data hiding scheme for wireless communication. *Wireless Communications and Mobile Computing* 2022: 6997190, 8 pages. https://doi.org/10.1155/2022/6997190.

20 Chanak, P. and Banerjee, I. (2020). Congestion free routing mechanism for IoT-enabled wireless sensor networks for smart healthcare applications. *IEEE Transactions on Consumer Electronics* 66 (3): 223–232. https://doi.org/10.1109/TCE.2020.2987433.

21 Ibarra, E., Antonopoulos, A., Kartsakli, E. et al. (2016). QoS-aware energy management in body sensor nodes powered by human energy harvesting. *IEEE Sensors Journal* 16 (2): 542–549. https://doi.org/10.1109/JSEN.2015.2483064.

22 Fengou, M.-A., Mantas, G., Lymberopoulos, D. et al. (2013). A new framework architecture for next generation healthcare services. *IEEE Journal of Biomedical and Health Informatics* 17 (1): 9–18. https://doi.org/10.1109/TITB.2012.2224876.

23 Khalifeh, A., Abou-Tair, D.E.D.I., Obermaisser, R. et al. (2023). A reliable system-of-systems healthcare monitoring framework. *IEEE Access* 11: 145679–145691. https://doi.org/10.1109/ACCESS.2023.3343414.

24 Rinchi, O., Nisbett, N., and Alsharoa, A. (2023). Patients Arms Segmentation and Gesture Identification Using Standalone 3-D LiDAR Sensors. *IEEE Sensors Letters* 7 (9): 1, 6005204–4. https://doi.org/10.1109/LSENS.2023.3303081.

25 Georgi, N., Corvol, A., and Le BouquinJeannès, R. (2018). Middleware architecture for health sensors interoperability. *IEEE Access* 6: 26283–26291. https://doi.org/10.1109/ACCESS.2018.2835644.

26 Liu, H.-W., Dubey, M., and Tseng, H.-W. (2023). LAEBLE: a lightweight authentication and encryption mechanism for the healthcare system in Bluetooth low energy. *IEEE Sensors Journal* 23 (21): 26712–26727. https://doi.org/10.1109/JSEN.2023.3307730.

27 Benharref, A. and Serhani, M.A. (2014). Novel cloud and SOA-based framework for healthcare monitoring using wireless biosensors. *IEEE Journal of Biomedical and Health Informatics* 18 (1): 46–55. https://doi.org/10.1109/JBHI.2013.2262659.

28 Kumar, M. and Chand, S. (2020). A secure and efficient cloud-centric internet-of-medical-things-enabled smart healthcare system with public verifiability. *IEEE Internet of Things Journal* 7 (10): 10650–10659. https://doi.org/10.1109/JIOT.2020.3006523.

29 Yan, H., Huo, H., Xu, Y., and Gidlund, M. (2010). Wireless sensor network based healthcare system - implementation and experimental results. *IEEE Transactions on Consumer Electronics* 56 (4): 2288–2295. https://doi.org/10.1109/TCE.2010.5681102.

20

Leveraging Generative Adversarial Networks for Image Augmentation in Deep Learning

Ravi Kumar[1,2], Akshay Kanwar[3], Amritpal Singh[1], and Aditya Khamparia[4]

[1] *Department of Computer Science Engineering, Lovely Professional University, Phagwara, 144411 Punjab, India*
[2] *Department of Computer Science Engineering (AIML), Jawaharlal Nehru Government Engineering college, University Hamirpur, Sundernagar, 175018, Himachal Pradesh, India*
[3] *Department of Electronics and Communication Engineering, Jawaharlal Nehru Government Engineering college, University Hamirpur, Sundernagar, 175018, Himachal Pradesh, India*
[4] *Department of Computer Science, Babasaheb Bhimrao Ambedkar University, Amethi Uttar Pradesh, 226025, India*

20.1 Introduction

In recent years, deep getting to know strategies have revolutionized diverse domain names via means of accomplishing high-quality overall performance in obligations inclusive of image classification and object detection. However, the efficacy of deep getting to know models closely is based on the availability and quality of training data [20]. In many real-world scenarios, acquiring annotated data in sufficient quantities can be challenging, leading to issues like overfitting and poor generalization. Image augmentation emerges as a fundamental strategy to address these challenges, enabling the generation of diverse training samples from existing data. While traditional augmentation methods like rotation and flipping provide limited variability, the advent of generative adversarial networks offers a paradigm shift by facilitating the creation of high-fidelity synthetic images closely resembling real data distributions [11, 22].

20.1.1 Evolution of GAN Architectures

The development of GAN architectures has been characterized by continuous innovation and refinement, spearheaded by pioneering works such as Goodfellow et al. [1] presented the concept of Original Adversarial Networks. Specialized variations, including deep-convolutional GAN (DC–GAN) by Radford et al.,

Generative Artificial Intelligence for Biomedical and Smart Health Informatics,
First Edition. Edited by Aditya Khamparia and Deepak Gupta.

which uses convolutional neural networks (CNNs) for enhanced stability and scalability, were introduced as a result of later developments [2]. Mirza and Osindero introduced conditional GANs, or C-GANs., enable conditional image generation by conditioning the generator on additional information, opening avenues for controlled synthesis tasks [3]. Wasserstein GANs (W-GANs) by Arjovsky et al. address training instability issues by introducing Wasserstein distance as a metric for measuring generator performance, thereby facilitating more stable training dynamics [4].

20.1.2 Applications of GANs

The versatility of GANs is exemplified through a plethora of applications spanning image generation, style transfer, super-resolution, and image-to-image translation. For instance, CycleGAN proposed by Zhu et al. [5] enables unsupervised image-to-image translation across different domains, showcasing its utility in tasks like artistic style transfer and domain adaptation. StarGAN [6] extends this capability to multiple domains, allowing unified image translation across diverse attributes such as age, gender, and facial expressions. Moreover, progressive growing of GAN (Pro-GAN) (Karras et al., 2018) [8] and to improve the quality and diversity of generated images, Style-GAN (Karras et al., 2019) [12] introduces progressive growth and style-based architectures, respectively.

20.1.3 GANs for Image Augmentation

In the context of deep learning, image augmentation plays a pivotal role in improving model generalization and robustness. By augmenting the training dataset with synthetically generated images, GANs offer a means to enrich the data manifold and expose the model to diverse variations present in real-world scenarios. This not only helps mitigate overfitting but also fosters better adaptation to unseen data distributions. Moreover, GAN-based augmentation techniques can be tailored to specific application domains, facilitating the generation of domain-specific features and enhancing model performance in target tasks.

20.1.4 Applications of GAN-Based Image Augmentation

The integration of GAN-based image augmentation has been instrumental across various domains, including healthcare, anomaly detection, and drug discovery. In medical imaging, GANs are employed to generate synthetic images augmenting limited datasets, thereby enhancing the robustness of deep learning models for tasks like lesion detection and classification [11, 20, 22]. Similarly, in anomaly detection, GAN-generated samples serve as representative outliers, aiding in the training of robust anomaly detection models. Furthermore, GANs contribute to drug discovery efforts by synthesizing molecular structures with desired properties, expediting the process of compound screening and optimization.

20.2 Literature Review

Image augmentation plays a pivotal role in improving model generalization and robustness. By augmenting the training dataset with synthetically generated images, GANs offer a means to enrich the data manifold and expose the model to diverse variations present in real-world scenarios. In the past researchers have applied GANs on various image datasets for generating good-quality synthetic images. In medical imaging, GANs are employed to generate synthetic images augmenting limited datasets, thereby enhancing the robustness of deep learning models for tasks like lesion detection and classification. In recent times, GANs are gaining popularity in generating medical image data as access to real medical data is very limited, and medical institutions do not share their data easily. The following studies show the usage and impact of GANs on medical image analysis.

The literature review encompasses a variety of GANs and their applications, offering insights into their methodologies, advantages, limitations, future scope, and results, which are presented in Tables 20.1 and 20.2. Starting with the foundational GANs introduced by Alan Johnson in 2014, these networks are lauded for their ability to produce realistic images, capture complex data distributions, and facilitate creative applications like art generation. However, challenges such as training instability and mode collapse persist. Nevertheless, ongoing research aims to enhance image generation quality, address stability issues, and integrate GANs with other modalities, such as text-to-image generation [1].

Moving to conditional generative adversarial nets (cGAN) proposed by Mehdi Mirza and Simon Osindero in 2014, this framework offers control over generated data distribution through conditioning, enabling tasks like generating MNIST digits conditioned on class labels or image tagging for multilabel predictions. While the flexibility in incorporating various factors into the model is appreciated, challenges related to hyperparameters and architecture choices persist, driving further exploration into improving experimental results and implementing joint training schemes for language models [1].

Further exploration reveals the GAN introduced by Ian J. Goodfellow and colleagues in 2014. This approach eliminates the need for Markov chains or unrolled inference networks, showcasing its ability to represent sharp distributions [1]. However, issues such as synchronization during training and the lack of explicit representation of generated distribution remain. Nonetheless, ongoing efforts

Table 20.1 Different GAN-based approaches and their results.

Reference number	Year	Methodology used	Applications	Result
[1]	2014	Adversarial Nets	Image generation, data augmentation	Adversarial networks excel at capturing precise, sometimes extreme distributions, unlike Markov chain methods which struggle with highly defined distributions and prefer blurrier ones for effective mode mixing.
[2]	2016	Deep convolutional generative adversarial networks (DCGANs)	Image generation, Feature extraction for supervised tasks, visualizing learned representations	While adversarial networks effectively learn image representations for tasks like supervised learning and generative modeling, there are lingering issues with model stability.
[3]	2014	Conditional Generative Adversarial Nets (cGAN)framework	Generating MNIST digits conditioned on class labels—Image tagging for multilabel predictions	The findings presented in this paper are in their early stages, yet they showcase the potential of conditional adversarial networks and hint at their promising applications.
[6]	2018	1. Generative Adversarial Networks (GANs) 2. Cycle-GANs, or Cycle-Consistent Adversarial Networks (CGAN)	Conversion of images across different domains	Effective and efficient multidomain image-to-image translation is achieved with a single model, demonstrating its versatility and applicability across various domains.
[9]	2019	Generative Adversarial Networks (GANs)	Image synthesis, data augmentation	Effective generation of high-resolution natural images with improved fidelity.

[10]	2023	U-Net architecture for lung and heart segmentation, progressive growing of GANs (Pro-GAN) for dataset generation	1. Cardiomegaly classification in chest X-ray images. 2. Automated measurement of cardiothoracic ratio (CTR)	Achieves high accuracy in cardiomegaly classification (94.61%)
[12]	2019	Generative adversarial Networks with style-based generator	1. Image generation: The model excels in generating high-quality images across various domains, including faces, animals, and landscapes. 2. Art creation: Artists and designers can leverage the model to produce novel and diverse artworks with fine-grained control over style and content.	Significant improvement in image quality, controllability, diversity, and scalability of image generation tasks using GANs.
[13]	2021	Generative adversarial networks (GANs)	CGAN to quantify the tissue traits applicable to tumor differentiation	The technique was carried out for prostate most cancers detection and acquired a F1 rating of 0.62 and an AUC of 0.9659.
[14]	2024	Generative adversarial networks (GANs)	This article proposes a generative adversarial network (GAN) for colorectal polyp classification using histopathology pictures based on a semisupervised framework.	Classification accuracy with 25% and 50% majority voting methods was 87.50% and 76.25%, respectively.

(Continued)

Table 20.1 (Continued)

Reference number	Year	Methodology used	Applications	Result
[15]	2022	Generative adversarial networks (GANs)	1. To identify undetected or easily overlooked polyps, a polyp detection method reflecting the morphological features of SSLs was proposed. 2. To create high-resolution complete endoscopic pictures, including sessile serrated lesions (SSL), a generative adversarial network (GAN) was employed.	The proposed system's sensitivity on SSLs was 17.5% higher when it was augmented with GAN-generated images.
[16]	2023	Semi-supervised generative adversarial network	Image augmentation for breast cancer classification	For the Aperio dataset, the model demonstrated a classification accuracy of 98.22% and an F1- score of 96.37%. On the Hamamatsu dataset, the model demonstrated accuracy of 98.44% and an F1-score of 97.47%.
[21]	2019	Generative adversarial networks (GANs)	Generating synthetic pathology images, representation learning for pathology images	Successful generation of synthetic pathology images with deep representations, enabling tasks such as data augmentation and representation learning.

Table 20.2 Pros, cons, and future scope of different GAN-based approaches.

Reference number	Year	Pros	Cons	Future scope
[1]	2014	1. No need for Markov chains or unrolled inference networks 2. Ability to represent sharp distributions	1. Requires synchronization between generator and discriminator during training 2. Lack of explicit representation of the generated distribution	Extensions to conditional generative models, learned inference, and semisupervised learning.
[2]	2016	Stable training with DCGAN architecture—Competes with other unsupervised algorithms in image classification tasks.	Previous instability issues in GANs addressed—Learned representations used for various tasks like image classification—Visualization of learned features.	Exploration of other domains like video and audio using similar frameworks—Further improvements in model stability and scalability
[3]	2014	Provides control over generated data distribution through conditioning—Flexibility in incorporating various factors and interactions into the model	Performance may vary based on hyperparameters and architecture choices—Potential for improvement in experimental results through further exploration.	Exploring the use of multiple tags simultaneously—Implementing joint training schemes for language models—Developing more sophisticated model architectures
[6]	2018	1. StarGAN is capable to perform image-to-image translation across multiple domains or styles. Unlike traditional image-to-image translation models that are trained for specific domain-to-domain mapping (e.g., translating images from one style to another), StarGAN can translate images among multiple domains in a single model.	May suffer from mode collapse	Improvement in model robustness and domain adaptation

(Continued)

Table 20.2 (Continued)

Reference number	Year	Pros	Cons	Future scope
		2. StarGAN model learns to perform image-to-image translation across multiple domains simultaneously. This means that during the training phase, the model is exposed to images from various domains and learns to translate between them without the need for separate training stages or models for each domain.		
[9]	2019	1. Produces high-fidelity natural images 2. Enables realistic image generation without artifacts 3. Scales to large datasets	1. Requires significant computational resources 2. Prone to mode collapse 3. Training instability	Optimization for efficiency, exploration of new architectures
[10]	2023	1. Utilization of ProGAN for dataset creation. 2. Achieves high accuracy in cardiomegaly classification (94.61%)	1. Dependency on accurate segmentation for CTR calculation. 2. Potential need for iterative refinement in real-world scenarios	1. Validation of CTR calculation in real-world scenarios. 2. Integration of user-editable iterations for inaccurate segmentations 3. Utilization of generated images for enhancing segmentation performance
[12]	2019	1. High-quality image generation: The model produces images with exceptional realism and diversity, often indistinguishable from real photographs. 2. The model enables users to manipulate various visual attributes	Computationally intensive: Training and inference require substantial computational resources, including powerful GPUs and significant time. The large model size and complex architecture demand significant memory and computational power.	Researchers are exploring techniques to reduce the computational cost and memory requirements of training and inference processes, making the model more accessible and scalable.

[13]	2021	The proposed approach is generic, and, accordingly, may be implemented to one of a kind styles of tissues and tumors	1. To better capture tissue properties and allow for limited, authorized use for reconstructing tissue images, benign GAN has to be improved. 2. Second, the intricate structural characteristics of tissues might not be entirely captured by the three similarity measures. 3. Third, since the basis for this study is image patches, the study's findings may differ depending on how the image patches are sampled.	1. A superior network optimization may have been attained by employing optimizers based on Sobolev gradients. 2. The proposed strategy will be contrasted with the patients' outcomes during an additional investigation.
[14]	2024	1. Enables generation of realistic histopathological images. 2. Potential to augment limited datasets for training models in pathology.	Limited control over generated images. 2. Accuracy can be further improved	To develop more advanced GAN architectures that can generate high-fidelity synthetic images closely resembling real histopathological images.
[15]	2022	The realistic images produced by GAN synthesize the endoscopic properties of polyps.	Requires large datasets for effective training.	Enhancing endoscopic resolution with real-time picture super-resolution can lead to the development of an advanced CADe system.
[16]	2023	Implemented and compared different GANs Generates realistic images,	The potential need for iterative refinement in real-world scenarios	It will be possible to create graph-based semisupervised GANs in the future that translate feature space into graph topologies.
[21]	2019	1. Enables generation of realistic pathology images. 2. Potential to augment limited datasets for training machine learning models in pathology.	1. Limited control over generated images. 2. Requires large datasets for effective training. 3. May generate unrealistic features	1. Integration with other machine learning models for enhanced diagnostic accuracy. 2. Medical education and virtual microscopy.

focus on extensions to conditional generative models, learned inference, and semisupervised learning [10, 21].

The DC–GANs presented by Alec Radford et al. in 2016 provide stable training and compete effectively in image classification tasks. Despite addressing previous instability issues, further exploration is warranted to enhance model stability and scalability, especially in domains like video and audio [2, 3].

Its capacity to generate high-fidelity natural images and scale to huge datasets is demonstrated in the 2019 study Large Scale—GAN Training for high fidelity Natural Image Synthesis by Andrew Brock et al. [9, 13]. However, computational resource requirements, mode collapse, and training instability remain challenges, driving research toward optimization for efficiency and the exploration of new architectures to improve fidelity [14, 15].

The Star-GAN proposed by Choi et al. in 2018 offers effective and efficient multidomain image-to-image translation with a single model, demonstrating versatility across various domains. Despite potential issues with mode collapse, ongoing research focuses on improving model robustness and domain adaptation [6].

The style-based architecture for GAN introduced by Tero Karras et al in 2019 significantly improves image quality, controllability, diversity, and scalability of image generation tasks using GANs [12]. However, computational intensity remains a challenge, prompting research into techniques to reduce computational cost and memory requirements for broader accessibility and scalability [16].

In this study, a semi-supervised GAN framework is proposed for enhancing colorectal polyp classification using histopathological images. The GAN enables the generation of realistic histopathological images and has the potential to augment limited datasets for ML model training in pathology [14]. However, drawbacks include limited control over generated images and room for improvement in accuracy. The aim is to develop more advanced GAN architectures capable of generating high-fidelity synthetic images that closely resemble real histopathological images [24, 26].

An additional study aimed to improve the identification of SSLs by means of a polyp detection technique that mirrors the morphological features of SSLs. This approach uses a GAN to create realistic, high-resolution entire endoscopic images, such as SSLs, that capture polyp endoscopic properties [15]. Challenges include the need for large datasets for effective training. Nevertheless, integrating GAN-synthesized images into a computer-aided detection (CADe) system demonstrated a significant improvement in sensitivity for SSL detection. This suggests the potential for developing an advanced CADe system by enhancing endoscopy resolution with real-time image super-resolution techniques [24, 25].

Overall, the reviewed literature underscores the diverse applications and advancements in GANs while also highlighting persistent challenges and avenues for future research and development.

20.3 Material and Method

Two datasets were considered for implementing GAN and creating synthetic images. The CVC-ClinicDB [17] dataset contains 612 images and CVC-ColonDB [18] dataset contains 2000 images. The dataset is created by combining two datasets. Normal images and polyps images were fed to GAN to generate other images. GAN is implemented to increase the samples. The dataset is created by combining original images from two datasets and images generated by the GAN.

20.3.1 Implementation

Implementation details will be divided into two parts: image augmentation by GAN and image classification by ResNet50 [19].

20.3.2 Image Augmentation by GAN

To increase the samples, GAN is employed. The generator module is in charge of creating artificial images, and the discriminator module is in charge of verifying that each generated image is unique. To achieve the best performance out of the GAN, the hyperparameters were adjusted fine. Hyperparameters are pivotal elements in the GAN framework, dictating its performance and stability. Key hyperparameters include the learning rate, determining the pace at which the model's parameters evolve through optimization algorithms like stochastic gradient descent (SGD) or Adam. Batch size, the number of examples processed in each training iteration, influences convergence speed and stability. Another crucial factor is the number of epochs, indicating how many times the entire dataset cycles through the GAN during training. The generator's input noise dimension plays a role in controlling the diversity of generated samples. Adjusting the discriminator and generator learning rates, along with the ratio of discriminator updates to generator updates, can fine-tune training dynamics. Activation functions, optimizer types, and loss functions, such as binary cross-entropy or Wasserstein loss, shape the learning process. Weight initialization schemes and

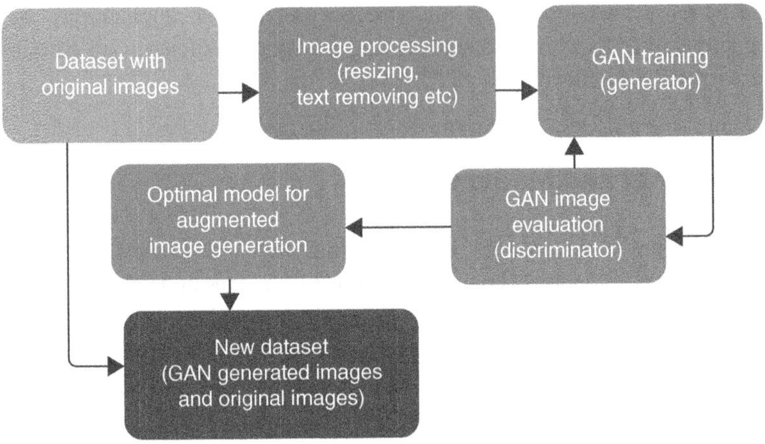

Figure 20.1 GAN workflow.

normalization techniques stabilize training by influencing initial parameter values and handling internal covariate shifts, respectively. In Wasserstein GANs, the gradient penalty coefficient modulates the impact of the gradient penalty term. Architectural choices, including the number of layers and their sizes, impact the model's capacity and expressiveness. Techniques like label smoothing and early stopping criteria are employed to prevent overconfidence in the discriminator and terminate training based on performance thresholds, respectively (Figure 20.1).

20.3.3 Image Classification by ResNet50

The dataset is divided 80:20 into training and testing portions. Next, a deep learning network (Resnet50) based on transfer learning was used to identify photos as either normal or polyps. The original dataset and the merged dataset were used to compare the model's performance. The hyperparameters implemented were adam optimizer, learning rate 0.001, batch size 32, epochs 100, dropout rate 0.2, and regularization L1 (Figure 20.2).

20.3.4 Model Evaluation

Model performance was evaluated using accuracy and F1 score. The equations for performance parameters are given by equations (20.1) and (20.2), respectively.

$$\text{Accuracy} = \frac{\text{TP} + \text{TN}}{\text{TP} + \text{TN} + \text{FP} + \text{FN}} \tag{20.1}$$

$$\text{F1 score} = 2 \times \frac{\text{Precision} \times \text{Recall}}{\text{Precision} + \text{Recall}} \tag{20.2}$$

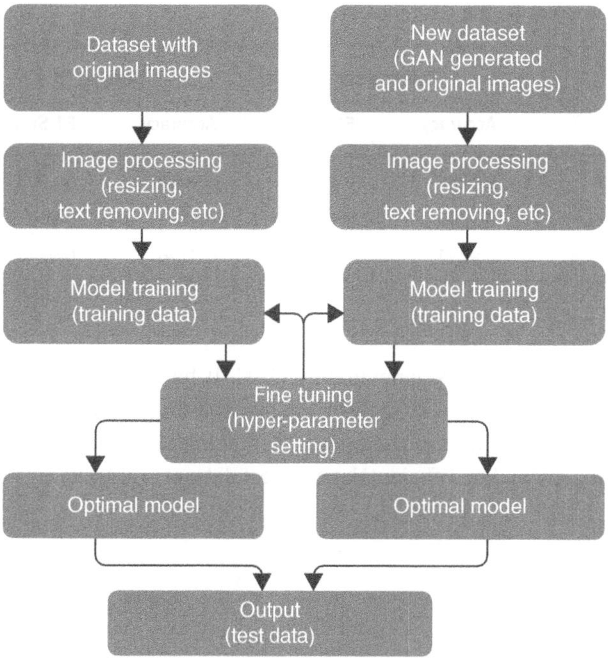

Figure 20.2 Image classification workflow.

20.4 Result and Discussion

The results on the original dataset constructed from CVS-ClinicDB and CVC-ColonDB are given in Table 20.3. The dataset contains original images without augmentation. The highest classification accuracy of 88.98% was achieved by EfficientNet on a test dataset.

The results of a combined dataset constructed from GAN-generated images, CVC-ClinicDB and CVC-ColonDB are given in Table 20.3. The dataset contains

Table 20.3 Model performance on original dataset.

Serial number	Model	Training set		Test set	
		Accuracy	F1 Score	Accuracy	F1 score
1	ResNet50	0.8999	0.8819	0.8759	0.876
2	DenseNet161	0.8985	0.8979	0.8873	0.8878
3	Efficient Net	0.8995	0.8985	0.8898	0.8899

Table 20.4 Model performance on the combined dataset

Serial number	Model	Training set		Test set	
		Accuracy	F1 Score	Accuracy	F1 Score
1	ResNet50	0.9295	0.9159	0.9049	0.9005
2	DenseNet161	0.9291	0.9271	0.9159	0.9151
3	Efficient Net	0.9293	0.9276	0.9176	0.9172

original images and synthetic images generated by GAN. It has been seen that GAN generated images were very close to realistic images, and the accuracy of the model is enhanced with the addition of these images. The highest classification accuracy of 91.76% was achieved by EfficientNet on a test dataset (Table 20.4).

20.5 Conclusion

GANs have emerged as a cornerstone within the realm of photo augmentation, providing exceptional abilities for synthesizing various and sensible images. By leveraging the improvements in GAN architectures and know-how of their programs throughout numerous domains, researchers, and practitioners can harness the electricity of GAN-primarily based total augmentation to decorate the overall performance and robustness of deep studying models. As the field continues to evolve, further research and exploration are warranted to unlock the full potential of GANs in addressing the challenges of limited data availability and improving the efficacy of deep learning systems.

References

1 Goodfellow, I., Pouget-Abadie, J., Mirza, M. et al. (2014). Generative adversarial nets. *Advances in Neural Information Processing Systems* 3 (11): https://doi.org/10.1145/3422622.

2 Radford, A., Metz, L., & Chintala, S. (2015). Unsupervised representation learning with deep convolutional generative adversarial networks. *arXiv preprint arXiv:1511.06434.*

3 Mirza, M., & Osindero, S. (2014). Conditional generative adversarial nets. *arXiv preprint arXiv:1411.1784.*

4 Gulrajani, I., Ahmed, F., Arjovsky, M. et al. (2017). Improved training of wasserstein gans. *Advances in neural information processing systems* 30: https://doi.org/10.48550/arXiv.1704.00028.

5 Zhu, J.Y., Park, T., Isola, P., & Efros, A.A. (2017). Unpaired image-to-image translation using cycle-consistent adversarial networks. *Proceedings of the IEEE international conference on computer vision*, pp. 2223–2232 Venice, Italy (22–29 October 2017). IEEE.

6 Choi, Y., Choi, M., Kim, M., et al. (2018). Stargan: Unified generative adversarial networks for multi-domain image-to-image translation. *Proceedings of the IEEE conference on computer vision and pattern recognition*, pp. 8789–8797. IEEE.

7 Rambow, F., Rogiers, A., Marin-Bejar, O. et al. (2018). Toward minimal residual disease-directed therapy in melanoma. *Cell* 174 (4): 843–855.

8 Karras, T., Aila, T., Laine, S., & Lehtinen, J. (2017). Progressive growing of gans for improved quality, stability, and variation. *arXiv preprint arXiv:1710.10196.*

9 Brock, A., Donahue, J., & Simonyan, K. (2018). Large scale GAN training for high fidelity natural image synthesis. *arXiv preprint arXiv:1809.11096.*

10 Kusakunniran, W., Saiviroonporn, P., Siriapisith, T. et al. (2023). Automatic measurement of cardiothoracic ratio in chest X-ray images with ProGAN-generated dataset. *Applied Computing and Informatics.* https://doi.org/10.1108/ACI-11-2022-0322.

11 Quiros, A.C., Murray-Smith, R., & Yuan, K. (2019). PathologyGAN: Learning deep representations of cancer tissue. *arXiv preprint arXiv:1907.02644.*

12 Karras, T., Laine, S., & Aila, T. (2019). A style-based generator architecture for generative adversarial networks. *Proceedings of the IEEE/CVF conference on computer vision and pattern recognition*, pp. 4401–4410, Long Beach, CA (15–20 June 2019). IEEE.

13 Vu, Q.D., Kim, K., and Kwak, J.T. (2020). Unsupervised tumor characterization via conditional generative adversarial networks. *IEEE Journal of Biomedical and Health Informatics* 25 (2): 348–357.

14 Sasmal, P., Sharma, V., Prakash, A.J. et al. (2024). Semi-supervised generative adversarial networks for improved colorectal polyp classification using histopathological images. *Information Sciences* 658: 120033.

15 Kim, B.S., Cho, M., Chung, G.E. et al. (2024). Density clustering-based automatic anatomical section recognition in colonoscopy video using deep learning. *Scientific Reports* 14 (1): 872.

16 Ryspayeva, M. (2023, May). Generative adversarial network as data balance and augmentation tool in histopathology of breast cancer. *2023 IEEE International Conference on Smart Information Systems and Technologies (SIST)*, pp. 99–104. IEEE.

17 Doansang CVC-ColonDB, Kaggle dataset, 21 March 2024, https://www.kaggle.com/datasets/doansang/cvc-colondb

18 Longvil, "CVS-ClinicDB, Kaggle dataset" 21 March 2024 https://www.kaggle.com/datasets/longvil/cvc-colondb

19 He, K., Zhang, X., Ren, S., & Sun, J. (2016). Deep residual learning for image recognition. *Proceedings of the IEEE conference on computer vision and pattern recognition*, pp. 770–778, Las Vegas, NV (27–30 June 2016). IEEE.

20 Kumar, R., Singh, A., & Khamparia, A. (2023). Multiclass classification of gastrointestinal colorectal cancer using deep learning. *International Conference On Innovative Computing And Communication*, pp. 625–636. Singapore: Springer Nature Singapore.

21 Kumar, R., Singh, A., and Khamparia, A. (2024). Deep learning-assisted techniques for detection and prediction of colorectal cancer from medical images and microbial modality. In: *Microbial Data Intelligence and Computational Techniques for Sustainable Computing* (ed. A. Khamparia, B. Pandey, D.K. Pandey, and D. Gupta), 151–169. Singapore: Springer Nature Singapore.

22 Goel, D., Kumar, R., and Kumar, S. (2024). AI-assisted methods for protein structure prediction and analysis. In: *Microbial Data Intelligence and Computational Techniques for Sustainable Computing* (ed. A. Khamparia, B. Pandey, D.K. Pandey, and D. Gupta), 365–391. Singapore: Springer Nature Singapore.

21

Exploring Trust and Mistrust Dynamics: Generative AI-Curated Narratives in Health Communication Media Content Among Gen X

Seema Shukla[1], Babita Pandey[2], Devendra Kumar Pandey[3], Brijendra Pratap Mishra[4], and Aditya Khamparia[2]

[1]*School of Modern Media, UPES, Dehradun, India*
[2]*Department of Computer Science, Baba Saheb Bhimrao Ambedkar (Central University), Lucknow, India*
[3]*School of Biotechnology, Lovely Professional University, Phagwara, Punjab, India*
[4]*Department of Biochemistry, Autonomous State Medical College, Bahraich, Atal Bihari Vajpayee Medical University, Lucknow, Uttar Pradesh, India*

21.1 Background

Chat Generative Pre-Trained Transformer (ChatGPT) is a generative artificial intelligence (GAI) interface that applies a large language model (LLM) to respond to queries from users [1]. Similarly, DALL-E 2 is a GAI interface for creating text-to-image [2]. Immediately after the launch of ChatGPT [3] and DALL-E 2 [2], the models received impressive public attention, with more than one million users signing up on the ChatGPT interface in the first week to test content creation [3], and DALL-E 2 gained significant popularity with 1.5 million active users [4]. The rapid uptake of ChatGPT and DALL-E 2 GAI models was attributed to their ability to generate responses in the form of text and images to the prompts given to them. Through these low entry barriers and user-friendly interfaces, users may produce content that closely resembles human-created content [5, 6]. The LLM provides ChatGPT with the ability to create new and original content based on available datasets of texts [7]. Similarly, DALL-E 2 uses diffusion models to generate new and original images based on available datasets, usually in response to a prompt or query. Both GAI models can generate new descriptions in the provided style, rewrite or summarize text in a different style, or generate images for specific audiences.

Generative Artificial Intelligence for Biomedical and Smart Health Informatics,
First Edition. Edited by Aditya Khamparia and Deepak Gupta.

Once trained, GAI models do not store the raw data on which they were trained and can be used in downstream tasks, including writing meaningful text or creating beautiful images in response to prompts [8]. However, there are major concerns that they may generate imprecise and incorrect information (text or images) that are not based on facts and could become sources of misinformation. Moreover, GAI-created content also generates doubt among users due to its etymology. In addition, several literatures advocate that GAI may fundamentally change how people interact with information and knowledge about various issues such as education, environment, coding, and health. In this context, Dwivedi and his team suggested that GAI tools will change the way people search for answers on online platforms, consume them, engage in peer learning, organize their lives, and turn their creative ideas into artwork [7]. While GAI may be used to improve and scale evidence-based health communications, users may also face unexpected consequences due to fictional information. An article published on the website "The Standard" also expresses concern about reducing readers' trust in online content due to the rising prevalence of GAI content.

In this viewpoint, it is crucial to consider the ways in which GAI tools might change the construction of health information, the types of health information users receive, and how marketing strategies might use misinformation with evidence or personalization, potentially introducing new misinformation risks. Therefore, the present research study measures the trust of 100 purposefully selected Generation X respondents with a previously established trust scale and examines the impact of displaying disclaimers on trust in content generated by AI. Through data analysis using SmartPLS, the results indicate that the three components of trust have a positive impact on individual trust. Semi-structured interviews further reinforce these findings.

This study sheds light on the adoption of new information technologies, focusing on how GAI tools such as LLMs, GANs, and VAEs may alter the production and consumption of health information. The study explores how these technologies may influence the content people encounter, the blending of marketing and misinformation with evidence, and the factors that influence trust.

21.2 Related Work

Health is a priority for everybody, and COVID-19 has created a scenario in which everybody is uncertain about their health, causing worries among common people and making them extremely active in gathering health-related information [9]. They are using various mediums (physical or online mode) to get health information [10]. These online platforms have no gatekeepers [11], and that's why there is no mechanism to check the authenticity of the content [12], leading to huge mistrust among users [13]. This mistrust is a matter of concern when the information is related to health issues. To address this concern, in 2023 Williamson and Prins conducted a cross-sectional survey among 544 respondents to test the medical mistrust of an individual in the situation of uncertainty and information seeking from online platforms. In another research study, Sillence and her team [14] conducted a study to examine Sidhartha the trust and mistrust of users of online health sites. Furthermore, the team also explored the trust factors involved in online health advice [15]. Bruzzese and his team [16] have established a relationship between individuals' confidence indicator and their trust in AI-generated content. The result indicates that the individual's confidence indicator influenced trust in a negative manner. Ribes et al. [17] explored the factors that influenced the trust of individuals in AI-generated news content (text and images). Hofeditz et al. [18] found that trust in AI-generated content depends on the credibility of the source of the information, like media companies or individual persons who generate information. This research study also explores how prior experiences with social media platforms and AI tools positively influence trust in GAI content. Karnouskos [19] discussed in their study how deep fakes create misinformation and fake information among users. They also advocated the requirement of awareness to reduce this misinformation. Siau and Wang [20] express concern about the accuracy of information, privacy breaches, cybersecurity, risk potential, and ethical use of AI. In a recent study, Fui-Hoon Nah and her team [21] opined that value creation is critical in the health industry, requiring a lot of accuracy and confidentiality. Therefore, relying too much on GAI content may lead to catastrophes, such as the mistreatment of patients based on wrong information. In addition, crucial and critical information may be leaked or compromised due to the use of AI in the healthcare sector. The literature has found that GAI is an emerging research area and content (text or images or both) generated through AI creates mistrust among users [7]. While the above-stated studies provide early evidence of mistrust of users in GAI content, there is no study available that has examined the mistrust of the most vulnerable age group, Gen X respondents, through an experimental study. Therefore, the purpose of this research study is to conduct an experimental study that explores the trust of Gen X Indians in AI-generated health advertisements and explores the factors affecting the trust level in GAI content. This research study is conducted to get the answers to the following research questions: • How do users rate the trustworthiness of GAI contents? • Why do users mistrust AI-generated content? • What factors influence the trust of an individual? This research study has seven sections: 1. Background, 2. Literature review, 3. Theoretical framework, Conceptual model and hypothesis, 4. Research methodology, 5. Data analysis, 6. Results, 7. Discussion, and conclusions.

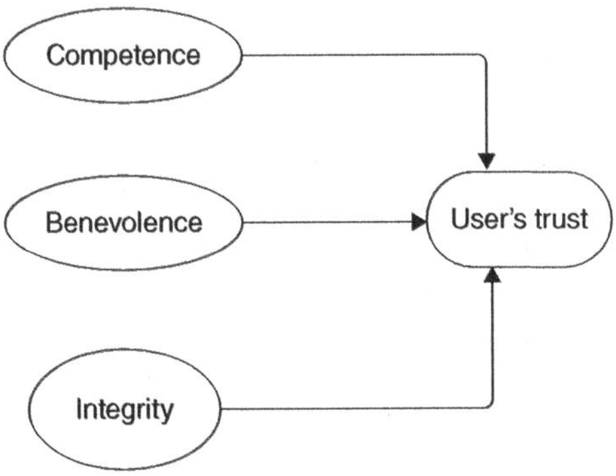

Figure 21.1 Conceptual model.

21.3 Theoretical Framework

In this research study, "Trust" is contemplated as a complex and cross-disciplinary construct. It encompasses trust in various aspects, including trust in oneself [22], trust in others [23], trust in organizations [24], trust in automation [25–27], trust in intelligent systems [28, 29], and trust in abstract entities such as money or political power [30]. Definitions of trust emphasize characteristics such as a willingness to be vulnerable, a confident and positive expectation, and a readiness to rely on others [31], as well as qualities like integrity, benevolence, and the ability to fulfill promises [24]. In the context of automation, Muir [26] focus on the expected behavior and its relation to reliability. Luhmann's definition of trust, as adopted by Muir et al. in the context of trust in automation, suggests that trust enables individuals to manage complexity and cope with risk [30]. Based on the above literature, the following conceptual model (Figure 21.1) and hypotheses have been proposed for this research study. Table 21.1 illustrates the meaning of competence, benevolence, and integrity.

21.3.1 Proposed Hypotheses

H1: The competence of an individual has a positive impact on trust.
H2: The benevolence of an individual has a positive impact on trust.
H3: The integrity of an individual has a positive impact on trust.
H4: Group 1 has a higher level of trust than group 2.

21.4 Research Methodology

To assess respondents' trust in GAI content, a quantitative study was conducted using a questionnaire consisting of 10-point closed-ended questions distributed among participants. Subsequently, to identify factors influencing respondents'

Table 21.1 Illustrates the meaning of competence, benevolence, and integrity.

Element	Representation	Abbreviation in this study	Definition	References
Competence	Some degree knowledge	SN	Ability to perform duty, responsibility, or task in an effective manner	[32]
Benevolence	Power of concern behavior	PBC	The foundation of social networking services that facilitate positive interaction between individuals is grounded in behaviors characterized by care, empathy, and genuine concern for others.	[33]
Integrity	Maintaining a positive attitude	ATT	The connection between integrity and trust entails the belief of the person placing trust (trustor) that the individual being trusted (trustee) abides by a set of principles deemed acceptable by the trustor.	[24]

trust, semi-structured interviews were conducted with the same participants. Figure 21.1 illustrates the steps of the research methodology.

For quantitative data analysis, multivariate data analysis was performed. Given the evolving nature of trust theory in the context of AI-generated content, partial least squares path modeling (partial least squares structural equation modeling—PLS-SEM) was employed to validate relationships between constructs [34]. Prior to the experimental study, the questionnaire underwent evaluation by a committee of five psychology specialists. Upon approval from this committee, the questionnaire was utilized to assess respondents' trust.

To measure trust and its relationship with competence, benevolence, integrity, and managing complexity in GAI health advertisements, Rotter's scales were adopted [25, 26, 30, 35]. The measurement instrument included 25 items from the Rotter Interpersonal Trust Scale [23] and three items from the Social Trust Scale [36].

To estimate the required sample size for the study, G*Power software version 3.1.9.7 was utilized [37]. The minimum required sample size, at a significance level (α) of 5%, with 0.95 statistical power and an average effect size (f^2) of 0.15, was determined to be 89 (see Figure 21.2). With the experimental study conducted on 100 respondents, the sample size is deemed suitable for estimation via PLS-SEM.

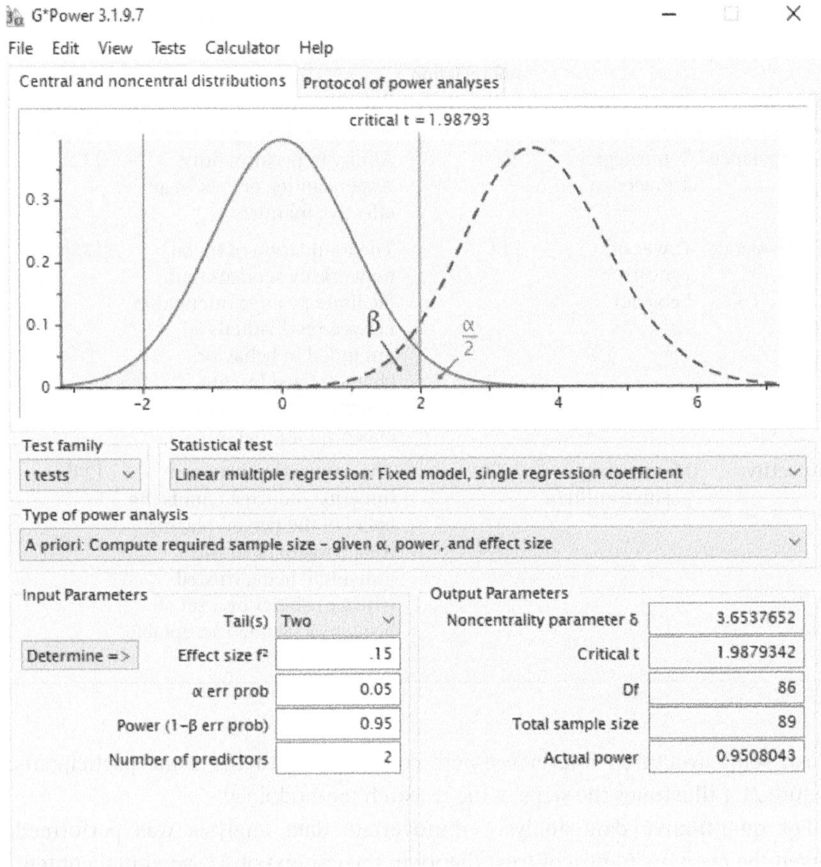

Figure 21.2 Required sample size: G*Power software (3.1.9.7 version).

21.4.1 Content and Material

For this research study, the researchers created five advertisements using ChatGPT 3.5 (a textual content creator) and DALL-E 2 (a text-to-image creator) AI-generated tools. After generating text and images separately, they were combined to create advertisements with the assistance of a professional graphic designer and Photoshop software.

21.4.2 Study Design

The experiment was conducted in Dehradun with purposefully selected 100 Gen X respondents. It took approximately 35 minutes to conduct the study. Before starting the experiment, the respondents were divided into two groups, each consisting of 50 respondents (24 males and 26 females). Both groups were

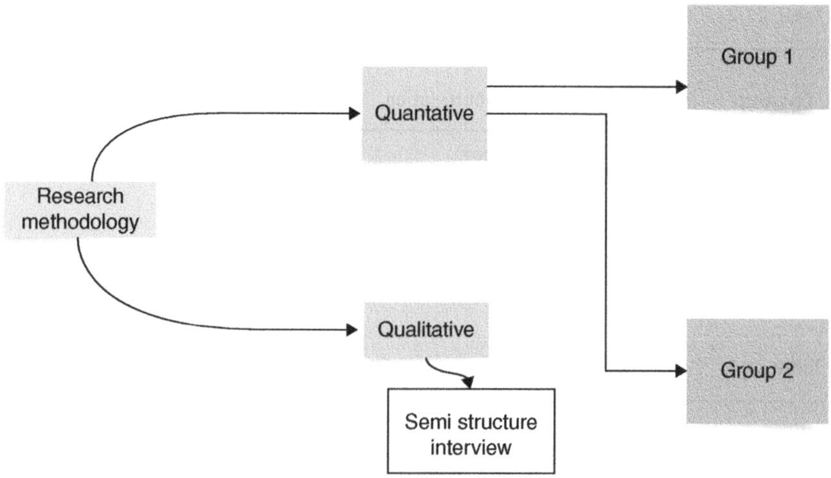

Figure 21.3 Initial steps of research methodology.

exposed to similar advertisements, with one group presented with a disclaimer (AI-generated) and the other group without a disclaimer. A total of 28 questions were circulated among the respondents. A 30-minute mandatory lecture was a prerequisite for each participant to participate in this study. This lecture served the purpose of showcasing the experimental stimulus and explaining the study to the respondents. During the lecture, the phenomenon of misinformation was illustrated using two examples: one on the COVID-19 case and the other on cancer treatment. Furthermore, to extend the study, a semi-structured interview was conducted with the respondents (Figure 21.3).

21.4.3 Participants

A total of 100 adults (age group 43–58 years) have been chosen through purposive sampling who are familiar with AI tools to conduct this research study. The selection of respondents was based on demographic criteria such as age, gender, marital status, income, education, and employment.

21.5 Data Analysis

21.5.1 Measurement: Scale Reliability and Validity Analysis of Data Received Through Quantitative Approach

All the measured items used in this study have been precisely taken from established scales [23, 36]. The Cronbach's alpha (see Table 21.2) for the constructs competence, benevolence, integrity, and trust was reported to be greater than 0.7 (suggested lower limit) [38, 39].

Table 21.2 Cronbach's alpha value of constructs.

Construct	Abbreviation	Cronbach's alpha (α)
Individual's trust	INT	0.903
Competence	SN	0.894
Benevolence	PBC	0.875
Integrity	ATT	0.752

Table 21.3 Demographic characteristics of the respondents.

Parameter	Categories	Frequency	Percentage
Gender	Female	52	52
	Male	48	48
Education	Graduate	29	29
	Postgraduate	61	61
	Above postgraduate	10	10
Salary status (Indian Rupees)	10K–20K	25	25
	21K–30K	7	7
	31K–40K	3	3
	41K–50K	65	65

21.6 Results

21.6.1 Demographic Profile

Table 21.3 illustrates the demographic profile of the respondents, which comprises gender, educational qualifications, and salary status. Respondents in the data constitute 48% males and 52% females. A large proportion of respondents are postgraduate 61%, 29% are graduate, and only 10% have qualifications above postgraduation. The monthly income of the majority of respondents, which is 65%, lies between 41K and 50K, 3% between 31K and 40K, 7% between 21K and 30K, and 25% belongs to 10K and 20K slabs in Indian rupees (Figure 21.4).

21.6.2 Assessment of Measurement Model

The researchers have checked the reliability and validity to examine the outer model specifications of the model. The appropriate values (above 0.70) of all

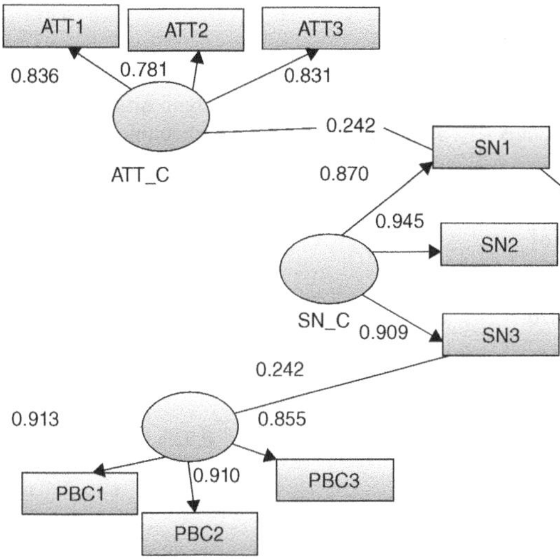

Figure 21.4 Structural model assessment results.

the indicators loading were received [40]. Researchers established the internal consistency among the items of the adopted scale through Cronbach's alpha coefficient (α) and composite reliability. An accepted value of average variance extracted that is greater than 0.5 established the convergent validity [34]. The discriminant validity was established through the Fornell–Larcker criterion [34]. Tables 21.4 and 21.5 illustrate the above-stated values.

21.6.3 Quantitative Approach: Hypothesis Testing

H1: Competence (SN) of an individual has a positive impact on trust (INT).
With respect to hypothesis H1, the results shown in Table 21.6 ($\beta = 0.298$, $p < 0.05$) indicate that competence has a significant influence in a positive direction on trust. Therefore, H1 is accepted.

H2: Benevolence (PBC) of an individual has a positive impact on trust (INT).
With respect to hypothesis H2, the results illustrated in Table 21.6 ($\beta = 0.242$, $p < 0.001$) indicate that benevolence has a significant influence on trust in a positive manner. Therefore, H2 is accepted.

H3: Integrity (ATT) of an individual has a positive impact on trust (INT).
Regarding hypothesis H3, the results shown in Table 21.6 suggested that integrity has significant positive effects on trust ($\beta = 0.242$, $p < 0.001$). Therefore, H3 is accepted.

H4: Group 1 has a higher level of trust than group 2.
To evaluate respondents in group 1, having higher trust than group 2, an independent one-tail t-test was applied. The Kolmogorov–Smirnov test satisfied

Table 21.4 Measurement model accuracy assessment.

Constructs of the research study	PLS code items	Outer loadings	Cronbach's alpha (α)	rhoA	Composite reliability	Average
Integrity	ATT1	0.836	0.752	0.763	0.857	0.666
	ATT2	0.781				
	ATT3	0.831				
Competence	SN1	0.870	0.894	0.901	0.934	0.825
	SN2	0.945				
	SN3	0.909				
Benevolence	PBC1	0.913	0.875	0.883	0.923	0.800
	PBC2	0.910				
	PBC3	0.859				
Individual's trust	INREP1	0.903	0.903	0.916	0.939	0.838
	INREP2	0.942				
	INREP3	0.900				

Table 21.5 Fornell–Larcker criterion: discriminant validity.

	ATT_C	INT	PBC_C	SN_C
ATT_C	0.815			
INT	0.374	0.915		
PBC_C	0.296	0.224	0.894	
SN_C	0.424	0.403	0.133	0.907

the normality condition of the data. Levine's test indicated that variances for the two groups (1 and 2) were equal, satisfying the assumption of homogeneity of variance. The SPSS does not have an inbuilt function available to calculate the one-tailed t-statistics. Therefore, the two-tailed independent t-test was performed, and later, the critical value was compared with the table value for testing the hypothesis. The mean score of trust of group 1 ($M = 6.38$; SD = 1.29) was significantly greater than the mean score of trust of group 2 ($M = 5.67$; SD = 1.67); $t\,(50) = 5.365$, $p = 0.000$, CV = 1.96 (two-tailed tailed). Hence, group 1 has a higher level of trust than group 2 (Table 21.7).

Table 21.6 Decision on the proposed hypothesis.

Hypothesis	Path relationship	Path coefficient	Sample mean (M)	*t*-values	Decisions
H_1	SN≫INT	0.298	0.298	4.084***	Supported
H_2	PBC≫INT	0.242	0.248	3.633***	Supported
H_3	ATT≫INT	0.242	0.250	3.642***	Supported

Path coefficient (*$p < 0.01$, **$p < 0.05$, ***$p < 0.001$).

Table 21.7 Group statistics.

Construct	Group	*N*	Mean	Standard deviation	Standard error mean
INT	1	50	6.38	1.29	0.082
	2	50	5.67	1.67	0.103

21.6.4 Qualitative Approach

A semi-structured interview was conducted with all the 21 (conveniently selected) respondents to get the answers to the questions, why do users mistrust AI-generated content? And what factors influence the trust of an individual? After the preparation of the transcript, the researchers used the constructivist grounded theory approach proposed by Charmaz [41], in which theory is generated from the analysis of data to analyze the data. After collecting the appropriate literature on the mistrust in AI-generated content, the researchers started the coding process [42].

In brief, the whole research followed the contemporary guidelines set forth by Charmaz [41], which suggested the repetitive process of data collection, coding of data, comparative analysis of data, and the concept of theoretical sampling till theoretical saturation is achieved [43, 44]. The purpose of the present analysis is to understand why users don't trust AI-generated content and what factors influence their mistrust. Table 21.8 shows the list of initial codes and the frequency of codes used by the respondents during the interviews.

Table 21.8 illustrates the frequency of codes used by the different respondents; it shows that respondents took terms like missing of human essence 97 times, lack of empathy 44 times, absence of the feeling of actual care 50 times, misinformation 89 times, biasness 73, and inaccuracies of the information 58 times in their conversation. The frequency count indicates that respondents use missing human touch maximum times (see Table 21.8). The majority of respondents thought that missing of human essence, lack of empathy, absence of the feeling of actual care, misinformation, biasness, and inaccuracy of the information are the

Table 21.8 Codes used by participants (frequency).

Code	Frequency of codes used by participants
Missing of human essence	97
Lack of empathy	44
Absence of the feeling of actual care	50
Misinformation	89
Biasness	73
Inaccuracy of the information	58

main factors that influence trust in AI-generated content and why users don't trust AI-generated content.

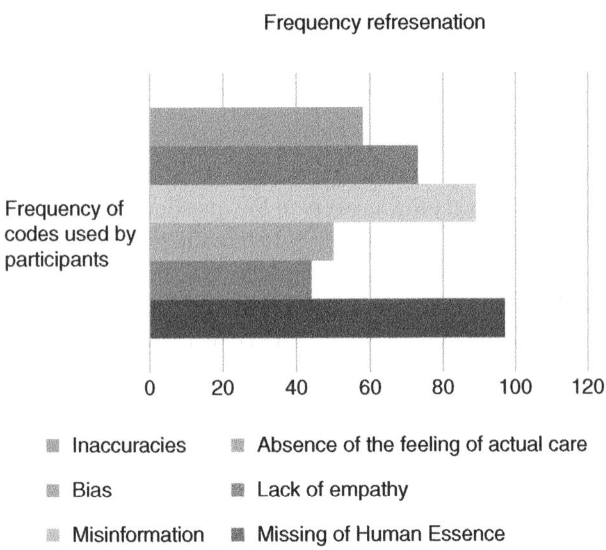

21.7 Conclusions and Discussion

The study aimed to investigate users' trust in AI-generated content, focusing on the factors influencing trust and the implications for health communications. The findings revealed that users' trust in AI-generated content is influenced by three key components: competence, benevolence, and integrity. Interestingly, while there was a general willingness among users to accept AI-generated content, trust varied significantly depending on the source of the content. This highlights the importance of understanding the factors contributing to trust imbalances and implementing measures to enhance the credibility of AI-generated content.

Moreover, respondents expressed mixed or unclear perceptions of AI, citing concerns about the absence of human touch, empathy, and genuine care in AI-generated content. Concerns about receiving misinformation or biased information also influenced users' trust. In addition, some respondents raised issues regarding content personalization, drawing parallels to algorithms used by popular search engines.

The study underscores the need for media literacy campaigns and user education on AI technologies to address trust-related concerns. While generative AI presents opportunities to enhance health communications, including supporting translation efforts and improving response quality, critical challenges remain. Establishing standard cues for assessing credibility and ensuring transparent explanations of AI-generated responses are essential steps to maximize the potential of generative AI in health communications.

21.7.1 Conclusion

In conclusion, the study sheds light on the complex relationship between users' trust and AI-generated content in health communications. While users generally demonstrate a willingness to accept AI-generated content, trust varies significantly depending on factors such as competence, benevolence, and integrity. Addressing trust-related challenges, such as establishing credibility cues and ensuring transparent explanations of AI-generated responses, is crucial to harnessing the full potential of GAI in health communications.

21.7.2 Limitations of the Study

Despite the valuable insights gained from this research study, several limitations should be acknowledged. Firstly, the study was conducted with a specific sample of Gen X respondents in Dehradun, which may limit the generalizability of the findings to other populations. In addition, the study focused primarily on users' perceptions and trust in AI-generated content, overlooking potential biases or limitations inherent in the AI models themselves. Furthermore, the study relied on self-reported data, which may be subject to biases or inaccuracies. Future research could explore these limitations further and investigate additional factors influencing trust in AI-generated content.

21.7.3 Further Recommended Research

Further recommendations stemming from the research study include the implementation of a longitudinal study to track changes in user trust over time, the adoption of user-centered design principles to tailor AI-generated content to user preferences, the exploration of personalized content delivery strategies, the establishment of robust quality assurance mechanisms, the integration of collaborative filtering techniques for content recommendations, continuous training and monitoring of AI models, enhancement of transparency and explanation features, and prioritization of ethical considerations. These recommendations aim to optimize the effectiveness, trustworthiness, and user experience of AI-generated content in health communications, ultimately empowering users to make informed decisions and improve health outcomes.

21.7.4 Statements and Declarations

This research study has not received any financial support from any organization. It is an independent work of researchers.

References

1 Vaishya, R., Misra, A., and Vaish, A. (2023). ChatGPT: Is this version good for healthcare and research? *Diabetes & Metabolic Syndrome: Clinical Research & Reviews* 17 (4): 102744.
2 Vayadande, K., Bhemde, S., Rajguru, V., et al. (2023). AI-based image generator web application using OpenAI's DALL-E system. *2023 International Conference on Recent Advances in Science and Engineering Technology (ICRASET)*, pp. 1–5, B G NAGARA, India (23–24 November 2023). IEEE.
3 Abdullah, M., Madain, A., & Jararweh, Y. (2022). ChatGPT: fundamentals, applications and social impacts. *2022 Ninth International Conference on Social Networks Analysis, Management and Security (SNAMS)*, pp. 1–8, Milan, Italy (29 November–1 December 2022). IEEE.
4 Benaich, N., and Hogarth, I. (2020). State of AI report. London, UK.
5 Guo, B., Zhang, X., Wang, Z., et al. (2023). How close is chatgpt to human experts? comparison corpus, evaluation, and detection. *arXiv preprint arXiv:2301.07597*.
6 Trivedi, A., Kaur, E.K., Choudhary, C., and Barnwal, P. (2023). Should AI technologies replace the human jobs? *2023 2nd International Conference for Innovation in Technology (INOCON)*, pp. 1–6, Bangalore, India (3–5 March 2023). IEEE.

7 Dwivedi, Y.K., Kshetri, N., Hughes, L. et al. (2023). "So what if ChatGPT wrote it?" Multidisciplinary perspectives on opportunities, challenges and implications of generative conversational AI for research, practice and policy. *International Journal of Information Management* 71: 102642.

8 Seneviratne, S., Senanayake, D., Rasnayaka, S., et al. (2022). DALLE-URBAN: capturing the urban design expertise of large text to image transformers. *2022 International Conference on Digital Image Computing: Techniques and Applications (DICTA)*, pp. 1–9. IEEE.

9 Khan, N. and Naushad, M. (2020). Effects of corona virus on the world community. *SSRN Electronic Journal* https://doi.org/10.2139/ssrn.3532001.

10 Cotten, S.R. and Gupta, S.S. (2004). Characteristics of online and offline health information seekers and factors that discriminate between them. *Social Science & Medicine* 59 (9): 1795–1806.

11 Mirza, M., Verma, M., Aggarwal, A. et al. (2024). Indian Model of Integrated Healthcare (IMIH): a conceptual framework for a coordinated referral system in resource-constrained settings. *BMC Health Services Research* 24 (1): 42.

12 Mahid, Z.I., Manickam, S., & Karuppayah, S. (2018). Fake news on social media: Brief review on detection techniques. *2018 Fourth International Conference on Advances in Computing, Communication & Automation (ICACCA)*, pp. 1–5, Subang Jaya, Malaysia (26–28 October 2018). IEEE.

13 Kim, Y.A. and Ahmad, M.A. (2013). Trust, distrust and lack of confidence of users in online social media-sharing communities. *Knowledge-Based Systems* 37: 438–450.

14 Sillence, E., Briggs, P., Fishwick, L., & Harris, P. (2004). Trust and mistrust of online health sites. *Proceedings of the SIGCHI conference on Human factors in computing systems*, pp. 663–670, Vienna Austria (24–29 April 2004). Association for Computing Machinery.

15 Sillence, E., Briggs, P., Harris, P., and Fishwick, L. (2006). A framework for understanding trust factors in web-based health advice. *International Journal of Human-computer Studies* 64 (8): 697–713.

16 Bruzzese, T., Gao, I., Dietz, G., et al. (2020). Effect of confidence indicators on trust in AI-generated profiles. *Extended Abstracts of the 2020 CHI Conference on Human Factors in Computing Systems*, pp. 1–8, Honolulu HI (25–30 April 2020). IEEE

17 Ribes, D., Henchoz, N., Portier, H., et al. (2021). Trust indicators and explainable AI: A study on user perceptions. *Human-Computer Interaction–INTERACT 2021: 18th IFIP TC 13 International Conference Proceedings, Part II 18*, pp. 662–671, Bari, Italy (30 August–3 September 2021). Springer International Publishing.

18 Hofeditz, L., Mirbabaie, M., Holstein, J., & Stieglitz, S. (2021). Do you trust an AI-journalist? A credibility analysis of news content with AI-authorship. *ECIS*. Marrakesh, Morocco.

19 Karnouskos, S. (2020). Artificial intelligence in digital media: the era of deepfakes. *IEEE Transactions on Technology and Society* 1 (3): 138–147.

20 Siau, K. and Wang, W. (2020). Artificial intelligence (AI) ethics: ethics of AI and ethical AI. *Journal of Database Management (JDM)* 31 (2): 74–87.

21 Fui-Hoon Nah, F., Zheng, R., Cai, J. et al. (2023). Generative AI and ChatGPT: applications, challenges, and AI-human collaboration. *Journal of Information Technology Case and Application Research* 25 (3): 277–304.

22 Marsh, S.P. (1994). *Formalizing trust as a computational concept*. PhD thesis, Department of Mathematics and Computer Science, University of Stirling, UK.

23 Rotter, J.B. (1967). A new scale for the measurement of interpersonal trust. *Journal of personality*. 35 (4): 651–665.

24 Mayer, R.C., Davis, J.H., and Schoorman, F.D. (1995). An integrative model of organizational trust. *Academy of Management Review* 20 (3): 709–734.

25 Lee, J.D. and See, K.A. (2004). Trust in automation: designing for appropriate reliance. *Human Factors* 46 (1): 50–80.

26 Muir, B.M. (1994). Trust in automation: Part I. Theoretical issues in the study of trust and human intervention in automated systems. *Ergonomics* 37 (11): 1905–1922.

27 Muir, B.M. and Moray, N. (1996). Trust in automation. Part II. Experimental studies of trust and human intervention in a process control simulation. *Ergonomics* 39 (3): 429–460.

28 Herlocker, J.L., Konstan, J.A., & Riedl, J. (2000). Explaining collaborative filtering recommendations. *Proceedings of the 2000 ACM Conference on Computer Supported Cooperative Work*, pp. 241–250, Philadelphia, PA. Association for Computing Machinery.

29 Tullio, J., Dey, A. K., Chalecki, J., and Fogarty, J. (2007). How it works: a field study of non-technical users interacting with an intelligent system. *Proceedings of the SIGCHI Conference on Human Factors in Computing Systems*, pp. 31–40, San Jose CA (28 April 2007–3 May 2007). Association for Computing Machinery.

30 Luhmann, N. (1979). *Trust and Power*. John Willey & Sons.

31 Rousseau, D.M., Sitkin, S.B., Burt, R.S., and Camerer, C. (1998). Not so different after all: a cross-discipline view of trust. *Academy of Management Review* 23 (3): 393–404.

32 Grzeda, M.M. (2005). In competence we trust? Addressing conceptual ambiguity. *Journal of Management Development* 24 (6): 530–545.

33 Svare, H., Gausdal, A.H., and Möllering, G. (2020). The function of ability, benevolence, and integrity-based trust in innovation networks. *Industry and Innovation* 27 (6): 585–604.

34 Hair, J.F., Hult, G.T.M., Ringle, C.M., and Sarstedt, M. (2017). *A Primer on Partial Least Squares Structural Equation Modeling (PLS-SEM).* Thousand Oaks, CA: Sage.

35 McKnight, D.H. and Chervany, N.L. (2001). What trust means in e-commerce customer relationships: an interdisciplinary conceptual typology. *International Journal of Electronic Commerce* 6 (2): 35–59.

36 Reeskens, T. and Hooghe, M. (2008). Cross-cultural measurement equivalence of generalized trust. Evidence from the European Social Survey (2002 and 2004). *Social Indicators Research* 85: 515–532.

37 Faul, F., Erdfelder, E., Buchner, A., and Lang, A.G. (2009). Statistical power analyses using G* Power 3.1: Tests for correlation and regression analyses. *Behavior Research Methods* 41 (4): 1149–1160.

38 Hair, J.F., Howard, M.C., and Nitzl, C. (2020). Assessing measurement model quality in PLS-SEM USING confirmatory composite analysis. *Journal of Business Research* 109: 101–110. https://doi.org/10.1016/j.jbusres.2019.11.069.

39 Nunnally, J.C. (1978). An overview of psychological measurement. In: *Clinical Diagnosis of Mental Disorders* (ed. B.B. Wolman), 97–146. Springer.

40 Hair, J.F., Risher, J.J., Sarstedt, M., and Ringle, C.M. (2019). When to use and how to report the results of PLS-SEM. *European Business Review* 31 (1): 2–24. https://doi.org/10.1108/ebr-11-2018-0203.

41 Charmaz, K. (2006). *Constructing Grounded Theory A Practical Guide through Qualitative Analysis*, 1e. London Sage Publications.

42 Rakhmawati, W. (2019). Understanding classic, Straussian, and constructivist grounded theory approaches. *Belitung Nursing Journal* 5 (3): 111–115. https://doi.org/10.33546/bnj.754.

43 Chun Tie, Y., Birks, M., and Francis, K. (2019). Grounded theory research: A design framework for novice researchers. *SAGE Open Medicine* 7: 2050312118822927.

44 Glaser, B. and Strauss, A. (1967). *The Discovery of Grounded Theory: Strategies for Qualitative Research.* Mill Valley, CA: Sociology Press.

22

Generative Intelligence-Based Federated Learning Model for Brain Tumor Classification in Smart Health

Niladri Maiti[1], Riddhi Chawla[1], Aadam Quraishi[2], Mukesh Soni[3], Maher Ali Rusho[4], and Sagar Dhanraj Pande[5]

[1] School of Dentistry, Central Asian University, Tashkent, Uzbekistan
[2] M. D. Research, Intervention Treatment Institute, Houston, TX, USA
[3] Dr. D. Y. Patil Vidyapeeth, Pune, Dr. D. Y. Patil School of Science & Technology, D Y Patil University, Mumbai, India
[4] Lockheed Martin Engineering Management, University of Colorado, Boulder, CO, USA
[5] School of Engineering and Technology, Pimpri Chinchwad University (PCU), Pune, Maharashtra, India

22.1 Introduction

In recent years, medical imaging technology has advanced significantly and is essential for diagnosing various medical conditions. Computed tomography (CT) is often used to analyze and monitor many medical conditions because it is inexpensive, easy to use, and noninvasive in smart healthcare. Medical imaging is important for the rapid diagnosis and evaluation of cancer [1], tumors [2], and osteonecrosis [3]. Many people agree that CT is an important tool in the diagnosis of brain disorders such as Alzheimer's disease (AD), supporting early diagnosis and treatment methods for sufferers. Recently, AD and brain tumors, commonly known as lesions, have become more common. Also, clinical diagnosis of this disease is a complex and lengthy process. This academic study conducts state-of-the-art research (HR) on brain disorders (such as brain tumors) and general health using data from brain CT imaging. Based on the aging process, the study divided brain CT pictures into three categories. Brain CT scans typically have higher noise and worse resolution when compared to scans of other anatomical regions like the liver and gallbladder. Because of this, categorizing brain pictures with greater precision is difficult to accomplish. As a result, it becomes more difficult to retrieve pertinent information, which lowers the accuracy of classification. Thus, brain disease early detection greatly depends on the procedure of excising brain tissue and detecting high-resolution characteristics in local CT images.

Generative Artificial Intelligence for Biomedical and Smart Health Informatics,
First Edition. Edited by Aditya Khamparia and Deepak Gupta.

Imaging pertaining to AD, brain lesions (including tumors), and normal aging are encompassed within this category. Please provide me with the precise topic or query you would like me to categorize. The structure of the model's residual mapping includes a hybrid residual attention module that is capable of concurrently estimating both brain-related tissue features and brain position inform categorization inside the image. The integration method effectively mitigates noise. Enhance the accuracy of the model's classification. When the number of samples is small, techniques like pooling and global averaging are commonly employed alongside label smoothing cross-entropy loss functions. This approach is employed to mitigate the issue of overfitting and enhance the model's capacity to generalize. A "series" refers to a compilation of objects or concepts that are systematically organized in a specific sequence. The empirical, experimental data unequivocally demonstrates that the residual hybrid attention module (RHAM)-MResNet-10 residual network model (RNM) is highly effective in classifying brain CT images. Our future research will prioritize the analysis of detrimental data collected from brain CT images. To accomplish this, we will employ a 3D convolutional neural network (CNN) to simultaneously handle this input.

Deep learning (DL), a crucial topic of machine learning, is extensively employed in several domains of medical picture analysis owing to its exceptional capacity to acquire intricate features. Some examples of applications include the screening of breast cancer and tumors [5, 6] as well as the classification of lung nodules [7]. The diagnosis of cardiac disease has been thoroughly examined, among other relevant subjects [8]. DL algorithms have gained significant attention in recent years for their application in analyzing CT and MRI brain images in the field of medical imaging. The paper cited above [9] presented a CNN design for the automated segmentation of brain tumors. This approach employs a diminutive convolution kernel to mitigate the issue of overfitting that arises from augmenting the depth of the model. The study integrates CNN to enhance the precision of brain cancer detection. This is accomplished by obtaining data at both the local and global levels. The researchers in this study [10] employed a comprehensive methodology to categorize medical photographs. By putting together different CNN models, researchers can get more than one layer of information from medical images like brain CT scans. This integration makes it easier to get complicated features from different image collections. According to an academic study [11], four different CNN models should be made. This model was created to divide brain scans using magnetic resonance imaging (MRI) into four separate groups: those with AD, mild cognitive impairment, serious cognitive impairment, and healthy people.

This study uses deep learning techniques to analyze brain CT imaging data sets. More precisely, a basic CNN model was created. The model achieved a classification accuracy of 86.32% for all three categories. To improve the classification accuracy in the data set provided, this study proposes a seven-layer CNN model [12].

By using a mixture of activation functions, the model achieved an accuracy of 88.67%. The classification accuracy of this data set is clearly not satisfactory.

CNN is well recognized as a prominent example within the field of deep learning. The utilization of deep convolutional neural networks (DCNNs) for extracting deep features from medical pictures has been found to enhance identification capabilities and improve resilience in image representation. Nevertheless, the current deep learning techniques acquire characteristics from the complete CT picture, encompassing not only aspects associated with brain lesions but also extraneous features like background regions. It is probable that the retrieved brain properties may comprise a combination of characteristics from different tissues present in the background region. Consequently, the characteristics that have been retrieved exhibit limited discriminatory power, leading to inaccuracies in the model's classification.

The visual attention mechanism has been shown to exhibit higher performance in visual tasks, such as picture classification [14–16] and target recognition [13]. This technique aligns with the functioning of the human visual system since it avoids attempting to comprehend the entirety of visual scene information simultaneously. Instead, it selectively engages when necessary. When directing attention toward the salient components within the entirety of the visual field. The inclusion of a visual attention module in the model facilitates the extraction of dynamic features from regions of the image that closely resemble brain-like structures. This is achieved by directing the model to focus on select sections of the image that contain relevant information. The research publication [13] introduced a residual attention module that utilizes down-sampling and up-sampling techniques for the extraction of attention feature maps. The study conducted by the authors [14] centered on investigating the relationship between individual channels inside the feature map. In addition, they introduced a channel attention module as a possible solution. This module is straightforward. The use of ground stacking in an attention network model significantly enhances the efficacy of classification. When doing feature extraction using a convolutional network, it is crucial to consider both the inter-channel correlation and the spatial relationship of the feature map. Hence, the study [15] aimed to integrate channel information and spatial information by introducing a hybrid attention module known as the Convolutional Block Attention Module (CBAM). To evaluate the efficacy of this integration, classification experiments were performed on the ImageNet dataset. Nevertheless, the attention module primarily employs pooling procedures to process feature maps, which can result in the loss of crucial information from these feature maps.

This article focuses on the classification problem of three distinct types of brain CT scans, namely, those related to AD, brain lesions (such as tumors), and healthy aging. The primary contributions of this study can be summarized as follows.

In this study, the authors propose the implementation of a RHAM. In contrast to the approach described in the article [15], the RHAM primarily employs convolution operations to extract the interdependence of feature maps. In addition, it incorporates a residual skip connection structure to mitigate the loss of crucial features during the process of capturing both the spatial and content-related information of brain tissue. The attention module exhibits favorable portability, and its integration into the network model has the potential to enhance the extraction of discriminative brain features, hence improving the accuracy of model classification.

In the ResNet-10 model [17], the global average pooling layer is better than the average pooling layer because it limits the input image size. Overfitting was reduced when the authors of this study [18] introduced a worldwide average pooling layer. This change created a new model called MResNet-10 [19–21].

This study uses the ResNet-10 CNN model to analyze three different brain CT images: classification problems related to AD, brain tumor-like lesions, and healthy aging. This model integrates RHAM into the residual network mapping structure to solve the problem of insufficient feature specificity identified by the original model. These improved models provide the ability to accurately capture spatial information and associated brain tissue content in CT images. The comprehensive series of experiments confirms the effectiveness of the improved ResNet-10 network model. The main contributions of the work are as follows:

- A: This study addresses the challenge of classifying CT images of the brain, with a focus on AD, brain injury, and healthy aging.
- b. Introducing the RHAM-MResNet-10 RNM with RHAM to improve the accuracy of feature extraction and classification.
- C. The model incorporates technologies such as global averaging pooling and dropout mechanisms to avoid overfitting during the training process.
- d. Label smoothing entropy loss functions can improve the model's generalization ability using limited training data.

22.2 Classification Model

Aiming at the problem of classifying brain CT images of AD, lesions and healthy aging, a CNN model RHAM-MResNet-10 based on the residual hybrid attention mechanism is proposed. This section details the design of this pattern [22].

This study introduces an innovative approach designed to help smart healthcare practitioners quickly identify atypical brain symptoms and reduce the variability inherent in manual diagnostic procedures. The suggested methodology entails the utilization of an RHAM-MResNet-10 RNM for the analysis of three unique types of brain CT images. These categories include images associated with AD, brain lesions (such as tumors), and healthy aging. Kindly specify a particular topic or issue that you would like me to categorize. The incorporation of the RHAM into the residual mapping structure of the model facilitates the concurrent consideration of both the positioning information of the brain in the image and the characteristic information of brain-related tissues. The integration process successfully reduces the impact of noise. Improve the categorization accuracy of the model. In situations where the available sample size is limited, it is customary to employ techniques such as global average pooling and dropout in combination with the label smoothing cross-entropy loss function. These tactics are utilized to address the problem of overfitting and improve the model's ability to generalize. The term "series" pertains to a sequential arrangement of items or concepts. In the conducted experiment, empirical data was obtained, which supports the effectiveness of the RHAM-MResNet-10 RNM in addressing issues related to the categorization of brain CT images. Our future research attempts will continue to prioritize the investigation of pathogenic data present in brain CT imaging. To achieve this, we will utilize 3D CNNs to process this information simultaneously. The inclusion of 20 slices per patient enables the recording of both static and gradient information, hence improving the capacity to predict the development of the disease.

22.2.1 RHAM-MResNet-10

At present, DCNNs have demonstrated their supremacy in the extraction of picture features. Nevertheless, as the complexity of the CNN model increases, there is a propensity for the gradient to either vanish or skyrocket, leading to a deterioration in the overall performance of the model. The effectiveness of the RNM lies in its unique skip connection structure, which effectively mitigates the issues of gradient disappearance or explosion. As a result, this model has found widespread use in diverse tasks [23–25]. DCNNs possess a larger number of parameters and exhibit exceptional performance when an ample amount of data samples, such as those found in ImageNet, are available for classification purposes. Nevertheless, it should be noted that the sample size of brain CT images utilized in this study is very limited, consisting of approximately 1100 samples for each class. The utilization of a deeper network model in a direct manner might readily result in overfitting, hence resulting in a decline in the overall performance of the model. Hence, this study presents the RHAM-MResNet-10 network model, seen in Figure 22.1, which integrates the RHAM into the MResNet-10 RNM. The objective is to effectively capture brain CT image information and enhance the classification accuracy of the model [26].

Figure 22.1 illustrates that the RHAM-MResNet-10 network model takes a brain CT image as input and produces the class probability for the CT image belonging

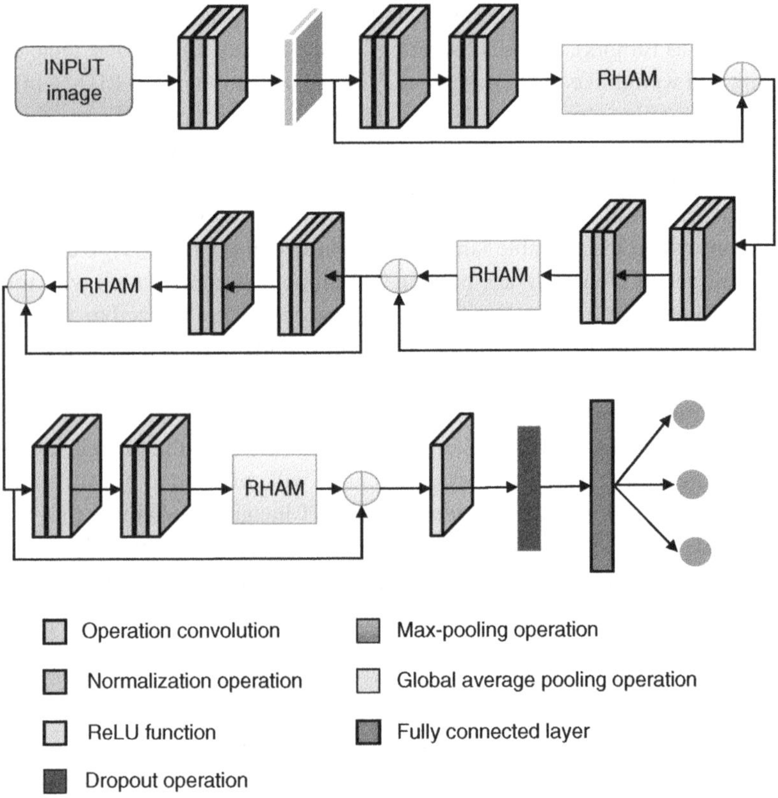

Figure 22.1 RHAM-MResNet-10 network model.

to categories such as AD, brain lesions (e.g., tumors), and healthy aging. The RHAM-MResNet-10 is a DL architecture that was developed initially, employing a single convolutional operation to process the input image. The dimensions of the filter are 7×7, the step size is set to 2, and the output feature map is reduced to half of its original dimension. Following each convolution operation, Batch Normalization [27] is employed to mitigate the issue of overfitting. In addition, the Leaky rectified linear unit (ReLU) activation function is utilized to effectively utilize gradient information and promote the continuous convergence of the model. Subsequently, the process of maximum pooling is employed with a filter size of 3×3 and a step size of 2. This operation serves to decrease the number of parameters within the feature map and lower its dimensionality to one-fourth of the original image. Next, the feature map undergoes four residual attention convolution groups in order to extract high-level features. Each residual attention convolution group is composed of two convolutional operations and one residual mixed attention operation. Each set of convolution operations uses a filter size of 3×3, with the number of filters being 64, 128, 256, and 512 in sequential order. Ultimately, global average pooling is employed. The layer is responsible for extracting the spatial information from the final convolution output feature map, hence decreasing the model's parameter count. In the present study (references [20] and [28]), the application of dropout is implemented afterward to mitigate the issue of overfitting. Following the fully connected layer, the SoftMax activation function is employed to generate the probability distribution for the classification outcome.

22.2.2 Residual Hybrid Attention Module

With an attention device built into a CNN, the network can pay more attention to certain areas of interest. This makes it easier for the network to focus on extracting important traits while ignoring ones that aren't important. The piece talks about an RHAM that is made up of a residual spatial attention (RSA) module and a residual channel attention (RCA) module. As shown in Figure 22.2, these modules are made to highlight both the spatial domain and channel domain information of the feature mapping [28, 29]. Figure 22.2 shows how the RCA module and the RSA modules are stacked to make the RHAM. It is possible for the RHAM to find useful information about a specific subject in an input feature map. It can also accurately find this target's location on the feature map while ignoring target features that aren't as important. In fact, the residual hybrid attention process doesn't help the model depth grow. Instead, it makes the general model architecture wider, which makes the model much faster [30–33]. We will talk about the RCA module and the residual space attention module in more depth in the next section.

The RCA block is a computational unit that is utilized in DL models to enhance the representation learning capabilities of the network. This paper introduces an RCA module, depicted in Figure 22.3, to investigate the correlation between feature mapping channels. The primary objective of the RCA module is to concentrate on the significant information included within the matrix. This module aims to extract extremely distinctive traits related to a given target. In conventional convolution procedures, the receptive field range imposes a constraint on the convolution kernel, limiting its ability to concentrate solely on

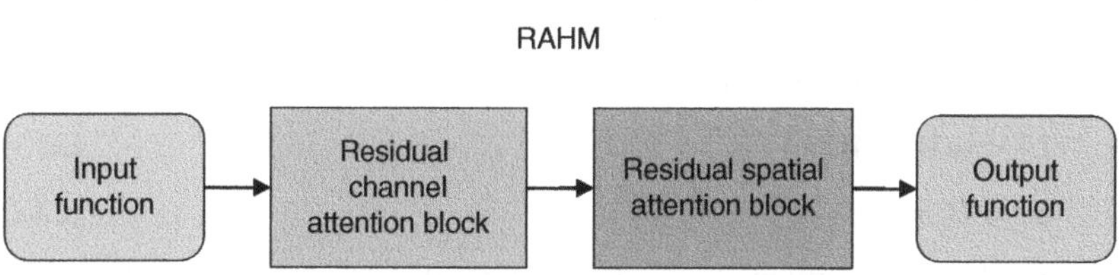

Figure 22.2 Residual hybrid attention module.

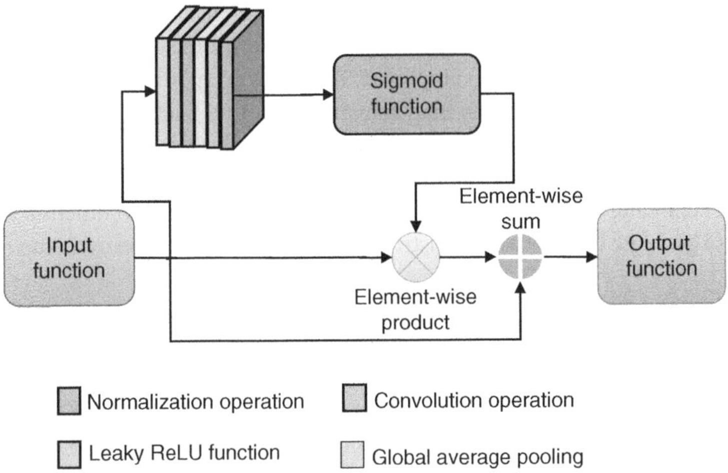

Figure 22.3 Residual channel attention block.

a certain local region inside the feature map. Consequently, it fails to capture contextual information beyond this local area. In this research, the input feature mapping $M \in R^{H\times W\times C}$ is transformed using a global average pooling operation to improve the exploration of semantic characteristics over the full spectrum of feature mappings. All of C's spatial information is included in the channel identification $I \in R^{1\times 1\times C}$. A channel identifier, represented by the notation $I \in R^{1\times 1\times C}$, can be extracted from a feature map by reducing its dimensionality from 2D to 1D. To effectively extract information from the channel identification, this article uses two convolution algorithms to capture the nonlinear relationship between the channels. The first convolution layer is set aside as a dimensionality-reduction layer to help handle the two convolution operations. To reduce the channel dimension of the channel identification, we use a dimensionality reduction ratio of 16 in accordance with articles [34, 35]. The second convolutional layer's job is to increase the feature map's dimension. After that, the sigmoid activation function is used to give the channel identifier some rudimentary gating control. U_c' memory, short for "logical channel information structure," is the product of this operation. After that, the well-coordinated spatial layout. The input feature map is subjected to a weighted sum operation in order to generate the channel attention feature matrix $U_c \in R^{H\times W\times C}$:

$$\boldsymbol{U}_c' = \sigma(\boldsymbol{W}_2 \mathrm{L}(\boldsymbol{W}_1 \boldsymbol{I})) \tag{22.1}$$

$$\boldsymbol{U}_c = \boldsymbol{U}_c' \times \boldsymbol{M} \tag{22.2}$$

Among the aforementioned elements, the symbol "L" (.) denotes the Leaky ReLU activation function. The weights of the first and second convolutions

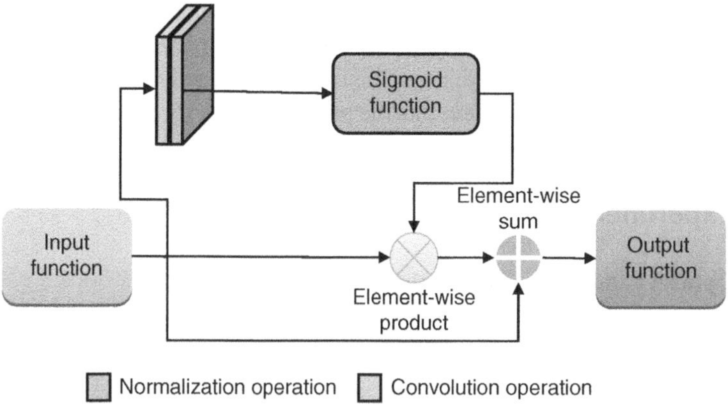

Figure 22.4 Residual spatial attention block.

are denoted by $W_1 \in \mathbb{R}^{\frac{c}{r} \times c} \in \mathbb{R}^{c \times \frac{c}{r}}$ and $W_2 \in \mathbb{R}^{\frac{c}{r} \times c} \in \mathbb{R}^{c \times \frac{c}{r}}$ correspondingly. In addition, the symbol "σ "(.) represents the sigmoid activation function, as referenced in [36].

To prevent too much data loss, the authors of this work present a strategy that uses a residual structure to combine the input feature map with the acquired channel attention feature map. $\tilde{U}_c \in \mathbb{R}^{H \times W \times C}$ is the final output, which is the channel attention feature map.

$$\tilde{U}_c = U_c + M \tag{22.3}$$

The RSA Block is a computational unit that has been developed for enhancing the performance of spatial attention mechanisms in deep learning models. This research introduces an RSA module, depicted in Figure 22.4, as a means to investigate the spatial interaction among local areas of feature mapping.

22.2.3 Loss Function

To make the model still have good generalization ability even when the brain CT data is limited when training the model, the classification labels are first smoothed, and then cross-entropy is used to calculate the loss of the model so that the model not only focuses on the correct classification labels. The loss value can also consider the loss of misclassified labels. The cross-entropy loss function after label smoothing is as follows [21]:

$$y'_k \& = (1 - v) \times y_k + v \times u(k)$$

$$\mathrm{H}(y', y) = \& - \sum_{k=1}^{K} y' \log(\hat{y}) \tag{22.4}$$

$$\mathrm{H}(y', y) = \& (1 - v)\mathrm{H}(y, \hat{y}) + vH(u, \hat{y}) \tag{22.5}$$

Among them, k represents the kth category; y_k represents the true value of the kth label; self-representation smoothing factor, v the value in this article is 0.1; $u(k)$ represents the uniform distribution, the value in this article is $1/3$; y_k' represents the kth smoothed label value; $\hat{y}$ represents the predicted category probability.

22.3 Experiment

22.3.1 Datasets and Evaluation Methods

The 3D brain CT data set used in this article comes from the literature [4]. The data set contains a total of 285 3D CT images. Among them, there are 57 AD types, 113 disease types, and 115 healthy aging types. Each 3D CT image contains 20 different 2D brain CT slices. This article uses 2D brain CT slices to train the model. Some sample pictures are shown in Figure 22.5.

For AD and healthy aging categories, all 2D brain CT slices are used to train the model. For lesion category data, only 2D slices containing lesion information (such as brain tumors) are used to train the model.

To verify the classification performance of the model, this paper still uses the same evaluation method as in the literature [4, 12]:

$$\text{Accuracy} = \frac{\text{TP} + \text{TN}}{\text{TP} + \text{TN} + \text{FP} + \text{FN}} \tag{22.6}$$

22.3.2 Model Parameter Settings

In the experimental procedure of brain CT image classification, the hyperparameters necessary for training the model are established as follows: The model is trained using a limited number of samples with a batch size of 32. The Adam

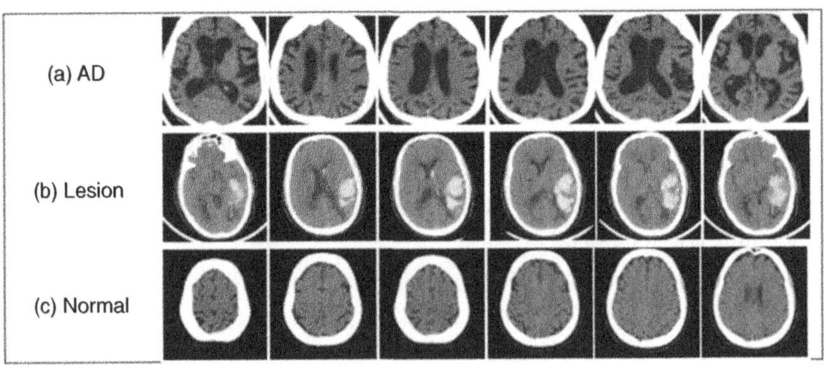

Figure 22.5 Partial brain CT image [4] / IEEE / CC BY 4.0.

Table 22.1 RHAM-MResNet-10 parameter settings.

Layer name	Output size	Parameters
Conv1	100×100	7×7, 64, *Stride2*
Max pool	50×50	3×3, *Stride2*
Residual unit 1	50×50	3×3, 64
Attention module	50×50	RHAM
Residual unit 2	25×25	3×3, 128
Attention module	25×25	RHAM
Residual unit 3	13×13	3×3, 256
Attention module	13×13	RHAM
Residual unit 4	7×7	3×3, 512
Attention module	7×7	RHAM
Global average pool	1×1	
Dropout	0.5	
FC, Softmax	3	

method [22] is employed to optimize the loss function, and an initial learning rate is specified. The weight parameters are subject to penalty constraints through the addition of L2 regularization, with a penalty factor of 0.0001 set at 0.0001. The learning rate is adjusted during the training phase using an exponential decay technique with a gamma value of 0.98. The remaining parameters remain unchanged. The settings are presented in a comprehensive manner in Table 22.1. Furthermore, the training data is augmented by the utilization of random horizontal flipping, random vertical flipping, and adjustments to brightness, contrast, and saturation. These techniques are employed to boost the model's generalization capability. All models discussed in this post were constructed utilizing PyTorch, a deep learning framework, and were trained on an NVIDIA 2080Ti GPU.

22.3.3 Experimental Results

At present, the mainstream residual CNN models include ResNet-10, ResNet-18, ResNet-34, and ResNet-50, and the depth of the models increases in sequence. To select a model that matches the complexity of the brain CT data in this article, the above-mentioned models are used, respectively. The RNM was trained on the brain CT image data set, and the classification results obtained are shown in Table 22.2.

Table 22.2 and Figure 22.6 shows that ResNet-10 has the best classification effect on the brain CT data set, indicating that the complexity of the model and the data

Table 22.2 Comparison of accuracy of residual network models.

Model	Accuracy (%)
Model _ResNet-50	87.12
Model _ResNet-34	88.45
Model _ResNet-18	89.95
Model _ResNet-10	91.51

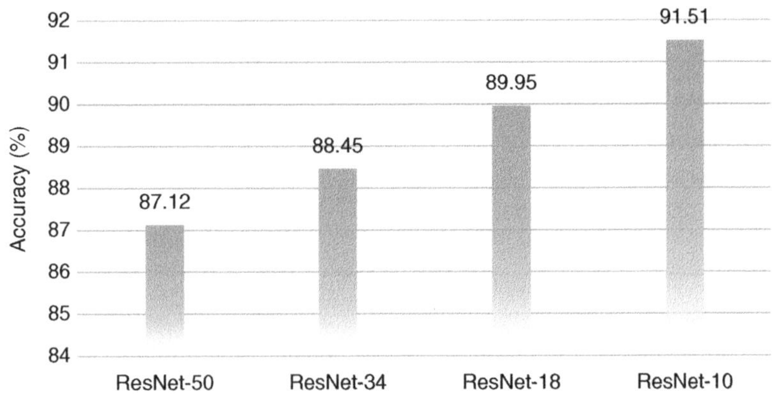

Figure 22.6 Comparisons of classification results of residual network models.

set basically match. Therefore, ResNet-10 was selected for improvement to obtain MResNet-10, which is used as the backbone network of this article Model.

Methods to suppress overfitting were added to the above RMMs to obtain backbone network models such as MResNet-10, MResNet-18, MResNet-34, and MResNet-50. These backbone network models were used to classify brain CT images, respectively. The classification results are shown in Table 22.3.

Table 22.3 Comparison of accuracy over benchmark network models.

Model	Accuracy (%)
Model _ResNet-50	88.64
Model _ResNet-34	89.86
Model _ResNet-18	90.02
Model _ResNet-10	92.41

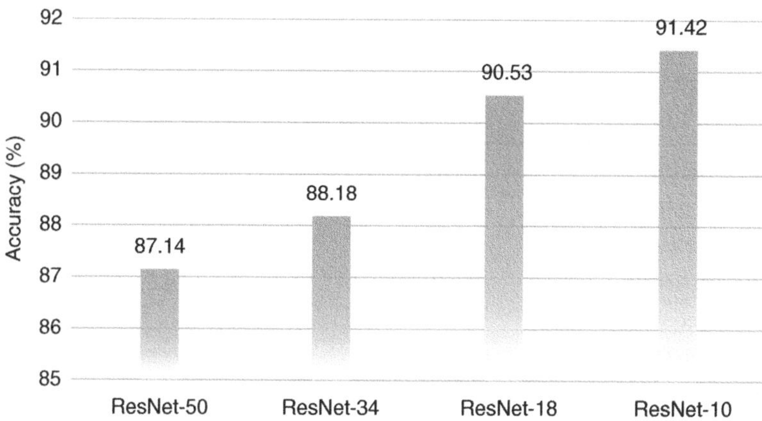

Figure 22.7 Comparison of classification results of backbone network models.

Table 22.3 and Figure 22.7 show that although DCNNs can show good classification results on large-scale data sets, they are prone to overfitting when faced with small-scale data sets, resulting in poor classification performance. Therefore, designing a network model that matches the complexity of the data set is particularly important. The RCA, RSA, RHAM, and CBAM [15] proposed in this article were added to the above-mentioned backbone network model, and the brain CT data were classified. The results are shown in Table 22.4.

We address weak feature distinctiveness in the original model by adding a residual mixed attention module to the network's residual mapping structure. This upgrade helps the model accurately collect brain tissue's spatial and content-related information in CT images for traditional categorization and brain tumor diagnosis utilizing federated learning and generative AI. In addition, we add a global average pooling layer to simplify the architecture. In addition, we drop out successive layers to prevent overfitting. The model uses a label-smoothed cross-entropy loss function during training to improve generalization, even with a few training examples. Our comprehensive studies confirm the upgraded ResNet-10 network model works. It classifies brain CT images with 97.47% accuracy, demonstrating its promise in federated learning and generative AI for brain tumor diagnosis.

The present research introduces the RHAM-MResNet-10 network model, which is utilized for the purpose of brain CT image classification. A comparative analysis is conducted between the suggested model and the methodologies put out by references [4, 12]. The comparative findings are presented in Table 22.5. Based on the comparison table displaying the classification accuracy of all models after five iterations, two conclusions may be inferred.

Table 22.4 Comparison of accuracy over existing attention modules.

Model	Accuracy (%)
RCA-MResNet-50	89.32
RSA-MResNet-50	89.60
CBAM-MResNet-50	89.71
RHAM-MResNet-50	89.89
RCA-MResNet-34	89.65
RSA-MResNet-34	89.95
CBAM-MResNet-34	90.48
RHAM-MResNet-34	90.18
RCA-MResNet-18	90.21
RSA-MResNet-18	90.42
CBAM-MResNet-18	90.76
RHAM-MResNet-18	90.91
RCA-MResNet-10	92.98
RSA-MResNet-10	93.02
CBAM-MResNet-10	95.20
RHAM-MResNet-10	97.47

Table 22.5 Comparison of accuracy over existing models.

Module	Accuracy (%)
2DSIFT	85.61
2D KAZE	86.31
2D CNN	86.32
Mixed LReLU/ELU CNN	87.12
GATED LReLU/ELU CNN	87.44
Mixed PReLU/PELU CNN	87.85
GATEDPReLU/PELU	88.59
$RHAM - MResNet - 10$	97.47

1) The findings indicate that including the attention mechanism in the conventional CNN model yields significant enhancements in model performance, as observed in the classification outcomes when compared to the results presented in [4]. In addition, the residual hybrid attention described in this article is validated. The utilization of the force module facilitates the model's ability to concentrate on the spatial and content characteristics of brain-related tissues. This enables the extraction of more distinct features, hence enhancing the accuracy of the model's categorization.

In contrast to the classification outcomes presented in reference [12], the findings indicate that including an attention mechanism and employing overfitting mitigation techniques yield superior enhancements in the classification performance of the model, as opposed to only altering the activation function.

The suggested method uses a RHAM-MResNet-10 RNM to interpret brain CT images of AD, brain lesions (such tumors), and healthy aging. Please name a topic for me to classify. The RHAM in the residual mapping structure of the model allows simultaneous attention to brain position in the image and brain-related tissue characteristics. Noise is reduced by this integration. Increase model categorization accuracy. When the sample size is limited, global average pooling, dropout, and the label smoothing cross-entropy loss function are used. These methods reduce overfitting and improve model generalization. The experiment showed that the RHAM-MResNet-10 RNM could categorize brain CT images. Future research will focus on pathogenic data in brain CT images, using 3D CNN to analyze this data. The 20 slices of each patient record both static and gradient information, improving disease progression prediction.

22.4 Conclusion

This study introduces an innovative approach to support medical professionals in the early detection of abnormal brain symptoms and to reduce the inconsistencies associated with manual diagnosis in smart healthcare. The proposed method uses the RHAM-MResNet-10 RNM to analyze brain CT images from three categories: AD, brain lesions (including tumors), and healthy aging. This approach aims to facilitate the process of identifying abnormal brain properties, especially in the context of associative learning and interpretable GAI. The RHAM can integrate into the residual mapping structure of the model the spatial information of the brain in the image and estimate the unique characteristics of brain-related tissues at the same time. This integration effectively reduces the effect of noise, thus improving the model's classification accuracy. When the number of samples is limited, joint strategies such as global mean clustering and dropout, combined with label smoothing cross-entropy loss functions, are used to solve the problem of overfitting and improve the model's generalization ability. Empirical evidence from the conducted experiments shows the effectiveness of the RHAM-MResNet-10 RNM in solving challenges related to brain CT image classification. In future research work, we will continue to investigate the presence of pathogen data in brain CT scans and, at the same time, process this data using 3D CNNs. In total, 20 slices per patient capture static information and gradient information between slices, increasing our ability to predict disease progression. This comprehensive approach integrates associative learning and demonstrable GAI to advance the field of brain imaging analysis in smart healthcare.

References

1 Mushtaq, M.F., Shahroz, M., Aseere, A.M. et al. (2021). BHCNet: neural network-based brain hemorrhage classification using head CT scan. *IEEE Access* 9: 113901–113916. https://doi.org/10.1109/ACCESS.2021.3102740.

2 Xu, Y., Holanda, G., Souza, L.F.d.F. et al. (2021). Deep learning-enhanced internet of medical things to analyze brain CT scans of hemorrhagic stroke patients: a new approach. *IEEE Sensors Journal* 21 (22): 24941–24951. https://doi.org/10.1109/JSEN.2020.3032897.

3 Negm, N., Aldehim, G., Nafie, F.M. et al. (2023). Intracranial haemorrhage diagnosis using willow catkin optimization with voting ensemble deep learning on CT brain imaging. *IEEE Access* 11: 75474–75483. https://doi.org/10.1109/ACCESS.2023.3297281.

4 Ramprasad, M.V.S., Rahman, M.Z.U., and Bayleyegn, M.D. (2022). A deep probabilistic sensing and learning model for brain tumor classification with fusion-Net and HFCMIK segmentation. *IEEE Open Journal of Engineering in Medicine and Biology* 3: 178–188. https://doi.org/10.1109/OJEMB.2022.3217186.

5 Khan, S., Sajjad, M., Hussain, T. et al. (2021). A review on traditional machine learning and deep learning models for WBCs classification in blood smear images. *IEEE Access* 9: 10657–10673. https://doi.org/10.1109/ACCESS.2020.3048172.

6 Subramanian, M., Cho, J., Sathishkumar, V.E., and Naren, O.S. (2023). Multiple types of cancer classification using CT/MRI images based on learning without forgetting powered deep learning models. *IEEE Access* 11: 10336–10354. https://doi.org/10.1109/ACCESS.2023.3240443.

7 Sun, L., Mo, Z., Yan, F. et al. (2020). Adaptive feature selection guided deep forest for covid-19 classification with chest CT. *IEEE Journal of Biomedical and Health Informatics* 24 (10): 2798–2805. https://doi.org/10.1109/JBHI.2020.3019505.

8 Wang, S., Nie, D., Qu, L. et al. (2020). CT male pelvic organ segmentation via hybrid loss network with incomplete annotation. *IEEE Transactions on Medical Imaging* 39 (6): 2151–2162. https://doi.org/10.1109/TMI.2020.2966389.

9 Yang, W., Shi, Y., Park, S.H. et al. (2020). An effective MR-guided CT network training for segmenting prostate in CT images. *IEEE Journal of Biomedical and Health Informatics* 24 (8): 2278–2291. https://doi.org/10.1109/JBHI.2019.2960153.

10 Zhang, L., Miao, W., Zhu, C. et al. (2023). A weakly supervised-guided soft attention network for classification of intracranial hemorrhage. *IEEE Transactions on Cognitive and Developmental Systems* 15 (1): 42–53. https://doi.org/10.1109/TCDS.2022.3141591.

11 Qian, X., Fu, H., Shi, W. et al. (2020). M^3Lung-Sys: a deep learning system for multi-class lung pneumonia screening from CT imaging. *IEEE Journal of Biomedical and Health Informatics* 24 (12): 3539–3550. https://doi.org/10.1109/JBHI.2020.3030853.

12 Arman, S.E., Rahman, S.S., Irtisam, N. et al. (2023). Intracranial hemorrhage classification from CT Scan using deep learning and Bayesian optimization. *IEEE Access* 11: 83446–83460. https://doi.org/10.1109/ACCESS.2023.3300771.

13 Ragab, M., Salama, R., Alotaibi, F.S. et al. (2023). Political optimizer with deep learning based diagnosis for intracranial hemorrhage detection. *IEEE Access* 11: 71484–71493. https://doi.org/10.1109/ACCESS.2023.3293754.

14 Tang, H. and Hu, Z. (2020). Research on medical image classification based on machine learning. *IEEE Access* 8: 93145–93154. https://doi.org/10.1109/ACCESS.2020.2993887.

15 Chabib, C.M., Hadjileontiadis, L.J., and Shehhi, A.A. (2023). DeepCurvMRI: deep convolutional curvelet transform-based MRI approach for early detection of Alzheimer's disease. *IEEE Access* 11: 44650–44659. https://doi.org/10.1109/ACCESS.2023.3272482.

16 Shukla, G.P., Kumar, S., Pandey, S.K. et al. (2023). Diagnosis and detection of Alzheimer's disease using learning algorithm. *Big Data Mining and Analytics* 6 (4): 504–512. https://doi.org/10.26599/BDMA.2022.9020049.

17 Zhou, Z., Siddiquee, M.M.R., Tajbakhsh, N., and Liang, J. (2020). UNet++: redesigning skip connections to exploit multiscale features in image segmentation. *IEEE Transactions on Medical Imaging* 39 (6): 1856–1867. https://doi.org/10.1109/TMI.2019.2959609.

18 Hussain, A., Yaseen, M.U., Imran, M. et al. (2022). An attention-based ResNet architecture for acute hemorrhage detection and classification: toward a health 4.0 digital twin study. *IEEE Access* 10: 126712–126727. https://doi.org/10.1109/ACCESS.2022.3225671.

19 Vaiyapuri, T., Mahalingam, J., Ahmad, S. et al. (2023). Ensemble learning driven computer-aided diagnosis model for brain tumor classification on magnetic resonance imaging. *IEEE Access* 11: 91398–91406. https://doi.org/10.1109/ACCESS.2023.3306961.

20 Byeon, H., Al-Kubaisi, M., Dutta, A.K. et al. (2024). Brain tumor segmentation using neuro-technology enabled intelligence-cascaded U-Net model. *Frontiers in Computational Neuroscience* 18: 1391025. https://doi.org/10.3389/fncom.2024.1391025.

21 Soni, M., Khan, I.R., Babu, K.S. et al. (2022). Light weighted healthcare CNN model to detect prostate cancer on multiparametric MRI. *Computational Intelligence and Neuroscience* 2022: 5497120. https://doi.org/10.1155/2022/5497120.

22 Gao, F. (2021). Integrated positron emission tomography/magnetic resonance imaging in clinical diagnosis of Alzheimer's disease. *European Journal of Radiology* 145: 110017.

23 Balwant, M.K. (2022). A review on convolutional neural networks for brain tumor segmentation: methods, datasets, libraries, and future directions. *IRBM* 43 (6): 521–537.

24 Chaddad, A., Lu, Q., Li, J. et al. (2023). Explainable, domain-adaptive, and federated artificial intelligence in medicine. *IEEE/CAA Journal of AutomaticaSinica* 10 (4): 859–876. https://doi.org/10.1109/JAS.2023.123123.

25 Arisdakessian, S., Wahab, O.A., Mourad, A. et al. (2023). A survey on IoT intrusion detection: federated learning, game theory, social psychology, and explainable AI as future directions. *IEEE Internet of Things Journal* 10 (5): 4059–4092. https://doi.org/10.1109/JIOT.2022.3203249.

26 Hou, B., Gao, J., Guo, X. et al. (2022). Mitigating the backdoor attack by federated filters for industrial IoT applications. *IEEE Transactions on Industrial Informatics* 18 (5): 3562–3571. https://doi.org/10.1109/TII.2021.3112100.

27 Riviera, W., Galazzo, I.B., and Menegaz, G. (2023). FeLebrities: a user-centric assessment of federated learning frameworks. *IEEE Access* 11: 96865–96878. https://doi.org/10.1109/ACCESS.2023.3312579.

28 Nehra, G., Bauer, B., and Hartz, A.M.S. (2022). Blood-brain barrier leakage in Alzheimer's disease: From discovery to clinical relevance. *Pharmacology & Therapeutics* 234: 108119.

29 Chen, Y., Zhang, D., Zhang, H., and Wang, Q.-G. (2022). Dual-path mixed-domain residual threshold networks for bearing fault diagnosis. *IEEE Transactions on Industrial Electronics* 69 (12): 13462–13472. https://doi.org/10.1109/TIE.2022.3144572.

30 Lan, Y. and Zhang, X. (2020). Real-time ultrasound image despeckling using mixed-attention mechanism based residual UNet. *IEEE Access* 8: 195327–195340. https://doi.org/10.1109/ACCESS.2020.3034230.

31 Lan, Y., Hao, Y., Xia, K. et al. (2020). Stacked residual recurrent neural networks with cross-layer attention for text classification. *IEEE Access* 8: 70401–70410. https://doi.org/10.1109/ACCESS.2020.2987101.

32 Ha, M.-H. and Chen, O.T.-C. (2021). Deep neural networks using residual fast-slow refined highway and global atomic spatial attention for action recognition and detection. *IEEE Access* 9: 164887–164902. https://doi.org/10.1109/ACCESS.2021.3134694.

33 Ma, X., Lv, W., and Zhao, M. (2023). A double stream person re-identification method based on attention mechanism and multi-scale feature fusion. *IEEE Access* 11: 14612–14620. https://doi.org/10.1109/ACCESS.2023.3243553.

34 Zhou, G., Li, Z., Fu, M. et al. (2021). Sequence-to-sequence load disaggregation using multiscale residual neural network. *IEEE Transactions on Instrumentation and Measurement* 70: 1, 2503310–10. https://doi.org/10.1109/TIM.2020.3034989.

35 Lakhan, A., Grønli, T.-M., Muhammad, G., and Tiwari, P. (2023). EDCNNS: federated learning enabled evolutionary deep CNN for Alzheimer disease detection. *Applied Soft Computing* 147: 110804.

36 Zhang, C., Meng, X., Liu, Q. et al. (2023). A robust multi-site brain network analysis framework based on federated learning for brain disease diagnosis. *Neurocomputing* 559: 126791.

23

AI-Based Emotion Detection System in Healthcare for Patient

Ati Jain[1] and Amiyavardhan Jain[2]

[1] *Institute of Advance Computing, SAGE University, Indore, India*
[2] *Consultant, Periodontology and Implantology, Noble Dental Care, Indore, India*

23.1 Introduction

For the biggest and revolutionary change in medical practices, one of the answerable applications of artificial intelligence (AI) is in healthcare which has nowadays become a popular and most needful one. AI has the capacity to analyze patients' data of medical, capture patterns that occur, and create insights that can help in decisions for clinical practices, recover patient consequences, and diminish healthcare costs of examination [1]. However, to reduce the potential harm and maximize the benefits of Emotion AI in healthcare, some factors to be taken care like ethical, transparency, legal, safety, social implications, and impartiality. With the great use of Emotion AI in the field of healthcare, its use in several applications will definitely play a vital role in shaping the future of medical diagnosis.

Emotion AI is single capable skilled technologies that may quicken the quality of online patient communications and diagnostics that mark higher. Emotion AI can know and assess emotional responses, such as anger, happy, boredom, contempt, fear, surprise, liking, sorrow, and sadness, by measuring expressions that are difficult for the human eye to record as it is too rapid and fast. It thus benefits in terms of sides of communication in a positive manner, generous with practical evidence to make cleverer decisions.

Smart health systems are fetching progressively significant deep learning technology as there is an advancement of many possibilities. There are several types of surveillance systems and diagnosis of diseases, possibly remote judgments, as many machine learning techniques help in healthcare for different age groups of human beings to realize patients' emotional states and sentiments.

Generative Artificial Intelligence for Biomedical and Smart Health Informatics,
First Edition. Edited by Aditya Khamparia and Deepak Gupta.

Early interventions are good as there will be a reduction in stress and unhappiness by detection of emotions at an early stage. These practices can be applied as an observation system like webcam and cameras that captures images and videos. The claims of AI emotion detection for patients are plentiful, and they include many significant features of regular routine, such as customer service, driving safely, mental health monitoring, education, marketing, social security, and so on [2]. There are several angles to look into different applications for the solution. Features that focus on AI emotions are postures, body gestures, visual expressions, voice expressions, and sound expressions while examining emotion recognition. Bi-models system helps in recognition using combinations of facial or speech with body signals and gestures to improve emotion recognition. Devices also help to recognize emotions; webcam and voice recorder are used as the most important that provide better results. Patients' emotional recognition has become an important part, as that helps doctors in identifying their patients' emotional and psychological issues, and as a result, it helps in early interventions. Worldwide, in many hospitals Emotion AI has been used to treat patients, and research on a daily basis in the field is being done on developing neural networks that can appreciate a patient's emotions [3]. This can be done through a variability of systems, such as investigating facial expressions, tone of voice, and other physiological pointers of emotion. Audio and video are major tools that help in finding human emotions.

23.2 Literature Survey

Researchers have discovered numerous methods, technologies, and applications to progress systems proficient in detecting and understanding emotions in healthcare settings. Emotional well-being is a crucial aspect of overall health, and detecting emotions in patients can aid in personalized healthcare. Effective emotion detection can contribute to early diagnosis, treatment adherence, and improved patient outcomes [4].

Natural Language Processing (NLP): Many studies focus on using NLP techniques to analyze text data from patient interactions, such as electronic health records, social media, and chat logs, to identify emotional cues.

Speech Analysis: Emotion detection through speech analysis, including prosody, pitch, and speech patterns, has been explored for its potential in assessing mental health and emotional states.

Facial Expression Recognition: Utilizing computer vision algorithms to analyze facial expressions in real time or from images to infer emotional states.

Physiological Sensors: Some researchers have investigated the use of physiological signals, such as heart rate variability, skin conductance, and EEG, to detect emotional states in patients [5].

Mental Health Monitoring: AI-based emotion detection systems are applied to monitor mental health conditions, including depression, anxiety, and stress.

Chronic Disease Management: Emotional monitoring can assist in the management of chronic diseases by identifying stressors and providing timely interventions.

Patient Engagement: Enhancing patient engagement and communication through emotion-aware systems to improve patient–doctor interactions [6]. Ongoing research emphasizes the need for multimodal approaches, combining data from various sources to improve the accuracy of emotion detection. Exploring the integration of AI systems with existing mental health interventions to create comprehensive and personalized treatment plans [7].

Dhuheir et al. [1] did an assessment of using convolutional neural networks (CNN) to analyze patients' emotions. Different significant applications of CNNs in emotion recognition were considered, are such as speech-based emotion recognition, facial-based emotion recognition [1], and audio–visual-based emotion recognition. Different approaches were used and tried for better accuracy. To identify overall expressions from the patient's medical report, some steps are used that cover preprocessing; second to select the features using feature selection and then extraction of best features for results, and at last classification method applied.

Swayam Badhe et al. (2022) [8] anticipated that the use of classification algorithms like CNN is presenting good outcomes by identifying sentiments from the real-time human video that is dynamic in nature while capturing. Some of the emotions like repulsions cannot be judged well but present diagnosis will help a lot in examination. More images for recognition of different emotions from the group of images to get exact acknowledgement of all several emotions from steal as well as current active images.

Yang and Yanbin [4] accomplish that the anticipated method is having the probability to improve the correctness of Smart Health Houses. For guidelines and future studies, examining the probability of merging various skills, including systems based on computer vision, wearable devices, and devices with sensors, to increase the accurateness and efficacy of Smart Health Houses. The learning grips extensive significance that helps us better understand the sentiment for recognition with facial expression investigation, and it also tends to have accurate results on the higher side.

Mutawa et al. [4] suggested an innovative multimodal method for patient emotion identification. It uses face expressions and EEG brain signals to precisely depict patients' true emotional state as, due to health issues, they are not exactly able to express themselves, or there may be a chance of getting the wrong treatment. A threefold cross-validation method was used to verify the training system for best results. When both face and EEG system were used, there was 99.3% accuracy.

Siddique et al. [7] deliberate on the proper challenges related to the ethics-related data and structures and highlight the preparations for prosocial [7] perspectives for future related applications. Also, projected strategies for scheming future prosocial AI Emotion Recognition solutions.

Suraj et al. [9] worked on recognition of emotions research in the field of retaining neural networks to that will be used in modeled systems [9]. Facial expressions recognition is the main motto behind the development of system that focuses on finding of seven standard emotions and imaging several slants for the implementation of said algorithms using classification algorithms. Methods for knowing emotions can be applied as an investigation system in healthcare centers to screening patients.

Bansal et al. [10] have given an idea by implementing a model using a deep learning method that scrutinizes language that appears in patterns, the pitch of voice, and facial expressions [10] that intended to recognize the utmost operative and multipurpose methods of emotion recognition to improve computer vision human–computer interaction in miscellaneous domains.

23.3 AI in Healthcare Sector

23.3.1 Autistic Child

Emotion AI, or artificial intelligence that identifies and replies to human emotions, can be an appreciated tool in supporting autistic children in several ways. Autism spectrum disorder (ASD) is a neurodevelopmental disorder that disturbs social interaction, communication, and behavior. Here are numerous ways in which Emotion AI can be beneficial for autistic children.

- **Facial Expression Recognition:** Emotion AI can analyze facial expressions and help autistic children understand emotions better. Many autistic individuals struggle with recognizing and interpreting facial cues, which are crucial for understanding social interactions. Emotion AI can provide real-time feedback on facial expressions, helping children learn to identify emotions and respond appropriately.
- **Social Skills Training:** Emotion AI can be integrated into social skills training programs [11]. By providing instant feedback on social interactions, such as tone of voice and body language, AI tools can help autistic children refine their social skills and enhance their ability to connect with others.
- **Personalized Learning:** Emotion AI can adapt to the individual needs of autistic children. By assessing their emotional states and preferences, AI systems can

tailor educational content and activities to suit the child's unique learning style. This personalized approach can improve engagement and overall learning outcomes.

- **Emotion Regulation:** Many autistic children struggle with emotional regulation. Emotion AI can be used to monitor and recognize signs of emotional distress in real time, providing timely interventions or suggesting coping strategies to help the child manage their emotions more effectively.
- **Communication Assistance:** For nonverbal or minimally verbal autistic children, Emotion AI can play a role in augmentative and alternative communication (AAC). By recognizing emotional cues and responses, AI tools can help build a more effective communication system, enabling children to express themselves and understand others.
- **Therapeutic Support:** Emotion AI can support therapeutic interventions for autistic children, such as behavioral therapy [12]. It can provide therapists and caregivers with data on the child's emotional responses during sessions, helping to tailor interventions and track progress over time.
- **Gaming and Engagement:** Interactive games and applications powered by Emotion AI can be designed to engage autistic children in learning and social scenarios. These tools can provide a safe and controlled environment for practicing social skills and emotional understanding.

23.3.2 Mental Health of Individual

Emotion AI's potential to distinguish both positive and negative emotional states may support the correct judgment and treatment of some specific mental health issues during virtual/offline consultations. In certain circumstances, the computers may also support clinicians, analyze, and forecast the varied degrees of anxiety and tension in distant patients through live video meetings [13]. Emotion AI plays a noteworthy role in auxiliary mental health by providing tools and technologies that can enhance emotional awareness, provide personalized interventions, and offer valuable insights. Here are several ways in which Emotion AI contributes to mental health.

- **Emotion Recognition and Monitoring:** Emotion AI can analyze facial expressions, vocal tone, and other physiological signals to recognize and monitor emotions in real time. Continuous monitoring helps individuals gain insights into their emotional states, providing awareness that can be valuable for self-reflection.
- **Early Detection of Mental Health Issues:** By analyzing patterns in emotional data, Emotion AI can contribute to the early detection of mental health issues or changes in emotional well-being. Early intervention can be crucial in preventing the escalation of mental health challenges.

- **Personalized Interventions:** Emotion AI can tailor interventions based on an individual's emotional needs and preferences. Personalized recommendations for coping strategies, mindfulness exercises, or therapeutic activities can be provided to help manage stress, anxiety, or other emotional concerns.
- **Mood Tracking and Trend Analysis:** Emotion AI can assist individuals in tracking their moods over time. Analyzing trends in emotional data can help identify potential triggers, patterns, or correlations with daily activities, facilitating a better understanding of one's mental health.
- **Virtual Mental Health Assistants:** Virtual assistants powered by Emotion AI can provide continuous emotional support and companionship. These virtual assistants can offer empathy, encouragement, and suggest coping mechanisms, helping individuals navigate challenging emotional periods.
- **Therapeutic Tools:** Emotion AI can be integrated into therapeutic tools and applications to enhance the effectiveness of mental health interventions. Virtual reality (VR) experiences or interactive applications using Emotion AI can provide immersive and engaging therapeutic environments.
- **Feedback for Mental Health Professionals:** Mental health professionals can benefit from Emotion AI by receiving additional data and insights about a patient's emotional well-being. This information can aid in treatment planning allowing therapists to make more informed decisions and adjustments to therapeutic approaches.
- **Stress Reduction and Relaxation Apps:** Emotion AI can power applications focused on stress reduction, relaxation, and mindfulness. These apps can offer personalized relaxation exercises, breathing techniques, or guided meditations based on the individual's emotional state [14].
- **Support for Neurodiverse Populations:** Emotion AI is definitely helpful for an individual having situations such as autism or ADHD, helping them better understand and regulate their emotions. Tailored interventions can address specific challenges related to emotional processing and social interactions.

23.3.3 Pregnancy Care

Experts have just begun to think about the potential utilization of Emotion Detection Tech in pregnancy care. Numerous research has previously pointed out that psychological responses (stress, anxiety, rage, etc.) might be an important risk factor throughout the pregnancy period [15]. This technology may surely assist in measuring the emotional health of pregnant females and take prompt action to help them cope with the mental disorders bothering them. Here are some ways in which Emotion AI can be beneficial in pregnancy care.

- **Stress and Emotional Monitoring:** Emotion AI can monitor the emotional well-being of pregnant individuals by analyzing expressions of facial, i.e., emotions, verbal tones, and other biological and psychological signals. Continuous monitoring will help identify symbols of stress of mind, anxiety of an individual, or mood changes, allowing for early intervention and support.

- **Mood Tracking and Self-awareness:** Pregnancy is a time of significant emotional and physical changes. Emotion AI can assist in tracking and analyzing mood fluctuations over the course of the pregnancy. This information can help individuals become more aware of their emotional well-being and take proactive steps to manage stress or emotional challenges.
- **Virtual Support and Education:** Virtual assistants powered by Emotion AI can provide emotional support, answer questions, and offer educational content related to pregnancy. These virtual support systems can offer reassurance, guidance on prenatal care, and information about physical and emotional changes during pregnancy.
- **Birth Preparation and Education:** Emotion AI can be utilized in virtual birth preparation programs to address emotional aspects of labor and delivery [16]. Providing information about coping strategies, relaxation techniques, and emotional preparation for childbirth can contribute to a more positive birth experience.
- **Monitoring Maternal Mental Health:** Emotion AI can assist in monitoring maternal mental health during and after pregnancy. Continuous emotional monitoring can help healthcare providers identify signs of perinatal mood disorders and tailor interventions accordingly.
- **Well-being Check-ins:** Emotion AI-powered applications can regularly check in on the emotional well-being of pregnant individuals, offering personalized content and resources based on their emotional states.

23.3.4 Patient Feedback and Experience Improvement

Emotion AI can be employed to gather and analyze patient feedback. Healthcare organizations can use this information to make improvements in communication, facilities, and overall care delivery. Emotion AI, or affective computing, involves the use of technology to detect and respond to human emotions [17]. Implementing Emotion AI in healthcare settings, such as patient feedback and experience improvement, can offer several benefits. Here's how Emotion AI can contribute to enhancing patient feedback and experience.

- **Real-time Emotion Monitoring:** Emotion AI can analyze facial expressions, voice tone, and other physiological signals to screen patients' emotive states in real time. This permits medical systems and healthcare benefactors to gauge patient emotions during interactions, helping them understand and address concerns promptly.

- **Automated Sentiment Analysis:** Emotion AI can be applied to analyze written feedback, online reviews, and survey responses to automatically identify sentiments expressed by patients. This automation allows healthcare organizations to quickly identify areas of satisfaction or dissatisfaction and prioritize improvements.
- **Personalized Patient Interactions:** Emotion AI can help in tailoring interactions based on individual patient emotions. By understanding the emotional context, healthcare providers can offer more personalized care, potentially improving the overall patient experience.
- **Improved Communication:** Analyzing emotions can enhance communication between healthcare providers and patients. Recognizing emotional cues can assist healthcare professionals in responding empathetically, leading to better rapport and understanding.
- **Identifying Pain and Discomfort:** Emotion AI can aid in the detection of pain and discomfort by analyzing facial expressions and other physiological signals. This information can be valuable for managing pain levels and adjusting treatment plans accordingly.
- **Enhanced Training for Healthcare Professionals:** Emotion AI can be utilized for training healthcare professionals in patient communication and empathy [18]. Simulations and feedback based on emotional cues can help practitioners develop better interpersonal skills.
- **Continuous Feedback Loop:** Implementing Emotion AI creates a continuous feedback loop, allowing healthcare organizations to monitor and adapt to evolving patient sentiments. Regular feedback can be used to make ongoing improvements to patient care processes and facilities.
- **Data-Driven Decision Making:** Emotion AI generates data that is further used to recognize patterns that help to know patient experiences that are in trend. Data-driven insights can guide strategic decisions aimed at enhancing overall patient satisfaction and well-being.

23.3.5 Training Healthcare Professionals

Emotion AI can be used in training programs for healthcare professionals to enhance their empathy and communication skills [19]. Simulations and feedback based on emotional analysis can help healthcare providers develop better bedside manners and patient-centered care.

- **Emotional Intelligence Development:** Emotion AI tools can help healthcare professionals develop their emotional intelligence by providing real-time feedback on their interactions with patients. Professionals can learn to recognize and respond appropriately to patient emotions, fostering better connections and understanding.

- **Simulated Patient Interactions:** Emotion AI can be integrated into simulation exercises, creating realistic scenarios for healthcare professionals to practice their communication skills. Simulations can include diverse emotional responses, helping professionals navigate various patient interactions and challenges.
- **Feedback and Coaching:** Emotion AI tools can provide detailed feedback on healthcare professionals' communication styles, tone of voice, and nonverbal cues during simulated or real interactions. This feedback can be used for coaching and improvement, guiding professionals toward more empathetic and effective communication [20].
- **Cultural Competence Training:** Emotion AI can aid in cultural competence training by simulating interactions with patients from diverse backgrounds and with different cultural norms. Professionals can learn to navigate cultural nuances in communication and understand how emotions may be expressed differently across cultures.
- **Stress Management Training:** Healthcare professionals often face high-stress situations. Emotion AI can simulate scenarios to help professionals manage their own stress and emotions during challenging patient encounters. By practicing stress management techniques in a controlled environment, professionals can enhance their resilience and maintain effective communication.
- **Patient-Centered Care Education:** Emotion AI can contribute to the education of patient-centered care by emphasizing the importance of understanding and addressing patient emotions. Professionals can learn to prioritize patients' emotional well-being alongside medical treatment, leading to a more holistic approach to healthcare.
- **Continuous Professional Development:** Emotion AI tools provide a platform for continuous professional development, allowing healthcare professionals to regularly assess and refine their communication skills. Professionals can use these tools throughout their careers to stay attuned to evolving patient expectations and communication dynamics.
- **Research and Insights:** Emotion AI-generated data from training sessions can be analyzed to identify trends and areas for improvement in healthcare professionals' emotional intelligence and communication skills. Research findings can inform the development of targeted training programs and resources.

23.3.6 Stress Reduction and Relaxation

Emotion AI-powered applications can offer stress reduction and relaxation exercises tailored to the state of an individual's emotions [21]. Such applications can be treasured tools for patients dealing with chronic conditions, undergoing treatments, or managing long-term health challenges.

- **Stress Detection and Monitoring:** Emotion AI systems can analyze various physiological signals for detecting stress signs with the help of expressions of the face, i.e., emotions, rate of heartbeat, skin factors, etc. Continuous monitoring allows for the early identification of stress triggers and the implementation of targeted interventions.
- **Personalized Relaxation Recommendations:** Based on real-time emotional data, Emotion AI can provide personalized recommendations for stress reduction techniques. Tailored suggestions may include breathing exercises, meditation, mindfulness practices, or other relaxation methods that align with an individual's current emotional state.
- **Wearable Devices Integration:** Emotion AI also helps to know stress levels, e.g., like real-time feedback by the use of wearable devices. Wearables can offer alerts or notifications to prompt users to engage in relaxation activities, helping them manage stress as it occurs.
- **Adaptive Meditation and Mindfulness Apps:** Emotion AI can enhance meditation and mindfulness applications by adjusting guided sessions based on the user's emotional state. Dynamic content, such as calming visualizations or soothing sounds, can be adapted in real time to optimize their effectiveness.
- **•VR and Augmented Reality (AR) Experiences:** Emotion AI in VR and AR environments can create immersive experiences aimed at inducing relaxation. Virtual scenarios can be adapted based on the user's emotional feedback, providing a personalized and engaging way to reduce stress.
- **Biofeedback and Neurofeedback Devices:** Emotion AI can be integrated into biofeedback and neurofeedback devices to help individuals gain awareness of their physiological responses to stress [22]. Real-time feedback on factors like heart rate variability or brainwave patterns can guide users in achieving a state of relaxation.
- **Chatbots for Emotional Support:** Emotion AI-powered chatbots can offer empathetic responses and provide emotional support to individuals experiencing stress. These chatbots can engage in conversations, offer encouragement, and suggest coping strategies based on the user's expressed emotions.
- **Customized Music and Audio Therapy:** Emotion AI can personalize music playlists or audio therapy sessions to align with an individual's emotional needs. Dynamic adjustments to tempo, volume, and genre can create a soothing auditory experience tailored to reduce stress.
- **Workplace Stress Management Programs:** In workplace settings, Emotion AI can be used to identify stress factors among employees. Employers can implement stress management programs, incorporating personalized interventions and wellness initiatives based on Emotion AI insights.
- **Educational and Training Tools:** Emotion AI can be integrated into educational tools to teach stress reduction techniques. Interactive modules can adapt based on users' emotional responses, offering a dynamic and effective learning experience (Figure 23.1).

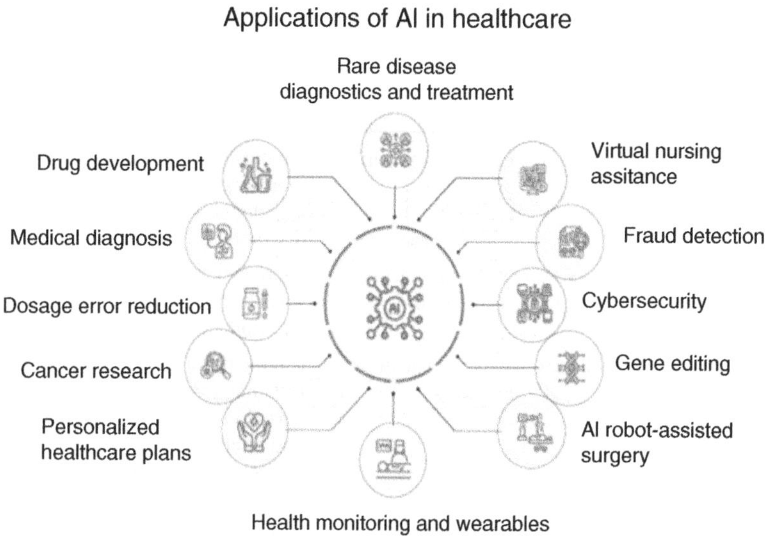

Figure 23.1 Applications of emotion AI in healthcare.

23.4 Methodology

Emotion AI in healthcare involves the application of technology and algorithms that are capable of recognizing, understanding, and answering to different human emotions that can occur [23]. Several key technologies and algorithms play a role in implementing Emotion AI in healthcare settings (Figure 23.2, Table 23.1). Here are some notable ones:

23.5 Conclusion

When it is a matter of the guts of AI in transmuting healthcare is enormous. This has various applications in several fields like pregnancy care, medical imaging, stress management, drug discovery, patient's diagnosis, personalized medicine, sentiment analysis, virtual health assistants, VR and AR, predictive analytics, Robotics surgery position to transfigure patient care, progress results, and consequences, and decrease costing in healthcare for examining. However, there are some challenges addressed related to the privacy of data, biasness, ethics, transparency for AI application for implementation. Joint efforts between AI experts, healthcare professionals, policymakers, and patients will pave the way for the successful integration of AI in healthcare, ultimately promoting society and forward-moving the park of medicine. AI's capability to augment diagnostic accuracy and simplify early detection of diseases has the probable to save immeasurable lives. Moreover, personalized medicine driven by AI algorithms grips the

Table 23.1 Technology and application for emotion AI in healthcare.

Serial number	Heads	Technology	Application
1	Facial Expression Recognition	Computer vision and facial recognition algorithms.	Analyzing facial expressions to identify emotions such as happiness, sadness, pain, or discomfort.
2	Speech and Voice Analysis	NLP and voice recognition	Analyzing tone, pitch, and speech patterns to detect emotional cues.
3	Physiological Signal Monitoring	Wearable devices and sensors	Gaging physiological signals like the rate of the heart and its variation with time, skin changes and related factors, or EEG system to infer emotional states.
4	Affective Computing	Affective computing frameworks and models.	Developing structures that can identify and answer to human emotional expressions using various moods that represent; e.g., text, images, speech, etc.
5	Sentiment Analysis	NLP and ML algorithms.	Analyzing written or verbal communication to determine the sentiment expressed (positive, negative, and neutral).
6	VR and AR	VR and AR platforms integrated with emotion-sensing capabilities.	Creating immersive environments that adapt based on the user's emotional responses.
7	Biometric Authentication and Emotional Access Control	Biometric recognition systems.	Integrating emotion recognition with biometric authentication for secure access.
8	ML for Predictive Analytics	ML algorithms trained on historical data.	Predicting patient outcomes, identifying potential mental health issues, or personalizing treatment plans based on emotional data.
9	Human–computer Interaction Design	User interface design principles.	Designing interfaces that consider emotional responses for improved user experience.
10	Robotics and Social Robots	Robotics integrated with emotion-sensing capabilities.	Creating socially intelligent robots for patient interaction and companionship.

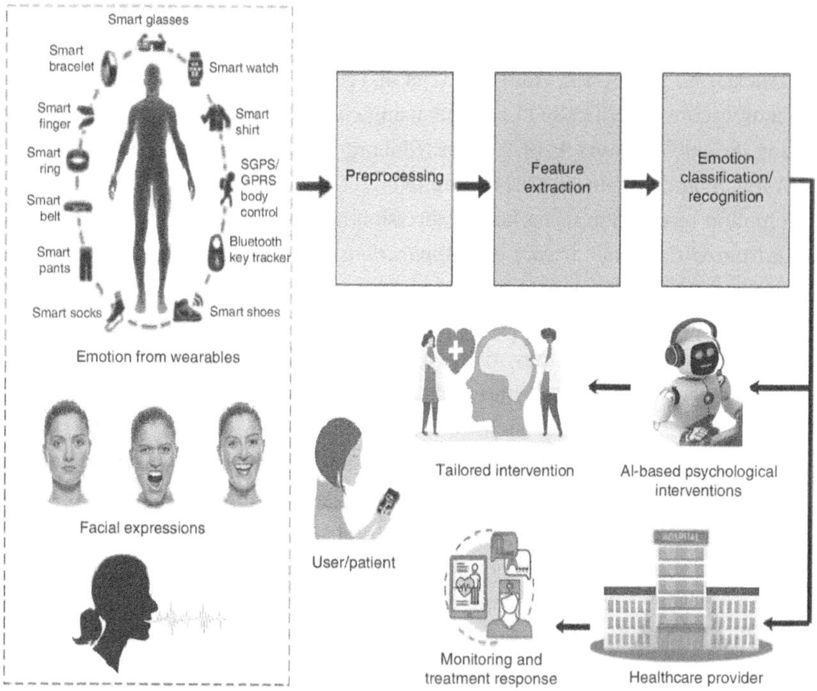

Figure 23.2 Methodology.

capacity of educating treatment usefulness and individualizing patient care. The appearance of virtual health supporters guarantees nonstop access to healthcare information, sanctioning patients and rationalization administrative tasks for healthcare providers. While AI's potential in healthcare is irrefutable, ethical considerations, data privacy, and regulatory compliance must be addressed to ensure responsible implementation.

References

1 Dhuheir, G.M., Albaseer, A., Baccour, E., et al. (2021). Emotion recognition for healthcare surveillance systems using neural networks: a survey. *2021 International Wireless Communications and Mobile Computing (IWCMC)*, pp. 681–687 Harbin City, China (28 June 2021–2 July 2021). IEEE. https://doi.org/10.1109/IWCMC51323.2021.9498861.

2 Sahoo, G.K., Das, S.K. and Singh, P. (2022). Deep learning-based facial emotion recognition for driver healthcare. *2022 National Conference on Communications*

(NCC), pp. 154–159, Mumbai, India (24–27 May 2022). IEEE. https://doi.org/10.1109/NCC55593.2022.9806751.

3 Shickel, B., Loftus, T.J., Adhikari, L. et al. (2019). DeepSOFA: a continuous acuity score for critically ill patients using clinically interpretable deep learning. *Scientific Reports* 9: 1879. https://doi.org/10.1038/s41598-019-38491-0.

4 Yang, S. and Yanbin, B. (2024). Improving of smart health houses: identifying emotion recognition using facial expression analysis. *International Journal of Advanced Computer Science and Applications (IJACSA)* 15 (1): http://dx.doi.org/10.14569/IJACSA.2024.0150121.

5 Santoni de Sio, F. and Mecacci, G. (2021). Four responsibility gaps with artificial intelligence: why they matter and how to address them. *Philosophy and Technology* 34: 1057–1084. https://doi.org/10.1007/s13347-021-00450-x.

6 Mutawa, A.M. and Hassouneh, A. (2024). Multimodal real-time patient emotion recognition system using facial expressions and brain EEG signals based on machine learning and log-sync methods. *Biomedical Signal Processing and Control* 91: 105942. https://doi.org/10.1016/j.bspc.2023.105942.

7 Latif, S., Ali, H., Usama, M., et al. (2022). AI-Based Emotion Recognition: Promise, Peril, and Prescriptions for Prosocial Path. 10.48550/arXiv.2211.07290.

8 Badhe, S. and Chaudhari, S. (2022). Deep learning based facial emotion recognition. *ITM Web of Conferences* 44: 03058.

9 Suraj, A., Kaushik, A., and Bai, K. (2022). Patient monitoring using emotion recognition. *International Journal for Research in Applied Science and Engineering Technology* 10: 1197–1201. https://doi.org/10.22214/ijraset.2022.46387.

10 Bansal, P.K. and Vishram, R.K. (2023). AI-driven emotion recognition for enhanced human-computer interaction: advancements, ethical considerations, and emotional intelligence. *European Chemical Bulletin* 12 (Special Issue 10): 4052–4059.

11 Abdullah, S.M., Abdullah, S., Ameen, S.Y. et al. (2021). Multimodal emotion recognition using deep learning. *Journal of Applied Science and Technology Trends* 2 (02): 52–58.

12 Ahmed, N., Al Aghbari, Z., and Girija, S. (2023). A systematic survey on multimodal emotion recognition using learning algorithms. *Intelligent Systems with Applications* 17: 200171.

13 Deng, J. and Ren, F. (2021). A survey of textual emotion recognition and its challenges. *IEEE Transactions on Affective Computing* 99: 1–1.

14 Lal, M. and Neduncheliyan, S. (2024). Enhanced V-Net approach for the emotion recognition and sentiment analysis in the healthcare data. *Multimedia Tools and Applications* 83 (29): https://doi.org/10.1007/s11042-024-18364-z.

15 Kumar, D., Bhavna, and Narzary, D. (2024). Exploring the utility of emotion recognition systems in healthcare. In: *Using Machine Learning to Detect Emotions and Predict Human Psychology* (ed. M. Rai and J.K. Pandey). IGI Global https://doi.org/10.4018/979-8-3693-1910-9.

16 Kumar, S., Prabha, R., and Samuel, S. (2022). Sentiment analysis and emotion detection with healthcare perspective. In: *Augmented Intelligence in Healthcare: A Pragmatic and Integrated Analysis* (ed. H.K. Tripathy, K. Shaalan, P. Mallick, and S. Mishra), 189–204. Springer https://doi.org/10.1007/978-981-19-1076-0_11.

17 Atlam, H., Shafik, M., Kurugollu, F., and ElKelany, Y. (2022). *Emotions in Mental Healthcare and Psychological Interventions: Towards an Inventive Emotions Recognition Framework Using AI*. IOS Press https://doi.org/10.3233/ATDE220609.

18 Kewalchand, P. (2024). AI in healthcare. *International Journal of Advanced Research in Science, Communication and Technology* 544–548. https://doi.org/10.48175/IJARSCT-15285.

19 Jayvir, S. (2024). *AI Automation in Healthcare: Revolutionizing Patient Care and Operational Efficiency AI Automation in Patient Care.*

20 Naqvi, W., Sundus, H., Mishra, G. et al. (2024). AI in medical education curriculum: the future of healthcare learning. *European Journal of Therapeutics* 30, 10.58600/eurjther1995 (2).

21 Rajkomar, A., Oren, E., Chen, K. et al. (2018). Scalable and accurate deep learning with electronic health records. *npj Digital Medicine* 1: 18. https://doi.org/10.1038/s41746-018-0029-1.

22 Topol, E.J. (2019). High-performance medicine: the convergence of human and artificial Intelligence. *Nature Medicine* 25: 44–56. https://doi.org/10.1038/s41591-018-0300-7.

23 Heaven, W.D. (2021). Hundreds of AI tools have been built to catch covid. None of them helped. https://www.technologyreview.com/2021/07/30/1030329/machine-learning-ai-failed-covid-hospitaldiagnosis-pandemic/

24

Leveraging Process Mining for Enhanced Efficiency and Precision in Healthcare

Parth Sharma[1], Sohan Kumar[1], Tanay Falor[2], Om Dabral[1], Abhinav Upadhyay[1], Rishik Gupta[1], and Vanshika Singh Andotra[1]

[1] *Manipal University, Jaipur*
[2] *IIIT, Allahabad*

24.1 Introduction

Efficiency and precision stand as the cornerstones within the ever-evolving sector of healthcare, where even incremental enhancements wield significant influence over patient well-being. What may seem like a trivial, recurring inconvenience for hospitals can, in reality, manifest as a life-or-death decision for a patient, compounded by the inherent human error embedded at every operational juncture. These human errors, occurring with such frequency and unpredictability, present a formidable challenge to our efforts. However, amid this complexity, a promising solution emerges: process mining.

Sitting at an intersection of data analytics and process science, process mining, a discipline within data science, involves analyzing event logs from information systems to derive insights about the underlying business processes. Utilizing a range of techniques and tools it enables the discovery, monitoring, and enhancement of real-world business processes by extracting knowledge from event logs, datasets, and other process-related information. By amalgamating process modeling techniques, data mining, and machine learning, process mining identifies and scrutinizes patterns, bottlenecks, and anomalies in process data. The primary aim of process mining is to provide an understanding of how processes are executed, uncover inefficiencies, and propose improvements to enhance process performance, reduce expenses, and boost customer satisfaction. Furthermore, in the healthcare sector, where stakes are high and margins for error are slim, process mining holds particular promise. By applying process mining techniques to healthcare data, organizations can gain deeper insights into patient pathways, clinical workflows, and resource utilization patterns.

Generative Artificial Intelligence for Biomedical and Smart Health Informatics,
First Edition. Edited by Aditya Khamparia and Deepak Gupta.

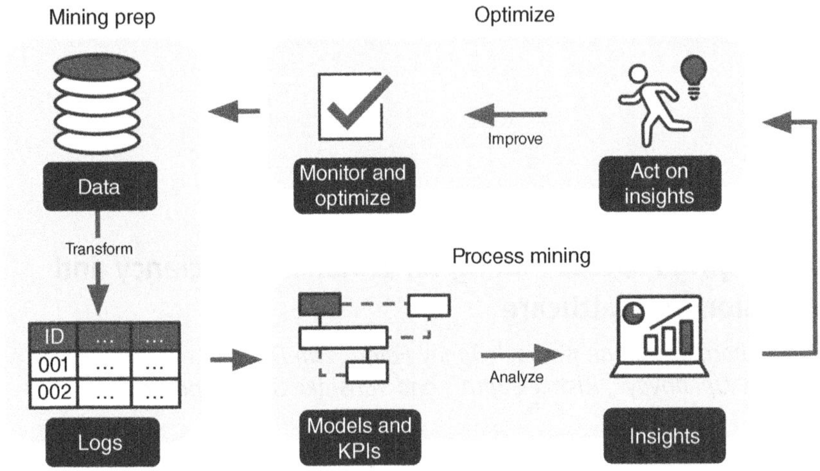

Figure 24.1 Process Mining Lifecycle: From Data to Actionable Insights [2].

This enables healthcare providers to identify areas for improvement, streamline care delivery processes, and ultimately enhance patient outcomes. In addition, by leveraging machine learning algorithms, process mining can adapt to the dynamic nature of healthcare operations, continuously optimizing processes to meet evolving patient needs and regulatory requirements [1]. Thus, in the pursuit of efficiency and precision in healthcare, process mining emerges as a vital tool for driving transformative change and improving the quality of care delivered to patients (Figure 24.1).

24.2 Process Mining

The roots of process mining stretch back to the late 20th century, coinciding with the rise of process management and workflow systems, which aimed to streamline business processes through automation [3].

In the early 2000s, process mining emerged as a research discipline pioneered by Wil van der Aalst and his colleagues, focusing on extracting process models from event logs and identifying patterns and bottlenecks.

The standardization of event logs, exemplified by the XES format, facilitated data exchange between process mining tools and enabled comparative analyses. Subsequent advancements led to the development of techniques for conformance checking, performance analysis, and predictive analytics, empowering organizations to pinpoint compliance issues, optimize processes, and anticipate outcomes.

Moreover, the integration of process mining with machine learning has further expanded its capabilities, allowing for the analysis of intricate event data and the discovery of hidden correlations. This synergy between machine learning and process mining has democratized the field, making it accessible across various domains and revolutionizing sectors previously untouched.

Broadly, process mining endeavours are classified into three primary categories: Discovery, conformance, and enhancement.

24.2.1 Discovery

During the discovery phase of process mining, event logs capturing the sequence of activities for each process instance, such as a customer order, are utilized to automatically construct a visual representation of the process. This method showcases the prowess of process mining by revealing the genuine flow of work and potentially highlighting any deviations from documented procedures within the resulting model.

24.2.2 Conformance

The stage of conformance checking emerges as a crucial step following the establishment of a process model. Its primary objective is to assess the alignment between the established model and the actual execution of processes. Through this analysis, deviations or exceptions, such as bypassed activities or rework loops, are identified, shedding light on discrepancies between documented procedures and real-world practices. Moreover, conformance checking plays a pivotal role in pinpointing bottlenecks, areas marked by high error rates, or activities that lack value addition within the overall process framework.

24.2.3 Enhancement

Enhancement represents a pivotal moment where insights garnered from the preceding discovery and conformance phases are harnessed to refine and optimize the overall process. Drawing upon the identified deviations and alignments, organizations can strategically streamline the flow, excise redundant steps, or redesign activities to bolster efficiency and efficacy. What distinguishes this phase is its reliance on data-driven insights gleaned from the meticulous analysis of event logs, eschewing conjecture in favor of informed decision-making. Process mining thus serves as a catalyst for continuous improvement, empowering stakeholders to enact meaningful changes that drive tangible enhancements in performance and outcomes (Figure 24.2).

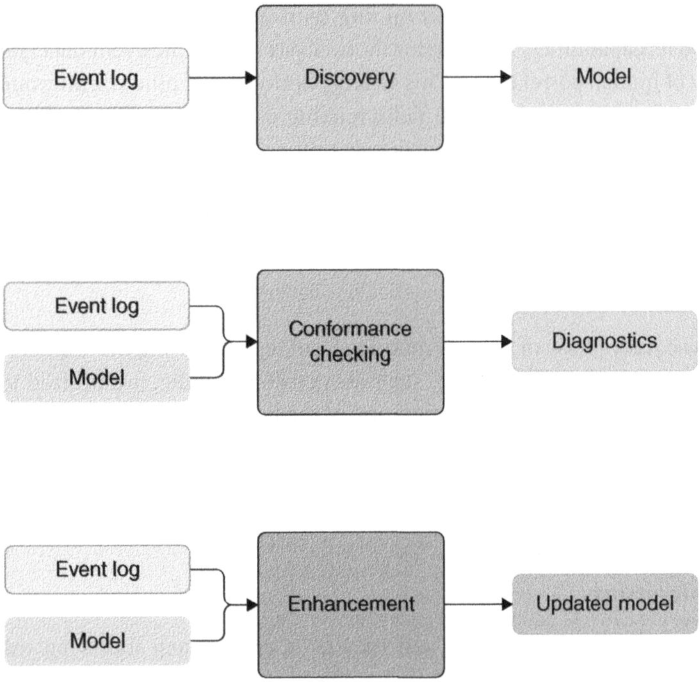

Figure 24.2 Steps in process mining [4].

24.3 Main Focus of the Chapter

In the contemporary digital era, the landscape of healthcare data management has undergone a profound transformation. With the advent of digital databases, the recording of patient files has become streamlined and efficient. This digitalization has not only facilitated the seamless storage of patient information but has also paved the way for a wealth of data to be harnessed for improving healthcare outcomes.

Within the vast expanse of hospital data lies a myriad of crucial elements, ranging from routine blood reports and entry-discharge times to intricate medical histories, allergies, and family backgrounds. Moreover, the repository encompasses a treasure trove of diagnostic tests such as X-rays, MRIs, CT scans, electrocardiograms (ECGs), and biopsies, alongside insurance details. Indeed, the breadth and depth of this data hold immense potential for enhancing patient care and operational efficiency.

Yet, the true power of this data transcends mere documentation. Through the conversion of these datasets into log files, wherein each step of the patient journey is carefully recorded, a digital twin of the patient emerges. This digital twin serves as a foundational cornerstone for the application of process mining-a methodology that delves deep into the intricacies of healthcare processes to unearth valuable insights.

By maintaining stringent privacy protocols, healthcare practitioners can leverage these data models to uncover patterns and trends, thus enabling informed decision-making and process optimization. These patterns not only offer granular insights into individual patient trajectories but also provide a broader understanding of healthcare delivery systems at large (Figure 24.3).

This chapter delves into an investigation of the hurdles faced when integrating process mining into the healthcare sector, alongside highlighting its numerous advantages. From navigating intricate regulatory landscapes to tapping into the vast potential of big data analytics, the path toward harnessing the transformative

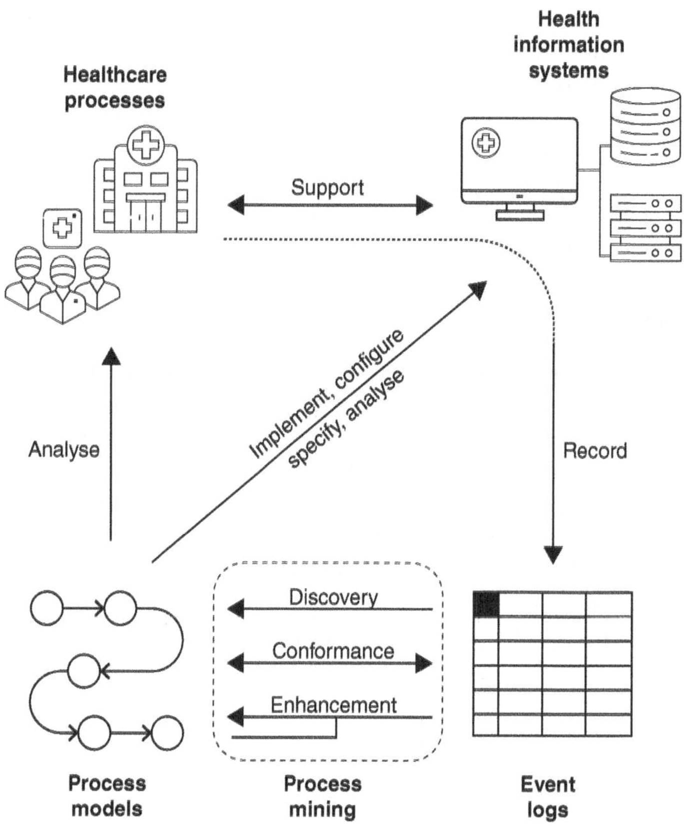

Figure 24.3 How process mining is implemented in healthcare? [5].

capabilities of process mining in healthcare is laden with challenges as well as opportunities.

24.4 Problems

While taking healthcare in picture we have divided the problems into two sects—**visible** and **invisible**.

24.4.1 Visible

Visible problems in the healthcare sector paint a stark picture of the challenges facing healthcare systems worldwide. Limited resources, poverty, create a tangible barrier to accessing and delivering essential care. Allocation of these resources is often swayed by social, economic, and political factors, further complicating equitable distribution. Government hospitals and healthcare centers, often in poor condition, struggle to meet the demands of burgeoning populations amidst environmental pollution and the lack of adequate health infrastructure [6]. Management issues plague the efficacy of healthcare delivery, compounded by insufficient medical research into emerging health threats such as antibiotic resistance and the health consequences of climate change. The rise in long-term conditions and a general lack of public awareness compound these visible problems, highlighting the urgent need for comprehensive solutions.

24.4.2 Invisible

Within the complex framework of the healthcare system lie invisible challenges that are equally consequential but often overlooked. The absence of standardized processes for healthcare services hampers efficiency and quality of care delivery [7]. Systematic patient journey management is lacking, leading to disjointed experiences for patients and inefficiencies in resource utilization. Specialized care units face unique demands that necessitate separate process models, yet the integration of these units into broader healthcare system remains a challenge. Addressing these invisible problems requires a paradigm shift toward comprehensive and integrated approaches to healthcare delivery, ensuring that every aspect of the patient experience is meticulously managed and optimized for better outcomes.

24.5 Solution

In this chapter, we are presenting a practically achievable method to resolve the m Process mining is particularly well-suited for the healthcare sector due to its inherent focus on operational business processes. Within healthcare, there are primarily two types of processes: **medical treatment processes** and **organizational processes**. Medical treatment processes encompass clinical activities which is directly involved in patient care, whereas organizational processes entail the broader activities necessary for the effective execution of medical treatment processes.

24.6 Tools

24.6.1 Software

Process mining software helps analyze, visualize, and improve how your business works. These tools use data collected by your computer systems to create a map of your processes [7, 8]. They then use clever algorithms to find patterns and areas for improvement.

24.6.1.1 Leading Process Mining Tools

- **Celonis:** A top provider, Celonis offers a toolbox for discovering, checking, and fixing your processes. Their platform uses artificial intelligence to analyze data and suggest ways to make things run smoother (Figure 24.4).
- **Disco:** Designed with ease of use in mind, Disco by Fluxicon makes process mining accessible. It lets you see how things flow, find where things go off track, and identify opportunities to improve (Figure 24.5).

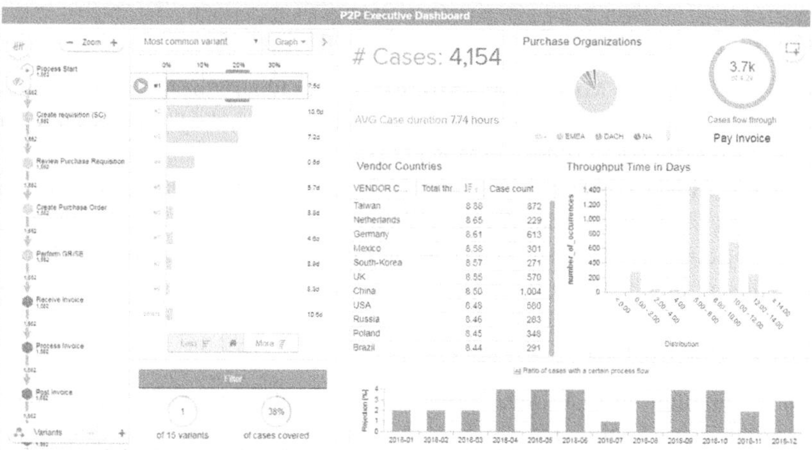

Figure 24.4 Celonis [9].

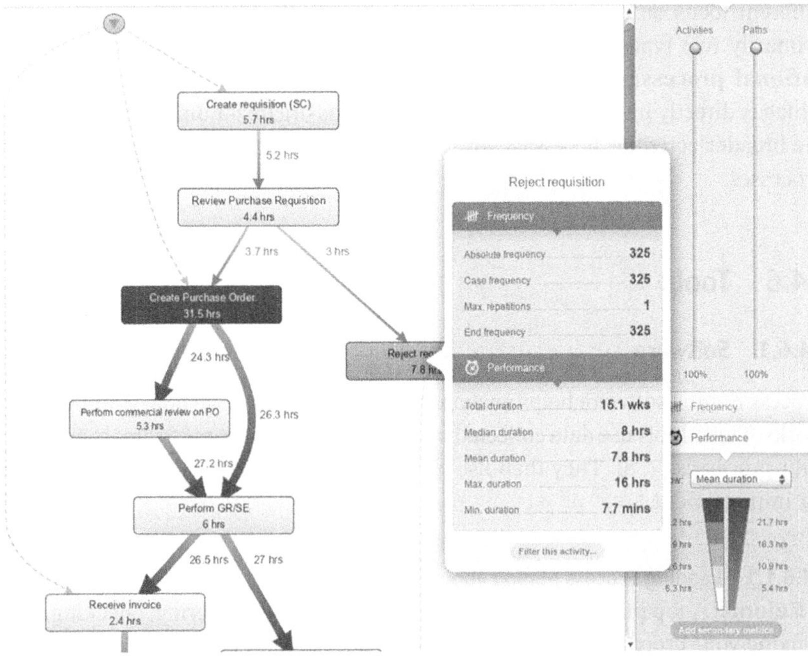

Figure 24.5 Disco [10].

- **ProM:** This free and open-source option from the Eindhoven University of Technology is a powerful toolkit for process mining. ProM offers a variety of tools for different tasks, giving advanced users more control (Figure 24.6).

24.6.2 Process Mining Powerhouses: Python Libraries

- **PM4Py (Process Mining for Python):** A go-to library for process mining in Python, PM4Py offers a wide range of algorithms, including popular ones like Heuristic Miner and Inductive Miner [12].
- **OCPA (Object-Centric Process Analysis):** As process mining evolves to focus on objects, OCPA steps in. This new library provides tools specifically designed for object-centric analysis, allowing you to explore your data from a different angle and gain deeper insights [13].

24.6.3 File Formats

Process mining relies on event logs stored in specific formats to analyze business processes. I order for a file to be called a log file we need three main columns—CaseID, Activity, Timestamp. Here's a breakdown of some common formats:

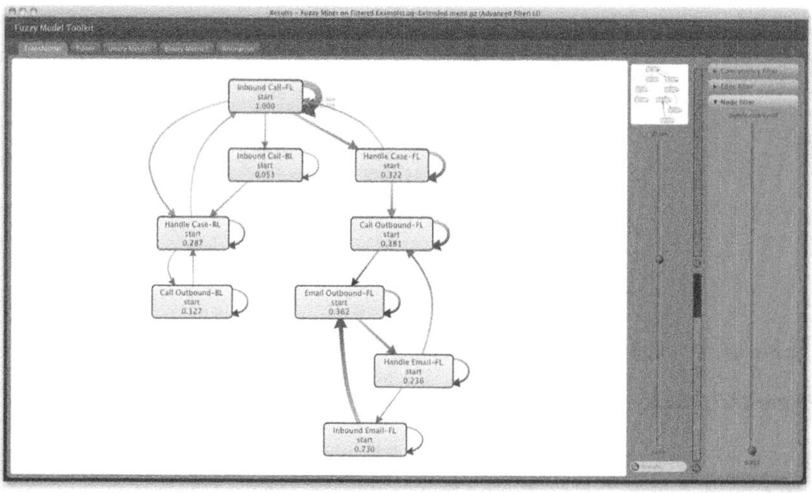

Figure 24.6 ProM [11].

- **Event Logs in XES Format:** The most widely used format, XES (eXtensible Event Stream), is the foundation for process mining. Its flexibility allows analysts to store a wide range of data, including event names, timestamps, case identifiers, and additional attributes. This richness enables exploring process data, uncovering hidden patterns, and identifying potential errors.
- **Event Logs in CSV Format:** While XES offers more features, CSV (comma-separated values) provides a simpler and easier-to-use alternative. Due to its widespread use and compatibility with many programs, CSV facilitates faster and more efficient data transfer during process mining analysis.
- **New Event Log Formats for Object-Centric Analysis:** As the focus in process mining shifts toward objects, new event log formats are emerging. These formats, such as JSON, XML, and SQLite, can store information specifically needed for object-centered analysis. This opens doors for novel discoveries and process improvements (Figure 24.7).

24.7 Ways Process Mining Solves Healthcare

24.7.1 Quality Improvement

Quality improvement is the cornerstone of effective healthcare. In this pursuit, process mining emerges as a powerful game-changer. By delving deep into the data trails of healthcare processes, organizations can uncover hidden inefficiencies,

patient	activity	timestamp	doctor	age	cost
5781	make X-ray	23-1-2014@10.30	Dr. Jones	45	70.00
5541	blood test	23-1-2014@10.18	Dr. Scott	61	40.00
5833	blood test	23-1-2014@10.27	Dr. Scott	24	40.00
5781	blood test	23-1-2014@10.49	Dr. Scott	45	40.00
5781	CT scan	23-1-2014@11.10	Dr. Fox	45	1200.00
5833	surgery	23-1-2014@12.34	Dr. Scott	24	2300.00
5781	handle payment	23-1-2014@12.41	Carol Hope	45	0.00
5541	radiation therapy	23-1-2014@13.57	Dr. Jones	61	140.00
5541	radiation therapy	23-1-2014@13.08	Dr. Jones	61	140.00
..	...			...	...

case id | activity name | timestamp | resource | other data

Figure 24.7 Basic structure of an event log [14].

deviations from established protocols, and errors that could potentially impact patient well-being. This newfound transparency empowers them to take targeted action [15, 16]. They can implement corrective measures to ensure better adherence to clinical guidelines, leading to a significant improvement in the quality and safety of healthcare delivery.

24.7.2 Identifying Redundant Steps

Efficiency is essential in healthcare. Every unnecessary step translates to delays in treatment, frustration for patients, and potential strain on resources. Process mining emerges as a powerful tool to identify and eliminate these inefficiencies.

By leveraging data from hospital information systems, process mining software like Celonis can transform raw information into a clear, visual representation of patient journeys. This unveils bottlenecks that impede patient flow, such as long wait times for approvals or delays in accessing diagnostic tests. Furthermore, it exposes redundancies that can be eliminated, like multiple layers of sign-off for routine procedures [17].

Equipped with these insights, hospitals can embark on data-driven process redesign. Redundant steps can be streamlined or eliminated, creating a smoother flow for patients. Process mining prioritizes areas for improvement, guiding resource allocation toward the most impactful changes. This continuous monitoring allows hospitals to iteratively enhance their process models, ensuring optimal patient care delivery.

24.7.3 Resource Allocation

Efficient resource allocation is a constant challenge in healthcare, where wasting vital supplies like medications can lead to stockouts, delays in treatment, and unnecessary costs. Process mining offers a groundbreaking solution to this problem by going beyond just analyzing past patient journeys. By delving into vast datasets, including EHRs, appointment logs, and medication databases, process mining can identify patterns and predict future needs. It can analyze historical "process chains," which map the typical steps in a specific treatment pathway. This predictive power allows hospitals to proactively allocate resources. For example, based on a patient's diagnosis and historical treatment patterns, medications can be prestaged or automatically ordered upon admission, eliminating the reactive scramble for supplies and the risk of delays due to stockouts [18].

The benefits extend beyond immediate patient care as process mining helps identify overused or underused medications, allowing for better inventory management and cost optimization. Healthcare institutions can leverage these insights to negotiate bulk purchasing discounts with suppliers, further reducing costs.

24.7.4 Predictive Analysis

Process mining becomes a game-changer in healthcare when combined with predictive analytics. By crunching historical data, it predicts future problems like patient readmissions, resource shortages, and equipment breakdowns. This goes beyond just looking back; it lets hospitals tackle issues before they even happen.

This foresight enables hospitals to strategically leverage predictive analytics in several impactful ways:

- **Reducing Readmissions:** By identifying high-risk patients, healthcare facilities can craft targeted care plans aimed at maintaining their well-being outside the hospital environment.
- **Optimizing Resources:** Anticipating surges in demand allows hospitals to ensure they are adequately stocked with the necessary supplies and equipment, thus enhancing operational efficiency.
- **Preventing Breakdowns:** Through predictive analytics, maintenance schedules for equipment can be arranged preemptively, mitigating the risk of disruptions in patient care due to equipment failures.

24.7.5 Bottlenecks

Identifying bottlenecks is crucial for efficient healthcare delivery. Process mining allows healthcare organizations to scrutinize the flow of patients, resources, and information through various processes. By visualizing these processes and pinpointing choke points, hospitals can eliminate inefficiencies that impede the system's smooth functioning. This proactive approach fosters a more streamlined and effective healthcare delivery system (Figure 24.8).

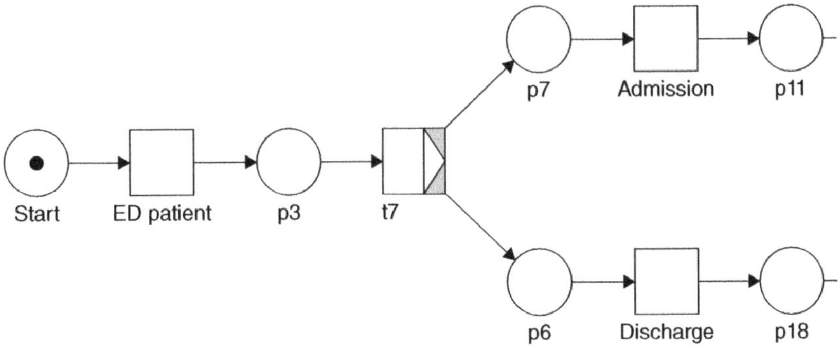

Figure 24.8 Process flow in hospitals [19].

24.8 One Solution: Robotic Process Automation (RPA)

Leveraging RPA alongside process mining techniques can significantly enhance efficiency in hospitals. Here's how RPA can be utilized [20]:

- **Data Extraction:** RPA bots can be programmed to extract data from various hospital systems and applications, including electronic health records (EHR), billing systems, and appointment scheduling software. This data can encompass patient information, treatment records, diagnostic reports, and billing details.
- **Event Log Generation:** RPA bots can automatically generate event logs based on activities performed within hospital systems. These logs capture timestamped information about each action taken, including task initiation and completion times, resource allocation, and interactions with different departments.
- **Process Discovery:** RPA can assist in discovering healthcare processes by continuously monitoring and recording the sequence of actions performed by healthcare staff and systems. By analyzing these logs using process mining techniques, hospitals can gain insights into the actual flow of activities, identify bottlenecks, and uncover variations in workflows.
- **Identifying Inefficiencies:** Process mining in conjunction with RPA can help identify inefficiencies and deviations from standard procedures in hospital workflows. By analyzing event logs, healthcare organizations can pinpoint areas where processes are slow, redundant, or prone to errors, enabling them to take corrective actions.
- **Automating Routine Tasks:** RPA bots can automate routine administrative tasks such as patient registration, appointment scheduling, and data entry. By automating these tasks, hospitals can free up staff time, reduce human errors, and ensure consistency in data entry and processing (Figure 24.9).

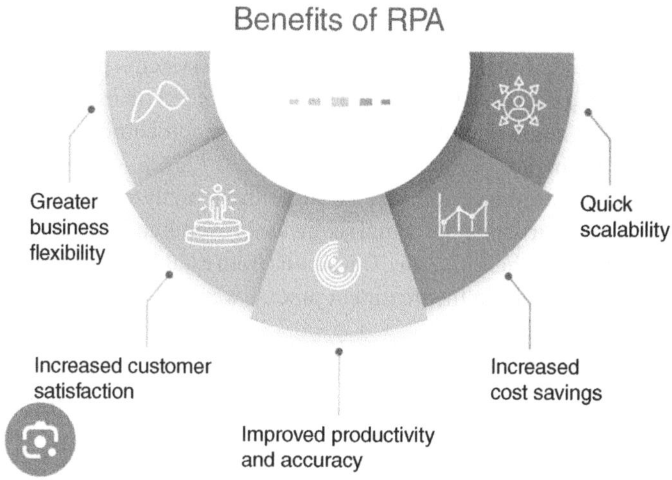

Figure 24.9 RPA [21].

- **Streamlining Billing and Claims Processing:** RPA can streamline billing and claims processing by automating tasks such as verifying insurance eligibility, coding diagnoses and procedures, and submitting claims to payers. This not only accelerates the revenue cycle but also reduces the likelihood of billing errors and denials.
- **Improving Patient Experience:** By automating administrative processes through RPA, hospitals can improve the overall patient experience. Patients may experience shorter wait times, smoother appointment scheduling, and faster access to medical services, leading to increased satisfaction and loyalty.
- **Enhancing Compliance and Audit Trails:** RPA can help ensure compliance with regulatory requirements and internal policies by enforcing standardized processes and generating detailed audit trails. This is particularly crucial in healthcare, where adherence to regulations such as HIPAA is essential for maintaining patient privacy and data security.

24.9 Case Study: Process Mining for Optimized COVID-19 ICU Care

The relentless surge of COVID-19 in 2021 demanded innovative approaches to patient care, particularly within the high-pressure environment of intensive care units (ICUs). Researchers at Uniklinik Aachen hospital in Germany leveraged the power of process mining to shed light on the intricacies of their COVID-19 ICU treatment process [22].

24.9.1 Methodology

- **Data Source:** Event data from the hospital's information systems provided a granular view of each patient's ICU journey. This data included timestamps for key events like patient admission, diagnostic tests, medication administration, ventilator use, and discharge.
- **Process Mining Techniques:** Sophisticated algorithms analyzed the event data, meticulously reconstructing the actual sequence of events each COVID-19 patient experienced during their ICU stay. Deviations from established protocols and potential bottlenecks within the treatment process were identified.

24.9.2 Key Findings and Impact

The process mining analysis yielded a treasure trove of insights (Figure 24.10):

- **Areas for Improvement:** The analysis revealed potential areas for streamlining the ICU treatment process for patients with COVID-19. This could involve optimizing medication administration schedules, reducing wait times for critical tests, and ensuring smoother transitions between different care stages [23, 24].
- **Bottleneck Identification:** Bottlenecks within the ICU treatment process were identified, such as delays in accessing specialized equipment or limited staffing during peak admission periods. Addressing these bottlenecks can significantly improve the efficiency of ICU care [25, 26].
- **Resource Allocation Optimization:** By understanding resource utilization patterns within the ICU, the study provided valuable data for optimizing resource allocation. This could involve ensuring the availability of critical equipment at the right time and making staffing adjustments based on patient acuity levels.
- **Standardized Protocols:** The analysis facilitated the development and implementation of standardized protocols for COVID-19 ICU care. This not only ensures consistency in treatment delivery but also helps in establishing best practices based on real-world data [27–29].

24.9.3 The Broader Significance

The Uniklinik Aachen study serves as a compelling example of how process mining can revolutionize ICU care for patients with COVID-19. By identifying bottlenecks, analyzing real-world treatment sequences, and providing insights for optimizing resource allocation and treatment protocols, process mining has the potential to:

- **Improved Patient Outcomes:** Streamlined processes, efficient resource utilization, and standardized protocols can all contribute to improved patient outcomes, potentially reducing ICU length of stay and mortality rates.

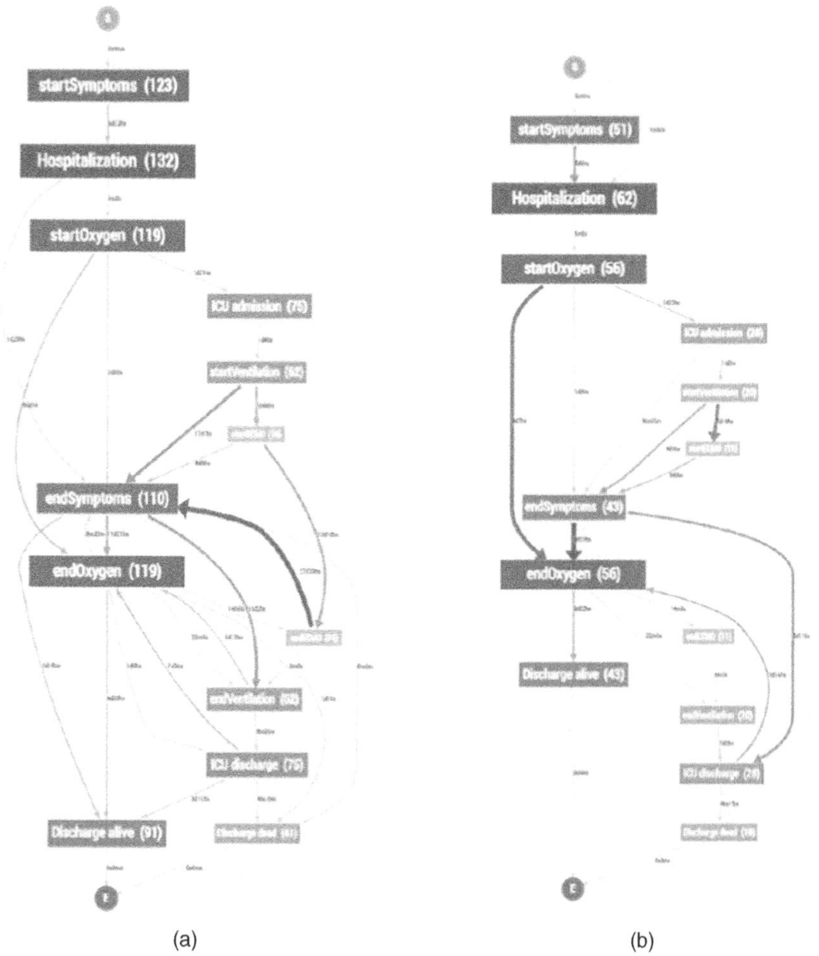

Figure 24.10 (a) Filtered directly follows graph related to the first wave of the COVID pandemic. (b) Filtered directly follows graph related to the second wave of the COVID pandemic.

- **Save Lives:** By ensuring timely access to critical care and optimizing treatment delivery, process mining can play a crucial role in saving lives during a pandemic.
- **Enhanced Decision-Making:** The data-driven insights gained from process mining empower healthcare administrators and clinicians to make informed decisions regarding resource allocation, staffing levels, and protocol development.

24.9.4 Challenges and Considerations

While process mining offers immense potential, it's important to acknowledge the challenges.

- **Data Quality:** The success of process mining hinges on the quality and completeness of the data within hospital information systems. Ensuring data accuracy is paramount.
- **Expertise Required:** Implementing and interpreting process mining analyses requires specialized skills and training for healthcare professionals. Collaboration with data scientists can bridge this gap.

24.9.5 Conclusion of Case Study

The Uniklinik Aachen study paves the way for utilizing process mining as a powerful tool to optimize ICU care for patients with COVID-19 and potentially other critical illnesses. By harnessing the power of data analysis, healthcare institutions can strive for continuous improvement in patient care delivery, ultimately saving lives and fostering a more efficient healthcare ecosystem.

24.10 Conclusion

The integration of process mining techniques into healthcare systems presents a transformative opportunity to revolutionize patient care delivery. By leveraging data analytics and process science, healthcare organizations can gain invaluable insights into their operations, identify areas for improvement, and optimize resource allocation. Through the discovery, conformance checking, and enhancement phases of process mining, hospitals can streamline workflows, eliminate redundancies, and enhance overall efficiency.

However, navigating regulatory landscapes and addressing hidden problems within healthcare systems pose challenges on this path to enhanced efficiency. Yet, with perseverance and innovation, these challenges can be transformed into opportunities for growth and improvement.

Furthermore, the integration of RPA with process mining offers a promising solution to enhance operational efficiency in healthcare. RPA can complement process mining efforts and drive tangible improvements in healthcare delivery by automating routine tasks, streamlining billing processes, and improving the overall patient experience.

In the pursuit of efficiency and precision in healthcare, process mining emerges as a powerful ally. By embracing this methodology alongside innovative technologies like RPA, healthcare organizations can navigate the complexities of modern healthcare delivery and ensure the highest standards of patient care. As we continue to harness the potential of process mining, we pave the way for a future where healthcare is not just efficient, but also patient-centric and truly transformative.

References

1 De Roock, E. and Martin, N. (2022). Process mining in healthcare–an updated perspective on the state of the art. *Journal of Biomedical Informatics* 127: 103995.

2 dos Santos Garcia, C., Meincheim, A., Junior, E.R.F. et al. (2019). Process mining techniques and applications–a systematic mapping study. *Expert Systems with Applications* 133: 260–295.

3 Geyer-Klingeberg, J., Nakladal, J., Baldauf, F., and Veit, F. (2018). Process mining and robotic process automation: a perfect match. *BPM (Dissertation/Demos/Industry)* 2196: 124–131.

4 Guo, C. and Chen, J. (2023). Big data analytics in healthcare. In: *Knowledge Technology and Systems: Toward Establishing Knowledge Systems Science*, 27–70. Springer.

5 Kaymak, U., Mans, R., van de Steeg, T., and Dierks, M. (2012). On process mining in health care. *2012 IEEE International Conference on Systems, Man, and Cybernetics (SMC)*, 1859–1864. IEEE.

6 Leno, V., Polyvyanyy, A., Dumas, M. et al. (2021). Robotic process mining: vision and challenges. *Business & Information Systems Engineering* 63: 301–314.

7 Mannhardt, F. (2018). Multi-perspective Process Mining.

8 Park, K., Cho, M., Song, M. et al. (2023). Exploring the potential of OMOP common data model for process mining in healthcare. *PLoS One* 18 (1): e0279641.

9 Pegoraro, M., Shankar, M., Benevento, E. et al. (2021). Analyzing medical data with process mining: a COVID-19 case study. *International Conference on Business Information Systems*, 39–44. Cham: Springer International Publishing.

10 Pika, A., Wynn, M.T., Budiono, S. et al. (2020). Privacy-preserving process mining in healthcare. *International Journal of Environmental Research and Public Health* 17 (5): 1612.

11 Pozharski, V. (2022). Streamlining operations: leveraging process mining for business enhancement. LinkedIn.

12 Pufahl, L., Zerbato, F., Weber, B., and Weber, I. (2022). BPMN in healthcare: challenges and best practices. *Information Systems* 107: 102013.

13 Rebuge, Á. and Ferreira, D.R. (2012). Business process analysis in healthcare environments: a methodology based on process mining. *Information Systems* 37 (2): 99–116.

14 Rojas, E., Munoz-Gama, J., Sepúlveda, M., and Capurro, D. (2016). Process mining in healthcare: a literature review. *Journal of Biomedical Informatics* 61: 224–236.

15 Rovani, M., Maggi, F.M., de Leoni, M., and van der Aalst, W.M.P. (2015). Declarative process mining in healthcare. *Expert Systems with Applications* 42 (23): 9236–9251.

16 Song, M., Günther, C.W., and van der Aalst, W.M.P. (2009). Trace clustering in process mining. *Business Process Management Workshops: BPM 2008 International Workshops*, Milano, Italy (1–4 September 2008). Revised Papers 6, 109–120. Berlin Heidelberg: Springer-Verlag.
17 EdgeVerve Systems (2022). Enhancing healthcare services through process mining. EdgeVerve Systems.
18 EdgeVerve Systems (2022). Process mining in healthcare - 5 winning initiatives to enhance patients' experiences. *Studies in Health Technology and Informatics* 332: 101–107.
19 Turner, C.J., Tiwari, A., Olaiya, R., and Xu, Y. (2012). Process mining: from theory to practice. *Business Process Management Journal* 18 (3): 493–512.
20 van der Aalst, W. (2012). Process mining: making knowledge discovery process centric. *ACM SIGKDD Explorations Newsletter* 13 (2): 45–49.
21 van der Aalst, W. (2012). Process mining: overview and opportunities. *ACM Transactions on Management Information Systems (TMIS)* 3 (2): 1–17.
22 van der Aalst, W. (2012). Service mining: using process mining to discover, check, and improve service behavior. *IEEE Transactions on Services Computing* 6 (4): 525–535.
23 van der Aalst, W. (2021). 12 Process mining and RPA. In: *Robotic Process Automation*, 223–240. De Gruyter Oldenbourg.
24 van der Aalst, W., Adriansyah, A., De Medeiros, A.K.A. et al. (2012). Process mining manifesto. *Business Process Management Workshops: BPM 2011 International Workshops*, Clermont-Ferrand, France (29 August 2011), Revised Selected Papers, Part I 9, 169–194. Springer.
25 van der Aalst, W.M.P. (2011). Using process mining to bridge the gap between BI and BPM. *Computer* 44 (12): 77–80.
26 van der Aalst, W.M.P. and Weijters, A.J.M.M. (2004). Process mining: a research agenda. *Computers in Industry* 53 (3): 231–244.
27 van Dongen, B.F., de Medeiros, A.K.A., Verbeek, H.M.W. et al. (2005). The prom framework: a new era in process mining tool support. *Applications and Theory of Petri Nets 2005: 26th International Conference*, ICATPN 2005, Miami, USA (20–25 June 2005). *Proceedings 26*, 444–454. Springer.
28 Weijters, A.J.M.M., van Der Aalst, W.M.P., and De Medeiros, A.K.A. (2006). Process mining with the HeuristicsMiner algorithm. (BETA publicatie: working papers; Vol. 166). Technische Universiteit Eindhoven.
29 Yang, W.-S. and Hwang, S.-Y. (2006). A process-mining framework for the detection of healthcare fraud and abuse. *Expert Systems with Applications* 31 (1): 56–68.

25

Transform Drug Discovery and Development With Generative Artificial Intelligence

Antonio Lavecchia

"Drug Discovery" Laboratory, Department of Pharmacy, University of Naples Federico II, Naples, Italy

25.1 Introduction

Drug discovery, a notoriously expensive and time-consuming process, is hindered by low success rates. On average, the development of a new drug incurs a staggering cost of $2.6 billion [129] and may extend beyond a decade. The probability of successfully bringing a drug to market from Phase I clinical trials is dishearteningly low, standing at less than 10% [36]. The formidable challenges in drug discovery arise from the expansive and discrete search space of chemical molecules. Specifically, the potential structures of drug-like compounds range between 10^{23} and 10^{60}, yet only a small fraction, approximately 10^{8}, holds therapeutic relevance ([167]). Conventional methods like high-throughput screening ([20]) prove inefficient due to an imbalance between the required resources and the limited number of hit compounds.

Traditional machine learning (ML) models played a pivotal role in virtual screening (VS) [98], addressing crucial tasks like predicting physico-chemical properties [169], drug-likeness [207], pharmacokinetic parameters [199], and pharmacodynamic properties [154]. These include probability-based classification models such as random forest (RF), logistic regression (LR), and Naive Bayes (NB), and score-based classification models like K-nearest neighbors (KNN) and support vector machines (SVM) [98]. Despite the successes of traditional ML models, deep neural networks (DNNs) have consistently outperformed them across a spectrum of tasks [122], paving the way for a paradigm shift in pharmaceutical science. Figure 25.1 showcases some of the pertinent applications in this domain.

Deep learning (DL), having proven successful in natural language processing (NLP) [69], computer vision ([109]), and diverse fields [175], has become a focal point in drug discovery [99]. DNNs, categorized into discriminative and

Generative Artificial Intelligence for Biomedical and Smart Health Informatics,
First Edition. Edited by Aditya Khamparia and Deepak Gupta.

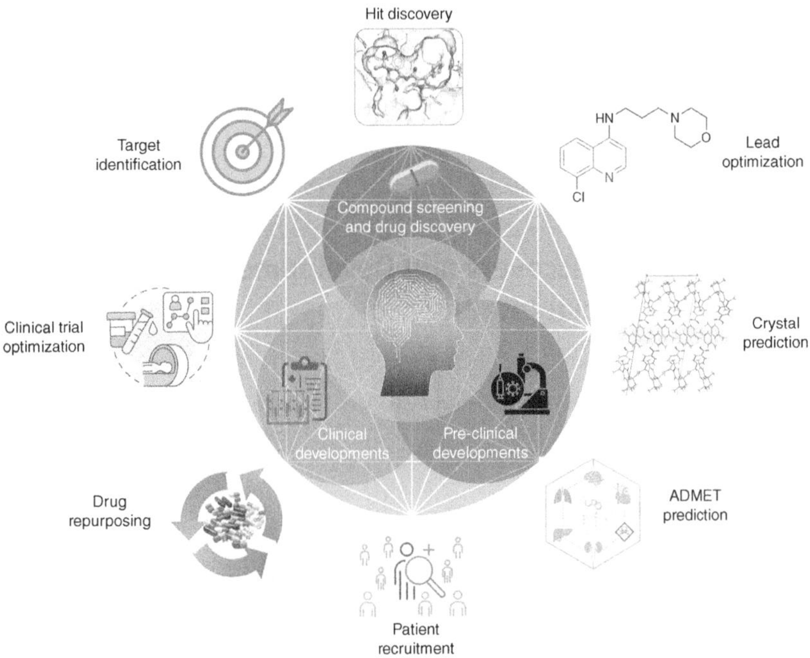

Figure 25.1 The multifaceted applications of AI-based methods in drug discovery and development encompass a broad spectrum of innovative techniques and technologies revolutionizing the pharmaceutical landscape.

generative models, offer distinct functionalities. Discriminative models aim to optimize classification by highlighting differences in heterogeneous data [99]. On the other hand, generative models, representing prior probabilities, indicate the similarity of congener data.

Deep generative models (DGMs) have seen rapid development in creating synthetic data, spanning text, images, and video. The analogy between molecular representations in silico and NLP texts or social network graphs has led to the extension of such models for de novo molecular design in drug discovery [19, 158]. Unlike discriminative models that screen databases and classify molecules as active or inactive, DGMs design new molecules with specific properties from scratch. The desire for automated molecule generation has been acknowledged in previous works [56] leading to a surge in DGMs dedicated to enhancing de novo molecular design. Two prevalent strategies have dominated this domain based on in silico molecular representations: sequence representation using a simplified molecular input line entry system (SMILES) [211] and graph-based representation ([220]). SMILES-based models leverage DGMs and text to generate molecular structures, while graph-based models encode molecular information into graphs, learning to aggregate features such as bond features and atoms.

This review centers on DGMs applied to molecular property prediction and molecule generation in drug discovery. It covers key aspects, including common data resources, molecular representation methods, and established benchmark platforms. Building on this foundational information, various related techniques are elaborated upon, including model architectures and learning paradigms. In addition, clinical-level assets produced by generative AI are explored, showcasing the increasing application of AI in drug discovery and development. Finally, challenges observed in the field are addressed to encourage new research initiatives and highlight potential future directions.

25.2 Dataset, Molecular Representation, and Benchmark Platforms in Molecular Generation

25.2.1 Public Data Resources

The foundational cornerstone of a DL-driven campaign lies in the quantity and quality of data, particularly molecular and biological data essential for developing generative chemistry models. Recently, there has been a significant surge in both the volume and scale of databases containing information on potential drug compounds. However, not all these databases are specifically tailored for substantial contributions to drug discovery and development. The extensive data available for DL-driven drug development can be categorized in various ways, encompassing databases of drugs, drug-like molecules, receptors, and ADMET data, among others. These databases collectively provide multidimensional information on drug candidates, including chemical structure, physico-chemical properties, and in vitro, in vivo, and clinical data. Categorized based on their application and relevance throughout different stages of drug discovery and development, these databases, whether public or private, fall into seven main categories: (i) comprehensive databases of chemical collections such as ChEMBL [51], PubChem [86], Zinc 15 [187], and Enamine REAL Database [89]; (ii) chemical databases tailored for drug/drug-like compounds, including DrugBank [213], AICD ([208]), and e-Drug3D [35]; (iii) collections of drug targets with genomics and proteomics data, like BindingDB [53], PDBbind ([113]), SuperTarget [62], and Ligand Depot [45]; (iv) databases storing biological data from assay screening, metabolism, and efficacy studies, such as HMDB [214], TTD [238], WOMBAT [133], and PKPB_DB [197]; (v) Information on drug liabilities and toxicities, seen in DrugMatrix [194], SIDER [94], OFFSIDES, TWO-SIDES, and LTKB Benchmark Dataset ([23]); and (vi) clinical databases including ClinicalTrials.gov [232], EORTC Clinical Trials Database (www.eortc.org/clinical-trials-database/), DILIrank ([22]), and PharmGKB [198]. Table 25.1 provides a list of commonly used databases documenting chemical and biological information.

Table 25.1 Illustrated cheminformatics databases available for drug discovery.

Datasets	Cpds	Description	Link	References
ZINC 15	750M	A free virtual scanning dataset of commercial compounds	http://Zinc15.docking.org/	[187]
ChEMBL	2M	Manage and edit biologically active molecules with drug-like properties	http://Zinc15.docking.org/	[51]
PubChem	115M	Unique structures with the largest and free chemical information	https://pubchem.ncbi.nlm.nih.gov/	[86]
DrugBank	16k	Information about drugs, drug targets, indications, etc.	https://www.drugbank.ca/	[213]
PDBbind	17k	Experimentally measured binding affinity data for PDB	http://www.pdbbind.org.cn/	[113]
Enamine Real Database	1.95B	A vendor to provide chemicals	https://enamine.net	[89]
QM9	134k	Small organic molecules with a maximum of nine atoms in four different types	https://doi.org/10.6084/m9.figshare.978904	[161]
ExCAPE-DB	1M	Aggregate PubChem and ChEMBL	https://solr.ideaconsult.net/search/excape/	[191]
GDB-13	977.5M	Chemical universe database	http://gdb.unibe.ch/downloads/	[13]
GDB-17	166.4B	Chemical universe database	http://gdb.unibe.ch/downloads/	[160]
MEGx	>4200	Natural products from plants and microorganisms	http://mb3is.megx.net	
MOSES	2M	A benchmarking dataset	https://github.com/molecularsets/moses	[140]
CEPDB	2.3M	The Harvard Clean Energy Project Database	http://cepdb.molecularspace.org	[114]

Table 25.1 (Continued)

Datasets	Cpds	Description	Link	References
L1000	3.7k	Contains mainly induced gene expression profiles	https://clue.io/	[190]
DUD-E	22k	Verified active compounds interacting with specific target proteins and carefully chosen decoys—inactive compounds with similar properties.	http://dude.docking.org/	[130]
MUV	1360	Contains 17 target proteins, with 30 active and 15,000 inactive molecules each, for testing various biological scenarios.	https://www.tu-braunschweig.de/pharmchem/forschung/baumann/muv	[157]
STITCH	430k	Stores data on how proteins and compounds interact, collected from predictions, databases like PubChem, and literature.	http://stitch.embl.de/	[195]
KEGG	19k	Provides multiple types of information centered on genes and genomes.	https://www.kegg.jp/	[82]

25.2.2 Molecular Representations

Chemical structures offer a myriad of representations, each pivotal in constructing datasets for developing predictive models. In addition to traditional Kekulé diagrams (Figure 25.2a), a variety of molecular descriptors capture varying levels of molecular information [200]. These descriptors fall into three categories: one-dimensional (1D), two-dimensional (2D), and three-dimensional (3D), categorized based on the molecular representations used to derive them [155]. 1D descriptors, including atom number, atom type count, and molecular weight, rely on the molecular formula. 2D descriptors derive from 2D structure representations like molecular graphs and connection tables, encompassing topological descriptors and computed descriptors that approximate molecular

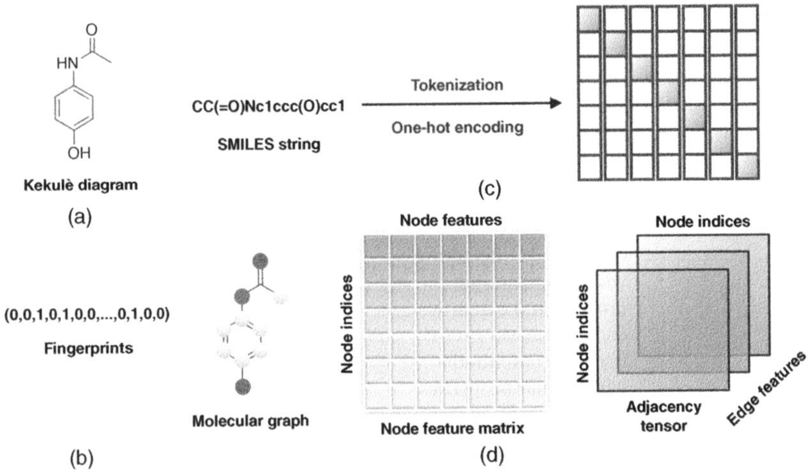

Figure 25.2 Different formats of small molecule representations include Kekulè Diagrams (a), Fingerprints (b), SMILES Strings (convertible to One-Hot Encoding) (c), and Molecular Graphs (d) constructed from adjacency, node, and feature matrices.

properties such as lipophilicity (e.g., Log *P*). 3D descriptors, derived from 3D molecular conformations, represent properties like molecular surface, shape, and volume.

Fingerprints (Figure 25.2b), popular bitstring representations, capture both structural features and physico-chemical properties. In binary fingerprints, each bit encodes the presence (1) or absence (0) of a specific feature. Descriptors include 1D representations for substituent atoms, chemical bonds, structural fragments, and functional groups, alongside 2D descriptors representing atom connectivity and molecular topology. Examples include keyed fingerprints (MACCS keys), path-based fingerprints (Day Light fingerprints), and circular fingerprints (ECFPs based on the Morgan algorithm) [127]. 3D descriptors encode structural information like steric properties, surface area, volume, and binding site properties.

Molecular descriptors, though vital in computational methods for drug discovery ([231]), are static and nonadaptive for improving model performance. The AI era has introduced various DL models, enabling end-to-end predictions by embedding molecules into a continuous latent space without handcrafted rules. Notably, two major representation formats in this context are SMILES strings and molecular graphs. SMILES notation (Figure 25.2c), utilizing ASCII strings, succinctly describes chemical structures and can be converted into a one-hot encoding or word embedding for ML and NLP methods. Each atom in SMILES is represented by a letter (e.g., C for carbon, N for nitrogen, and O for oxygen), with uppercase for aliphatic and lowercase for aromatic environments. Implicit single bonds, double bonds represented by "=," and triple bonds by "#." Rings are labeled by joining atoms, and sidechains are enclosed in brackets. Grammar rules within the SMILES language define a unique representation for any molecule. The SMILES sequence can be converted into a one-hot matrix, where columns correspond to positions in the SMILES sequence, rows denote token types in SMILES language, and matrix elements are binary values indicating token presence. This one-hot matrix serves as input for various neural network architectures used in structural generation. It's noteworthy that one molecule may correspond to multiple SMILES strings [31], necessitating canonicalization methods [211] to designate a unique SMILES string for each molecule. The conversion of molecular structure to text in SMILES facilitates computer processing, offering convenience for chemists and serving as an ideal input for training ML models [39]. To overcome the validity limitations of SMILES, alternative text representations have been proposed, including Deep SMILES [132] and SELFIES [92]. These approaches aim to streamline the generation of valid strings and provide a more robust pathway for mapping to small molecules, eliminating the necessity to learn intricate details of SMILES syntax.

Graph-based representations provide graphical expressions of molecular structural connectivity, with atoms as nodes and intramolecular bonds as edges (Figure 25.2d). Each molecule is represented as an undirected graph G, with nodes (atoms) and edges (bonds). Atom types and bond types are encoded into T-dimensional one-hot vectors and represented as $y \in \{1, \ldots, Y\}$, respectively. Molecular graphs offer valuable information on connectivity, substructures, symmetry, and functional groups, aiding in predicting molecular properties (e.g., toxicity, solubility) or explaining their origins (e.g., alert structures). To be processed by ML models, a molecule is transformed into a node matrix, an adjacency matrix indicating connections among atoms. Graph-based neural networks use additional matrices for node and edge attributes to enhance learning efficiency. Edge attribute matrices provide information on bond types, while node attribute matrices include molecular characteristics (e.g., element, orbital hybridization, charge status). Various graph-based DL architectures, such as ECFP [156] and graph-embedding features [43], fully exploit the potential of molecular graphs. Graph representations excel in carrying more structural information and direct mapping to chemical substructures, making them highly interpretable ([78]). However, a drawback is the significant disk space and memory requirements during computation, potentially impacting efficiency in molecule generation [31].

After collecting and vectorizing data, the process advances to chemical data analysis and the implementation of DL-based applications. Cheminformatics tools like the Chemistry Development Kit (CDK) or the open-source toolkit RDKit facilitate chemical data analysis either directly from databases or derived from SMILES.

Numerous open-source DL frameworks and popular higher-level Application Programming Interfaces (API) support the quick training of DNNs with billions of parameters. Table 25.2 illustrates examples of frequently considered cheminformatics toolkits and ML packages.

25.2.3 Benchmark Datasets and Tools

Evaluation of automated chemical structure generation and molecular property prediction relies on standard benchmark packages Despite the use of various open-source chemoinformatics datasets for model evaluation and comparison, their impact on DL method development remains limited due to small dataset sizes, limited options for splitting training and testing sets, and the absence of a standardized assessment platform [191]. In addition, these datasets often include both active and inactive molecules, where the status of inactivity is provisional until validated through biological tests [71]. To address these limitations, benchmarking datasets like the Directory of Useful Decoys-Enhanced (DUD-E), aim to provide refined decoy compounds that prevent false negatives in prediction techniques [151]. They also strive to maintain physico-chemical equivalence to known ligands [130]. However, concerns about hidden biases in DUD-E ([21]) have led to the development of Maximum Unbiased Validation (MUV), datasets [157], and Demanding Evaluation Kits for Objective In Silico Screening (DEKOIS) [7]. These datasets address limitations in decoy exploration and challenges posed by artificially high enrichment during an assessment. Researchers have additionally created Unbiased Ligand Sets (ULS) and Unbiased Decoy Sets (UDS) for specific targets, such as G protein-coupled receptors (GPCRs) ([219]). Novel datasets like LIT–PCBA, designed with an asymmetric validation embedding approach for PubChem bioassays, have also been introduced [201]. Common parameters used to assess DGMs are outlined in Table 25.3, with a focus on evaluating how well these models navigate chemical space, conduct focused searches, and leverage available information.

MoleculeNet, inspired by pioneering work like WordNet and ImageNet, includes quantum mechanics (QM7, QM7b, QM8, QM9), physico-chemical chemistry (ESOL, FreeSolv, and Lipophilicity), biophysics (PCBA, MUV, HIV, PDDBind, BACE), and physiological (BBBP, Tox21, ToxCast, SIDER, ClinTox) datasets [218] offering convenient access to DL algorithms through the open-source DeepChem package (https://deepchem.io). Notably, MoleculeNet addresses imbalanced datasets in molecular property prediction by considering positive rates when selecting evaluation metrics, such as favoring the area under the precision-recall curve (AUPRC) over the area under the receiver operating characteristic curve (AUROC) in cases of low-positive rates [218]. It also offers various splitting methods, including scaffold split, stratified split, and time split

Table 25.2 Commonly used cheminformatics tools and ML packages.

Name	Description	Link	References
CDK	A collection of Java libraries for handling cheminformatics.	https://cdk.github.io/	[185]
RDKit	A free software, offering tools like descriptor creation, molecular database functions, and operations in various dimensions.	https://www.rdkit.org/	
PyTorch	A Python package offering rapid GPU support for tensor computation and DNN via an autograd system.	https://pytorch.org/	[186]
TensorFlow	An open-source platform for ML with a wide range of tools, libraries, and community support.	https://www.tensorflow.org/	[1]
CNTK	An open-source high-level DL framework using directed graphs to show NN computations.	https://github.com/Microsoft/CNTK/	[41]
Keras	An open-source Python neural network library compatible with TensorFlow, Microsoft Cognitive Toolkit, Theano, and PlaidML.	https://keras.io/	
Scikit-Learn	An efficient data prediction tool crafted with NumPy, SciPy, and matplotlib.	https://scikit-learn.org/stable/	[137]
Theano	A Python library for defining, optimizing, and evaluating math equations.	http://deeplearning.net/software/theano/	[2]
KNIME	A user-friendly software for creating and deploying data science projects, enabling stakeholders to focus on their strengths.	https://www.knime.com/	[9]

Table 25.3 Some common parameters in use to assess DGMs.

Type	Assessment parameters
Molecule Set	Validity
	Novelty
	Uniqueness
	Controllability
	Nearest neighbor similarity
	Scaffold similarity
	Internal diversity
	Fragment similarity
	Fréchet ChemNet Distance [144]
	Completeness, Uniformity, Closedness [5]
Molecules	Physicochemical property
	Synthetic accessibility score (SA score)
	Natural product likeness score
	QED
	Jointly score ([225])
Integrated Benchmark	GuacaMol [16]
	MOSES [140]

for different datasets. However, MoleculeNet's limitation lies in the absence of explicit training, validation, and test folds for datasets [42], prompting the release of the ChemBench package from MolMapNet for improved reproducibility [174]. MolMapNet expands MoleculeNet by adding pharmacokinetics-related datasets, including PubChem CYP inhibition and liver microsomal clearance data. Another benchmarking tool, Chemprop, was proposed for benchmarking learned molecular representations, systematically comparing fixed molecular descriptors with learned molecular representations across 19 public and 16 proprietary industrial datasets ([224]).

In the context of molecule generation models, both REINVENT and its updated version, REINVENT 2.0, utilize SMILES strings for sequence-based generative modeling [11, 134]. Another model, GraphINVENT, proposed by Mercado et al. in 2020 [124], focuses on benchmarking the generation of molecules using molecular graphs. To standardize molecule generation assessment, GuacaMol [16] employs diverse tests for correctness, originality, and variety, including goal-directed techniques to evaluate the precision of DGMs in targeting chemical space The MOSES benchmark [140] offers distribution learning tasks that assess molecular validity, uniqueness, and diversity by linking the generated chemical space with known molecular frameworks. Fréchet ChemNet Distance (FCD) sheds light on how well the generated molecules align with a target distribution, revealing potential biases [144]. A lower FCD value indicates similar distributions of molecules. The Coverage Score [216] quantifies the model's ability to sample from larger datasets. The #Circles Metric [221] takes a comprehensive approach, assessing structural diversity between chemical sets and the impact of introducing new molecules to the sampling range. Kullback–Leibler (KL) divergence measures the difference between probability distributions, indicating how well-generated molecules approximate the targeted property in the training set [28]. Models for goal-directed design receive scores based on predefined criteria, such as containing specific substructures, presenting certain physico-chemical properties, or exhibiting similarity or dissimilarity to certain molecules. Evaluation metrics like similarity and rediscovery gauge the model's proficiency in generating molecules that are similar or dissimilar to given ones. Finally, to assess the real-world synthesizability of generated molecular structures, Gao and Coley introduced an approach using retrosynthetic analysis tools [49].

25.3 Deep Generative Model Architectures

25.3.1 Recurrent Neural Networks

Recurrent neural networks (RNNs) are pivotal for processing sequential data [99, 100], originally designed for signal and NLP. Their applicability extends to molecular property prediction and molecule generation (Figure 25.3), using SMILES strings as input [74]. The RNN iteratively receives a vector of numbers and a hidden state matrix containing information from previous steps, producing output vectors and updated hidden state matrices for subsequent iterations until all input sequences are processed. However, the long-term dependency of RNNs poses challenges in parameter learning due to the gradient explosion or vanishing problem [99, 100]. To mitigate this, variants like long short-term memory (LSTM) [64] and gated recurrent unit (GRU) [27] include a memory module for enhanced network capabilities.

In molecular property prediction, RNNs generate a final output after processing all steps. SmilesLSTM [122] excels in drug–target interaction (DTI) prediction, outperforming traditional ML models. In addition, SMILES2Vec [54] utilizes RNNs to learn features from SMILES and predict various chemical properties. RNNs also contribute to molecule generation, functioning akin to language models for text generation [134, 173]. Output is generated at each step in an autoregressive manner, dependent on input from previous steps. This involves producing a probability

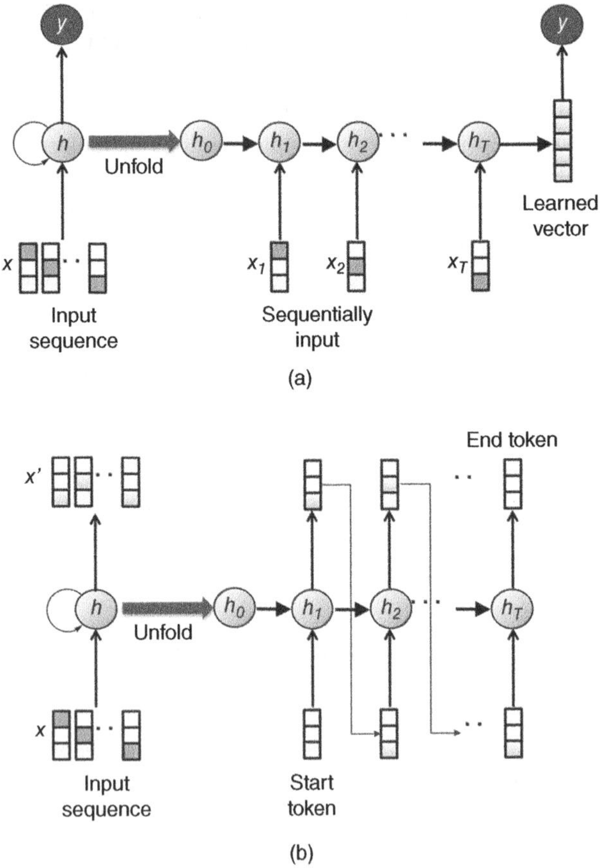

Figure 25.3 Depiction of RNNs in prediction mode (a) and generation mode (b).

distribution over possible tokens based on current and prior steps, with a token sampled as the current step's output and used to predict the next token. However, regular RNNs struggle to capture algorithmic patterns in the "SMILES language," resulting in invalid strings due to syntax complexities. Memory-augmented versions like Stack-RNN [142], and bidirectional RNNs like bidirectional LSTM [183, 235] address this issue.

Beyond string-based molecule production, RNNs contribute to developing graph-based DGMs. GraphNet ([105]), using a message-passing neural network (MPNN), generates molecules by adding atoms or bonds based on computed probabilities. MolMP and MolRNN, akin to GraphNet, enhance diversity by incorporating constraints as auxiliary information. GraphRNN [228], a hierarchical RNN-based model, estimates joint probability at both graph and edge levels, constructing molecular structures using adjacency vectors. MolecularRNN

[143], a modification of GraphRNN, ensures output molecule validity through valency-based rejection sampling.

Importantly, RNNs are integral components in other DNN architectures, functioning as generators in generative adversarial networks (GANs) [163] or autoencoder (AE)-based GANs [12, 141]. In addition, RNN-learned hidden states provide the foundation for encoding molecules in a latent space within variational AEs (VAEs) [10, 56].

25.3.2 Convolutional Neural Networks

Originally designed for image recognition, CNNs have demonstrated remarkable performance in major artificial vision competitions [100], thanks to their parameterized convolution implementation. These architectures employ 2D or 3D kernels, enabling pattern recognition across various scales and locations in the input. By replacing fully connected layers with small kernels, CNNs share weights among units from the previous layer, reducing parameters and preventing overfitting. A typical CNN layer involves a sublayer for convolution transformation, performing an affine transformation to the output of the previous layer, usually based on several parallel convolutions [98]. Outputs are nonlinearly transformed, typically with a ReLU function, and summarized through a pooling layer, often using the maxpool operator (Figure 25.4).

In drug discovery, CNNs find application in elucidating bioactivity profiles from microscopy images [65] and are extensively utilized for molecular property prediction [38]. The application of CNNs to circular fingerprints has enabled the creation of a differentiable fingerprint, marking a notable shift toward data-driven representation learning for molecular property prediction, departing from fixed chemical descriptors [38]. Beyond fingerprints, CNNs exhibit proficiency in extracting features from images of molecular structures. One pioneering approach that applied CNNs to molecular graph drawings is exemplified by Chemception [55], drawing inspiration from Google's Inception-ResNet. In this framework, molecular graphs were treated as images, without explicit chemical

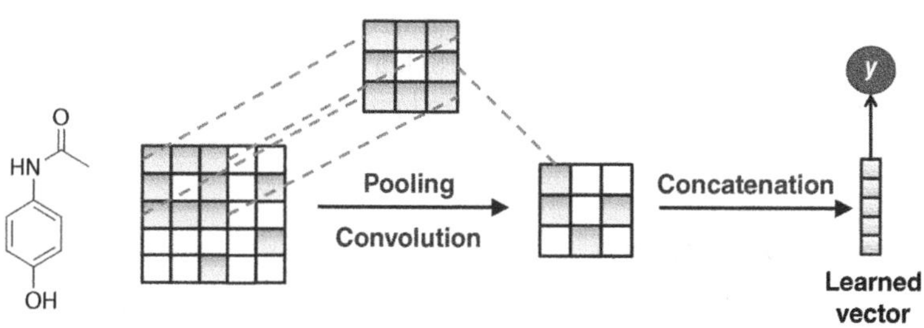

Figure 25.4 Depiction of CNNs.

knowledge provided to the network. Chemception demonstrated success in both binary classification tasks, such as determining the activity and toxicity of a compound, and regression tasks, including predicting the free energy of solvation. A parallel strategy was employed in the DeepScreen method [192], where researchers constructed a large-scale drug-target interaction system exclusively utilizing 2D images of known drugs, proving effective in identifying new targets for existing drugs. Toxic Colors [46] represents another instance where CNNs applied to molecular graph drawings were employed for toxicity prediction, enhancing molecular graph drawings by coloring specific areas based on the electrical charge at each position. In addition, Meyer et al. [125] utilized CNNs to predict MeSH-therapeutic-use classes based on compound images, surpassing previous predictions reliant on transcriptomic data. Existing CNN architectures [e.g., VGG-19 [179], ResNet152 [63], DenseNet-201 ([70]), and AlexNet [93]] were then extended to Kekulé structure images (KekuleScope) for molecular property prediction [29], demonstrating comparable performance to RF and DNNs on ECFPs. The evolution of molecular property prediction with images as input aligns with progress in computer vision, enabling automatic extraction of chemical structures from literature and patents [149, 184]. The chemical structure recognition model can integrate with NLP models like DECIMER [150] and DECIMER 1.0 [149], translating bitmap images into SMILES strings, akin to an image captioning task [68].

As regards molecular generation, Li et al. introduced DeepScaffold, a novel comprehensive tool for scaffold-based drug discovery that utilizes CNNs and 2D graphs of molecular structures [103]. This method enables the creation of new molecules by leveraging a diverse array of scaffolds including Bemis–Murcko scaffolds, cyclic skeletons, and side chain properties. One of its key advantages lies in its ability to extend preexisting scaffolds by applying generalized chemical rules to add atoms and bonds. The resulting molecules generated by DeepScaffold have been evaluated using molecular docking against corresponding macromolecular targets, yielding promising results. Furthermore, DeepGraphMolGen employs a multiobjective approach integrating graph CNN and reinforcement learning (RL) to generate molecules [85]. Represented as 2D graphs, this methodology offers a computationally inexpensive framework based on a graph generational model [106]. In addition, Song et al. proposed DeepFusion [181], a CNN-based model for generating structural similarity features for drugs and proteins, successfully applied in developing therapeutic agents against SARS-CoV-2 [182].

25.3.3 Graph Neural Networks

Graph neural networks (GNNs) constitute a specialized subset of ML algorithms tailored for drug discovery, uniquely equipped to analyze graph data composed of

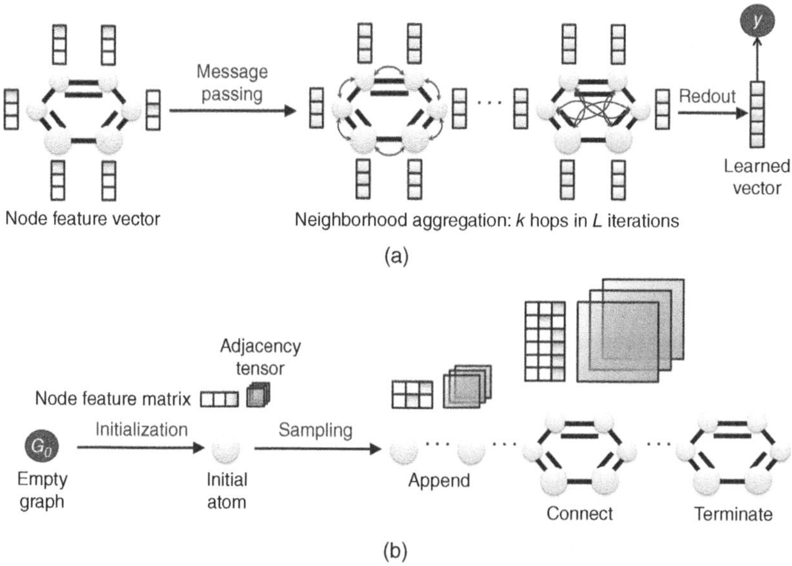

Figure 25.5 GNNs operate in prediction mode (a) for learning embeddings from molecular data to predict properties and generation mode (b), where molecules are built step by step with graph transitions such as appending, connecting, or terminating atoms.

nodes and edges [217]. This framework effectively captures relationships among entities such as chemical compounds and proteins [166], encoding pairwise connectivity within a non-Euclidean space and furnishing a structured representation of atomistic data.

A standard GNN consists of layers that aggregate node features and neighboring nodes' information [73] through recursive message passing until reaching stability (Figure 25.5). Node features, representing properties like mass, electron number, and charge, are organized into a matrix and multiplied by the adjacency tensor to capture the graph structure. Increasing the power of the adjacency tensor extends feature propagation to distant nodes, akin to expanding receptive fields in images. These acquired embeddings are valuable for both molecular property prediction and molecule ration tasks.

Two prominent types of GNNs include recurrent GNNs [217] and convolutional GNNs (GCNs). Recurrent GNNs employ recurrent neural architectures like the graph-gated neural network (GGNN) ([104]) to learn node representations, while GCNs generalize grid-to-graph data convolution by transforming node representation into a spectral domain using the graph Fourier transform ([102]). Many sophisticated GNN models rely on GCNs for their construction, including spectral-based and spatially based MPNN, graph attention network (GAT), and graph isomorphism network (GIN) [204].

In drug discovery, GNNs find extensive application in bioactivity or physico-chemical property prediction. Several studies have demonstrated the superiority of GCNs as 3D descriptors over SMILES strings, excelling in prediction tasks and offering better interpretability [177, 229]. Models like Chemi-net utilize GCNs for molecular representation, comparing single-task and multitask DNNs' performances on internal QSAR datasets ([111]). Weave, another graph-based model, leverages graph structure information by treating each molecule as an undirected graph [84]. The MPNN [52] enhances information flow between atoms using a unique message transmission method for undirected graphs. MPNN stacks multiple message-passing and updating blocks to extract abstract neural representations of nodes, followed by merging node features in the readout phase to form graph features. In addition, the directed message-passing neural network (D-MPNN) adopts a directed message-passing paradigm, outperforming traditional 3D descriptors in most datasets ([224]). Notably, this model facilitated the discovery of halicin, an antibiotic, through large-scale chemical space exploration [188]. Moreover, attentive FP, derived from GCN, employs an attention mechanism to learn nonlocal intramolecular interactions and capture hidden edges for specific tasks [222]. Further advancements include the attention message passing neural network (AMPNN) [215] and the edge memory neural network (EMNN), which integrate attention mechanisms into the MPNN framework for improved performance on standardized missing data from benchmark sets. Several other models have contributed to enhancing molecular property prediction, including DimeNet [50], PotentialNet [44], and SchNet [172] among others.

GNNs also play a crucial role in molecule generation, enabling common drug design applications such as scaffold-based molecule design. RL is often integrated with GNNs or graph CNN in frameworks like MolDQN [237], Graph Convolutional Policy Network (GCPN) [227], MNCE-RL [223], and DeepGraphMolGen [85] to generate molecules with desired attributes while ensuring chemical validity and uncovering novel compounds.

25.3.4 Variational Autoencoders

VAEs represent a probabilistic adaptation of traditional AE architectures [88]. While standard AEs comprise encoder and decoder models with mirrored layers, VAEs take a different approach. They learn the mean and variance for each latent variable, defining a probability distribution rather than deterministically mapping inputs. This probabilistic framework ensures a continuous latent space, crucial

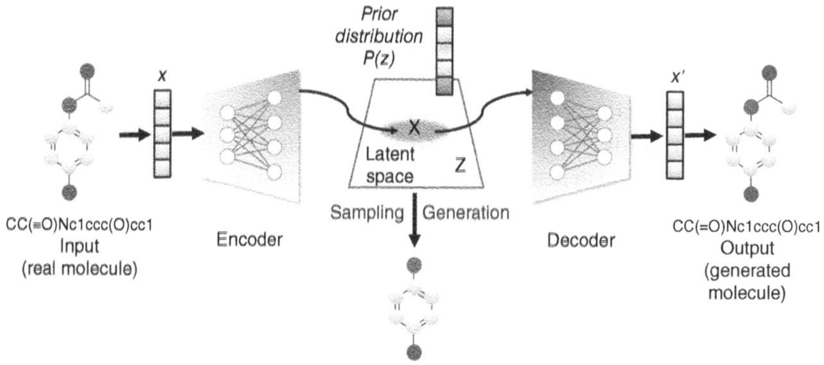

Figure 25.6 Depiction of VAEs.

for VAEs' generative capability, enabling the sampling of latent representations to generate entirely new observations (Figure 25.6).

The first molecular DGM for SMILES-formatted structures, ChemicalVAE, was pioneered by Gómez-Bombarelli et al. [56]. This model transforms SMILES strings into one-hot matrices, utilizing a CNN-based encoder and a GRU-based decoder. However, SMILES syntax can lead to sparse latent spaces in AEs, with "dead areas" representing invalid molecules. To address this, Kusner et al. [95] developed Grammar-directed VAE (GVAE), which predicts the likelihood of predefined production rules to ensure syntactic correctness and generate valid SMILES strings. Expanding on this approach, Dai et al. [30] further improved GVAE with the Syntax-Directed VAE (SD-VAE) [30], integrating stochastic elements to enhance string validity through offline syntax and semantic evaluations. Several related variants, including semisupervised VAE (SSVAE) [83], conditional VAE (CVAE) [108], constrained graph VAE (CGVAE) ([112]), GTM VAE [165], NeVAE [162], and CogMol [25] have been explored. Another notable variant is the adversarial AE (AAE) [119], employing adversarial training to shape the latent space by introducing a discriminator network to differentiate between encoded points and samples from a predefined distribution. AAEs have shown promise in molecule generation [12, 80, 141], improving reconstruction quality and the validity of generated molecules. Graph-based representations have also been leveraged in VAE-based models for molecule generation, including Graph-VAE [178], JT-VAE (W. [76]), Regularized VAE ([117]), MHG-VAE [81], MGCVAE [101], and ScaffoldVAE [107]. However, VAEs face challenges in accurately predicting substructures and handling computational complexity, especially with larger molecules. Fu et al. addressed this by proposing the copy and refine strategy named CORE [48], improving decoding efficiency by predicting substructure copying probability and selection. In addition, Kwon et al. [97] introduced a compressed graph representation to reduce computational complexity without sacrificing the validity or diversity of generated molecules. Furthermore, Jin et al. ([77]) introduced a hierarchical graph VAE named HierG2G, which used larger and more flexible graph motifs as building blocks for molecules. This hierarchical approach significantly improved reconstruction accuracy and generation quality by modeling the strong dependency between the successive addition and selection of substructures in the decoding process.

25.3.5 Generative Adversarial Networks

GANs [58] have revolutionized the generation of realistic synthetic samples. Unlike VAEs, GANs comprise two adversarial networks: the generator, which produces random SMILES strings, and the discriminator, which distinguishes between generated molecules and those in the training set (Figure 25.7) [57]. Through iterative training, the generator improves progressively, generating molecular structures that closely resemble the target molecules. Training halts when the discriminator can no longer differentiate between the generator's molecules and the target molecules, enabling the generator to produce desired molecules. To generate molecules with specific properties, GAN training is augmented with an auxiliary task, where the generator produces SMILES strings with desired attributes, and RL optimizes the generator during GAN training. Algorithms such as objective-reinforced GANs (ORGAN) [61] and objective-reinforced GANs for inverse-design chemistry (ORGANIC) [163] utilize GAN+RL-based training for chemical space exploration. ORGAN generates molecules in SMILES strings while optimizing various domain-specific metrics. The generator, based on

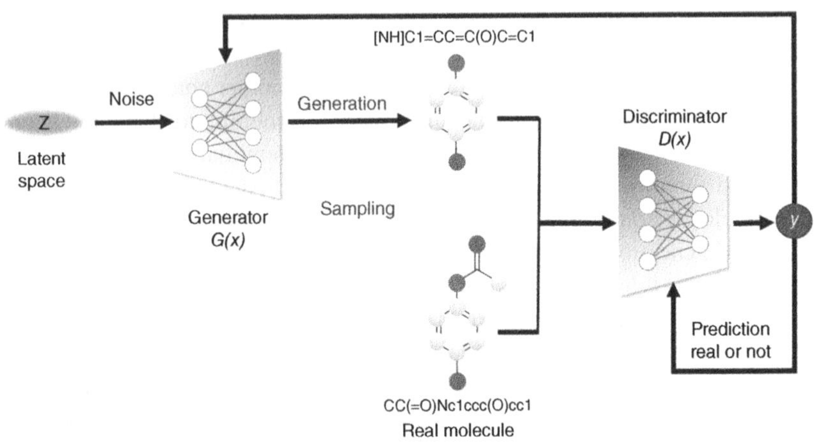

Figure 25.7 Depiction of GANs.

LSTM, functions as a stochastic policy in an RL setting, while the discriminator (a CNN model) is trained using Wasserstein loss. Experimental results demonstrate that the generated molecules exhibit drug-like structures and show improvement in evaluation metrics. ORGANIC can generate molecules with a biased distribution towards specific attributes for drug discovery and material design but faces challenges in optimizing discrete values from Lipinski's rule of five heuristic score while successfully optimizing the QED score. RANC (Reinforced Adversarial Neural Computer) [147] and ATNC (Adversarial Threshold Neural Computer) [146] also employ GAN+RL-based training, using a differential neural computer (DNC) [59] as a substitute for the central RNN. DNC-based architectures excel in handling longer SMILES sequences and yield greater output diversity compared to the ORGANIC implementation. LatentGAN [145], a novel approach, combines an AE with the GAN algorithm for molecular design tasks. Unlike the ORGANIC model, which directly utilizes SMILES as GAN input, LatentGAN uses the hidden variables generated by the AE as GAN input, showing promising results.

GANs can also be applied to molecular graphs for molecule generation. MolGAN [32] is an implicit, likelihood-free DGM for small molecular graph generation, bypassing expensive graph-matching procedures. MolGAN follows the GraphVAE approach in generating graphs based on their adjacency matrix and attributes but employs GANs instead of VAEs. The architecture, consisting of a generator, discriminator, and reward networks, optimizes molecules for target properties through RL. Despite mode collapse susceptibility, MolGAN generates nearly 100% valid molecules, outperforming ORGAN on the QM9 dataset [161].

25.3.6 Normalizing Flow Models

Unlike GANs and VAEs, flow-based DGMs, such normalizing flow (NF) models [90], explicitly learn the probability density function of all possible real data values through a sequence of invertible transformations (Figure 25.8). Leveraging exact likelihood estimation for training, these models enable efficient one-shot inference and complete reconstruction of training data [123]. Notable examples include RealNVP [33], Glow [87], and MAF [136], which perform precise distribution approximation via invertible transformations. Compared to VAE and GAN, NF models offer distinct advantages such as not requiring noisy output data, creating robust local variance models, and achieving enhanced training stability and convergence. Another key advantage of these models is their ability to precisely reconstruct input data without duplicates, making them valuable for molecule generation tasks, especially in scenarios sensitive to minor structural changes, such as activity cliffs [189]. However, they also have limitations,

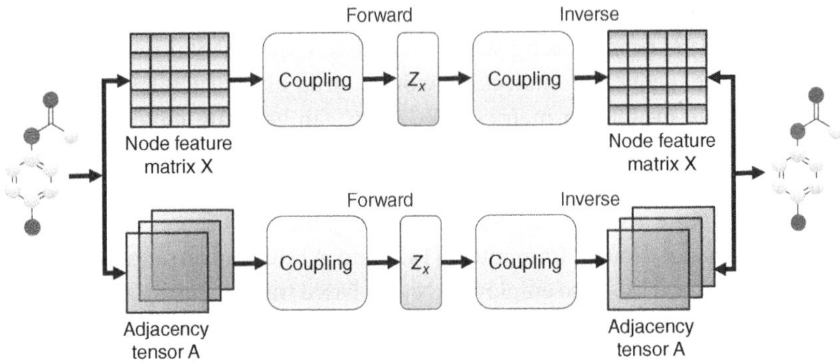

Figure 25.8 Illustrations of NF models.

including reduced interpretability and challenges in ensuring the synthesizability of generated molecules.

NF models find successful applications in various molecule generation tasks, particularly on molecular graphs. For example, GraphNVP [118] learns the latent space to generate molecules with desired properties by inverting graph components containing adjacency tensors and dequantized node attributes. Similarly, graph residual flow [66] achieves comparable performance using residual flows for molecular graph generation, offering more flexible and complex nonlinear mappings. However, both approaches may suffer from low validity due to their one-shot generation strategy. Shi et al. combined autoregression modeling with NF to create GraphAF [176], ensuring 100% structural validity using valency constraints. MoFlow ([230]), an alternative one-shot generator, combines modified Glow models for bonds, a novel graph conditional flow for atoms, and validity checking rules, demonstrating robust performance but slower generation due to validity constraints. MolGrow [96], characterized by hierarchical NF, generates molecular graphs with gradually expanding sizes during sampling. MolGrow's generation phase involves a recursive division process, where one node is split into two. This model demonstrated higher performance when trained on a fixed atom ordering. FastFlows [47], a robust nonautoregressive model, produces novel SELFIES-formatted structures with desired attributes using very small dataset. FFLOM ([75]), a flow-based autoregressive model, generates novel molecules by modifying reconstructed structures with additional molecular fragments, achieving higher binding affinity compared to parental molecules.

25.3.7 Transformer-Based Models

The Transformer architecture [203] revolutionized NLP, especially for sequence transduction and machine translation tasks. Over the past five years, it has gained significant traction, with breakthroughs like Generative Pretrained Transformer (GPT) models excelling in NLP tasks [135]. Similarly, Bidirectional Encoder Representations from Transformers (BERT) and Bidirectional Autoregressive Transformer (BART) models have been pivotal in learning embeddings of small molecule string representations.

Transformers come in various forms: encoder-only (e.g., BERT), decoder-only (e.g., GPT), or combined encoder and decoder modules trained together. Alternatively, BERT-style Transformers employ multiple sequential encoder blocks without decoders, returning embeddings to string inputs via a simple classifier layer. For molecular representation, bidirectional Transformer training often includes masking, where SMILES string representations undergo tokenization with random element hiding (Figure 25.9). The Transformer then predicts the unmasked original string as output, learning the general ruleset of valid strings and producing chemically informed embeddings. A key feature of the Transformer is its attention mechanism ([110]), which rapidly learns contextual information about input sequence data. This mechanism weights each input sequence element based on its relative position, akin to how atoms' positions or neighboring atoms affect molecular properties. Transformers typically comprise attention layers with normalization and dense layers in "blocks," boasting billions of trainable parameters

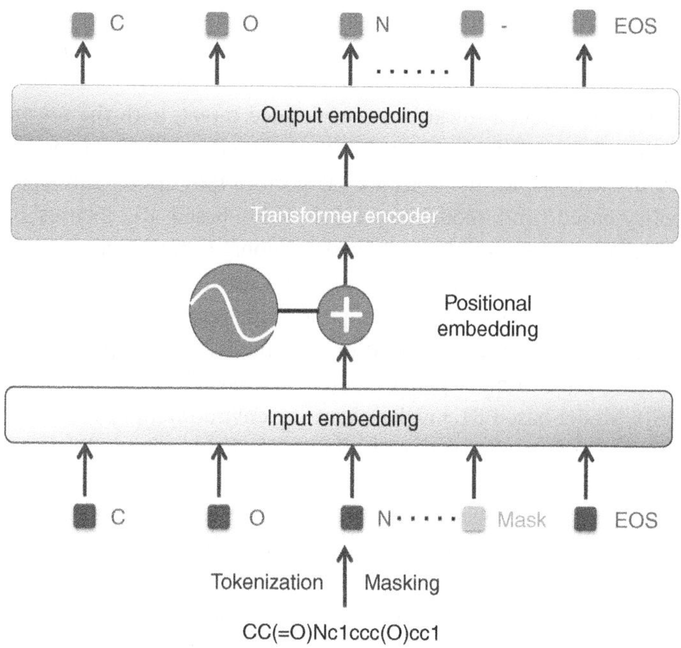

Figure 25.9 Depiction of Transformers.

considering both element identities and relative positions. Learned embeddings reside in a highly organized latent space, with similar molecules clustering closely due to unsupervised training [139]. AEs and Transformers encode molecules into this latent space and decode vectors back into small molecules, facilitating generative exploration in small molecule design and drug discovery [79]. Notably, models like SMILES–BERT [210], SMILES Transformer [67], ChemBERTa [26], and MolBERT [42] have excelled in molecular property prediction, achieving improved performance compared to traditional methods. Moreover, Transformers find utility in molecular graphs, as demonstrated by GROVER [159], which achieves superior performance via self-supervised contextual property prediction and graph-level motif tasks. They're also applied in protein-specific molecule generation [60], utilizing amino acid sequences to produce ligands in SMILES format. In addition, Transformers power molecular generation tools like MoleculeChef [14], generating reactants for specified products, similar to machine translation.

25.3.8 Reinforcement Learning

RL is a methodological framework aimed at optimizing behavior in a given environment to achieve maximum reward [193]. In drug design, the agent acts as a DGM, producing molecules to maximize specific reward functions. The environment reflects the intricate chemical space, with the reward function based on properties like drug-likeness, bioactivity, or synthetic feasibility. The goal is to optimize the agent's behavior towards a user-defined target, with the reward function evaluating the quality of selected actions based on domain-specific rules, guiding future actions. RL methods are categorized into three main types: value-based, policy-based, and model-based [4]. Value-based RL focuses on determining value functions and their optimal versions, exemplified by deep Q-learning variants like double deep Q-learning and dueling deep Q-learning [18]. Policy-based RL aims to find an optimal policy, stochastic or deterministic, for better convergence in high-dimensional or continuous action spaces, with examples such as deep deterministic policy gradient and asynchronous advantage actor critic ([236]). Model-based RL involves learning environment functionality and dynamics from previous observations to find efficient solutions, illustrated by imagination-augmented agents and model-based value expansion.

RL has been successfully applied in molecule generation. Zhou et al. [237] employed value-based algorithms such as double deep Q-learning to optimize generated molecules. Other works, such as REINVENT [11], ORGAN [61], and ORGANIC [164] predominantly utilized the policy-gradient algorithm REINFORCE [212] for gradient estimation. Proximal policy optimization (PPO) [171] has gained popularity, offering improved performance over traditional methods like trust region policy optimization (TRPO) [170] due to its lower sample complexity. Studies leveraging PPO in drug design include those by Neil et al. [131], as well as those employing MNCE–RL [223], DeepGraphMolGen [85], and GCPN [226]. Hybrid actor-critic methods, like off-policy deterministic policy gradient (DPG) and deep deterministic policy gradient (DDPG), mitigate the high variance associated with policy-gradient algorithms [4]. DDPG utilizes neural networks for high-dimensional spaces, as seen in MolGAN [32]. In addition, the advantage actor-critic (A2C) algorithm, utilized by Neil et al. [131], minimizes variance by subtracting estimated rewards from true rewards to accelerate convergence. A significant challenge in RL is the exploration-exploitation trade-off, where the agent must balance exploring new actions while exploiting known ones to maximize cumulative reward. Active learning presents a potential solution, allowing the model to query experts during learning [74]. Another issue arises with RL training, where chemical libraries are expected to evolve towards desired properties, posing a multiobjective optimization dilemma ([168]). Techniques like nondominated sorting or pair-based comparisons help prioritize molecules based on predefined goals, achieving Pareto optimal solutions [34].

25.4 AI Applications in Drug Discovery and Development

25.4.1 Emerging AI-Powered Drug Discovery Companies

The potential of ML and advanced AI algorithms in the field of drug discovery and development is increasingly recognized. AI-driven drug discovery platforms have made significant leaps forward in recent years, harnessing sophisticated technologies like neural networks for drug design and knowledge graphs for deciphering target biology. These breakthroughs have led to the successful progression of molecules into clinical trials with unprecedented efficiency, leading to shortened development timelines and heightened cost-effectiveness. Moreover, collaborations between traditional pharmaceutical companies and AI-focused firms have surged, fostering a fertile ground for innovation and cross-pollination of expertise. Yet, amidst these strides, the true magnitude and trajectory of AI's impact in drug discovery and development remain subjects of ongoing exploration, promising to revolutionize productivity, widen the scope of molecular exploration, and elevate clinical success rates.

A comprehensive analysis of AI's influence on drug discovery and development, with a predominant focus on small molecules, unveils a striking growth trajectory among "AI-native" companies. Spanning the years from 2010 to 2021, these companies have witnessed a meteoric expansion of their pipelines, boasting an impressive average annual growth rate of approximately 36%. Within their combined pipeline lie around 160 preclinical candidates and 15 clinical candidates. Notably, these companies often gravitate towards established target classes such as enzymes, notably kinases, potentially driven by a strategic approach to risk mitigation through the pursuit of targets with validated biological significance. Given the pressing unmet medical needs and the plethora of well-characterized targets, AI-powered discovery programs tend to gravitate towards oncology and central nervous system indications. A summary of AI-native companies, their platforms, and the number of clinical candidates is provided in Table 25.4.

25.4.2 Success Stories of AI-Discovered Molecules in Clinical Trials

The integration of AI into the pharmaceutical industry has sparked a significant transformation in drug discovery and development. This essay explores successful examples of AI-assisted drug discovery that have advanced to clinical trials, highlighting AI's potential to expedite and enhance the drug development process.

DSP-1181, the first AI-designed drug, entered Phase I clinical trials in early 2020 for treating obsessive–compulsive disorder. Developed through a collaboration between Sumitomo Dainippon Pharma and Exscientia, DSP-1181, a potent serotonin 5-HT1A receptor agonist, owes its existence to Exscientia's AI platform, "CentaurAI systems." This platform not only generated novel molecules but also optimized drug targets, compressing the exploratory phase from 4 to 5 years to just 12 months. Similarly, DSP-2230, another product of this collaboration, is currently under investigation for obsessive–compulsive disorder treatment, with AI algorithms scrutinizing biological data to pinpoint compounds modulating specific brain receptors associated with the disorder.

Furthermore, Exscientia, in partnership with Evotec, introduced EXS-21546, an AI-designed small molecule antagonist for the A2A receptor, into clinical trials in 2020 as a potential cancer immunotherapy (Clinical trial ID: NCT05920408). In addition, they developed a pioneering small molecule inhibitor of Protein Kinase C theta, EXS-4318, targeting inflammation and immunology. LegoChem Biosciences utilized AI models to formulate Delpazolid (LCB-010371), a promising antibiotic targeting drug-resistant bacteria strains like Methicillin-resistant Staphylococcus aureus (MRSA) and Vancomycin-resistant Enterococci (VRE). Berzosertib, a hopeful cancer medication developed by Merck KGaA and C4X Discovery [138, 196], underscores AI's pivotal role in identifying novel therapeutic candidates by dissecting genetic and molecular data. Likewise, Amarin Corporation's AI-driven analysis of clinical trial data expedited the approval process for Icosapent Ethyl [126] intended for reducing cardiovascular risk in patients with elevated triglyceride levels [6]. Evinacumab, a prospective therapy for cholesterol regulation disorders, developed by Regeneron Pharmaceuticals

Table 25.4 AI platforms for drug discovery and development.

Company	AI application	Platform name(s)	Preclinical	Clinical	Website
Atomwise	VS through molecular recognition, structure-guided molecule generation and optimization	AtomNet®	2	0	https://www.atomwise.com
BenevolentAI	Bioinformatics target discovery	Benevolent platform™	2	1	https://www.benevolent.com
	Molecule generation and optimization				
C4X discovery	Genomics-based bioinformatics target discovery	Taxonomy3®	4	1	https://www.c4xdiscovery.com
	Structure-guided molecule generation and optimization	Conformetrix			
Berg/BPGBio	Bioinformatics target discovery	Interrogative biology®	1	5	https://bpgbio.com
Denovicon therapeutics	Bioinformatics target discovery		2	0	https://www.denovicontx.com
	VS Molecular optimization ADMET predictions				
A2A Pharmaceuticals	Molecule generation and optimization	Sculpt™	6	0	https://www.a2apharma.com
Exscientia	Bioinformatic target discovery Phenotypic screening Molecule generation and optimization ADMET prediction Clinical prediction based on patient tissue	CentaurAI systems	2	2	https://www.exscientia.ai

(*continued*)

Table 25.4 (Continued)

Company	AI application	Platform name(s)	Preclinical	Clinical	Website
Frontier medicines	Protein hotspot mapping Generation of compound libraries Molecule optimization		3	0	https://www.frontiermeds.com
Auransa	Bioinformatics target discovery	SMarTR ENGINE*	5	1	https://www.auransa.com
Healx	Bioinformatics to discover novel drug-target relationships/repurposing	Healnet	9	0	https://healx.ai
Insilico medicine	Bioinformatics in novel target discovery	PandaOmics*	11	6	https://insilico.com
	Molecule generation and optimization with ADMET prediction	Chemistry42*			
	Clinical trial prediction	InClinico*			
Nimbus Therapeutics	Molecular dynamics ADME predictions		4	1	https://www.nimbustx.com
Pharos iBio	Bioinformatic target discovery		4	2	https://www.pharosibio.com/en
	Protein structure characterization				
	Molecule optimization and ADMET prediction	Chemiverse			
Aria Pharmaceuticals	Bioinformatics target discovery Polypharmacology		25	0	https://ariapharmaceuticals.com
Recursion pharmaceuticals	Bioinformatic target discovery		2	5	https://www.recursion.com
	Experimental target validation and hit identification with phenotypic	Recursion operating			

Collaborations pharmaceuticals	Bioinformatics drug repurposing	MegaPredict	13	0	https://www.collaborationspharma.com
	Molecule generation and optimization	MegaSyn			
	Mechanism, ADMET prediction	AssayCentral, MegaTox, MegaTrans			
Insitro	Disease modeling Deconvolution of in vitro phenotypic disease models		2	0	https://insitro.com
Turbine AI	Predictive cell behavior modeling to interrogate the mechanism of action	Simulated cell™	3	0	https://turbine.ai
Cyclica12	Polypharmacology	Ligand express®	2	0	https://cyclicarx.com
	Molecule generation and optimization	Ligand design™			
	Off-target interaction prediction	MatchMaker™			
	ADMET predictions	Poem™			
Verge genomics	Genomic-based bioinformatics in novel target discovery		0	1	https://www.vergegenomics.com
Roivant sciences	Molecular dynamics	Silicon therapeutics	6	1	https://www.roivant.com
Relay therapeutics	Molecular dynamics	Dynamo™ platform	0	3	https://relaytx.com
	Molecule identification				
	Protein degrader deep learning models	VantAI			

using AI [121], showcases how AI algorithms can sift through vast datasets to identify pertinent targets and pathways involved in cholesterol regulation. Moreover, in 2023, Insilico Medicine administered the first dose of INS018_055, an AI-developed antifibrotic small molecule inhibitor, in Phase II clinical trials for idiopathic pulmonary fibrosis patients (Clinical trial ID: NCT05938920), further highlighting AI's impact on accelerating drug development processes. INS018_055 works by inhibiting the discoidin domain receptor 1 (DDR1), an epithelial cell-expressed proinflammatory receptor tyrosine kinase involved in fibrosis. Another AI-generated drug from the same company, ISM3312, currently undergoing Phase I clinical trials, demonstrated efficacy in reducing viral load in lung tissue in patients with COVID-19. In 2023, Ren et al. reported a new inhibitor for cyclin-dependent kinase 20 (CDK20), utilizing multiple AI-based tools for target prediction and structure modeling [152], showcasing the rapid identification of potential therapeutic candidates through AI-driven approaches. Pembrolizumab (Keytruda), developed by Merck & Co., stands as an AI-discovered drug utilized in the treatment of various cancers, including melanoma, lung cancer, and head and neck cancers. In addition, the UK Medicines and Healthcare Products Regulatory Agency (MHRA) received a clinical trial application for BEN-8744 from BenevolentAI, a small molecule phosphodiesterase 10 (PDE10) inhibitor intended for ulcerative colitis treatment [3], indicating AI's adaptability in addressing diverse medical needs. Sotorasib (AMG 510), an AI-optimized drug developed by Amgen, specifically targets nonsmall cell lung cancer with specific genetic mutations, showcasing AI's prowess in analyzing cancer genomic data to identify potential compounds inhibiting the mutated protein responsible for tumor growth.

The utilization of AI technologies in these processes empowers the design of molecules imbued with unique attributes, deviating from the conventional approach adopted by medicinal chemists. This opens up avenues for exploring uncharted territories within the vast expanse of chemical space. As Alan Lipkus from Chemical Abstracts Service elaborates, AI serves as a catalyst for breaking away from the confines of traditional scaffolds commonly utilized in drug design. This, in turn, catalyzes the development of novel and distinct molecular structures, heralding a paradigm shift in pharmaceutical innovation.

25.5 Challenges and Future Outlooks

Over the past decade, the integration of AI into drug discovery has experienced a significant surge, a trend that continues to gain momentum. However, this advancement is accompanied by a spectrum of challenges and constraints that necessitate acknowledgment and strategic resolution to ensure its effective application.

Among the primary hurdles lies the issue of data quality and quantity. Both predictive and generative AI models necessitate a substantial amount of high-quality data for adequate training. Insufficient data can significantly impair their performance and reliability, elevating the risk of overfitting [120]. Indeed, the limited availability of labeled data poses a formidable barrier to the progression of AI-driven drug discovery. Employing TL algorithms [17] and focusing on smaller, curated datasets are emerging strategies to mitigate this challenge, emphasizing the importance of extracting meaningful insights from limited yet relevant data to enhance model precision and applicability in the intricate domain of drug discovery. Knowledge graphs (KGs) have emerged as a powerful tool in this context. KGs are multirelational networks that store interlinked descriptions of various entities, facilitating a deep understanding of complex biological systems and pathologies [234]. By integrating KGs into molecular representation learning, AI models can capture the nuanced relationships between different entities, enhancing their ability to represent crucial structural and functional relationships between molecules. Recent studies have underscored the efficacy of incorporating KG pretraining strategies to address challenges posed by small training sets, achieving remarkable generalization capabilities even with limited data [148]. Furthermore, prior knowledge derived from diverse sources, including proteomics, metabolomics, and phenotypic features, can enrich AI models [37]. Moreover, the combination of AI with physical simulations [24] holds promise in overcoming limitations associated with small or nonexistent datasets owing to enhanced understanding of biological systems and the availability of advanced hardware acceleration tools such as supercomputers, GPUs, TPUs, and other quasi-ASIC devices. While encoding molecular information into descriptors, fingerprints, and DL models remains challenging, combining different representations through multiview techniques [116] can mitigate biases inherent to individual representations.

However, challenges extend beyond data quality and quantity. The vast chemical space poses significant hurdles, with many benchmark datasets lacking in representativeness for real-world drug discovery [205]. Furthermore, datasets are often imbalanced [91], and the data collected can vary widely depending on the biological assays, conditions, or methods used, coupled with data originating from disparate biological assays, conditions, or methods. This variability complicates the direct comparison of results and necessitates sophisticated strategies for data preprocessing and model evaluation. Strategies aimed at filtering raw inputs to eliminate noise, outliers, or irrelevant data, along with the automation of data entry can significantly improve model performance and reliability. Techniques such as noise reduction algorithms, outlier detection methods like Z-scores and box plots, and cross-validation experiments are instrumental in ensuring model robustness and generalization across diverse datasets. Consequently, the evaluation of models necessitates the acquisition of appropriate datasets, consideration of data balancing techniques, and the utilization of comprehensive evaluation metrics, including accuracy, precision, recall, F1 score, AUC, and AUPR ([168]).

Sequence- and graph-based DL methods, while powerful in molecular representation learning across various molecular sizes, lack interpretability and transparency, often termed as "black boxes" [209]. Employing visualization tools such as Local Interpretable Model-agnostic Explanations (LIME) [153], Activation Maximization [40] and Shapley Additive exPlanations (SHAP) [115] can shed light on the decision-making process of these models, providing insights into the most influential features. Moving forward, there is a continuous need to develop robust models with high interpretability.

Another challenge arises in AI-based prediction of "activity cliffs," where pairs of structurally similar molecules exhibit significantly different potencies. A study by van Tilborg et al. [202] found that all tested ML and DL methods struggled with activity cliffs. However, ML approaches demonstrated a slight advantage over more complex DL approaches, indicating the necessity for improved metrics and algorithms to address these challenges effectively.

Technical concerns also persist, especially regarding the representation learning on molecular graphs. For instance, traditional fingerprints can still outperform representations derived from GNNs for molecular property prediction. Moreover, the absence of a unified protocol for AI-driven drug discovery studies leads to inconsistency in benchmark datasets, evaluation metrics, split folds, and hyper-parameter tuning, training, and evaluation procedures [73]. While initial guidelines exist for molecule generation [206], further protocols are essential for accurate molecular property prediction.

Another critical aspect to consider is the intensification of expert interaction in the development and application of AI models for molecule generation [72, 128]. While AI models can generate numerous potential molecules, engaging medicinal chemists in the evaluation and selection process ensures their synthetic feasibility and likelihood of success in subsequent drug discovery stages. This collaborative effort can be facilitated through the development of interactive platforms, enabling experts to provide feedback on generated molecules and steer the model toward more promising candidates. Moreover, integrating expert knowledge in the form of medicinal chemistry rules and heuristics can further enhance the performance of AI models in molecule generation.

At last, the use of large language models (LLMs) for molecule generation is a promising area of research in drug discovery [15, 180, 233]. LLMs have the potential to analyze extensive scientific literature, extracting insights to fuel novel ideas for molecular design. This approach enables the discovery of overlooked rules, mechanisms, and chemical structures, complementing traditional methods. By encoding chemical data in text, LLMs streamline molecule generation with desired properties, facilitating efficient exploration of the chemical space. However, further research is necessary to optimize LLM performance and integrate expert knowledge and medicinal chemistry rules into these models.

Beyond technical limitations, the use of AI in drug discovery faces various regulatory and societal challenges. For example, regulatory agencies like the FDA are still working to evaluate and approve AI tools for drug discovery, but this process creates uncertainty and slows down their adoption. It's important to note the gap between the high expectations for AI in drug discovery and the practical challenges it faces. While AI has made significant advancements, it still relies on traditional methods for validation, which need to be considered [8]. Ethical issues, such as data privacy, consent, and bias in algorithms, add further complexity to the integration of AI in healthcare. However, despite these challenges, the potential and ongoing progress of AI in drug discovery is clear. Continued investment in research and innovation is necessary to overcome existing barriers and fully realize the transformative potential of AI in revolutionizing drug discovery. These challenges underscore areas requiring further attention and development.

In summary, the application of AI in drug discovery presents numerous promising opportunities alongside significant challenges. To successfully leverage AI in this domain, it is imperative to grasp the fundamental concepts and consider various factors such as the task at hand, the nature of the data, the nuanced representation of molecules, the sophistication of model architectures, and the dynamics of the learning paradigm as a cohesive whole. Throughout this comprehensive survey, we have meticulously explored myriad aspects surrounding AI-driven drug discovery, illuminating the multifaceted nature of this evolving field. By cultivating a deep understanding of these intricacies, we can unlock a wealth of opportunities for innovation and advancement. With a solid grasp of these fundamentals, we are poised to make substantial strides, catalyzing a transformative shift in the landscape of drug discovery.

Acknowledgments

A.L. acknowledges funding from the Italian Ministry of Education Progetti di Rilevante Interesse Nazionale (PRIN) grant 2022P5LPHS.

References

1 Abadi, M., Agarwal, A., Barham, P., et al. (2016). Tensorflow: Large-scale machine learning on heterogeneous distributed systems. arXiv Preprint arXiv:1603.04467.

2 Al-Rfou, R., Alain, G., Almahairi, A., et al. (2016). Theano: A Python framework for fast computation of mathematical expressions. arXiv E-Prints, arXiv: 1605.02688.

3 Arnold, C. (2023). Inside the nascent industry of AI-designed drugs. *Nature Medicine* 29 (6): 1292–1295.

4 Arulkumaran, K., Deisenroth, M.P., Brundage, M., and Bharath, A.A. (2017). A brief survey of deep reinforcement learning. *IEEE Signal Processing Magazine* 34 (6): 26–38. https://doi.org/10.1109/MSP.2017.2743240.

5 Arús-Pous, J., Johansson, S.V., Prykhodko, O. et al. (2019). Randomized SMILES strings improve the quality of molecular generative models. *Journal of Cheminformatics* 11 (1): 71. https://doi.org/10.1186/s13321-019-0393-0.

6 Ballantyne, C.M., Manku, M.S., Bays, H.E. et al. (2019). Icosapent ethyl effects on fatty acid profiles in statin-treated patients with high triglycerides: The randomized, placebo-controlled ANCHOR study. *Cardiology and Therapy* 8: 79–90.

7 Bauer, M.R., Ibrahim, T.M., Vogel, S.M., and Boeckler, F.M. (2013). Evaluation and optimization of virtual screening workflows with DEKOIS 2.0–a public library of challenging docking benchmark sets. *Journal of Chemical Information and Modeling* 53 (6): 1447–1462.

8 Bender, A. and Cortés-Ciriano, I. (2021). Artificial intelligence in drug discovery: What is realistic, what are illusions? Part 1: Ways to make an impact, and why we are not there yet. *Drug Discovery Today* 26 (2): 511–524.

9 Berthold, M.R., Cebron, N., Dill, F. et al. (2009). KNIME-the Konstanz information miner: Version 2.0 and beyond. *AcM SIGKDD Explorations Newsletter* 11 (1): 26–31.

10 Bjerrum, E.J. and Sattarov, B. (2018). Improving chemical autoencoder latent space and molecular de novo generation diversity with heteroencoders. *Biomolecules* 8 (4): 131. https://doi.org/10.3390/biom8040131.

11 Blaschke, T., Arús-Pous, J., Chen, H. et al. (2020). REINVENT 2.0: An AI tool for de novo drug design. *Journal of Chemical Information and Modeling* 60 (12): 5918–5922. https://doi.org/10.1021/acs.jcim.0c00915.

12 Blaschke, T., Olivecrona, M., Engkvist, O. et al. (2018). Application of generative autoencoder in de novo molecular design. *Molecular Informatics* 37 (1–2): 1700123. https://doi.org/10.1002/minf.201700123.

13 Blum, L.C. and Reymond, J.-L. (2009). 970 million druglike small molecules for virtual screening in the chemical universe database GDB-13. *Journal of the American Chemical Society* 131 (25): 8732–8733.

14 Bradshaw, J., Paige, B., Kusner, M.J., Segler, M.H.S. and Hernández-Lobato, J.M. (2019). A Model to Search for Synthesizable Molecules (arXiv:1906.05221). arXiv. https://doi.org/10.48550/arXiv.1906.05221.

15 Bran, A.M., Cox, S., Schilter, O., et al. (2023). Augmenting large language models with chemistry tools. NeurIPS 2023 AI for Science Workshop.

16 Brown, N., Fiscato, M., Segler, M.H.S., and Vaucher, A.C. (2019). GuacaMol: Benchmarking models for de novo molecular design. *Journal of Chemical Information and Modeling* 59 (3): 1096–1108. https://doi.org/10.1021/acs.jcim.8b00839.

17 Cai, C., Wang, S., Xu, Y. et al. (2020). Transfer learning for drug discovery. *Journal of Medicinal Chemistry* 63 (16): 8683–8694.

18 Celard, P., Iglesias, E.L., Sorribes-Fdez, J.M. et al. (2023). A survey on deep learning applied to medical images: From simple artificial neural networks to generative models. *Neural Computing and Applications* 35 (3): 2291–2323. https://doi.org/10.1007/s00521-022-07953-4.

19 Cerchia, C. and Lavecchia, A. (2023). New avenues in artificial-intelligence-assisted drug discovery. *Drug Discovery Today* 103516.

20 Chen, H., Engkvist, O., Wang, Y. et al. (2018). The rise of deep learning in drug discovery. *Drug Discovery Today* 23 (6): 1241–1250.

21 Chen, L., Cruz, A., Ramsey, S. et al. (2019). Hidden bias in the DUD-E dataset leads to misleading performance of deep learning in structure-based virtual screening. *PloS One* 14 (8): e0220113.

22 Chen, M., Suzuki, A., Thakkar, S. et al. (2016). DILIrank: The largest reference drug list ranked by the risk for developing drug-induced liver injury in humans. *Drug Discovery Today* 21 (4): 648–653. https://doi.org/10.1016/j.drudis.2016.02.015.

23 Chen, M., Vijay, V., Shi, Q. et al. (2011). FDA-approved drug labeling for the study of drug-induced liver injury. *Drug Discovery Today* 16 (15): 697–703. https://doi.org/10.1016/j.drudis.2011.05.007.

24 Chen, P., Chen, J., Yan, H. et al. (2022). Improving material property prediction by leveraging the large-scale computational database and deep learning. *The Journal of Physical Chemistry C* 126 (38): 16297–16305.

25 Chenthamarakshan, V., Das, P., Hoffman, S. et al. (2020). CogMol: Target-specific and selective drug design for COVID-19 using deep generative models. *Advances in Neural Information Processing Systems* 33: 4320–4332.

26 Chithrananda, S., Grand, G., & Ramsundar, B. (2020). ChemBERTa: Large-scale self-supervised pretraining for molecular property prediction. arXiv Preprint arXiv:2010.09885.

27 Chung, J., Gulcehre, C., Cho, K., & Bengio, Y. (2014). Empirical evaluation of gated recurrent neural networks on sequence modeling. arXiv Preprint arXiv:1412.3555.

28 Contreras-Reyes, J.E. and Arellano-Valle, R.B. (2012). Kullback–Leibler divergence measure for multivariate skew-normal distributions. *Entropy* 14 (9): 1606–1626.

29 Cortés-Ciriano, I. and Bender, A. (2019). KekuleScope: Prediction of cancer cell line sensitivity and compound potency using convolutional neural networks trained on compound images. *Journal of Cheminformatics* 11 (1): 41. https://doi.org/10.1186/s13321-019-0364-5.

30 Dai, H., Tian, Y., Dai, B., et al. (2018). Syntax-directed variational autoencoder for structured data. arXiv Preprint arXiv:1802.08786.

31 David, L., Thakkar, A., Mercado, R., and Engkvist, O. (2020). Molecular representations in AI-driven drug discovery: A review and practical guide. *Journal of Cheminformatics* 12 (1): 56.

32 De Cao, N., & Kipf, T. (2022). MolGAN: An implicit generative model for small molecular graphs (arXiv:1805.11973). arXiv. https://doi.org/10.48550/arXiv.1805.11973

33 Dinh, L., Sohl-Dickstein, J., & Bengio, S. (2016). Density estimation using real nvp. arXiv Preprint arXiv:1605.08803.

34 Domenico, A., Nicola, G., Daniela, T. et al. (2020). De novo drug design of targeted chemical libraries based on artificial intelligence and pair-based multiobjective optimization. *Journal of Chemical Information and Modeling* 60 (10): 4582–4593. https://doi.org/10.1021/acs.jcim.0c00517.

35 Douguet, D. (2018). Data sets representative of the structures and experimental properties of FDA-approved drugs. *ACS Medicinal Chemistry Letters* 9 (3): 204–209. https://doi.org/10.1021/acsmedchemlett.7b00462.

36 Dowden, H. and Munro, J. (2019). Trends in clinical success rates and therapeutic focus. *Nature Reviwes Drug Discovery* 18 (7): 495–496.

37 Duran-Frigola, M., Pauls, E., Guitart-Pla, O. et al. (2020). Extending the small-molecule similarity principle to all levels of biology with the chemical checker. *Nature Biotechnology* 38 (9): 1087–1096.

38 Duvenaud, D.K., Maclaurin, D., Iparraguirre, J., et al. (2015). Convolutional networks on graphs for learning molecular fingerprints. Advances in Neural Information Processing Systems, 28. https://proceedings.neurips.cc/paper_files/paper/2015/hash/f9be311e65d81a9ad8150a60844bb94c-Abstract.html

39 Elton, D.C., Boukouvalas, Z., Fuge, M.D., and Chung, P.W. (2019). Deep learning for molecular design—A review of the state of the art. *Molecular Systems Design & Engineering* 4 (4): 828–849.

40 Erhan, D., Bengio, Y., Courville, A., and Vincent, P. (2009). Visualizing higher-layer features of a deep network. *University of Montreal* 1341 (3): 1.

41 Etaati, L. (2019). Deep learning tools with cognitive toolkit (CNTK). In: *Machine Learning with Microsoft Technologies: Selecting the Right Architecture and Tools for Your Project*, 287–302.

42 Fabian, B., Edlich, T., Gaspar, H., et al. (2020). Molecular representation learning with language models and domain-relevant auxiliary tasks. arXiv Preprint arXiv:2011.13230.

43 Fang, X., Liu, L., Lei, J. et al. (2022). Geometry-enhanced molecular representation learning for property prediction. *Nature Machine Intelligence* 4 (2): 127–134.

44 Feinberg, E.N., Sur, D., Wu, Z. et al. (2018). PotentialNet for molecular property prediction. *ACS Central Science* 4 (11): 1520–1530.

45 Feng, Z., Chen, L., Maddula, H. et al. (2004). Ligand Depot: A data warehouse for ligands bound to macromolecules. *Bioinformatics* 20 (13): 2153–2155. https://doi.org/10.1093/bioinformatics/bth214.

46 Fernandez, M., Ban, F., Woo, G. et al. (2018). Toxic colors: the use of deep learning for predicting toxicity of compounds merely from their graphic images. *Journal of Chemical Information and Modeling* 58 (8): 1533–1543. https://doi.org/10.1021/acs.jcim.8b00338.

47 Frey, N.C., Gadepally, V., & Ramsundar, B. (2022). Fastflows: Flow-based models for molecular graph generation. arXiv Preprint arXiv:2201.12419.

48 Fu, T., Xiao, C., and Sun, J. (2020). Core: Automatic molecule optimization using copy & refine strategy. *Proceedings of the AAAI Conference on Artificial Intelligence* 34 (01): 638–645.

49 Gao, W. and Coley, C.W. (2020). The synthesizability of molecules proposed by generative models. *Journal of Chemical Information and Modeling* 60 (12): 5714–5723.

50 Gasteiger, J., Groß, J., & Günnemann, S. (2003). Directional message passing for molecular graphs. arXiv. 2020 doi: 10.48550. Arxiv.

51 Gaulton, A., Hersey, A., Nowotka, M. et al. (2017). The ChEMBL database in 2017. *Nucleic Acids Research* 45 (D1): D945–D954. https://doi.org/10.1093/nar/gkw1074.

52 Gilmer, J., Schoenholz, S.S., Riley, P.F. et al. (2017). Neural message passing for quantum chemistry. *International Conference on Machine Learning* 70: 1263–1272.

53 Gilson, M.K., Liu, T., Baitaluk, M. et al. (2016). BindingDB in 2015: A public database for medicinal chemistry, computational chemistry and systems pharmacology. *Nucleic Acids Research* 44 (D1): D1045–D1053. https://doi.org/10.1093/nar/gkv1072.

54 Goh, G.B., Hodas, N.O., Siegel, C., & Vishnu, A. (2017). Smiles2vec: An interpretable general-purpose deep neural network for predicting chemical properties. arXiv Preprint arXiv:1712.02034.

55 Goh, G.B., Siegel, C., Vishnu, A., Hodas, N.O., & Baker, N. (2017). Chemception: a deep neural network with minimal chemistry knowledge matches the performance of expert-developed QSAR/QSPR models (arXiv:1706.06689). arXiv. https://doi.org/10.48550/arXiv.1706.06689

56 Gómez-Bombarelli, R., Wei, J.N., Duvenaud, D. et al. (2018). Automatic chemical design using a data-driven continuous representation of molecules. *ACS Central Science* 4 (2): 268–276. https://doi.org/10.1021/acscentsci.7b00572.

57 Goodfellow, I., Bengio, Y., and Courville, A. (2016). *Deep Learning*. MIT Press.

58 Goodfellow, I., Pouget-Abadie, J., Mirza, M. et al. (2014). Generative adversarial nets. *Advances in Neural Information Processing Systems* 27: https://doi.org/10.1145/3422622.

59 Graves, A., Wayne, G., Reynolds, M. et al. (2016). Hybrid computing using a neural network with dynamic external memory. *Nature* 538 (7626): https://doi.org/10.1038/nature20101.

60 Grechishnikova, D. (2021). Transformer neural network for protein-specific de novo drug generation as a machine translation problem. *Scientific Reports* 11 (1): 321.

61 Guimaraes, G.L., Sanchez-Lengeling, B., Outeiral, C., et al. (2018). Objective-reinforced generative adversarial networks (ORGAN) for sequence generation models (arXiv:1705.10843). arXiv. https://doi.org/10.48550/arXiv.1705.10843

62 Günther, S., Kuhn, M., Dunkel, M. et al. (2008). SuperTarget and Matador: Resources for exploring drug-target relationships. *Nucleic Acids Research* 36 (suppl_1): D919–D922. https://doi.org/10.1093/nar/gkm862.

63 He, K., Zhang, X., Ren, S., & Sun, J. (2016). Deep Residual Learning for Image Recognition. 2016 IEEE Conference on Computer Vision and Pattern Recognition (CVPR), pp. 770–778, Las Vegas, NV (27-30 June 2016). IEEE.

64 Hochreiter, S. and Schmidhuber, J. (1997). Long short-term memory. *Neural Computation* 9 (8): 1735–1780.

65 Hofmarcher, M., Rumetshofer, E., Clevert, D.-A. et al. (2019). Accurate prediction of biological assays with high-throughput microscopy images and convolutional networks. *Journal of Chemical Information and Modeling* 59 (3): 1163–1171. https://doi.org/10.1021/acs.jcim.8b00670.

66 Honda, S., Akita, H., Ishiguro, K., et al. (2019). Graph residual flow for molecular graph generation. arXiv Preprint arXiv:1909.13521.

67 Honda, S., Shi, S., & Ueda, H. R. (2019). Smiles transformer: Pre-trained molecular fingerprint for low data drug discovery. arXiv Preprint arXiv:1911.04738.

68 Hossain, M.D.Z., Sohel, F., Shiratuddin, M.F., and Laga, H. (2019). A comprehensive survey of deep learning for image captioning. *ACM Computing Surveys* 51 (6): 1, 36–118. https://doi.org/10.1145/3295748.

69 Hsu, S.T., Moon, C., Jones, P., and Samatova, N. (2018). An interpretable generative adversarial approach to classification of latent entity relations in unstructured sentences. *Proceedings of the AAAI Conference on Artificial Intelligence* 32 (1): https://doi.org/10.1609/aaai.v32i1.11972.

70 Huang, G., Liu, Z., van der Maaten, L., & Weinberger, K. Q. (2017). Densely connected convolutional networks. 2017 IEEE Conference on Computer Vision and Pattern Recognition (CVPR), pp. 4700–4708, Honolulu, HI (21–26 July 2017). IEEE.

71 Irwin, J.J. (2008). Community benchmarks for virtual screening. *Journal of Computer-Aided Molecular Design* 22: 193–199.

72 Ivanenkov, Y.A., Polykovskiy, D., Bezrukov, D. et al. (2023). Chemistry42: An AI-driven platform for molecular design and optimization. *Journal of Chemical Information and Modeling* 63 (3): 695–701.

73 Jiang, D., Wu, Z., Hsieh, C.-Y. et al. (2021). Could graph neural networks learn better molecular representation for drug discovery? A comparison study of descriptor-based and graph-based models. *Journal of Cheminformatics* 13: 1–23.

74 Jiménez-Luna, J., Grisoni, F., and Schneider, G. (2020). Drug discovery with explainable artificial intelligence. *Nature Machine Intelligence* 2 (10): 573–584.

75 Jin, J., Wang, D., Shi, G. et al. (2023). FFLOM: A flow-based autoregressive model for fragment-to-lead optimization. *Journal of Medicinal Chemistry* 66 (15): 10808–10823.

76 Jin, W., Barzilay, R., and Jaakkola, T. (2018). Junction tree variational autoencoder for molecular graph generation. *Proceedings of the 35th International Conference on Machine Learning*, 2323–2332. https://proceedings.mlr.press/v80/jin18a.html

77 Jin, W., Barzilay, R., and Jaakkola, T. (2020a). Hierarchical generation of molecular graphs using structural motifs. *International Conference on Machine Learning*, 4839–4848.

78 Jin, W., Barzilay, R., and Jaakkola, T. (2020b). Multi-objective molecule generation using interpretable substructures. *International Conference on Machine Learning*, 4849–4859.

79 Joo, S., Kim, M.S., Yang, J., and Park, J. (2020). Generative model for proposing drug candidates satisfying anticancer properties using a conditional variational autoencoder. *ACS Omega* 5 (30): 18642–18650.

80 Kadurin, A., Nikolenko, S., Khrabrov, K. et al. (2017). druGAN: an advanced generative adversarial autoencoder model for de novo generation of new molecules with desired molecular properties in silico. *Molecular Pharmaceutics* 14 (9): 3098–3104.

81 Kajino, H. (2019). Molecular hypergraph grammar with its application to molecular optimization. *International Conference on Machine Learning*, 3183–3191.

82 Kanehisa, M., Furumichi, M., Tanabe, M. et al. (2017). KEGG: new perspectives on genomes, pathways, diseases and drugs. *Nucleic Acids Research* 45 (D1): D353–D361.

83 Kang, S. and Cho, K. (2018). Conditional molecular design with deep generative models. *Journal of Chemical Information and Modeling* 59 (1): 43–52.

84 Kearnes, S., McCloskey, K., Berndl, M. et al. (2016). Molecular graph convolutions: moving beyond fingerprints. *Journal of Computer-Aided Molecular Design* 30: 595–608.

85 Khemchandani, Y., O'Hagan, S., Samanta, S. et al. (2020). DeepGraphMolGen, a multi-objective, computational strategy for generating molecules with desirable properties: A graph convolution and reinforcement learning approach. *Journal of Cheminformatics* 12: 1–17.

86 Kim, S., Chen, J., Cheng, T. et al. (2019). PubChem 2019 update: Improved access to chemical data. *Nucleic Acids Research* 47 (D1): D1102–D1109. https://doi.org/10.1093/nar/gky1033.

87 Kingma, D.P. and Dhariwal, P. (2018). Glow: Generative flow with invertible 1x1 convolutions. *Advances in Neural Information Processing Systems*, 31.

88 Kingma, D.P. and Welling, M. (2013). Auto-encoding variational bayes. arXiv Preprint arXiv:1312.6114.

89 Klingler, F.-M., Gastreich, M., Grygorenko, O.O. et al. (2019). SAR by space: enriching hit sets from the chemical space. *Molecules* 24 (17): https://doi.org/10.3390/molecules24173096.

90 Kobyzev, I., Prince, S.J.D., and Brubaker, M.A. (2021). Normalizing flows: an introduction and review of current methods. *IEEE Transactions on Pattern Analysis and Machine Intelligence* 43 (11): 3964–3979. https://doi.org/10.1109/TPAMI.2020.2992934.

91 Korkmaz, S. (2020). Deep learning-based imbalanced data classification for drug discovery. *Journal of Chemical Information and Modeling* 60 (9): 4180–4190.

92 Krenn, M., Häse, F., Nigam, A. et al. (2020). Self-referencing embedded strings (SELFIES): A 100% robust molecular string representation. *Machine Learning: Science and Technology* 1 (4): 045024. https://doi.org/10.1088/2632-2153/aba947.

93 Krizhevsky, A., Sutskever, I., and Hinton, G.E. (2012). ImageNet classification with deep convolutional neural networks. Advances in Neural Information

Processing Systems, 25. https://proceedings.neurips.cc/paper/2012/hash/c399862d3b9d6b76c8436e924a68c45b-Abstract.html

94 Kuhn, M., Letunic, I., Jensen, L.J., and Bork, P. (2016). The SIDER database of drugs and side effects. *Nucleic Acids Research* 44 (D1): D1075–D1079. https://doi.org/10.1093/nar/gkv1075.

95 Kusner, M.J., Paige, B., and Hernández-Lobato, J. M. (2017). Grammar variational autoencoder. *International Conference on Machine Learning*, 1945–1954. http://proceedings.mlr.press/v70/kusner17a.html?ref=https://githubhelp.com

96 Kuznetsov, M. and Polykovskiy, D. (2021). MolGrow: A graph normalizing flow for hierarchical molecular generation. *Proceedings of the AAAI Conference on Artificial Intelligence* 35 (9): 8226–8234.

97 Kwon, Y., Lee, D., Choi, Y.-S. et al. (2020). Compressed graph representation for scalable molecular graph generation. *Journal of Cheminformatics* 12: 1–8.

98 Lavecchia, A. (2015). Machine-learning approaches in drug discovery: methods and applications. *Drug Discovery Today* 20 (3): 318–331.

99 Lavecchia, A. (2019). Deep learning in drug discovery: opportunities, challenges and future prospects. *Drug Discovery Today* 24 (10): 2017–2032.

100 LeCun, Y., Bengio, Y., and Hinton, G. (2015). Deep learning. *Nature* 521 (7553): 436–444. https://doi.org/10.1038/nature14539.

101 Lee, M. and Min, K. (2022). MGCVAE: multi-objective inverse design via molecular graph conditional variational autoencoder. *Journal of Chemical Information and Modeling* 62 (12): 2943–2950.

102 Li, G., Muller, M., Thabet, A., and Ghanem, B. (2019). Deepgcns: Can gcns go as deep as cnns? *Proceedings of the IEEE/CVF International Conference on Computer Vision*, 9267–9276. http://openaccess.thecvf.com/content_ICCV_2019/html/Li_DeepGCNs_Can_GCNs_Go_As_Deep_As_CNNs_ICCV_2019_paper.html

103 Li, Y., Hu, J., Wang, Y. et al. (2019). DeepScaffold: A comprehensive tool for scaffold-based de novo drug discovery using deep learning. *Journal of Chemical Information and Modeling* 60 (1): 77–91.

104 Li, Y., Tarlow, D., Brockschmidt, M., & Zemel, R. (2015). Gated graph sequence neural networks. arXiv Preprint arXiv:1511.05493.

105 Li, Y., Vinyals, O., Dyer, C., et al. (2018). Learning deep generative models of graphs. arXiv Preprint arXiv:1803.03324.

106 Li, Y., Zhang, L., and Liu, Z. (2018). Multi-objective de novo drug design with conditional graph generative model. *Journal of Cheminformatics* 10 (1): 33. https://doi.org/10.1186/s13321-018-0287-6.

107 Lim, J., Hwang, S.-Y., Moon, S. et al. (2020). Scaffold-based molecular design with a graph generative model. *Chemical Science* 11 (4): 1153–1164.

108 Lim, J., Ryu, S., Kim, J.W., and Kim, W.Y. (2018). Molecular generative model based on conditional variational autoencoder for de novo molecular design.

Journal of Cheminformatics 10 (1): 31. https://doi.org/10.1186/s13321-018-0286-7.

109 Lin, J., Pang, Y., Xia, Y., (2020). Tuigan: Learning versatile image-to-image translation with two unpaired images. *Computer Vision–ECCV 2020: 16th European Conference*, pp. 18–35, Glasgow, UK, (23–28 August 2020), Proceedings, Part IV 16.

110 Lin, T., Wang, Y., Liu, X., and Qiu, X. (2022). A survey of transformers. *AI Open* 3: 111–132.

111 Liu, K., Sun, X., Jia, L. et al. (2019). Chemi-Net: A molecular graph convolutional network for accurate drug property prediction. *International Journal of Molecular Sciences* 20 (14): 3389.

112 Liu, Q., Allamanis, M., Brockschmidt, M., & Gaunt, A.L. (2019). Constrained graph variational autoencoders for molecule design (arXiv:1805.09076). arXiv. https://doi.org/10.48550/arXiv.1805.09076

113 Liu, Z., Li, Y., Han, L. et al. (2015). PDB-wide collection of binding data: Current status of the PDBbind database. *Bioinformatics* 31 (3): 405–412. https://doi.org/10.1093/bioinformatics/btu626.

114 Lopez, S.A., Pyzer-Knapp, E.O., Simm, G.N. et al. (2016). The Harvard organic photovoltaic dataset. *Scientific Data* 3 (1): 1–7.

115 Lundberg, S.M., and Lee, S.-I. (2017). A unified approach to interpreting model predictions. *Advances in Neural Information Processing Systems*, 30.

116 Ma, H., Bian, Y., Rong, Y., et al. (2020). Multi-view graph neural networks for molecular property prediction. arXiv Preprint arXiv:2005.13607.

117 Ma, T., Chen, J., & Xiao, C. (2018). Constrained generation of semantically valid graphs via regularizing variational autoencoders (arXiv:1809.02630). arXiv. https://doi.org/10.48550/arXiv.1809.02630

118 Madhawa, K., Ishiguro, K., Nakago, K., & Abe, M. (2019). GraphNVP: An Invertible Flow Model for Generating Molecular Graphs (arXiv:1905.11600). arXiv. https://doi.org/10.48550/arXiv.1905.11600

119 Makhzani, A., Shlens, J., Jaitly, N., et al. (2015). Adversarial autoencoders. arXiv Preprint arXiv:1511.05644.

120 Mamoshina, P., Vieira, A., Putin, E., and Zhavoronkov, A. (2016). Applications of deep learning in biomedicine. *Molecular Pharmaceutics* 13 (5): 1445–1454.

121 Markham, A. (2021). Evinacumab: first approval. *Drugs* 81 (9): 1101–1105.

122 Mayr, A., Klambauer, G., Unterthiner, T. et al. (2018). Large-scale comparison of machine learning methods for drug target prediction on ChEMBL. *Chemical Science* 9 (24): 5441–5451.

123 Mercado, R., Rastemo, T., Lindelöf, E. et al. (2020). Practical notes on building molecular graph generative models. *Applied AI Letters* 1 (2).

124 Mercado, R., Rastemo, T., Lindelöf, E. et al. (2021). Graph networks for molecular design. *Machine Learning: Science and Technology* 2 (2): 025023.

125 Meyer, J.G., Liu, S., Miller, I.J. et al. (2019). Learning drug functions from chemical structures with convolutional neural networks and random forests. *Journal of Chemical Information and Modeling* 59 (10): 4438–4449. https://doi.org/10.1021/acs.jcim.9b00236.

126 Miller, M., Tokgozoglu, L., Parhofer, K.G. et al. (2022). Icosapent ethyl for reduction of persistent cardiovascular risk: a critical review of major medical society guidelines and statements. *Expert Review of Cardiovascular Therapy* 20 (8): 609–625.

127 Morgan, H.L. (1965). The generation of a unique machine description for chemical structures-a technique developed at chemical abstracts service. *Journal of Chemical Documentation* 5 (2): 107–113.

128 Mosqueira-Rey, E., Hernández-Pereira, E., Alonso-Ríos, D. et al. (2023). Human-in-the-loop machine learning: a state of the art. *Artificial Intelligence Review* 56 (4): 3005–3054.

129 Mullard, A. (2014). New drugs cost US $2.6 billion to develop. *Nature Reviews Drug Discovery* 13 (12): 877–877.

130 Mysinger, M.M., Carchia, M., Irwin, J.J., and Shoichet, B.K. (2012). Directory of useful decoys, enhanced (DUD-E): Better ligands and decoys for better benchmarking. *Journal of Medicinal Chemistry* 55 (14): 6582–6594.

131 Neil, D., Segler, M., Guasch, L. et al. (2018). Exploring deep recurrent models with reinforcement learning for molecule design. In *6th International Conference on Learning Representations.*

132 O'Boyle, N., & Dalke, A. (2018). DeepSMILES: An adaptation of SMILES for use in machine-learning of chemical structures. ChemRxiv. https://doi.org/10.26434/chemrxiv.7097960.v1

133 Olah, M., Rad, R., Ostopovici, L. et al. (2007). WOMBAT and WOMBAT-PK: Bioactivity Databases for Lead and Drug Discovery. In: *Chemical Biology* (ed. S.L. Schreiber, T.M. Kapoor, and G. Wess), 760–786. John Wiley & Sons, Ltd. https://doi.org/10.1002/9783527619375.ch13b.

134 Olivecrona, M., Blaschke, T., Engkvist, O., and Chen, H. (2017). Molecular de-novo design through deep reinforcement learning. *Journal of Cheminformatics* 9 (1): 48. https://doi.org/10.1186/s13321-017-0235-x.

135 OpenAI, Achiam, J., Adler, S., et al. (2024). GPT-4 Technical Report (arXiv:2303.08774). arXiv. https://doi.org/10.48550/arXiv.2303.08774

136 Papamakarios, G., Pavlakou, T., and Murray, I. (2017). Masked autoregressive flow for density estimation. *Advances in Neural Information Processing Systems*, 30.

137 Pedregosa, F., Varoquaux, G., Gramfort, A. et al. (2011). Scikit-learn: Machine learning in Python. *The Journal of Machine Learning Research* 12: 2825–2830.

138 Plummer, R., Dean, E., Arkenau, H.-T. et al. (2022). A phase 1b study evaluating the safety and preliminary efficacy of berzosertib in combination with gemcitabine in patients with advanced non-small cell lung cancer. *Lung Cancer* 163: 19–26.

139 Polanski, J. (2022). Unsupervised learning in drug design from self-organization to deep chemistry. *International Journal of Molecular Sciences* 23 (5): 2797.

140 Polykovskiy, D., Zhebrak, A., Sanchez-Lengeling, B. et al. (2020). Molecular sets (MOSES): A benchmarking platform for molecular generation models. *Frontiers in Pharmacology* 11: 565644.

141 Polykovskiy, D., Zhebrak, A., Vetrov, D. et al. (2018). Entangled conditional adversarial autoencoder for de novo drug discovery. *Molecular Pharmaceutics* 15 (10): 4398–4405. https://doi.org/10.1021/acs.molpharmaceut.8b00839.

142 Popova, M., Isayev, O., and Tropsha, A. (2018). Deep reinforcement learning for de-novo drug design. *Science Advances* 4 (7): eaap7885. https://doi.org/10.1126/sciadv.aap7885.

143 Popova, M., Shvets, M., Oliva, J., & Isayev, O. (2019). MolecularRNN: Generating realistic molecular graphs with optimized properties (arXiv:1905.13372). arXiv. https://doi.org/10.48550/arXiv.1905.13372

144 Preuer, K., Renz, P., Unterthiner, T. et al. (2018). Fréchet ChemNet distance: A metric for generative models for molecules in drug discovery. *Journal of Chemical Information and Modeling* 58 (9): 1736–1741.

145 Prykhodko, O., Johansson, S.V., Kotsias, P.-C. et al. (2019). A de novo molecular generation method using latent vector based generative adversarial network. *Journal of Cheminformatics* 11 (1): 74. https://doi.org/10.1186/s13321-019-0397-9.

146 Putin, E., Asadulaev, A., Ivanenkov, Y. et al. (2018). Reinforced adversarial neural computer for de novo molecular design. *Journal of Chemical Information and Modeling* 58 (6): 1194–1204. https://doi.org/10.1021/acs.jcim.7b00690.

147 Putin, E., Asadulaev, A., Vanhaelen, Q. et al. (2018). Adversarial threshold neural computer for molecular de novo design. *Molecular Pharmaceutics* 15 (10): 4386–4397. https://doi.org/10.1021/acs.molpharmaceut.7b01137.

148 Qiu, J., Xie, J., Su, S. et al. (2022). Selective functionalization of hindered meta-C–H bond of o-alkylaryl ketones promoted by automation and deep learning. *Chem* 8 (12): 3275–3287.

149 Rajan, K., Brinkhaus, H.O., Sorokina, M. et al. (2021). DECIMER-Segmentation: automated extraction of chemical structure depictions from scientific literature. *Journal of Cheminformatics* 13 (1): 20. https://doi.org/10.1186/s13321-021-00496-1.

150 Rajan, K., Zielesny, A., and Steinbeck, C. (2020). DECIMER: towards deep learning for chemical image recognition. *Journal of Cheminformatics* 12 (1): 65. https://doi.org/10.1186/s13321-020-00469-w.

151 Réau, M., Langenfeld, F., Zagury, J.-F. et al. (2018). Decoys selection in benchmarking datasets: overview and perspectives. *Frontiers in Pharmacology* 9: 328937.

152 Ren, F., Ding, X., Zheng, M. et al. (2023). AlphaFold accelerates artificial intelligence powered drug discovery: efficient discovery of a novel CDK20 small molecule inhibitor. *Chemical Science* 14 (6): 1443–1452.

153 Ribeiro, M.T., Singh, S., and Guestrin, C. (2016). "Why should i trust you?" Explaining the predictions of any classifier. *Proceedings of the 22nd ACM SIGKDD International Conference on Knowledge Discovery and Data Mining*, 1135–1144.

154 Riddick, G., Song, H., Ahn, S. et al. (2011). Predicting in vitro drug sensitivity using Random Forests. *Bioinformatics* 27 (2): 220–224.

155 Rifaioglu, A.S., Atas, H., Martin, M.J. et al. (2019). Recent applications of deep learning and machine intelligence on in silico drug discovery: Methods, tools and databases. *Briefings in Bioinformatics* 20 (5): 1878–1912.

156 Rogers, D. and Hahn, M. (2010). Extended-connectivity fingerprints. *Journal of Chemical Information and Modeling* 50 (5): 742–754.

157 Rohrer, S.G. and Baumann, K. (2009). Maximum unbiased validation (MUV) data sets for virtual screening based on PubChem bioactivity data. *Journal of Chemical Information and Modeling* 49 (2): 169–184.

158 Romanelli, V., Cerchia, C., and Lavecchia, A. (2024). Unlocking the potential of generative artificial intelligence in drug discovery. In: *Applications of Generative AI* (ed. Z. Lyu), 37–63. Springer.

159 Rong, Y., Bian, Y., Xu, T., et al. (2020). Grover: Self-supervised message passing transformer on large-scale molecular data. arXiv Preprint arXiv:2007.02835, 2(3), 17.

160 Ruddigkeit, L., Van Deursen, R., Blum, L.C., and Reymond, J.-L. (2012). Enumeration of 166 billion organic small molecules in the chemical universe database GDB-17. *Journal of Chemical Information and Modeling* 52 (11): 2864–2875.

161 Salimans, T., Goodfellow, I., Zaremba, W., et al. (2016). Improved techniques for training gans. *Advances in Neural Information Processing Systems*, 29.

162 Samanta, B., De, A., Jana, G., et al. (2019). NeVAE: A deep generative model for molecular graphs (arXiv:1802.05283). arXiv. https://doi.org/10.48550/arXiv.1802.05283

163 Sanchez-Lengeling, B., Outeiral, C., Guimaraes, G.L., & Aspuru-Guzik, A. (2017a). Optimizing distributions over molecular space. An Objective-

Reinforced Generative Adversarial Network for Inverse-design Chemistry (ORGANIC). ChemRxiv. https://doi.org/10.26434/chemrxiv.5309668.v3

164 Sanchez-Lengeling, B., Outeiral, C., Guimaraes, G. L., & Aspuru-Guzik, A. (2017b). Optimizing distributions over molecular space. An objective-reinforced generative adversarial network for inverse-design chemistry (ORGANIC). https://chemrxiv.org/engage/chemrxiv/article-details/60c73d91702a9beea7189bc2

165 Sattarov, B., Baskin, I.I., Horvath, D. et al. (2019). De novo molecular design by combining deep autoencoder recurrent neural networks with generative topographic mapping. *Journal of Chemical Information and Modeling* 59 (3): 1182–1196. https://doi.org/10.1021/acs.jcim.8b00751.

166 Scarselli, F., Gori, M., Tsoi, A.C. et al. (2008). The graph neural network model. *IEEE Transactions on Neural Networks* 20 (1): 61–80.

167 Schneider, G. (2018). Automating drug discovery. *Nature Reviews Drug Discovery* 17 (2): 97–113.

168 Schneider, P., Walters, W.P., Plowright, A.T. et al. (2020). Rethinking drug design in the artificial intelligence era. *Nature Reviews Drug Discovery* 19 (5): 353–364. https://doi.org/10.1038/s41573-019-0050-3.

169 Schroeter, T., Schwaighofer, A., Mika, S. et al. (2007). Machine learning models for lipophilicity and their domain of applicability. *Molecular Pharmaceutics* 4 (4): 524–538.

170 Schulman, J., Levine, S., Abbeel, P., et al. (2015). Trust region policy optimization. *Proceedings of the 32nd International Conference on Machine Learning*, 1889–1897. https://proceedings.mlr.press/v37/schulman15.html

171 Schulman, J., Wolski, F., Dhariwal, P., et al. (2017). Proximal policy optimization algorithms (arXiv:1707.06347). arXiv. https://doi.org/10.48550/arXiv.1707.06347

172 Schütt, K., Kindermans, P.-J., Sauceda Felix, H.E., et al. (2017). Schnet: A continuous-filter convolutional neural network for modeling quantum interactions. *Advances in Neural Information Processing Systems*, 30.

173 Segler, M.H.S., Kogej, T., Tyrchan, C., and Waller, M.P. (2018). Generating focused molecule libraries for drug discovery with recurrent neural networks. *ACS Central Science* 4 (1): 120–131. https://doi.org/10.1021/acscentsci.7b00512.

174 Shen, W.X., Zeng, X., Zhu, F. et al. (2021). Out-of-the-box deep learning prediction of pharmaceutical properties by broadly learned knowledge-based molecular representations. *Nature Machine Intelligence* 3 (4): 334–343.

175 Sheng, N., Cui, H., Zhang, T., and Xuan, P. (2021). Attentional multi-level representation encoding based on convolutional and variance autoencoders for lncRNA–disease association prediction. *Briefings in Bioinformatics* 22 (3): 1–14. https://doi.org/10.1093/bib/bbaa067.

176 Shi, C., Xu, M., Zhu, Z., et al. (2020). GraphAF: A flow-based autoregressive model for molecular graph generation (arXiv:2001.09382). arXiv. https://doi.org/10.48550/arXiv.2001.09382

177 Shin, B., Park, S., Kang, K., and Ho, J.C. (2019). Self-attention based molecule representation for predicting drug-target interaction. *Machine Learning for Healthcare Conference*, 230–248.

178 Simonovsky, M. and Komodakis, N. (2018). GraphVAE: towards generation of small graphs using variational autoencoders (arXiv:1802.03480). arXiv. https://doi.org/10.48550/arXiv.1802.03480

179 Simonyan, K., and Zisserman, A. (2015). Very deep convolutional networks for large-scale image recognition (arXiv:1409.1556). arXiv. https://doi.org/10.48550/arXiv.1409.1556

180 Singh, R., Sledzieski, S., Bryson, B. et al. (2023). Contrastive learning in protein language space predicts interactions between drugs and protein targets. *Proceedings of the National Academy of Sciences* 120 (24): e2220778120.

181 Song, T., Zhang, X., Ding, M. et al. (2022). DeepFusion: A deep learning based multi-scale feature fusion method for predicting drug-target interactions. *Methods* 204: 269–277.

182 Srinivasan, S., Batra, R., Chan, H. et al. (2021). Artificial intelligence-guided De novo molecular design targeting COVID-19. *ACS Omega* 6 (19): 12557–12566.

183 Ståhl, N., Falkman, G., Karlsson, A. et al. (2019). Deep reinforcement learning for multiparameter optimization in de novo drug design. *Journal of Chemical Information and Modeling* 59 (7): 3166–3176. https://doi.org/10.1021/acs.jcim.9b00325.

184 Staker, J., Marshall, K., Abel, R., and McQuaw, C.M. (2019). Molecular structure extraction from documents using deep learning. *Journal of Chemical Information and Modeling* 59 (3): 1017–1029. https://doi.org/10.1021/acs.jcim.8b00669.

185 Steinbeck, C., Han, Y., Kuhn, S. et al. (2003). The Chemistry Development Kit (CDK): An open-source Java library for chemo-and bioinformatics. *Journal of Chemical Information and Computer Sciences* 43 (2): 493–500.

186 Steiner, B., DeVito, Z., Chintala, S., et al. (2019). Pytorch: An imperative style, high-performance deep learning library.

187 Sterling, T. and Irwin, J.J. (2015). ZINC 15–ligand discovery for everyone. *Journal of Chemical Information and Modeling* 55 (11): 2324–2337.

188 Stokes, J.M., Yang, K., Swanson, K. et al. (2020). A deep learning approach to antibiotic discovery. *Cell* 180 (4): 688–702. e13.

189 Stumpfe, D., Hu, Y., Dimova, D., and Bajorath, J. (2014). Recent progress in understanding activity cliffs and their utility in medicinal chemistry: Miniperspective. *Journal of Medicinal Chemistry* 57 (1): 18–28.

190 Subramanian, A., Narayan, R., Corsello, S.M. et al. (2017). A next generation connectivity map: L1000 platform and the first 1,000,000 profiles. *Cell* 171 (6): 1437–1452. e17.

191 Sun, J., Jeliazkova, N., Chupakhin, V. et al. (2017). ExCAPE-DB: an integrated large scale dataset facilitating big data analysis in chemogenomics. *Journal of Cheminformatics* 9: 1–9.

192 Sureyya Rifaioglu, A., Nalbat, E., Atalay, V. et al. (2020). DEEPScreen: High performance drug–target interaction prediction with convolutional neural networks using 2-D structural compound representations. *Chemical Science* 11 (9): 2531–2557. https://doi.org/10.1039/C9SC03414E.

193 Sutton, R.S. and Barto, A.G. (2018). *Reinforcement Learning: An Introduction*, 2e. MIT Press.

194 Svoboda, D.L., Saddler, T., and Auerbach, S.S. (2019). An overview of national toxicology program's toxicogenomic applications: DrugMatrix and ToxFX. In: *Advances in Computational Toxicology: Methodologies and Applications in Regulatory Science* (ed. H. Hong), 141–157. Springer International Publishing https://doi.org/10.1007/978-3-030-16443-0_8.

195 Szklarczyk, D., Santos, A., Von Mering, C. et al. (2016). STITCH 5: Augmenting protein–chemical interaction networks with tissue and affinity data. *Nucleic Acids Research* 44 (D1): D380–D384.

196 Terranova, N., Jansen, M., Falk, M., and Hendriks, B.S. (2021). Population pharmacokinetics of ATR inhibitor berzosertib in phase I studies for different cancer types. *Cancer Chemotherapy and Pharmacology* 87: 185–196.

197 Thompson, C.M., Johns, D.O., Sonawane, B. et al. (2009). Database for physiologically based pharmacokinetic (PBPK) modeling: physiological data for healthy and health-impaired elderly. *Journal of Toxicology and Environmental Health, Part B* 12 (1): 1–24. https://doi.org/10.1080/10937400802545060.

198 Thorn, C.F., Klein, T.E., and Altman, R.B. (2010). Pharmacogenomics and bioinformatics: PharmGKB. *Pharmacogenomics* 11 (4): 501–505. https://doi.org/10.2217/pgs.10.15.

199 Tian, S., Li, Y., Wang, J. et al. (2011). ADME evaluation in drug discovery. 9. Prediction of oral bioavailability in humans based on molecular properties and structural fingerprints. *Molecular Pharmaceutics* 8 (3): 841–851.

200 Todeschini, R. and Consonni, V. (2009). *Molecular Descriptors for Chemoinformatics: Volume I: Alphabetical Listing/Volume II: Appendices, References*. John Wiley & Sons.

201 Tran-Nguyen, V.-K., Jacquemard, C., and Rognan, D. (2020). LIT-PCBA: an unbiased data set for machine learning and virtual screening. *Journal of Chemical Information and Modeling* 60 (9): 4263–4273.

202 van Tilborg, D., Alenicheva, A., and Grisoni, F. (2022). Exposing the limitations of molecular machine learning with activity cliffs. *Journal of Chemical Information and Modeling* 62 (23): 5938–5951.

203 Vaswani, A., Shazeer, N., Parmar, N., et al. (2017). Attention is all you need. *Advances in Neural Information Processing Systems*, 30.

204 Veličković, P., Cucurull, G., Casanova, A., et al. (2017). Graph attention networks. arXiv Preprint arXiv:1710.10903.

205 Walters, W.P. and Barzilay, R. (2021). Critical assessment of AI in drug discovery. *Expert Opinion on Drug Discovery* 16 (9): 937–947.

206 Walters, W.P. and Murcko, M. (2020). Assessing the impact of generative AI on medicinal chemistry. *Nature Biotechnology* 38 (2): 143–145.

207 Walters, W.P. and Murcko, M.A. (2002). Prediction of 'drug-likeness'. *Advanced Drug Delivery Reviews* 54 (3): 255–271.

208 Wang, K., Xiao, J., Liu, X. et al. (2019). AICD: An integrated anti-inflammatory compounds database for drug discovery. *Scientific Reports* 9 (1): 7737. https://doi.org/10.1038/s41598-019-44227-x.

209 Wang, L., Ding, J., Pan, L. et al. (2019). Artificial intelligence facilitates drug design in the big data era. *Chemometrics and Intelligent Laboratory Systems* 194: 103850.

210 Wang, S., Guo, Y., Wang, Y., et al. (2019). Smiles-bert: Large scale unsupervised pre-training for molecular property prediction. *Proceedings of the 10th ACM International Conference on Bioinformatics, Computational Biology and Health Informatics*, 429–436.

211 Weininger, D. (1988). SMILES, a chemical language and information system. 1. Introduction to methodology and encoding rules. *Journal of Chemical Information and Computer Sciences* 28 (1): 31–36. https://doi.org/10.1021/ci00057a005.

212 Williams, R.J. (1992). Simple statistical gradient-following algorithms for connectionist reinforcement learning. *Machine Learning* 8 (3): 229–256. https://doi.org/10.1007/BF00992696.

213 Wishart, D.S., Feunang, Y.D., Guo, A.C. et al. (2018). DrugBank 5.0: A major update to the DrugBank database for 2018. *Nucleic Acids Research* 46 (D1): D1074–D1082. https://doi.org/10.1093/nar/gkx1037.

214 Wishart, D.S., Guo, A., Oler, E. et al. (2022). HMDB 5.0: The human metabolome database for 2022. *Nucleic Acids Research* 50 (D1): D622–D631. https://doi.org/10.1093/nar/gkab1062.

215 Withnall, M., Lindelöf, E., Engkvist, O., and Chen, H. (2020). Building attention and edge message passing neural networks for bioactivity and physical–chemical property prediction. *Journal of Cheminformatics* 12 (1): 1.

216 Woodward, D.J., Bradley, A.R., and van Hoorn, W.P. (2022). Coverage score: a model agnostic method to efficiently explore chemical space. *Journal of Chemical Information and Modeling* 62 (18): 4391–4402.

217 Wu, Z., Pan, S., Chen, F. et al. (2020). A comprehensive survey on graph neural networks. *IEEE Transactions on Neural Networks and Learning Systems* 32 (1): 4–24.

218 Wu, Z., Ramsundar, B., Feinberg, E.N. et al. (2018). MoleculeNet: A benchmark for molecular machine learning. *Chemical Science* 9 (2): 513–530.

219 Xia, J., Jin, H., Liu, Z. et al. (2014). An unbiased method to build benchmarking sets for ligand-based virtual screening and its application to GPCRs. *Journal of Chemical Information and Modeling* 54 (5): 1433–1450.

220 Xia, X., Hu, J., Wang, Y. et al. (2019). Graph-based generative models for de Novo drug design. *Drug Discovery Today: Technologies* 32–33: 45–53. https://doi.org/10.1016/j.ddtec.2020.11.004.

221 Xie, Y., Xu, Z., Ma, J., and Mei, Q. (2021). How much space has been explored? Measuring the chemical space covered by databases and machine-generated molecules. arXiv Preprint arXiv:2112.12542.

222 Xiong, Z., Wang, D., Liu, X. et al. (2019). Pushing the boundaries of molecular representation for drug discovery with the graph attention mechanism. *Journal of Medicinal Chemistry* 63 (16): 8749–8760.

223 Xu, C., Liu, Q., Huang, M., and Jiang, T. (2020). Reinforced molecular optimization with neighborhood-controlled grammars. *Advances in Neural Information Processing Systems* 33: 8366–8377.

224 Yang, K., Swanson, K., Jin, W. et al. (2019). Analyzing learned molecular representations for property prediction. *Journal of Chemical Information and Modeling* 59 (8): 3370–3388.

225 Yang, X., Zhang, J., Yoshizoe, K. et al. (2017). ChemTS: an efficient python library for de novo molecular generation. *Science and Technology of Advanced Materials* 18 (1): 972–976.

226 You, J., Liu, B., Ying, R., et al. (2019). graph convolutional policy network for goal-directed molecular graph generation (arXiv:1806.02473). arXiv. https://doi.org/10.48550/arXiv.1806.02473

227 You, J., Liu, B., Ying, Z., et al. (2018). Graph convolutional policy network for goal-directed molecular graph generation. *Advances in Neural Information Processing Systems*, 31.

228 You, J., Ying, R., Ren, X., et al. (2018). GraphRNN: generating realistic graphs with deep auto-regressive models. *Proceedings of the 35th International Conference on Machine Learning*, 5708–5717. https://proceedings.mlr.press/v80/you18a.html

229 Yu, Y., Si, X., Hu, C., and Zhang, J. (2019). A review of recurrent neural networks: LSTM cells and network architectures. *Neural Computation* 31 (7): 1235–1270.

230 Zang, C., and Wang, F. (2020). MoFlow: an invertible flow model for generating molecular graphs. *Proceedings of the 26th ACM SIGKDD International Conference on Knowledge Discovery & Data Mining*, 617–626. https://doi.org/10.1145/3394486.3403104

231 Zang, Q., Mansouri, K., Williams, A.J. et al. (2017). In silico prediction of physicochemical properties of environmental chemicals using molecular fingerprints and machine learning. *Journal of Chemical Information and Modeling* 57 (1): 36–49.

232 Zarin, D.A., Tse, T., Williams, R.J. et al. (2011). The ClinicalTrials.gov results database—update and key issues. *New England Journal of Medicine* 364 (9): 852–860. https://doi.org/10.1056/NEJMsa1012065.

233 Zhao, W.X., Zhou, K., Li, J., et al. (2023). A survey of large language models. arXiv Preprint arXiv:2303.18223.

234 Zheng, S., Rao, J., Song, Y. et al. (2021). PharmKG: a dedicated knowledge graph benchmark for bomedical data mining. *Briefings in Bioinformatics* 22 (4): bbaa344.

235 Zheng, S., Yan, X., Yang, Y., and Xu, J. (2019). Identifying structure–property relationships through SMILES syntax analysis with self-attention mechanism. *Journal of Chemical Information and Modeling* 59 (2): 914–923. https://doi.org/10.1021/acs.jcim.8b00803.

236 Zheng, Y., Xu, Z., and Xiao, A. (2023). Deep learning in economics: A systematic and critical review. *Artificial Intelligence Review* 56 (9): 9497–9539. https://doi.org/10.1007/s10462-022-10272-8.

237 Zhou, Z., Kearnes, S., Li, L. et al. (2019). Optimization of molecules via deep reinforcement learning. *Scientific Reports* 9 (1): 10752.

238 Zhu, F., Han, B., Kumar, P. et al. (2010). Update of TTD: therapeutic target database. *Nucleic Acids Research* 38 (suppl_1): D787–D791. https://doi.org/10.1093/nar/gkp1014.

26

Medical Image Analysis and Morphology with Generative Artificial Intelligence for Biomedical and Smart Health Informatics

Dharmendra Dangi[1], Arish Mallick[2], Amit Bhagat[3], and Dheeraj Kumar Dixit[4]

[1] *Indian Institute of Information Technology (IIITB), Bhopal*
[2] *Queens University Belfast, UK*
[3] *Maulana Azad National Institute of Technology (MANIT), Bhopal*
[4] *Madhav Institute of Science and Technology (MITS), Gwalior*

26.1 Introduction

The advancement of processors and the increase in processing speed have always been strongly correlated with the evolution of computer systems. High performance [1] is attained by transistors by combining several chips onto a single chip. However, this strategy is constrained by the physical limitations of silicon, which leads to high energy usage and CPU overheating [2]. Recent developments in this field have led to the development of modern processor architecture, which is utilized for the following purposes:

- General-Purpose Computing on Graphics Processing Units (GPGPU), also known as "many-core architecture"
- Multicore CPUs have more than one processing core.

The many multicore architectures have taken advantage of parallel features that magnify the performance enhancements and lead to more rapid computing.

High-performance computing demands have historically been met by expensive computing equipment. Research fields have evolved tremendously as a result of the decreasing cost of processing systems due to graphics processing units (GPUs) and the advent of concurrent computing approaches. Life sciences [3], scientific modeling [4], statistical modeling [3], ray tracing [3], visualization [3] and digital design automation, signal processing [5], medical image processing and analysis [6–8], and computer vision [9] are a few examples of these fields.

Generative Artificial Intelligence for Biomedical and Smart Health Informatics,
First Edition. Edited by Aditya Khamparia and Deepak Gupta.

Medical imaging facilities help doctors by extracting information for disease diagnosis, surgical operations, therapy, and follow-up on treatments, as well as by helping them develop superior rehabilitation programs. To extract the pertinent clinical information from images and analyze them reliably and consistently in the shortest run-time, advanced computational methods are required.

Enhancing the barely noticeable structural elements to the human eye is one of the many scientific difficulties posed by the quantitative interpretation of the plethora of complex biomedical images. Some methods of enhancing contrast have been developed using rotational morphological processing (RMP), a kind of mathematical morphology. This technique is applied to medical imaging to improve structural aspects.

Structural features are obtained by image processing and are quantitatively quantified in the analysis of images. Contrast enhancement, which automatically extracts structural characteristics those are barely perceptible to the eyes of human, is one of the main components of image processing. Many techniques have been developed for enhancing contrast, such as filtering in the frequency and spatial domains and modifying histograms. Nevertheless, these techniques improved a biomedical image's whole structure without making any distinctions. To properly identify a region of concern, particular structures need to be altered, but the surrounding items should remain unchanged. Mathematical morphology is used in the contrast enhancement technique to enable the selective amplification of specific components. Set theory states that in mathematical morphology, shape data is used in image processing.

Medical picture morphological contrast enhancement techniques have been developed and implemented in a number of ways. A set of morphological operations, where we use tiny visuals as structuring elements, are used to operate mathematical morphology; usually, only one structuring component is utilized. It functions as a moving probe that samples all the pixels in the image. Certain complex images (notably those whose structural features include an array of directional variables) may not process correctly because the structuring components motion in a fixed direction. As such, an artifact in the form of structuring elements may emerge at the periphery of the component. Given that objects in biological imaging are made up of delicate structural characteristics, this limitation is quite significant.

RMP, an expansion of traditional mathematical morphology, is the method used to tackle this problem. This technique's morphological filters are widely used on a broad range of biomedical pictures, including light and electron micrographs, as well as medical imaging like chest X-rays and mammographs.

In this chapter, we will examine an RMP-based contrast enhancement technique. The top-hat contrast operator, an established and often applied morphological operation, is going to be employed in this method to acquire specific characteristics from a low-contrast image. White top-hat (WTH) and black top-hat (BTH) are the two varieties of top-hat operations.

WTH and BTH, respectively, extract structures that are more vibrant and gloomier than the surrounding environment. This approach computes these RMP-based top-hat operators concurrently. Three key steps make up the method's functioning:

i) Target features are extracted selectively using top-hat techniques.
ii) The top-hat pictures were converted to grayscale.
iii) Merging the original image with a greyscale version of the top-hat image.

In particular, this contributes to the enhancement of intended structures from complicated environments and inconsistent background intensity. Using a synthetic image, the contrast improvement ratio (CIR) is utilized to assess this procedure both objectively and subjectively. Next, it is used on two real medical pictures: a radiographic visual of the chest and visuals of the mammography.

26.2 Medical Imaging

Another name for medical imaging is radiology. It refers to the area of medicine where medical practitioners recreate different body parts visuals for treatment or diagnosis. Among these techniques are nonintrusive diagnostics that enable medical professionals to identify illnesses and injuries without causing discomfort.

One of the main contributors to the observably better results [8] in contemporary medicine has been medical imaging. Various kinds of imaging methods used in medicine involve the following:

- X-rays
- Magnetic resonance imaging (MRI)
- Ultrasounds
- Endoscopy
- Tactile imaging
- Computerized tomography (CT) scan

Functional imaging methods in nuclear medicine, such as positron emission tomography (PET) scans, are additional advantageous medical imaging treatments. Medical imaging, such as scans, is used to observe how our bodies react to disease or fracture treatments.

Innovations from the radiography industry are utilized in medical imaging. The use of ionizing radiation in CT and X-ray scans means that they should be used with caution. Ionizing radiation aggravates the chance of developing cancer, cellular mutations, aberrant fetal development, and cataracts. MRIs, which include nuclear magnetic resonance (NMR), have minimal danger because they don't use ionizing radiation. Ultrasound is the most secure method of medical imaging since it produces images via ultrasonic vibrations.

Another secure kind of medical imaging is electroencephalography (EEG) and electrocardiography (ECG), which employ surface-mounted sensors to assess electrical activity and provide a variation over time graph instead of a graphical image.

The ability to evaluate and understand the data in a number of medical imaging systems is being improved by artificial intelligence (AI). There is a growing trend in the use of computer vision to visually assess problems that are not yet discernible to the human eye.

26.2.1 Who Is Using Medical Imaging Facilities?

Other titles for radiographers include radiology technologist and medical imaging technologist. The management of medical imaging methods falls under their authority. Radiographers are well-versed in the anatomy of the human body and how various illnesses and traumas impact it. In addition to the above-mentioned techniques, such as MRIs and CT scans, they are typically experts in the following fields:

- **Angiography:** This entails evaluating the individual's heart and blood arteries.
- **Mobile radiography:** This involves using specialized equipment to provide imaging services to patients who are unfit to make it to a hospital.
- **Fluoroscopy:** An X-ray that looks within the patient's body and shows moving pictures on a screen akin to a movie.
- **Trauma radiography:** This often entails working in emergency rooms.

Medical imaging techniques are performed by radiographers upon receiving a request from radiologists. Medical imaging technologies are used by radiologists to detect and cure illnesses. Radiologists treat conditions including cancer and heart disease with radiation or minimally intrusive, image-guided surgery.

The radiographer gives images to the radiologists once all procedures have been completed. After analyzing the data, the radiologist diagnoses the illness or impact and decides on the patient's best course of treatment.

26.2.2 Importance of Medical Imaging

Medical professionals are using noninvasive medical imaging on a larger scale to evaluate patients' bones, organs, tissue, and blood arteries. Finding tumors for expulsion or medication, locating clots of blood or additional clogs, guiding physicians in the replacement of joints or fracture treatment, and supporting other operations that involve the implantation of devices like stents or catheters within the body are all examples of tasks that involve medical diagnostics.

Overall, medical imaging has enhanced the process of treatment and diagnosis by reducing the need for guesswork on the part of doctors and enabling them to treat patients' illnesses and injuries more quickly.

26.3 Various Types of Modalities

The analysis of medical images serves a critical role in the scientific understanding of the illness, tracking, and comprehension of patients' responses to certain types of treatments, all of which support ongoing medical planning. Various healthcare imaging modalities employ distinct methods to generate pictures for different objectives. These diagnostic pictures either evaluate several organs at once (MRI, CT, etc.) or are focused on one organ alone (retinal scans, mammograms, dermoscopy, and colonoscopy). Different data volumes are generated by all of them. We go through a few types of medical imaging modalities here.

26.3.1 CT Scanners

The CT scan, employs X-rays and computers that don't actually look like X-rays as it is used for producing cross-sectional pictures of the human anatomy that can then be used to [6] create detailed views of the body's interior components (Figure 26.1).

Advantages

- As CT scans are nonintrusive, they are harmless.
- These are employed for more accurate examination of soft tissues and complex areas of the picture that may be challenging to analyze with X-rays.
- Inspection and imaging of blood arteries, internal organs, bones, the brain, neck, spine, and chest are often accomplished using these.
- These aid healthcare providers in the detection of tumors and fractures and keeping tabs on the impact of treatment on patients with cancer.

26.3.2 MRI Scanners

Similar to a CT scan, an MRI scan provides a thorough cross-sectional representation of a body component and is thus of a higher standard (Figure 26.2).

Advantages

- Because magnetic fields and radio waves are not harmful to clients, MRIs, similar to CT scans, are secure and uncomplicated procedures.
- These are used to visualize the internal anatomy of numerous bodily organs, including the heart, blood arteries, bones, brain, and spinal cord.
- Like CT scans, they are used for evaluation, tracking the impact of treatment, and helping medical professionals determine subsequent courses of action.

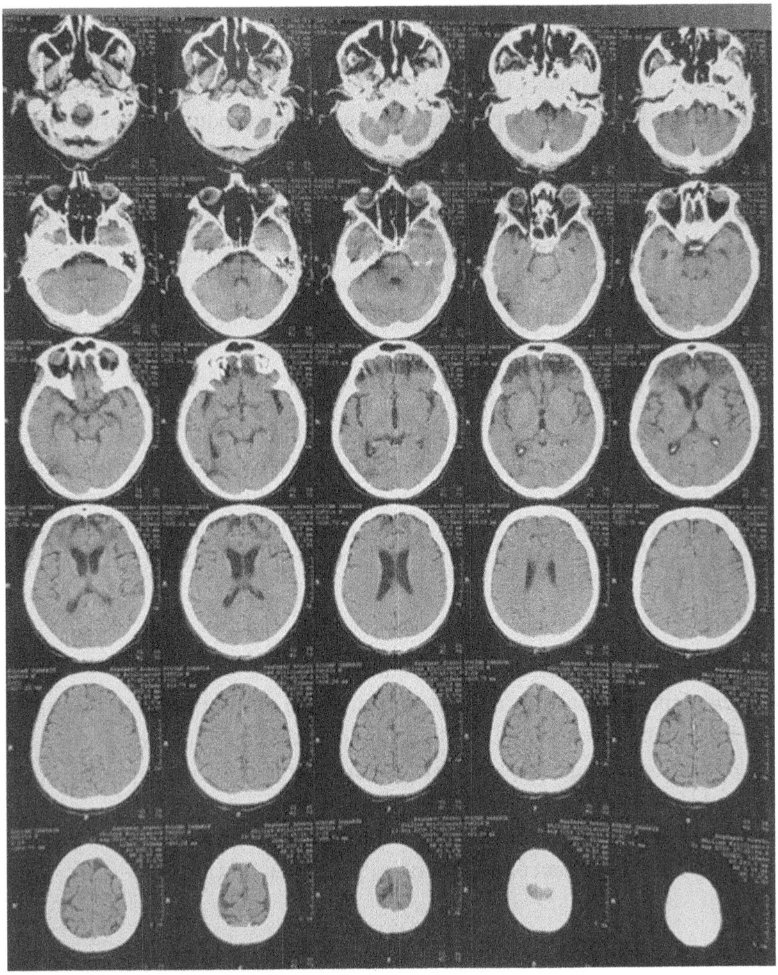

Figure 26.1 Brain CT scan. Source: Romanian Balneology Association.

Disadvantage

- Individuals who have particular implants, such as pacemakers, are incapable of going through an MRI scanner because of its responsiveness to metal.

26.3.3 PET Scanners

The interior components of the body can be visualized in three dimensions using a PET scan. By concentrating on a specific body area, these are utilized to determine how well that part is operating (Figure 26.3).

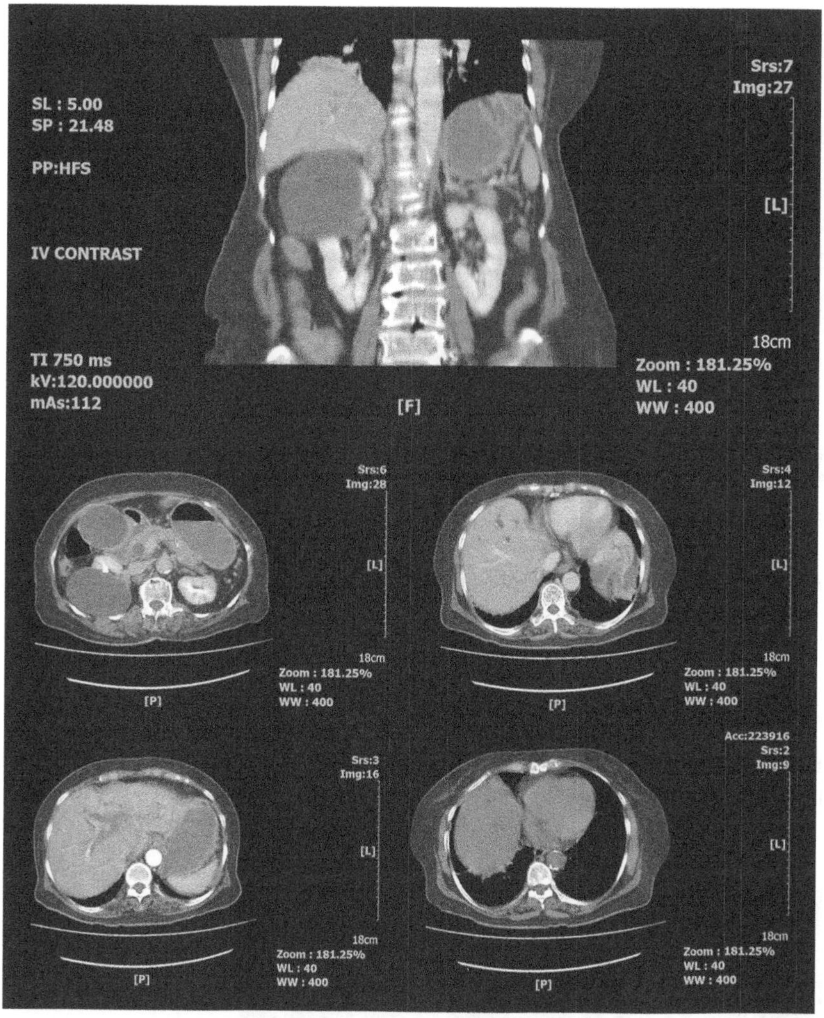

Figure 26.2 Abdomen MRI scan.

Advantages

- They are especially useful for forecasting the course of cancer and for creating high-resolution pictures of the brain.
- These are used on patients with cancer because they can show how far along the disease has progressed and how the patient is responding to chemotherapy.
- Employed for planning the brain or heart surgery, among other applications.

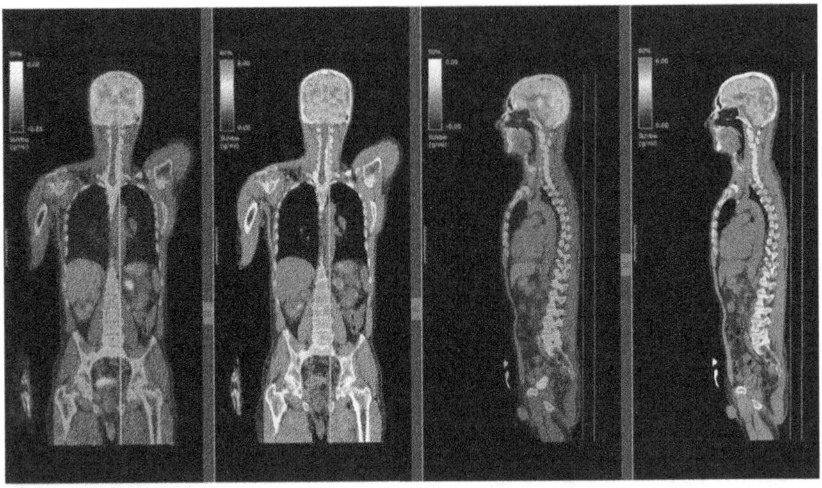

Figure 26.3 PET image.

- As it makes it evident whether or not the brain's functionality has changed, it can also be utilized for its diagnosis.

26.3.4 Ultrasound

Ultrasound are also called a sonogram. It demonstrates the internal part of the body by use of high-frequency waves (Figure 26.4).

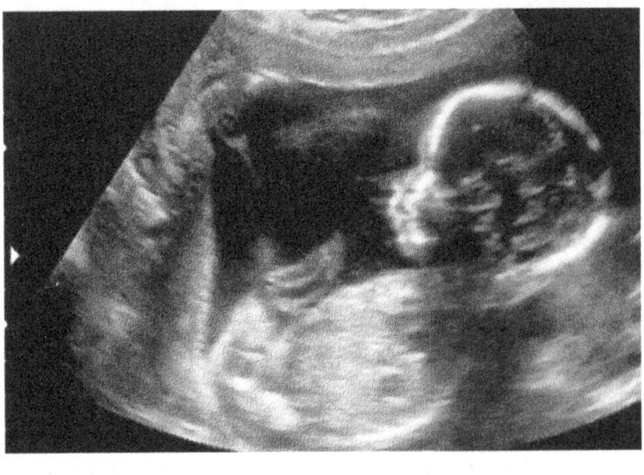

Figure 26.4 Ultrasound showing unborn baby in womb. Source: Jovannig/Adobe Stock.

Advantages

- It is used to monitor the growth of unborn babies by producing real-time images.

26.3.5 X-Rays

X-rays are used to illustrate the interior parts of the body (Figure 26.5).

Advantages

- These are utilized to check if there are breakages in bones or not by using images of bones.
- These are used to have an excellent visualization of the teeth by dentists and orthodontists.

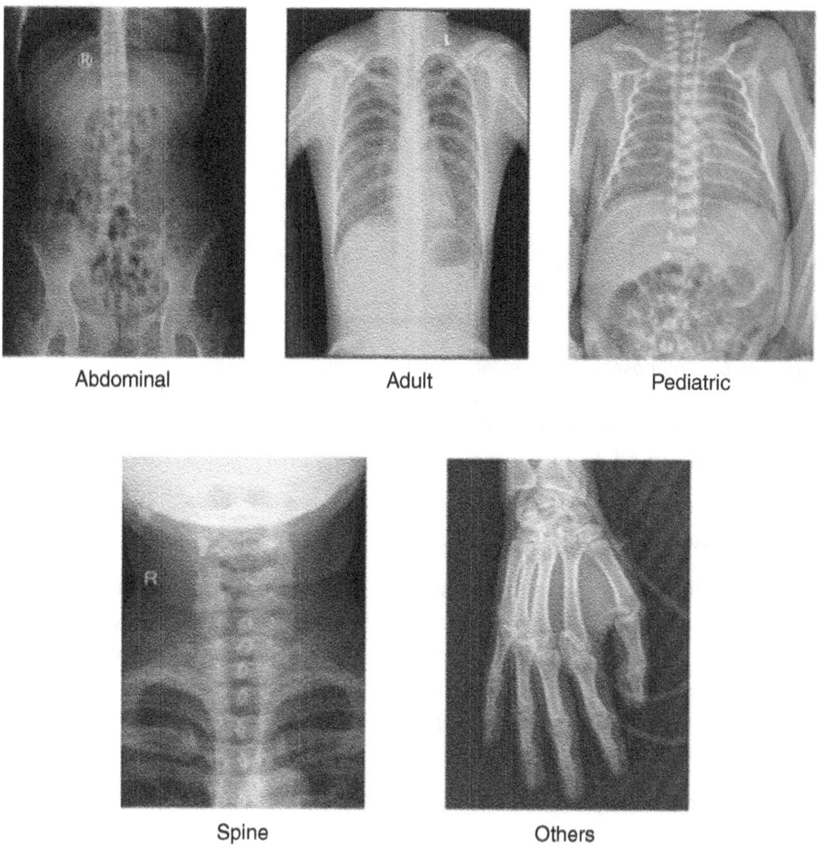

Figure 26.5 X-rays of different body parts. Source: VinLab.io.

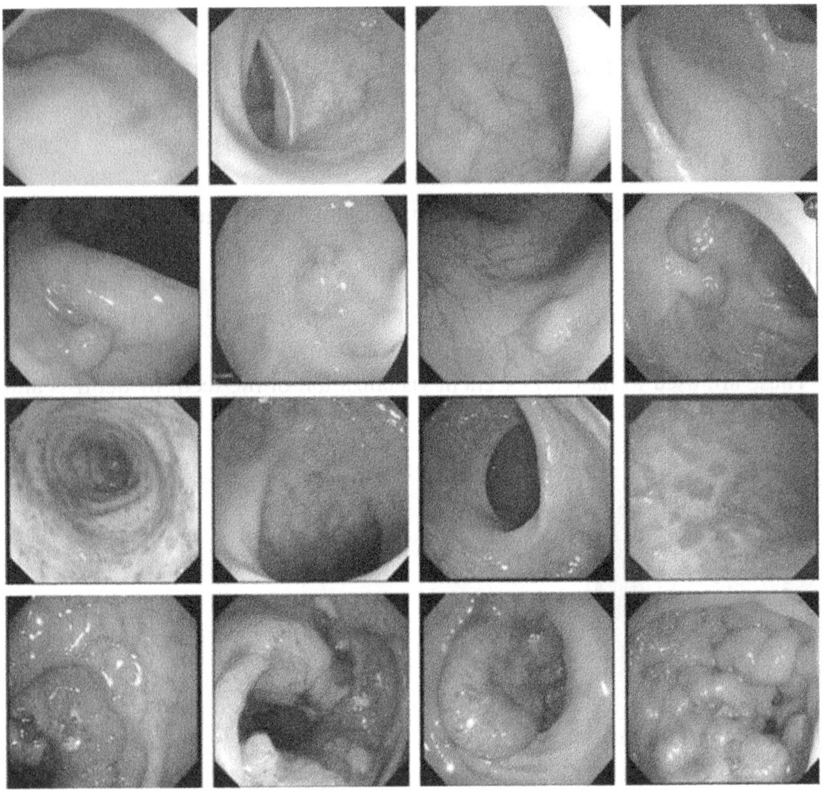

Figure 26.6 Colonoscopy. Source: John Wiley & Sons / CC BY 4.0.

- These can also be used for the detection of tumors on bone.
- They are also used during surgery to guide surgeons.

26.3.6 Colonoscopy

Medical professionals can examine the large intestinal tract for tumors known as polyps and colon or rectal cancer through the use of virtual colonoscopy or CT colonoscopy. A little flexible tube is passed through the rectum during the large intestine inspection to enable gas supplementation while colon and rectum CT scans are being obtained (Figure 26.6).

26.3.7 Dermoscopy

Dermoscopy is a minimally invasive form of skin imaging that facilitates the visualization of pigmented melanocytic neoplasm features that are not noticeable with

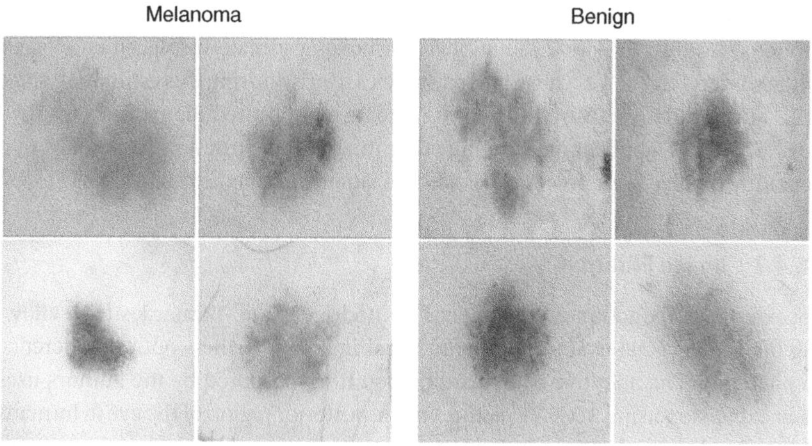

Figure 26.7 Dermoscopy. Source: Athanasios–Valavanidis / National and Kapodistrian University of Athens.

the sight of the naked eye. Dermoscopy refers to the investigation of the skin by using skin surface microscopy. These are typically utilized to evaluate tumors of the pigmented skin. Medical professionals are able to evaluate melanoma tumors via these photos. Dermoscopy, which allows for simpler and better study of skin lesions and patterns, requires the Dermatoscope, an exceptionally high-quality amplifying lens with a powerful illumination system (Figure 26.7).

26.4 Medical Imaging Analysis

The initial stage in medical imaging is gathering the data with an appropriate imaging equipment and rebuilding relevant images. Subsequently, a variety of image processing and analysis techniques, including image segmentation, image registration, image reconstruction, and image filtering, can be utilized.

26.4.1 Image Reconstruction

The act of creating 2D or 3D images of a component using data that is, signals which are obtained by an imaging instrument is called image reconstruction. Imaging devices are responsible for translating anatomical and physiological data into digital information during the data-gathering phase [10]. Nevertheless, the digital information is readily distorted by the noise generated by the imaging device's mechanical and electronic parts. Furthermore, there are many noise source displacements during the capturing of MRE [11] images. In areas with low signal noise rates, common ambiguity errors are caused by long, protracted motions, leading to poor estimations. Erroneous estimate displacements occur when susceptible factors cause inconsistencies to arise during this estimation stage [12]. Massive data sets are utilized to recreate complicated 3D pictures in MRI, SPECT, and CT applications, among other image reconstruction techniques that generally involve high processing costs and significant memory capacities [13].

26.4.2 Image Filtering

Speckle noise reduction was enhanced by Rodrigues and Bernardes [14], allowing for better visual examination of medical imaging, such as optical coherence tomography. The adaptive complex-diffusion filter proposed by the authors uses filter expansion using 3D OCT pictures of the posterior region of the eye in humans to retain edges and other vital characteristics. An environment setup step and four further, so-called iterative stages made up their implementation. CUDA kernels have been taken into account for element-wise arithmetic operations over the inputs, parallel reductions, and parallel convolutions.

A hybrid parallelization approach was presented by Nguyena et al. [15] to speed up the NL-Means filter algorithm. The authors separated the input 3D MRI volume into subvolumes to narrow down the search region at the outermost region. Next, the image was divided into overlaid images, and the search region radius was superposed. Several different parallel technologies were employed during execution: GPUs, MPI, and multithreading on multicore systems. Every cluster was able to communicate with one another via MPI. The authors' primary objective was to provide a methodology that called for several implementation strategies and the option to use MPI technology either exclusively or in combination with POSIX Threads and GPUs [16]. However, as it consumed three times as much memory as the previous technique, the use of large memory became an issue.

26.4.3 Image Segmentation

One of the many crucial steps in image processing and analysis is image segmentation, which is accountable for locating and defining items of interest in input images [17–19]. To attain the most effective results in activities like 3D visualization, interpolation, filtering, classification, and even registration, there is typically a strong reliance on the outcomes of picture segmentation. There are various methods for segmenting images, such as thresholding [8, 20], clustering [21], and deformable models [22].

To cut down on the overhead of communication between processes, Daggett and Greenshields [23] employed a PC cluster to generate a parallel algorithm that can be employed for automatic image categorization in 24 orders to segment MRI images. The aforementioned parallel algorithm known as the virtual shared memory method allows processes to interact directly by exchanging data as if it were present in a universally available shared memory space. The primary goal of the study was to segment anatomical photographs to get quantifiable characteristics and geometrically shaped representations of the items under investigation [24].

26.4.4 Image Registration

To compare or fuse visual data acquired at various points in time or with different imaging modalities or equipment, a uniform geometrical reference frame between two or more image datasets is generated using a computational procedure known as image registration [25, 26]. Because intensity-based registration methods rely on the search space, an optimization [27, 28] strategy, an intensity metric, and an interpolation scheme, they are reliable, accurate, and efficient. As a result, these methods rely on similarity metrics [29, 30], optimization techniques [27], and geometric changes [31].

26.5 Conventional Morphological Image Processing

A mathematical morphology [32] method is useful for extracting structural information from images and describing shape information as well. Set theory is the basis of mathematical morphology. With the help of structuring elements that are acted on by a collection of nonlinear operators, images can be classified as a function (greyscale image) or a set (binary image). Structuring elements are typically simple binary images that show the shape characteristics of an image, such as discs, squares, and lines. Dilation and erosion are two types of morphological operators.

- **Dilation:** This maximum operator chooses the most radiant value in the vicinity of the structuring element.
- **Erosion:** This minimal operator chooses the gloomiest value in the vicinity of the structuring element.

These operators serve as the foundation for a variety of further operations. The following definitions of dilation and erosion are applied to a greyscale picture f and a structuring component B:

- **Dilation** : $\delta_B(f)_{(x,\ y)} = \max\{f(x-s,\ y-t)+b(s,\ t) \mid (x-s),(y-1)\ \varepsilon\ D_f;(s,t)\ \varepsilon\ D_b\}$ (26.1)

- **Erosion** : $\varepsilon_B(f)_{(x,\ y)} = \min\{f(x+s,\ y+t)-b(s,\ t) \mid (x+s),(y+1)\ \varepsilon\ D_f;(s,t)\ \varepsilon\ D_b\}$ (26.2)

Here, the positions of the coordinate for the pairs for images f and B are (x, y) and (s, t), respectively. In addition, the corresponding domains of functions f and B are D_f and D_b. The following opening and shutting operations are used in conjunction with these procedures.

- **Opening** : $\gamma_B(f)_{(x,y)} = \delta_B[\varepsilon_B(f)_{(x,y)}]$ (26.3)

- **Closing** : $\varphi_B(f)_{(x,y)} = \varepsilon_B[\delta_B(f)_{(x,y)}]$ (26.4)

These opening and closing procedures are performed on features that are narrower than the structuring component's breadth. The opening is described as erosion followed consequently by dilation occurring inside a single structural component. Closing is the opposite of opening; so, it involves dilation consequently followed by erosion within a single structural component. Radiant characteristics like spikes and crests are eliminated by the opening operation, and gloomy regions such as troughs, holes, and voids are stuffed up with the close operation. These processes' properties allow for easy processing, and when coupled, they can produce morphological filters with a range of functions.

A morphological technique called the top-hat transform [33] is used to extract structures locally from images. Grey-level extraction and background brightness have no effect on the extraction process of structures. As a result of which, we are able to separate desired structures from an inconsistent background. We are already aware that the WTH and BTH operators are utilized, respectively, to extract bright and dark characteristics. The retrieved structures' size is smaller than the structuring component in both instances. The WTH takes the original greyscale image f and then reduces it using the opening image $\gamma_B(f)$.

- **White top-hat** : $\mathrm{WTH}(f) = f - \gamma_B(f)$ (26.5)

WTH produces an image that includes every remaining structure that is, all of the crest and spikes that the opening procedure has removed. The dimensions of the retrieved structures are dictates the dimensions of the structuring component.

On the contrary, BTH eliminates the initial grayscale picture f from the final picture $\varphi_B(f)$.

- **Black top-hat** : $\mathrm{BTH}(f) = \varphi_B(f) - f$ (26.6)

BTH facilitates in the extraction of the gloomy areas, such as troughs, holes, and voids, that are closed during the closing procedure. The dimensions of the retrieved structures are determined by dimensions of the structuring element, identical to that of WTH.

If the background and target structures in an image have comparable greyscale levels, the target characteristics are difficult for the human eye to distinguish between. Nonetheless, top-hat can be used to optimize and retrieve low-contrast objects.

26.6 Rotational Morphological Processing

As is well known, during a specific procedure, the structuring component is applied in a particular direction in conventional morphological operations. The technique's deployment in images with simple directional structures is restricted by the unidirectional fitting of the structuring component to image components. Images with more intricate directional modifications, such as those found in biomedical imaging, are more likely to have aberrations brought on by inadequate morphological processing.

Morphological filters are used by RMP [34, 35] to allow isotropic processing with only one structuring component. One structural component is created using constant rotation of the original image via the RMP algorithm. For every rotational image, conventional morphological operators (such as opening and closing) are used. Finally, the processed images make use of a maximum or minimum operator of the image pixel value to combine it into an output image (Figure 26.8).

Phases of the method are outlined below:

- **Phase 1:** Rotate the original picture f clockwise (with regard to the image frame's center). For each $i = 0, 1, \dots, N-1$, let f_i indicate the rotary motion of the original picture f by the angle $\theta_i = \pi i \mid N$ [rad].
- **Phase 2:** A single structural component B is used for interpreting the rotated visuals (either by closing or opening operations). $\varphi_B(f_i)$ and $\gamma_B(f_i)$ are the associated results of closing and opening operations on the rotated visuals f_i within B.
- **Phase 3:** Rotation of the processed images anticlockwise by θ_i [rad] is done. h_i^{Clsn} and h_i^{Opn} are used as notations for the ith rotated closed and opened visuals, respectively.
- **Phase 4:** The final product is created through the combination of the processed photos. The output image produced by RMP opening (closing) computation has pixels at each place that record the highest (lowest) amount across all treated visuals.

The descriptions of the opening $\gamma_{B'}(f)$ and closing $\varphi_{B'}(f)$ operators under RMP are as follows:

- **RMP opening** : $\gamma_B{}'(f)_{(x,y)} = \max\left\{h_i^{Opn}(x, y)\right\}$ (26.7)

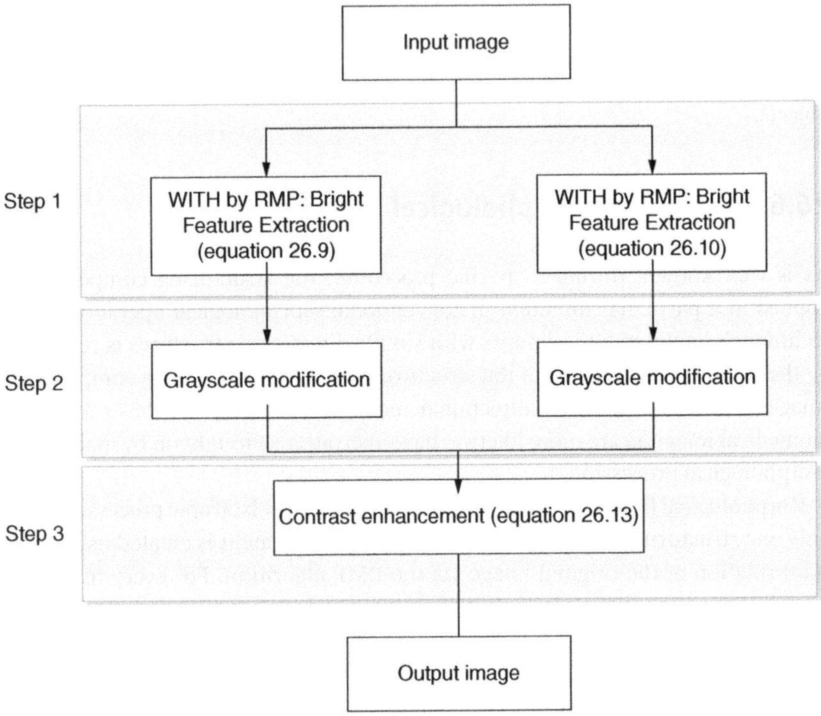

Figure 26.8 Diagram showing the RMP method's flow.

- **RMP closing** : $\varphi_{B'}(f)_{(x,y)} = \min\left\{\mathrm{h_i}^{\mathrm{Clsn}}(\mathrm{x}, \mathrm{y})\right\}$ (26.8)

The aforementioned operations are identical to the conventional operations for $N = 1$. The structural component's form has an impact on the choice of N. The optimum value for N for either a disc or square structuring component is 8, and the optimum value for a line-segment structuring component is 36. The artifacts caused by an individual structuring element's unidirectional raster are substantially decreased by RMP. For instance, geometrical smoothing of a chaotic image using RMP results in a reasonable decrease in noise while maintaining edges and additional information.

The top-hat operators are represented in the following manner with regard to RMP:

- **RMP white top-hat** : $\mathrm{WTH}'(f) = f - \gamma_B{}'(f)$ (26.9)

- **RMP black top-hat** : $\mathrm{BTH}'(f) = \varphi_B{}'(f) - f$ (26.10)

Top-hat techniques based on RMP have previously been utilized on a number of distinct biological structures. We have retrieved glowing regions from fluorescence microscope pictures using enhanced WTH. Spots that are grouped together or accumulated are also able to employ it. We utilize RMP-based BTH to obtain the actin filament's surface structural pattern, which is the primary cytoskeleton constituent recorded by electron microscopy (EM).

26.6.1 RMP-Based Top-Hat Contrast Enhancement Operator

We employ the top-hat contrast enhancement operator by processing BTH and WTH in parallel. We subtract BTH from the final image to enhance gloomy features and add WTH to the original image to improve dazzling features [36]. Following is how this operator describes itself:

- $K = f + \text{WTH} - \text{BTH}$ (26.11)

Likewise, we describe the top-hat contrast operator on the basis of RMP in the following manner:

- $K' = f + \text{WTH}' - \text{BTH}'$ (26.12)

Low contrast target structures have no potential for enhancement by top-hat operations as their greyscale values are too minimal to make an important distinction. As a result of this, we are unable to make improvements to low-contrast structures by utilization of equations (26.11) and (26.12).

For a solution to overcome this problem, an appropriate greyscale transformation approach is needed. Two new greyscale transformation methods are added to the top-hat contrast operation.

In particular, after the patterns intended to be improved via top-hat operations are carefully extracted, two greyscale transformation approaches are applied to improve the contrast of the derived patterns. Histogram equalization [37] and linear contrast stretching are the processes that improve the contrast in the top-hat image. The histogram of a picture is manipulated using the histogram equalization approach, which involves dispersing the amount of pixels with varying brightness to equal frequencies. In linear contrast stretching, the greyscale levels are first standardized by figuring out the image's minimum and maximum greyscale values. Next, we increase this range linearly so that output intensities can be applied across the full range (e.g., 0–255 for 8-bit greyscale image).

The terms "$\nu_{\text{BTH}}{}'$ and $\nu_{\text{WTH}}{}'$" symbolize BTH′ and WTH′-based contrast enhancement (i.e., BTH′ and WTH′ accompanied through the two greyscale modification procedures). The suggested contrast enhancement operator λ is expressed in the following manner in terms of $\nu_{\text{BTH}}{}'$ and $\nu_{\text{WTH}}{}'$:

- **Contrast enhancement operator** : $\lambda = f + \nu_{WTH}{}' - \nu_{BTH}{}'$ (26.13)

Once the original image has been merged with $\nu_{WTH}{}'$ and $\nu_{BTH}{}'$, the greyscale values generally either reside inside or outside of the range of variation. Consequently, the range of the picture display is specified as the resulting greyscale range for λ (e.g. [0:255] to display an 8-bit greyscale image). With this technology, $\nu_{WTH}{}'$ and $\nu_{BTH}{}'$ enhance processed images sequentially, with a high level of contrast augmentation anticipated.

26.6.2 Contrast Improvement Ratio

The impact of contrast augmentation on picture quality is determined by the contrast improvement ratio, or CIR [38].

The contrast ratio that exists between improved and unimproved pictures within the region of relevance R is referred to as CIR as follows:

- $$\text{CIR} = \frac{\sum_{(\mathrm{x,y}\,\varepsilon\,\mathrm{R})} |C(x,y) - C(x,y)|^2}{\sum_{(\mathrm{x,y}\,\varepsilon\,\mathrm{R})} C(x,y)^2} \tag{26.14}$$

The values at local contrast at (x, y) of the improved and unimproved pictures are $C(x, y)$ and $C(x, y)$, respectively. The following equation is used to calculate the values at local contrast $C(x, y)$:

- $$C(x, \ y) = \frac{|(p - a)|}{|(p + a)|} \tag{26.15}$$

where p and a indicate the mean contrasts in the neighboring region (R_N) and central region (R_C), consequently.

26.6.3 Assessing Contrast Improvement Using a Fictitious Test Image

To assess the contrast improvement provided by RMP [39], it was compared to two traditional techniques of contrast enhancement: contrast-limited adaptive histogram equalization (CLAHE) [40] and multiscale retinex (MSR) [41]. We are using a 238 × 218-pixel synthetic test image to conduct our assessment.

The picture improvements obtained by both the traditional and proposed approaches are shown in Figure 26.9. The artificial test image and associated greyscale intensity distribution histogram are displayed in Figure 26.9a. The enhancement result obtained by MSR is displayed in Figure 26.9b. MSR computes the output picture values as the difference between the original and distorted pictures in the logarithmic domain, applying the usual retinex theory to image contrast improvement. This approach used three convolutions scaling with

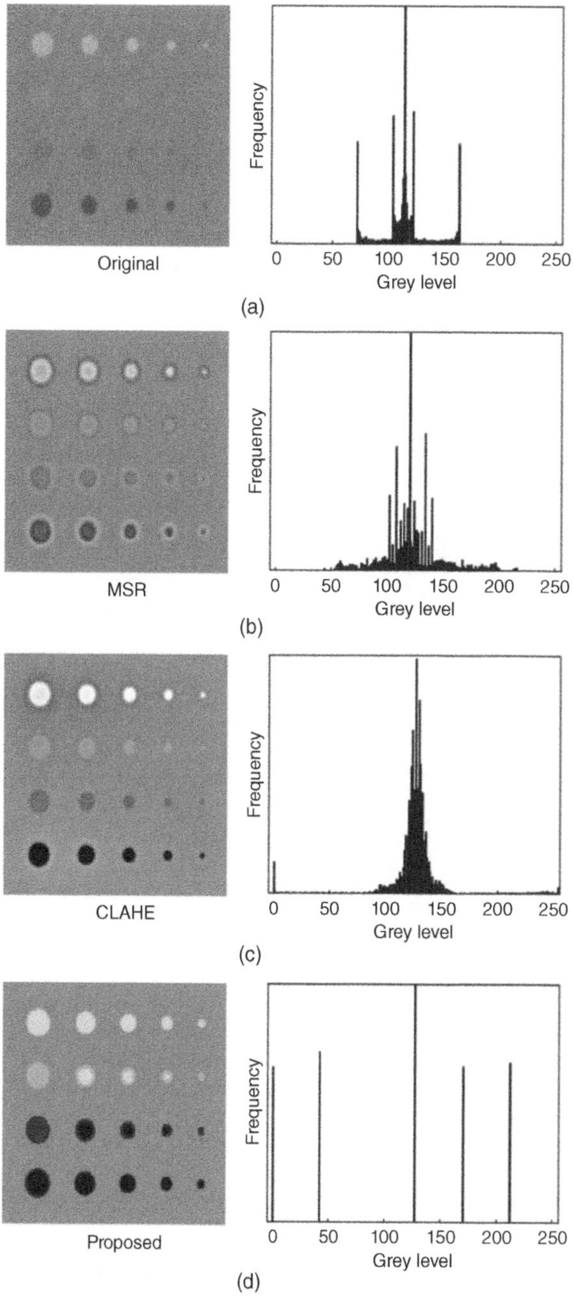

Figure 26.9 Contrast enhancement techniques are compared on a fictitious test visual. (a) The artificial test is visual on the left, and the associated grey-level distribution histogram on the right. (b)–(d) The following techniques were used to obtain the contrast enhancement images and accompanying histograms: multiscale retinex (b), contrast-limited adaptive histogram equalization (c), and the suggested method (d).

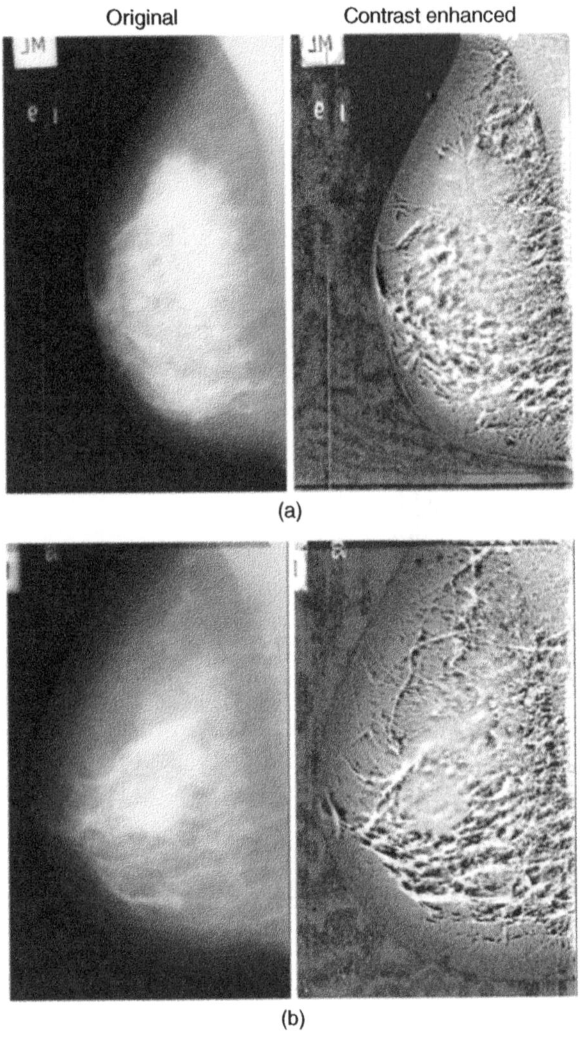

Figure 26.10 Original mammographic images are shown in the left-hand panels. Images on the right side are contrast-enhanced using the suggested technique. Source: Yoshitaka Kimori / International Union of Crystallography / CC BY 2.0.

standardized deviations of five, fifteen, and twenty-five pixels. For every scale, the weights have been set to 1/3.

The modified output of CLAHE, a flexible image contrast enhancement method based on histogram modification, is displayed in Figure 26.9c. This technique works with discrete areas, or blocks, inside an image. The block size

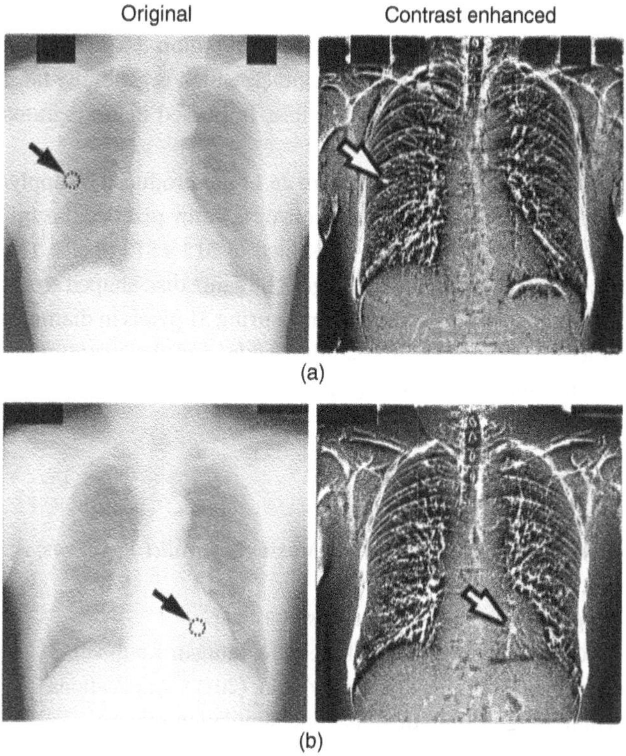

Figure 26.11 Improved radiography images of the chest using the suggested technique. Original radiography images of the chest in the left-hand panels. In every picture, the pointer points to a nodule. Boxes on the right hand: contrast-enhanced photos produced by the suggested technique. Source: Yoshitaka Kimori / International Union of Crystallography / CC BY 2.0.

applied to this experiment is 9×9 pixels. Based on a disc-shaped structuring element with a diameter of 31 pixels, the enhancements achieved by the proposed contrast enhancement operator λ are shown in Figure 26.9d. For each intended characteristic, the disc diameter is specified to be greater than the base diameter.

26.6.4 Application Results

By employing the suggested technique, improved mammography images are shown in Figure 26.10. The original pictures are displayed at half their original size in [Figure 26.10, left-hand panel]. 400 μm pixel^{-1} is the spatial resolution as a result. In the right-hand panel, a disc-shaped structuring component having a diameter of 31 pixels, or 12.4 mm, has been used to improve the mammary gland

25 Rohlfing, T. and Maurer, C.R. Jr., (2003). *Nonrigid image registration in shared-memory multiprocessor environments with application to brains, breasts, and bees. IEEE Transactions on Information Technology in Biomedicine* 7 (1): 16–25.

26 Ur Rehman, T., Haber, E., Pryor, G. et al. (2009). *3D nonrigid registration via optimal mass transport on the GPU. Medical Image Analysis* 13 (6): 931–940.

27 Wachowiak, M. and Peters, T. (2006). *High-Performance Medical Image Registration Using New Optimization Techniques. IEEE Transactions on Information Technology in Biomedicine* 10: 344–353.

28 Dangi, D., Bhagat, A., and Dixit, D. (2021). Sentiment analysis on social media using genetic algorithm with CNN. *Computers, Materials & Continua* 70 (3): 5399–5419.

29 Dandekar, O. and Shekhar, R. (2007). *FPGA-accelerated deformable image registration for improved target-delineation during CT-guided interventions. IEEE Transactions on Biomedical Circuits and Systems* 1 (2): 116–127.

30 Ellingwood, N.D., Yin, Y., Smith, M., and Lin, C.-L. (2016). *Efficient methods for implementation of multi-level nonrigid mass-preserving image registration on GPUs and multi-threaded CPUs. Computer Methods and Programs in Biomedicine* 127: 290–300.

31 Christensen, G. (1998). MIMD vs. *SIMD parallel processing: a case study in 3D medical image registration. Parallel Computing* 24: 1369–1383.

32 Serra, J. (1983). *Image Analysis and Mathematical Morphology*. Academic Press, Inc.

33 Meyer, F. (1979). *Iterative image transformations for an automatic screening of cervical smears. Journal of Histochemistry and Cytochemistry* 27 (1): 128–135.

34 Kimori, Y., Oguchi, Y., Ichise, N. et al. (2007). *A procedure to analyze surface profiles of the protein molecules visualized by quick-freeze deep-etch replica electron microscopy. Ultramicroscopy* 107 (1): 25–39.

35 Kimori, Y., Baba, N., and Morone, N. (2010). *Extended morphological processing: a practical method for automatic spot detection of biological markers from microscopic images. BMC Bioinformatics* 11: 1–13.

36 Soille, P. (1999). *Morphological Image Analysis: Principles and Applications*, vol. 2. Springer.

37 Mora-González, M., Munoz-Maciel, J., Rodríguez, J.C. et al. (2011). Image processing for optical metrology. In: *MATLAB–A Ubiquitous Tool for the Practical Engineer*, 1e, 523–546. Rijeka, Croatia: InTech.

38 Oh, J. and Hwang, H. (2010). *Feature enhancement of medical images using morphology-based homomorphic filter and differential evolution algorithm. International Journal of Control, Automation and Systems* 8: 857–861.

39 Kimori, Y. (2013). *Morphological image processing for quantitative shape analysis of biomedical structures: effective contrast enhancement. Journal of Synchrotron Radiation* 20 (Pt 6): 848–853.

40 Pizer, S.M., Amburn, E.P., Austin, J.D. et al. (1987). *Adaptive histogram equalization and its variations. Computer Vision, Graphics, and Image Processing* 39 (3): 355–368.

41 Jobson, D.J., Rahman, Z.-u., and Woodell, G.A. (1997). *A multiscale retinex for bridging the gap between color images and the human observation of scenes. IEEE Transactions on Image Processing* 6 (7): 965–976.

42 Dangi, D., Dixit, D., and Bhagat, A. (2021). *Cloud Based Security Analysis in Body Area Network for Health Care Applications.* CRC Press.

27

Machine Learning Applications in the Prediction of Polycystic Ovarian Syndrome

Ardra Nair, Virrat Devaser, and Komal Arora

School of Computer Science, Lovely Professional University, Phagwara Punjab, India

27.1 Introduction

In recent years, machine learning (ML) has emerged as a powerful tool in healthcare, revolutionizing disease detection and diagnosis. A patient's well-being and the planning of appropriate treatment depend heavily on the diagnosis of their illness. Accurately and quickly interpreting medical information is a difficult cognitive task. The effectiveness and accuracy of diagnostics can be greatly improved by ML. A thorough analysis of the domains in which ML has been used is required, as is information on how well it has identified newly developed digitalized healthcare services. In addition to discussing the state of ML in diagnostics, this chapter offers a research agenda to direct future efforts. Healthcare professionals are aware of how ML can enhance diagnosis and improve patient outcomes. To achieve successful use in illness detection, however, a few obstacles must be overcome, especially regarding promoting early detection. The promise of ML to transform healthcare by improving diagnosis speed and accuracy makes it crucial for medical diagnosis. It makes it possible to spot patterns and trends that human practitioners could miss, which could result in the early discovery of conditions like polycystic ovary syndrome (PCOS). In addition, ML-driven diagnostic tools frequently offer greater affordability, accessibility, and user-friendliness, enabling people to take charge of their health. In contrast to traditional methods requiring costly blood tests and scans, our ML-based PCOS detection model offers a cost-effective, noninvasive approach through user-provided answers, enabling early identification and intervention without the need for extensive medical procedures. In this work, a highly effective model was constructed to predict the existence or absence of PCOS using a labeled historical dataset. To help with early identification and prompt consultations,

Generative Artificial Intelligence for Biomedical and Smart Health Informatics,
First Edition. Edited by Aditya Khamparia and Deepak Gupta.

users can forecast medical issues by answering questions [1–4]. By enhancing early detection and healthcare delivery, this research will help individuals and healthcare clinics through data selection, sophisticated analysis, and practical implementation. In the end, the health and well-being of women everywhere are improved by this research's contribution to the ongoing efforts to enhance the early detection and management of PCOS. This chapter explores the role of ML in healthcare and its significance in early disease detection, with a focus on PCOS.

27.1.1 Overview of PCOS

PCOS is a heterogeneous endocrine disorder characterized by the manifestation of ovarian cysts, anovulation, and variations in reproductive hormones. These disruptions in hormone levels often lead to menstrual irregularities such as oligomenorrhea and amenorrhea. PCOS affects approximately 116 million women worldwide, according to estimates by the World Health Organization. The condition presents with hyperandrogenism, menstrual irregularities, and varying ovarian cyst sizes, though individual differences exist.

The condition known as PCOS is brought on by an excess of male hormones produced by the ovaries, which is the organ responsible for producing and releasing eggs. The production of androgens by the ovaries is abnormally high in PCOS. This leads to an imbalance in the hormones that control reproduction. Due to a lack of ovulation, small cysts (fluid-filled sacs) may form on the ovaries. Nevertheless, despite the label "polycystic," PCOS may not necessarily involve ovarian cysts. Most typical signs and symptoms of PCOS include irregular periods include missing periods or not menstruating at all. It could also result in significant bleeding during periods [6–8]. Excessive facial hair and thick hair growth on the arms, chest, and belly are examples of abnormal hair growth (hirsutism). Up to 70% of women with PCOS are impacted by this [11]. PCOS can lead to acne, particularly on the back, chest, and face. Acne may persist throughout the adolescent years and be challenging to cure. Obesity: Around 80% of PCOS-affected women are overweight or obese and struggle to lose weight. Skin discoloration: Dark skin patches, particularly in the creases of the neck, armpits, groyne, and beneath the breasts. Cysts: Small fluid pockets are common in PCOS patients' ovaries of fluid are common in the ovaries of patients with PCOS. Skin tags: Skin tags are tiny skin flaps that protrude. In PCOS-afflicted women, they are frequently located on the neck or in the armpits. Hair loss: People with PCOS may experience patches of hair loss or begin to grow bald. Female infertility is most frequently caused by PCOS. Lack of ovulation or decreased ovulation frequency can prevent conception. PCOS can exist without any obvious symptoms. Many individuals don't even recognize they have the illness until they experience difficulties becoming pregnant or start accumulating weight for unexplained reasons. It's also possible to have mild PCOS, in

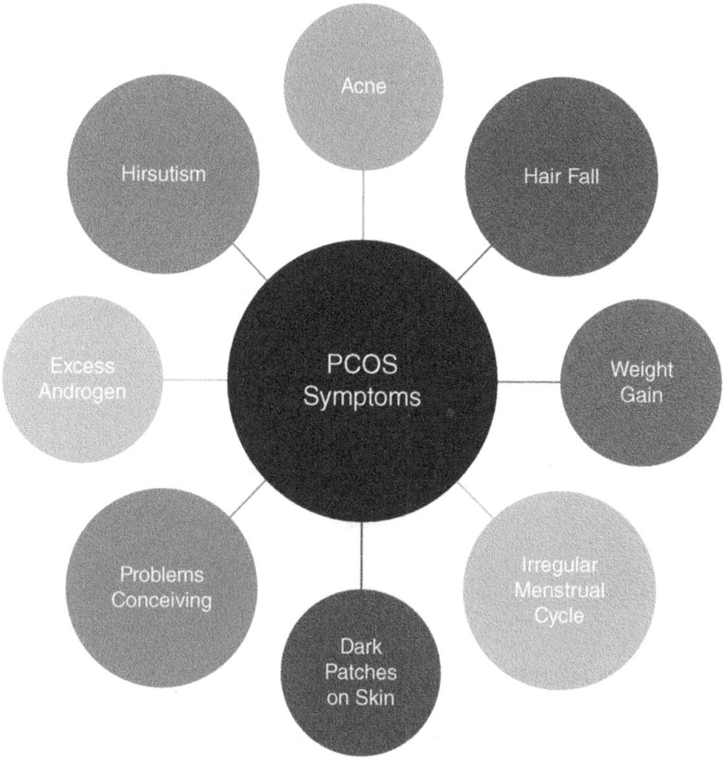

Figure 27.1 Common symptoms of PCOS.

which case your symptoms might go unnoticed. There is no recognized cause for PCOS. There is proof that genetics are involved. Figure 27.1 shows the common symptoms of PCOS [15–19].

Diagnosis involves a combination of medical history assessment, physical examination, pelvic examination, ultrasound imaging to assess ovarian size and cyst presence, and blood tests to measure hormone levels and assess for insulin resistance. Diagnosing PCOS relies on clinical criteria, with the rotterdam criteria/international PCOS criteria being widely accepted. PCOS is identified by a combination of hyperandrogenism, ovulatory irregularities, and PCOM. The complex clinical picture is further complicated by genetic and environmental factors like obesity or lifestyle choices, impacting presentation [23–28]. Diagnosis based on criteria is hindered by variations in assessing hyperandrogenism and menstrual irregularities. In addition, differences in normative standards for PCOM add to these challenges. It's estimated that diagnosis is delayed by over two years in a significant portion of women with PCOS, though this figure

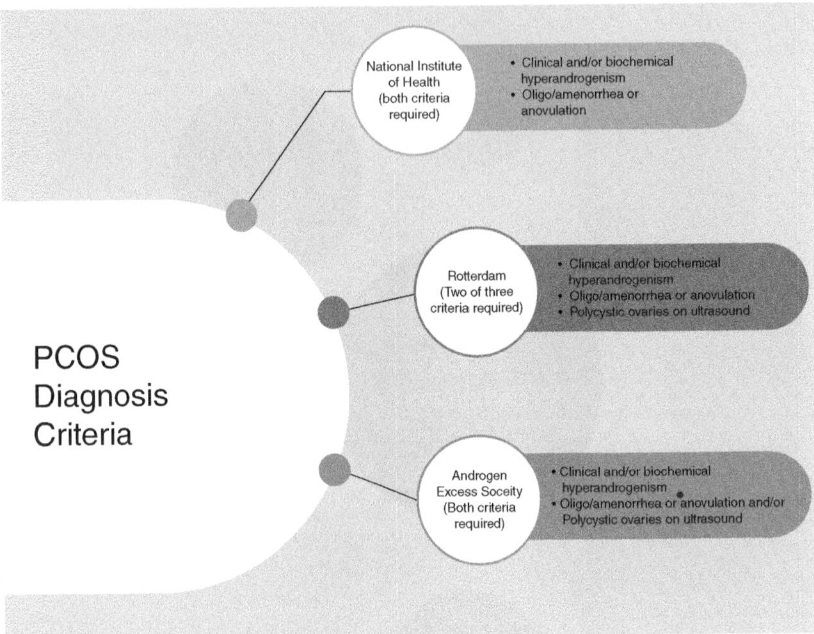

Figure 27.2 PCOS diagnosis criteria.

likely underrepresents the true extent of the issue. Treatment for PCOS typically involves medication to manage symptoms and prevent associated health problems. Options may include lifestyle modifications such as diet and exercise, medications to induce ovulation, birth control pills to regulate menstrual cycles and lower androgen levels, diabetes medications to address insulin resistance, and medications to manage other symptoms like excessive hair growth or acne [29–31]. Early diagnosis and appropriate management are crucial in reducing the risk of complications and improving long-term health outcomes for individuals with Figure 27.2 illustrates the PCOS Diagnosis Criteria, including the National Institute of Health, Rotterdam, and Androgen Excess Society criteria.

27.1.2 Role of ML in Healthcare and Disease Detection

Ensuring good health is paramount for every individual, with regular health check-ups being essential for prevention and maintenance. Unfortunately, many people neglect their health due to busy schedules and other priorities. Healthcare professionals, despite their dedication, often sacrifice their own well-being to save lives. Furthermore, remote areas often lack adequate medical facilities. The recent fear of COVID-19 has exacerbated reluctance to seek medical attention.

However, technology, particularly in the field of ML, offers a solution. ML enables machines to learn from past data, making it highly efficient in healthcare. By developing a user-friendly interface to gather symptoms, ML models like Naive Bayes (NB) and Decision Trees can accurately diagnose diseases. The output includes the disease identified, the model's accuracy, its definition, and recommended treatments based on the symptoms provided. Recent studies investigating ML in PCOS have demonstrated impressive sensitivity and accuracy in detecting the condition. These findings suggest that a carefully developed AI/ML program could substantially improve early PCOS diagnosis, leading to cost savings and alleviating the burden on both patients and the healthcare system.

In essence, this approach emphasizes the importance of early disease detection, enabling individuals to seek timely medical assistance and maintain their well-being.

27.2 Literature Review

This literature survey offers a summary of current research on ML-based prediction of PCOS. These studies employ a variety of approaches and methodologies and seek to get important insights from patient data. Every research project advances the knowledge and use of ML in interpreting patient symptoms, from new classifier proposals to in-depth investigations of feature extraction and preprocessing. The studies were published from 2011 to 2023. The data from the paper is extracted and integrated into Table 27.1.

27.3 ML Techniques for Polycystic Ovarian Syndrome

ML enables the detection of PCOS by analyzing diverse patient data. This brief overview outlines the process, including data collection, preprocessing, feature selection, classification algorithms, and evaluation metrics, contributing to accurate PCOS prediction models (Figure 27.3).

27.3.1 ML Architecture for PCOS Diagnosis

ML architecture offers a comprehensive approach to diagnosing PCOS by leveraging advanced algorithms and data analytics techniques. By integrating various stages such as data collection, preprocessing, feature extraction, model development, and evaluation, this architecture aims to accurately predict PCOS risk in individuals. Through the deployment of predictive models into clinical practice, this architecture seeks to enhance early detection and personalized

Table 27.1 Summary of reviewed literature.

Author	Year	Method	Findings
Mehrotra, P et al. [23]	2011	Bayesian classifier, Logistic regression	Bayesian classifier outperformed logistic regression with an accuracy of 93.93%.
A. Denny, A. Raj, A. Ashok, C. M. Ram, and R. George [13]	2019	NB, KNN, Classification and Regression Trees (CART), Random Forest, SVM	Random Forest gave the highest accuracy of 89.02%. Integration of clinical tests and ultrasound scans for prediction used.
Thomas, N., & Kavitha, A. [41]	2020	KNN, SVM, linear regression.	SVM had the peak accuracy at 91%, while KNN was at 75%, K-means at 72%, and linear regression at 85%.
Bharati, S et al. [7]	2020	Hybrid RF and logistic regression (RFLR), Gradient boosting, random forest, logistic regression	Through the utilization of 40-fold cross-validation to divide the data into training and testing portions, RFLR was found to have the highest accuracy of 91.01%.
Neto C et al. [30]	2021	Logistic regression, multilayer perceptron, neural networks, RF, and GNB	The best model, which made use of RF, produced acceptable results, with an accuracy of 0.95.
Katarya, R., Srivastava, G., & Chauhan, N. [17]	2021	Ensemble model	The proposed system achieved 90.74% accuracy.
Chauhan, P. Patil, N. Rane, P. Raundale and H. Kanakia [10]	2021	KNN, NB, L R, Decision Tree, Flask	Decision tree gave highest accuracy of 81%, mobile app developed to predict PCOS.
Nabi, Nusrat, et al. [27]	2021	Random Forest, NB Classification, Decision Tree Classification, Super Vector Machine Learning, KNN, Logistic Regression, XGBoost Classifier, Gradient Boosting	Among all classifications SVM has the highest accuracy of 99.09%
Y. A. Abu Adla et al. [43]	2021	Hybrid Feature Selection with Classification Algorithms	Support Vector Machine (SVM) was chosen, as it performed best with an accuracy of 91.6%.

Table 27.1 (Continued)

Author	Year	Method	Findings
Sinthia, G., Poovizhi, T., & Khilar, R. [37]	2022	Linear Regression, K-means, SVM	The SVM algorithm was the most effective with an accuracy of 91%.
Nasim, S., Hussain, M. A., Riaz, F., Iqbal, N., & Qazi, A. [29]	2022	Gaussian Naive Bayes (GNB)	The GNB algorithm attained 100% accuracy and a minimum computation time of 0.002 s
Hdaib, D et al.	2022	SVM, Neural Network (NN), Naïve Bayes (NB), classification tree, logistic regression, linear discriminant	The most effective classifier, in terms of accuracy, precision, and specificity, was the linear discriminant classifier.
Suriya P.T., Reka, S. and Elakkiya, R. [39]	2022	Raman Spectroscopy with advanced ML algorithms	Model using Raman spectra and advanced ML algorithms achieved 100% accuracy using follicular fluid samples.
Nasim, Shazia, et al. [29]	2022	GNB using CS (optimized chi-squared)-PCOS feature selection approach	The GNB model achieved 100% accuracy
Hdaib, Dana, et al.	2022	KNN, Neural Network (NN), NB, SVM, classification tree, logistic regression, and linear discriminant	Linear discriminant classifier exhibits the best performance in terms of accuracy (93.55%)
Nandipati, S. C., C. X. Ying, and Khaw Khai Wah	2022	KNN, SVM, NB, RF, bagging, boosting, neural network	The highest accuracy was shown by RF (93.12%, RapidMiner)
A. Karia, A. Poojary, A. Tiwari, L. Sequeira and M. K. Sokhi [16]	2023	Decision Tree, RF, KNN, NLP, NN	RF gave the highest accuracy of 90.44%, and app with the period tracker, PCOS diagnosis, built-in Chatbot, and medically valid information blogs
Chitra, P., et al. [12]	2023	Transfer learning techniques like Alexnet, Inception V3, Resnet50, VGG16, and Hybrid Models	Hybrid model exhibits the best accuracy of 95%
Meena, K., M. Manimekalai, and S. Rethinavalli	2023	SNM, artificial neural network, NB, classification tree	Artificial Neural Networks gave the highest accuracy with 82.75%

Table 27.1 (Continued)

Author	Year	Method	Findings
Sethi, Rithwick, et al. [36]	2023	RF Classifier (RFC), SVM, XGBoost, and Ensemble Learning	XGBoost outperformed with an accuracy of 89.63% before PCA. After PCA, RFC and SVC performed similarly, achieving 91.11%
Jyothi, R., et al. [15]	2023	LGBM (Light Gradient Boosting Machine)	LGBM classifier achieved 95% accuracy in categorizing PCOS. A Flask web app provides predictions, remedies, and additional information.

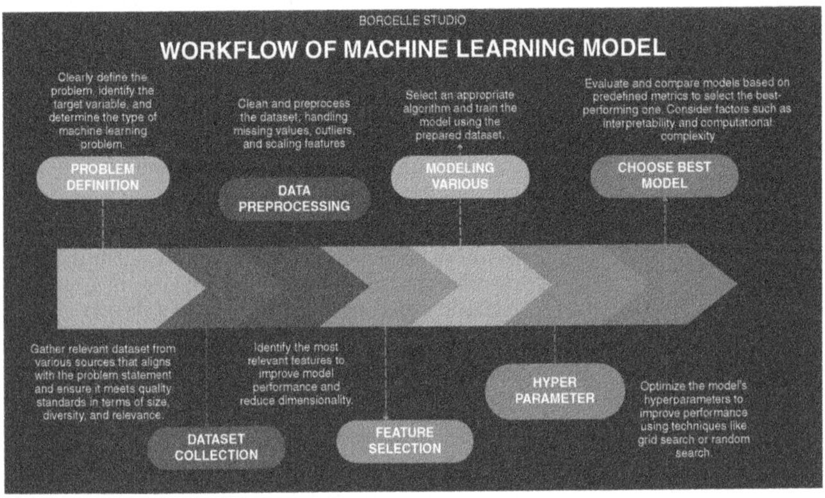

Figure 27.3 Workflow of machine learning model.

treatment strategies, ultimately improving healthcare outcomes for individuals affected by PCOS. Figure 27.4 illustrates the ML architecture for PCOS diagnosis. The basic parts of the same is given below.

Data Collection: Gather information related to PCOS from various sources such as medical databases, research articles, patient forums, and social media platforms where individuals discuss their experiences with PCOS. APIs and web scraping techniques can be employed to collect structured or unstructured data. Collecting comprehensive data related to PCOS is essential. This may include medical records, hormone levels, patient demographics, symptoms, and potentially genetic information.

Preprocessing: Clean and prepare the collected data for analysis. This involves tasks like removing duplicates, handling missing values, standardizing formats, and dealing with noise, such as irrelevant information or unrelated topics preprocessing involves cleaning the data, handling missing values, and standardizing formats. Feature engineering may include creating new features or transforming existing ones to better represent the data.

Data Visualization: Visualize key insights from the preprocessed data to gain a better understanding of PCOS-related trends, patterns, and correlations. Visualization techniques such as histograms, scatter plots, heatmaps, and word clouds can be utilized to explore various aspects of the data.

Feature Extraction: Extract relevant features from the preprocessed data to facilitate predictive modeling. Features may include demographic information (e.g., age, gender), medical history (e.g., menstrual irregularities, hormonal levels), lifestyle factors (e.g., diet, exercise), symptoms (e.g., hirsutism, acne), genetic predispositions, and psychological aspects (e.g., anxiety, depression).

Data Splitting: Split the dataset into training, validation, and testing sets to assess the performance of predictive models accurately. The training set is used to train the model, the validation set helps optimize model hyperparameters, and the testing set evaluates the model's generalization ability on unseen data.

Model for PCOS Prediction: Develop a predictive model to classify individuals based on their likelihood of having PCOS. Various ML algorithms such as logistic regression, random forests (RF), support vector machines (SVMs), gradient boosting machines, and neural networks can be employed for this task. The model should be trained on the labeled dataset, where each sample is associated with a binary label indicating the presence or absence of PCOS.

Evaluation and Tuning of Model: Evaluate the performance of the predictive model using appropriate metrics such as accuracy, precision, recall, F1-score, and area under the receiver operating characteristic curve (AUC–ROC). Evaluation metrics help assess the performance of the PCOS prediction model. Common metrics for binary classification tasks include: • Accuracy: The proportion of correctly predicted instances. • Precision: The ratio of true positive predictions to the total predicted positives. • Recall (Sensitivity): The ratio of true positive predictions to the total actual positives. • F1-score: The harmonic mean of precision and recall, providing a balance between the two. • ROC Curve and AUC: ROC curve and AUC measure the trade-off between true positive rate and false positive rate.

Integration and Deployment: Integrate the trained model into a user-friendly application or platform that allows healthcare providers and individuals to assess the risk of PCOS based on input features such as symptoms, medical

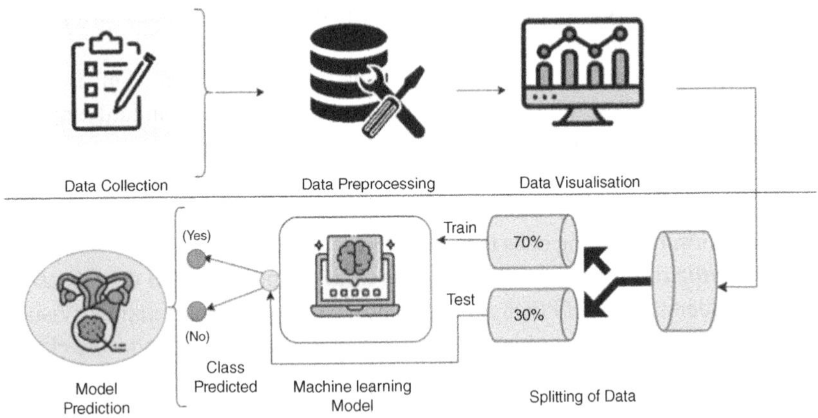

Figure 27.4 Machine learning architecture for PCOS diagnosis.

history, and lifestyle factors. Ensure that the deployment environment complies with relevant regulations and standards for data privacy and security. Continuously monitor and update the model as new data becomes available or clinical guidelines evolve.

27.3.2 ML Techniques Outline

ML algorithms in the modern era have demonstrated encouraging outcomes in diverse healthcare domains, encompassing the field of disease diagnostics. ML models possess the capability to analyze vast datasets, discern patterns, and generate predictions with a high degree of accuracy. Within the domain of PCOS, ML models have the potential to undergo training utilizing a fusion of clinical, laboratory, and imaging data. This training process aims to ascertain the capability of these models to forecast the likelihood of PCOS occurrence in a given patient.

By optimizing the precision and efficacy of PCOS diagnosis, healthcare practitioners have the potential to enhance the overall well-being of individuals affected by PCOS and mitigate the likelihood of enduring health difficulties in the long run. ML has the potential to make a valuable contribution towards the development of universally accepted diagnostic criteria for PCOS and assist the seamless incorporation of ML methods into regular clinical procedures. This, in turn, might lead to a transformative phase in the diagnosis and treatment of PCOS.

Data mining is the process of extracting valuable patterns and insights from large datasets using computational techniques. The core of the data mining process consists of many sub processes. The essential information is extracted from the given data sets using various prediction and classification data mining

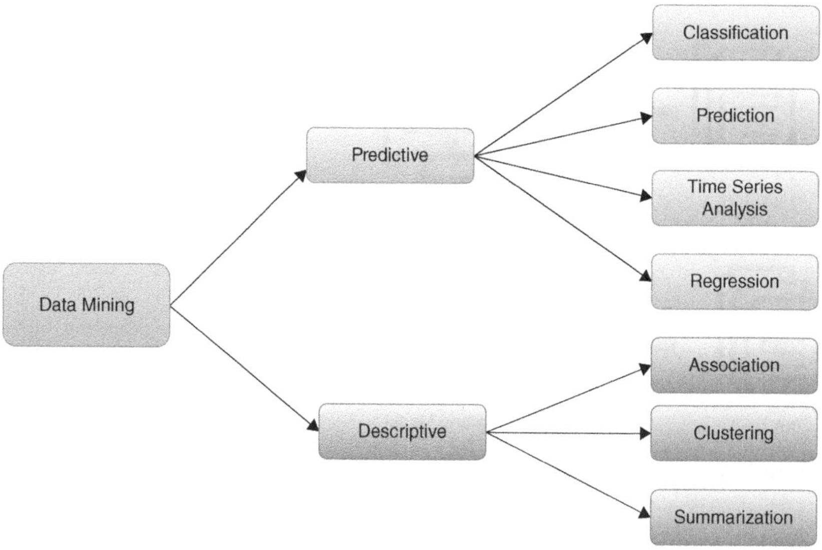

Figure 27.5 Data mining tasks.

techniques. The data mining tasks help uncover meaningful information from the given raw data. In general, two types of data mining tasks may be distinguished depending on the objectives of each. These two types of tasks are descriptive and predictive. While predictive data mining jobs use inference on the current data set to forecast how a new data set will behave, descriptive data mining activities define the general qualities of data. Some examples of data mining tasks encompass classification, prediction, time-series analysis, association, grouping, and summarization. They all come under one of two categories: descriptive and predictive data Figure 27.5 presents a flowchart depicting the classification of various data mining tasks.

The following are some of the different data mining tasks.

27.3.2.1 Classification

Finding a model that adequately represents the various data classes or ideas is the process of classification. The goal is to be able to forecast the class of objects whose class label is unknown using this model. This model was developed by the examination of training data sets. Figure 27.6 shows a general structure of ML based predictive model considering both the training and testing phase.

The following forms can be used to convey the generated model.

KNN: K-Nearest Neighbors, commonly referred to as KNN, is a fundamental and intuitive ML algorithm that belongs to the category of supervised learning. It is

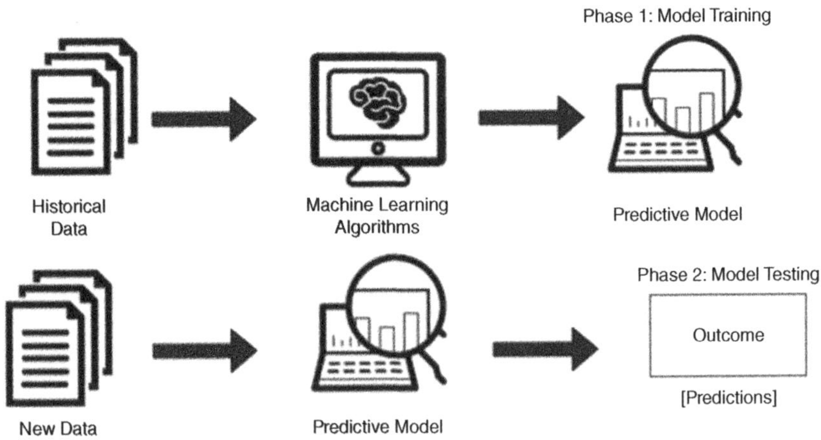

Figure 27.6 Machine learning predictive model structure-training and testing phase.

widely used for classification and regression tasks, making it an essential tool in the field of pattern recognition and data analysis. KNN operates on the principle of similarity, where it classifies or predicts the target value of a data point based on the majority class or average of its KNN in a feature space. This algorithm's simplicity and effectiveness make it a valuable choice for both beginners and experienced data scientists in various domains, from recommendation systems to image recognition and beyond. In this introduction, we will explore the underlying principles, advantages, and potential applications of the KNNs algorithm, shedding light on its significance in the world of ML.

Adaboost: AdaBoost is an ML algorithm that enhances the performance of weak classifiers by combining their outputs. Developed in 1996, it assigns weights to training examples, prioritizing misclassified ones in each iteration. The algorithm adapts and focuses on challenging instances, producing a robust and accurate final model. AdaBoost is widely used in applications such as face detection and object recognition due to its ability to improve predictive power.

Linear Discriminant Analysis: Linear discriminant analysis (LDA) is a statistical method for dimensionality reduction and classification. Unlike other techniques, LDA considers class labels, aiming to maximize the distance between class means while minimizing within-class variance. It transforms input features into a new space, highlighting class differences, and is especially effective in multiclass problems like facial recognition and medical diagnosis. LDA enhances class discrimination and is valuable for improving ML model efficiency.

SVM: SVMs are a powerful and widely used ML algorithm that falls under the category of supervised learning. They are primarily employed for classification and regression tasks, making them versatile tools in the field of data analysis and pattern recognition. One of the key concepts in SVM is the use of support vectors, which are the data points closest to the decision boundary and play a crucial role in determining the hyperplane's position. SVM can handle linear and nonlinear data separations using different kernel functions, allowing it to be adaptable to various real-world problems. In summary, SVM is a valuable tool in ML, known for its ability to find an optimal decision boundary that maximizes the margin between classes, making it a popular choice for classification and regression tasks.

Logistic Regression: Regression is a statistical method to model the relationship between dependent and independent variables. Linear regression predicts continuous outcomes assuming a linear relationship. Logistic regression, used for categorical dependent variables, predicts probabilities of class membership using the logistic function. Unlike linear regression, it models the probability of class membership rather than predicting exact outcomes. Logistic regression is a statistical method for binary classification, predicting the probability of an observation belonging to one of two classes. It uses the logistic function to transform a linear combination of input features into a probability between 0 and 1. The model is trained by adjusting weights to maximize the likelihood of observed outcomes. Logistic regression is widely used for its simplicity and efficiency in various fields like finance, medicine, and ML. In Figure 27.7, the dashed line represents a linear boundary that separates the two classes in classification, while in regression, it illustrates the linear relationship between the two variables. Regression predicts continuous outcomes, while classification predicts categorical outcomes.

Random Forest: RF is an ensemble learning algorithm used for classification and regression. It builds multiple decision trees during training, introducing randomness in data and feature selection to enhance robustness and prevent overfitting. By combining predictions from various trees, RF delivers accurate results, especially effective with large datasets. It also provides insights into feature importance for better interpretability.

CatBoost: CatBoost is a high-performance open-source ML library tailored for gradient boosting on decision trees. Noteworthy for its seamless handling of categorical features, it eliminates the need for extensive preprocessing. Developed by Yandex, CatBoost supports GPU acceleration, speeding up training, and employs ordered boosting for optimized tree sequence construction. Its robustness to overfitting, ability to handle missing data, and out-of-the-box support for multiclass classification make it a versatile choice for various ML tasks.

Naïve Bayes: NB is a probabilistic ML algorithm used for classification and spam filtering. It assumes feature independence, making computations efficient. Despite its simplicity, it often performs well in practice, especially for text-based

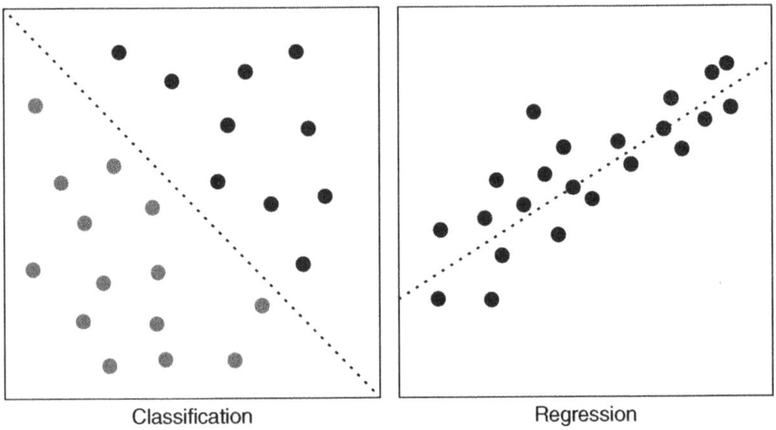

Figure 27.7 Comparison of classification and regression.

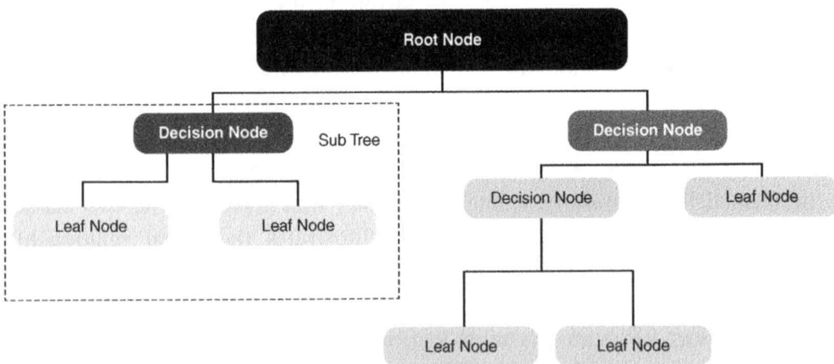

Figure 27.8 An example of decision tree structure.

tasks like spam detection and sentiment analysis. Its ease of implementation, computational efficiency, and minimal tuning requirements make it a popular choice in various applications.

Decision Tree: A decision tree is an ML algorithm that models decisions by dividing input data into subsets based on features. Its tree structure comprises nodes (decision points), branches (outcomes), and leaves (final decisions). The algorithm selects features at each node to maximize information gain or minimize impurity. Decision trees are versatile for classification and regression tasks, known for interpretability, and widely applied in finance, healthcare, and marketing. Their simplicity extends to use in ensemble methods like RF, making them popular in ML (Figure 27.8).

27.3.2.2 Prediction

The task of prediction involves anticipating future or unknown data values. To begin with, a model is built using the available data, which is then utilized to predict future values for a new and exciting dataset. Prediction analysis is applied in various fields, such as fraud detection and medical diagnostics.

27.3.2.3 Correlation Analysis

A mathematical method known as correlation may be used to assess whether and how strongly two qualities are connected. It refers to the numerous kinds of data structures that may be joined with an item set, such as trees and graphs. It determines how closely two continuous variables with numerical measurements are related. This kind of analysis may be used by researchers to check for potential connections between study variables.

27.3.2.4 Association

Discovering a relationship or connection between a group of things is called association. Association reveals the connections between various elements. Commodity management, advertising, catalogue design, direct marketing, etc. all employ association analysis [33].

27.3.2.5 Clustering

Data items that are similar to one another are found via clustering. A multitude of variables, including purchasing patterns, reactivity to certain activities, geographic regions, and other considerations, can be used to determine the degree of resemblance [36]. Popular clustering algorithms include:

- Means
- DB Scan

27.3.2.6 Summarization

Summarization is the process of generalizing data. It involves condensing a collection of relevant data into a smaller set that provides aggregated information. Sales or customer relationship teams might find high-level summaries of information useful for examining customer and purchase behavior in depth. To summarize data, one can use different levels of abstraction and perspectives [38–40].

27.3.2.7 Outlier Analysis

An outlier refers to a data point that deviates from the typical behavior or pattern of the rest of the data. Such data points can lead to inaccurate results in data analysis. However, outlier analysis can help identify unusual or suspicious activity, analyze rare events, and make predictions.

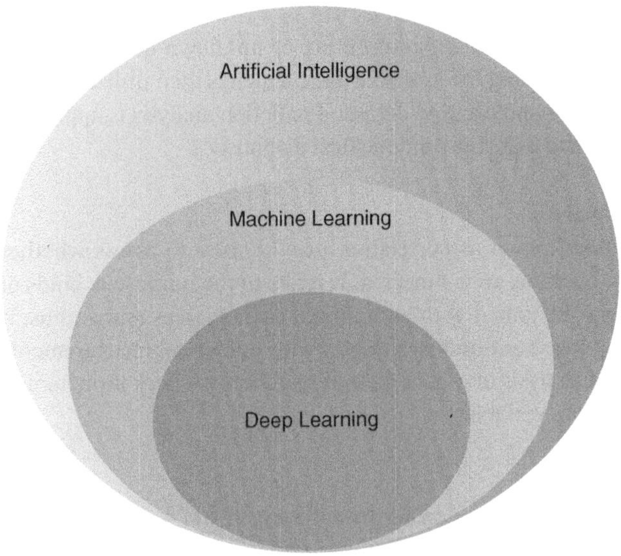

Figure 27.9 Relation between deep learning, machine learning, and artificial intelligence.

27.4 Artificial Neural Network and Deep Learning

Deep learning (DL) is a subset of artificial neural networks (ANN) within ML, characterized by representation learning. It leverages computational architectures comprising multiple processing layers, including input, hidden, and output layers, to learn from data. Compared to traditional ML methods, DL exhibits superior performance, particularly when dealing with large datasets (Figure 27.9).

The most common DL algorithms include.

Multilayer Perceptron (MLP): MLP, also known as the feed-forward ANN, serves as the foundational architecture of DL. It consists of an input layer, one or more hidden layers, and an output layer. Each node in one layer connects to every node in the following layer, with weight adjustments made internally using the "Backpropagation" technique [43]. MLP requires careful tuning of hyperparameters, such as the number of hidden layers and neurons, which can lead to computationally expensive models [44].

Convolutional Neural Network (CNN or ConvNet): CNN enhances the design of standard ANNs by incorporating convolutional layers, pooling layers, and fully connected layers. It excels in processing two-dimensional (2D) input data and finds broad applications in image and video recognition, medical image analysis, and natural language processing. Despite its computational complexity, CNN automatically detects important features without manual intervention, making it more powerful than conventional ANNs. Various advanced DL models based on CNN, such as AlexNet, Xception, and ResNet, are widely utilized across different domains [47].

Long Short-Term Memory Recurrent Neural Network (LSTM–RNN): LSTM is an artificial recurrent neural network architecture suited for sequential data analysis. Unlike feed-forward neural networks, LSTM incorporates feedback links and is adept at processing time series data. It finds applications in time-series analysis, natural language processing, and speech recognition, among others.

In addition to these common DL methods, several others exist for various purposes.

Self-Organizing Map (SOM): Utilizes unsupervised learning to represent high-dimensional data on a 2D grid map, facilitating dimensionality reduction.

Autoencoder (AE): Widely used for dimensionality reduction and feature extraction in unsupervised learning tasks.

Restricted Boltzmann Machines (RBM): Suitable for dimensionality reduction, classification, regression, collaborative filtering, feature learning, and topic modeling.

Deep Belief Network (DBN): Comprises simple, unsupervised networks such as RBMs or AE, along with a backpropagation neural network, facilitating various learning tasks.

Generative Adversarial Network (GAN): Capable of generating data with characteristics similar to actual input data, facilitating tasks like data generation.

Transfer Learning: Reuses pretrained models to train deep neural networks with relatively low amounts of data.

In summary, the diverse range of ML techniques, including classification, regression, clustering, and DL, and offer significant potential across various applications. Each technique possesses unique capabilities, making it suitable for specific tasks within different domains. The discussion of these ANN and DL models highlights their versatility and applicability in addressing complex problems across various fields.

27.4.1 Some PCOS Diagnosis Applications Using ML Techniques

27.4.1.1 Imaging Analysis

Ultrasound imaging is commonly used to detect ovarian cysts and other morphological features indicative of PCOS. ML algorithms trained on image data can automate the analysis of ultrasound scans, assisting radiologists in identifying characteristic PCOS features accurately. AI-driven follicle counting in ultrasound images aids in quantifying the presence of multiple small follicles, a characteristic feature of PCOS.

Purnama et al. [5] proposed a method for classifying PCOS using ultrasound (USG) images via follicle detection. They utilized 80 ultrasound images, 60 normal and 20 indicative of PCOS. Preprocessing involved noise reduction and segmentation, followed by feature extraction using Gabor wavelets. Classification with NN–LVQ, KNN, and SVM–RBF Kernel achieved the highest accuracy with SVM–RBF Kernel at $C = 40$, distinguishing PCOS-affected follicles effectively.

The paper by P. B and Khilar [32] addresses the classification of PCOS using ultrasound images of ovaries with the aid of ML algorithms. The study employs ML algorithms such as SVM, KNN, and CNN for classification. The CNN algorithm achieves the highest accuracy of 0.99 among the tested methods. The paper utilizes a large dataset for training, providing improved results compared to existing systems. Preprocessing techniques including grayscale conversion, normalization, and noise removal are applied to the ultrasound images before classification.

27.4.1.2 Predictive Models

Predictive models are utilized to analyze data patterns for identifying PCOS.

Risk Scoring Models: These models evaluate an individual's risk of PCOS by considering factors like age, weight, hormonal levels, family history, and other relevant risk factors. By drawing from past cases, these models calculate the probability of PCOS occurrence.

Symptom-Based Models: Predictive models incorporate PCOS symptoms alongside additional data to forecast the likelihood of PCOS development.

App-Based Predictive Tools: Some AI-powered apps allow users to input their symptoms and health information. The app's predictive model then generates a probability score indicating the likelihood of PCOS based on the provided information.

The paper by Tanwar et al. [40] propose a flask web app for predicting PCOS likelihood using easily measurable clinical features. It addresses the challenges of PCOS diagnosis and emphasizes early detection. By analyzing the dataset, the authors identify key features like skin darkening, hair growth, and weight gain using feature selection techniques. Results show prediction accuracies ranging from 85.15% to 92.59%. The highlight is the development of a user-friendly web app for accessible and noninvasive initial diagnosis, particularly beneficial in regions where PCOS diagnosis is stigmatized or inaccessible (Figure 27.10).

Although these models offer valuable assistance, the expertise of a medical professional remains vital for interpreting the predictions and reaching a conclusive

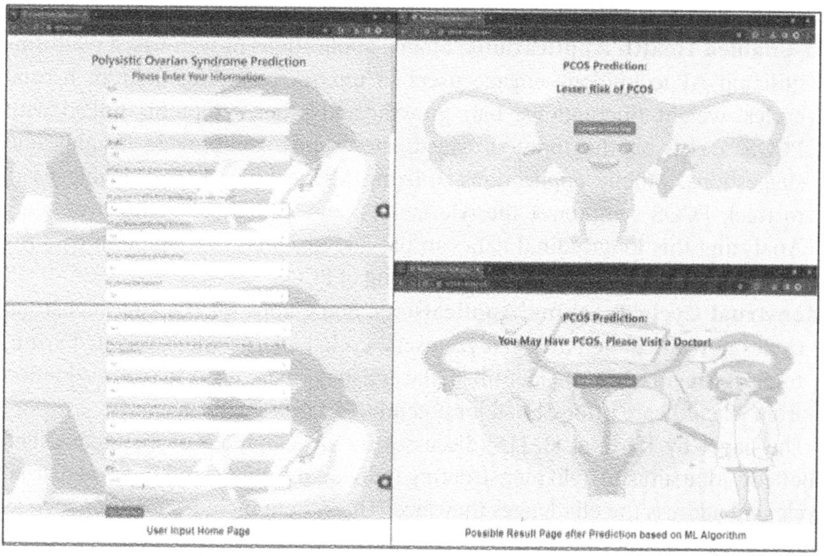

Figure 27.10 Illustration of a website model for predicting PCOS risk based on symptom analysis.

diagnosis. Furthermore, the accuracy of predictive models relies on the quality and diversity of the training data, emphasizing the necessity for continuous research and validation efforts.

27.4.1.3 Chatbots and Symptom Checkers

Chatbots and symptom checkers can lead users through a series of inquiries and then offer recommendations for the next steps, such as advising further medical assessment.

Telemedicine Platforms: Certain telemedicine services utilize chatbots to gather initial details from patients prior to a virtual consultation. These chatbots may inquire about PCOS symptoms, which are later discussed by healthcare providers during the appointment.

Virtual Health Assistants: Educational chatbots provide users with accurate information regarding PCOS, its symptoms, and when to seek medical assistance. Users can engage with the chatbot to enhance their understanding of the condition.

Voice-Activated Assistants: Smart speakers and other voice-controlled devices are capable of providing information about PCOS symptoms and suggesting whether an individual should seek advice from a healthcare professional based on the symptoms described.

27.4.1.4 App-Based Models

AI-Enabled Health Applications: Mobile applications or web-based platforms utilizing AI technology engage users in queries regarding their menstrual cycles, weight fluctuations, hair growth, and other symptoms linked with PCOS. Based on the input provided, these apps can provide insights and suggestions. Mobile applications utilizing ML techniques can enable users to track PCOS symptoms, lifestyle factors, and menstrual cycles over time. Analyzing this longitudinal data can provide insights into symptom patterns and facilitate early detection or monitoring of PCOS.

Menstrual Cycle Tracking Applications: Some apps for tracking menstrual cycles now integrate AI to analyze users' cycle patterns and associated symptoms. If irregularities are identified, the app may advise users to seek evaluation from a healthcare professional for potential PCOS.

The paper by Karia et al. [16] discusses the development of a system called "BeRedy" that aims to help menstruating individuals understand their menstrual cycle and address the challenges they face. The system includes features such as period cycle tracking, PCOS/PCOD diagnosis, a chatbot for personalized advice and support, and access to informative blogs. It also provides the option to purchase menstrual products from trustworthy websites. The system aims to provide accurate information and support to individuals, especially those who may lack access to resources and education about mesturation.

27.5 Challenges

While ML models hold promise in assisting with the prediction of conditions like PCOS, it's essential to acknowledge that they are not a substitute for the expertise of medical professionals. Interpretation of predictions and reaching a conclusive diagnosis still requires the knowledge and judgment of trained healthcare providers. Moreover, the accuracy and reliability of predictive models are contingent upon the quality and diversity of the training data. The use of sensitive health data for training ML models raises ethical and privacy concerns. Ensuring the confidentiality and security of patient data while also obtaining informed consent for data usage is essential but can be challenging to navigate. Before deploying ML models for PCOS prediction in clinical practice, rigorous validation studies are necessary to assess their performance, reliability, and safety. Clinical validation requires collaboration with healthcare professionals and adherence to regulatory standards, which can be time-consuming and resource-intensive. In addition, the interpretation of model outputs and integration into existing clinical workflows pose logistical challenges that must be addressed to ensure seamless adoption and effective utilization in real-world healthcare settings. Continuous research and validation efforts are necessary to ensure that these models perform effectively across different populations and settings. By integrating ML technology with ongoing medical research and clinical practice, we can harness the potential of predictive models to enhance diagnostic capabilities while maintaining the critical role of medical professionals in patient care.

27.6 Conclusion

In conclusion, this chapter has explored the landscape of ML algorithms for PCOS detection across healthcare domains. It emphasized the importance of robust feature engineering, meticulous data preprocessing, and algorithm selection to enhance accuracy. The significance of leveraging diverse data sources underscores the multifaceted nature of PCOS diagnosis. Moving forward, the chapter anticipates further advancements in ML models, to improve the early detection and management of PCOS.

References

1 Dhileep, P. and Kesavamurthy, T. (2015). Diagnostic tool for pcos classification. In: *7th WACBE World Congress on Bioengineering 2015* (ed. J. Cho and C.T. Lim), 182–185. Springer.

2 Barber, T.M., McCarthy, M.I., Wass, J.A.H., and Franks, S. (2006). Obesity and polycystic ovary syndrome. *Clinical Endocrinology* 65 (2): 137–145.

3 Barrera, F.J., Brown, E.D.L., Rojo, A. et al. (2023). Application of machine learning and artificial intelligence in the diagnosis and classification of polycystic ovarian syndrome: a systematic review. *Frontiers in Endocrinology* 14: 1106625.

4 Bedrick, B.S., Eskew, A.M., Chavarro, J.E., and Jungheim, E.S. (2020). Self-administered questionnaire to screen for polycystic ovarian syndrome. *Women's Health Reports* 1 (1): 566–573.

5 Purnama, B., Wisesti, U.N., Nhita, F., et al. (2015). A classification of polycystic ovary syndrome based on follicle detection of ultrasound images. *2015 3rd International Conference on Information and Communication Technology (ICoICT)*, pp. 396–401, Nusa Dua, Bali (27–29 May 2015). IEEE.

6 Bharathi, R.V., Swetha, S., Neerajaa, J. et al. (2017). An epidemiological survey: effect of predisposing factors for PCOS in Indian urban and rural population. *Middle East Fertility Society Journal* 22 (4): 313–316.

7 Bharati, S., Podder, P. and Mondal, M.R.H. (2020). Diagnosis of polycystic ovary syndrome using machine learning algorithms. *2020 IEEE Region 10*

Symposium (TENSYMP), pp. 1486–1489, Dhaka, Bangladesh (05–07 June 2020). IEEE.

8 Bulsara, J., Patel, P., Soni, A., and Acharya, S. (2021). A review: brief insight into polycystic ovarian syndrome. *Endocrine and Metabolic Science* 3: 100085.

9 Chandra, S. and Kaur, M. (2015). Creation of an Adaptive Classifier to enhance the classification accuracy of existing classification algorithms in the field of Medical Data Mining. *2015 2nd International Conference on Computing for Sustainable Global Development (INDIACom)*, pp. 376–381, New Delhi, India (11–13 March 2015). IEEE.

10 Chauhan, P. Patil, N. Rane, P.R. and Kanakia, H. (2021). Comparative analysis of machine learning algorithms for prediction of PCOS. *2021 International Conference on Communication information and Computing Technology (ICCICT)*, pp. 1–7, Mumbai, India (25–27 June 2021). IEEE. https://doi.org/10.1109/ICCICT50803.2021.9510128

11 Cheng, J.J. and Mahalingaiah, S. (2019). Data mining polycystic ovary morphology in electronic medical record ultrasound reports. *Fertility Research and Practice* 5 (1): 1–7.

12 Chitra, P., Srilatha, K., Sumathi, M. et al. (2023). Classification of Ultrasound PCOS Image using Deep Learning based Hybrid Models. *2023 Second International Conference on Electronics and Renewable Systems (ICEARS)*, Tuticorin, India (02–04 March 2023). IEEE.

13 Denny, A., Raj, A., Ashok, A. et al. (2019). i-HOPE: detection and prediction system for polycystic ovary syndrome (PCOS) using machine learning techniques. *TENCON 2019 – 2019 IEEE Region 10 Conference (TENCON)*, pp. 673–678, Kochi, India (17–20 October 2019). IEEE https://doi.org/10.1109/TENCON.2019.8929674.

14 Hdaib, D., Alkafaween, E., Alzoubi, K., & Khalayleh, W. (2022). Detection of polycystic ovary syndrome (PCOS) using machine learning algorithms. *2022 5th International Conference on Engineering Technology and its Applications (IICETA)*, pp. 1–6, Al-Najaf, Iraq (31 May–01 June 2022). IEEE.

15 Jyothi, R., Shivani, H.C., Yashaswi, R. et al. (2023). Detection of polycystic ovary syndrome (PCOS) using machine learning techniques. *2023 International Conference on Computational Intelligence for Information, Security and Communication Applications (CIISCA)*. IEEE.

16 Karia, A. Poojary, A. Tiwari, L.S., and Sokhi, M.K. (2023). BeRedy (Period Tracker & PCOS Diagnosis). *2023 International Conference on Communication System, Computing and IT Applications (CSCITA)*, Mumbai, India (31 March–1 April 2023). IEEE

17 Katarya, R., Srivastava, G., & Chauhan, N. (2021). A novel polycystic ovarian syndrome diagnostic system using machine learning. *Proceedings of 3rd*

International Conference on Computing Informatics and Networks: ICCIN 2020, pp. 333–343). Springer Singapore.

18 Khan, A., Karim, N., Ainuddin, J.A., and Fahim, M.F. (2019). Polycystic ovarian syndrome: correlation between clinical hyperandrogenism, anthropometric, metabolic and endocrine parameters. *Pak J Med Sci.* 35 (5): 1227–1232. https://doi.org/10.12669/pjms.35.5.742.

19 Lizneva, D., Suturina, L., Walker, W. et al. (2016). Criteria, prevalence, and phenotypes of polycystic ovary syndrome. *Fertility and Sterility* 106 (1): 6–15.

20 Makhdoomi, A., Jan, N., Palak, P., and Goel, N. (2022). Machine learning techniques for medical images in PCOS. *2022 4th International Conference on Artificial Intelligence and Speech Technology (AIST)*, Delhi, India (09–10 December 2022). IEEE.

21 Mallela, R.C., Bhavani, R.L., and Ankayarkanni, B. (2021). Disease prediction using machine learning techniques. *2021 5th International Conference on Trends in Electronics and Informatics (ICOEI)*, Nagpur, India (29–30 April 2022). IEEE.

22 Meena, K., Manimekalai, M., and Rethinavalli, S. (2015). Correlation of artificial neural network classification and NFRS attribute filtering algorithm for PCOS data. *International Journal of Research in Engineering and Technology* 4 (3): 519–524.

23 Mehrotra, P., Chatterjee, J., Chakraborty, C., et al. (2011). Automated screening of polycystic ovary syndrome using machine learning techniques. *2011 Annual IEEE India Conference*, pp. 1–5, Hyderabad, India (16–18 December 2011). IEEE.

24 Mirbabaie, M., Stieglitz, S., and Frick, N.R.J. (2021). Artificial intelligence in disease diagnostics: A critical review and classification on the current state of research guiding future direction. *Health and Technology* 11: 693–731.

25 Mittapalli, J.S., Khanna, K., Mutha, J.A., and Nair, S. (2023). A cloud-based prediction and self-diagnosis system for PCOS using machine learning models. In: *Futuristic Communication and Network Technologies*, Lecture Notes in Electrical Engineering, vol. 966 (ed. N. Subhashini, M.A.G. Ezra, and S.K. Liaw). Singapore: Springer.

26 Munjal, A., Khandia, R., and Gautam, B. (2020). A machine learning approach for selection of polycystic ovariansyndrome (PCOS) attributes and comparing different classifier performance with the help of weka and pycaret. *International Journal of Scientific Research* 9: 1–5.

27 Nabi, N., Islam, S., Khushbu, S.A., and Masum, A.K.M. (2021). Machine learning approach: detecting polycystic ovary syndrome & it's impact on Bangladeshi women. *2021 12th International Conference on Computing Communication and Networking Technologies (ICCCNT)*, Kharagpur, India (6–8 July 2021). IEEE.

28 Nandipati, S.C., Ying, C.X., and Wah, K.K. (2020). Polycystic Ovarian Syndrome (PCOS) classification and feature selection by machine learning techniques. *Applied Mathematics and Computational Intelligence* 9: 65–74.

29 Nasim, S., Hussain, M.A., Riaz, F. et al. (2022). A novel approach for polycystic ovary syndrome prediction using machine learning in bioinformatics. *IEEE Access* 10: 97610–97624.

30 Neto, C., Silva, M., Fernandes, M. et al. (2021). Prediction models for Polycystic Ovary Syndrome using data mining. In: *Advances in Digital Science: ICADS 2021* (ed. T. Antipova), 210–221. Springer International Publishing.

31 Nichols, J.A., Herbert Chan, H.W., and Baker, M.A.B. (2019). Machine learning: applications of artificial intelligence to imaging and diagnosis. *Biophysical Reviews* 11 (1): 111–118. https://doi.org/10.1007/s12551-018-0449-9.

32 B, P. and Khilar, R. (2023). Classification of PCOS using machine learning algorithms based on ultrasound images of ovaries. *2023 Eighth International Conference on Science Technology Engineering and Mathematics (ICONSTEM)*, Chennai, India, pp. 1–7. https://doi.org/10.1109/ICONSTEM56934.2023.10142359.

33 Pedersen, S.D., Brar, S., Faris, P., and Corenblum, B. (2007). Polycystic ovary syndrome: validated questionnaire for use in diagnosis. *Canadian Family Physician* 53 (6): 1041–1047.

34 Suriya, P.T., Reka, S. and Elakkiya, R. (2022). Early diagnosis of poly cystic ovary syndrome (PCOS) in young women: a machine learning approach. *2022 IEEE International Symposium on Mixed and Augmented Reality Adjunct (ISMAR-Adjunct)*, pp. 286–288, Singapore (17–21 October 2022). IEEE.

35 Sarker, I.H. (2021). Machine learning: algorithms, real-world applications and research directions. *SN Computer Science* 2: 160.

36 Sethi, R., Vishwakarma, D.K., Ganguly, S., and Ray, R. (2023). A comparative study on different machine learning algorithms to detect PCOS. *2023 14th International Conference on Computing Communication and Networking Technologies (ICCCNT)*, Delhi, India (6–8 July 2023). IEEE.

37 Sinthia, G., Poovizhi, T., & Khilar, R. (2022). Analysis on polycystic ovarian syndrome and comparative study of different machine learning algorithms. *Advances in Intelligent Computing and Communication: Proceedings of ICAC 2021*, pp. 191–196. Springer Nature Singapore.

38 Soni, P. and Vashisht, S. (2018). Exploration on polycystic ovarian syndrome and data mining techniques. *2018 3rd International Conference on Communication and Electronics Systems (ICCES)*, pp. 816–820, Coimbatore, India (15–16 October 2018). IEEE.

39 Subha, R., Nayana, B.R., Radhakrishnan, R., and Sumalatha P. (2022). Computerized Diagnosis of Polycystic Ovary Syndrome Using Machine Learning and Swarm Intelligence Techniques. https://doi.org/10.21203/rs.3.rs-2027767/v2

40 Tanwar, A., Jain, A., and Chauhan, A. (2022). Accessible polycystic ovarian syndrome diagnosis using machine learning. *2022 3rd International Conference for Emerging Technology (INCET)*, pp. 1–544, Belgaum, India (27–29 May 2022). IEEE.

41 Thomas, N. and Kavitha, A. (2020). Prediction of polycystic ovarian syndrome with clinical dataset using a novel hybrid data mining classification technique. *International Journal of Advanced Research in Engineering and Technology* 11 (11): 1872–1881.

42 Vijayalakshmi, N. and Uma Maheshwari, M. (2016). Data mining to elicit predominant factors causing infertility in women. *International Journal of Computer Science and Mobile Computing* 5 (8): 5–9.

43 Adla, Y.A.A., Raydan, D.G., Charaf, M.-Z.J., et al. (2021). Automated detection of polycystic ovary syndrome using machine learning techniques. *2021 Sixth International Conference on Advances in Biomedical Engineering (ICABME)*, pp. 208–212, Werdanyeh, Lebanon (7–9 October 2021). IEEE.

28

Diagnosis and Classification of Skin Cancer Using Generative Artificial Intelligence (Gen AI)

Niveditha N. Reddy and Pooja Agarwal

Computer Science, PES, Bangalore, Karnataka

28.1 Introduction

Technology and artificial intelligence (AI) are becoming increasingly significant in dermatology. Convolutional neural networks (CNNs) and image processing techniques are widely studied for their ability to distinguish specific features in photos of skin lesions, which could help detect suspicious lesions and diagnose diseases such as melanoma. Cancer of the skin is the most common kind of cancer worldwide [1]. Over the previous decade, the annual diagnosis of severe melanoma cases has climbed by a startling 27%. Nonmelanoma skin cancer kills approximately 5,400 individuals every month, which is disturbing. Carcinoma basal cells are the most common kind of skin cancer, followed by squamous cell carcinoma and melanoma, which are the most aggressive and deadly. Merkel cell carcinoma is also distinct among aggressive tumors [2]. It has become difficult to identify due to obvious similarities. Melanoma, a well-known kind of skin cancer, has been responsible for a large number of deaths in recent years. According to recent polls, the number of skin cancer patients is increasing each year, unlike other kind of cancer. It affects melanocytes, which are the skin's surface cells. It has various cell kinds, which cause the skin to become darker. It is more deadly and hazardous because it spreads quickly. Melanoma is found anywhere in the human body, yet it most commonly develops on the rear of the lower limbs. Traditionally, skin cancer was diagnosed through physical examination and visual inspection. Lesion photography is time-consuming, complicated, and error-prone. Melanomas are typically recognized using the ABCDE criterion (asymmetry, borders, color, diameter, and evolving). Melanoma diagnosis is based on the observation of these warning signals. The first warning indicator is an asymmetrical or irregularly bordered mole, or one bigger than 6 mm in

Generative Artificial Intelligence for Biomedical and Smart Health Informatics,
First Edition. Edited by Aditya Khamparia and Deepak Gupta.

diameter and unusually colored. Deep learning-enabled CNNs outperformed dermatologists in diagnosing skin cancer through picture analysis. Segmentation is crucial in developing an automated melanoma detection system. Region of interest or thresholding-based algorithms are effective when image contrast and lighting vary minimally.

28.2 Factors Affecting Skin Cancer Detection

Skin type and pigmentation: People with lighter skin tones and less pigmentation are more likely to develop skin cancer, and they may have milder lesions that require deeper examination.

Personal History: A personal history of sunburn, sun exposure, or prior skin cancers raises the chance of acquiring new skin cancers. A family history of skin cancer increases an individual's risk and emphasizes the significance of regular check-ups.

Awareness and Self-Examination: Regularly inspecting your skin for changes and understanding the signs and symptoms of skin cancer can lead to earlier detection and a better prognosis.

28.3 Different Types of Skin Cancer

28.3.1 Nonmelanoma Skin Cancers

Basal and squamous cell carcinomas are nonmelanoma cancers. These are rarely fatal, although surgeries are painful and disfiguring. Analysis of the temporal trends in the incidence of nonmelanoma skin cancers is challenging since these tumors have not yet been effectively registered. There is a direct correlation in certain countries between rising nonmelanoma skin cancer incidence and falling latitude, or higher UV radiation levels.

28.3.2 Malignant Melanoma

Since the early 1970s, the incidence of malignant melanoma increased considerably, by an average of 4.

28.4 How Common Is Skin Cancer?

The occurrence of the two nonmelanoma and melanoma skin cancers has risen in recent decades. Every year, around 2M to 3M nonmelanoma cancers in the skin and 132,000 melanoma skin cancers are diagnosed worldwide. Ozone levels fall, the atmosphere's protective filter function deteriorates, and more amount of solar UV radiation reaches the Earth's surface. It was predicted that an additional 300,000 cases of nonmelanoma and 4,500 cases of melanoma skin cancer would occur for every 10 melanoma is a type of skin cancer that can appear anywhere on the skin. It is also referred to as cutaneous melanoma or malignant melanoma. Melanoma arises from the mutation of melanocytes, which are cells responsible for producing melanin, a dark pigment, and their excessively fast growth. Though it usually begins on the soles of the feet in women and the chest and back in men, it can appear anywhere on the skin. The cheeks and neck are other common places. Although it can also happen in the mouth, sexual organs, anal region, and eyes, the likelihood of melanoma growing there is far lower than that of the skin (Figure 28.1).

Classification of skin cancer detection: Melanoma, basal cell carcinoma (BCC), and squamous cell carcinoma (SCC), which are considered as dangerous. Other types consist of melanocytic nevi, actinic keratosis (AK), benign keratosis, dermatofibromas, and vascular lesions. Melanoma is the most dangerous form and can recur even after treatment. Several articles have been published on diagnostic breakthroughs in the classification of skin cancer (Figure 28.2). No reviews have addressed breakthrough challenges similar to data imbalance, realm adaptability, model strength, and efficiency. This article reviews new advances in the arrangement of skin using dermoscopy images. A comprehensive study that used convolution neural networks (CNNs) to classify skin lesions. A study [8] demonstrated the effectiveness of using CNNs for skin cancer detection. There are algorithms for

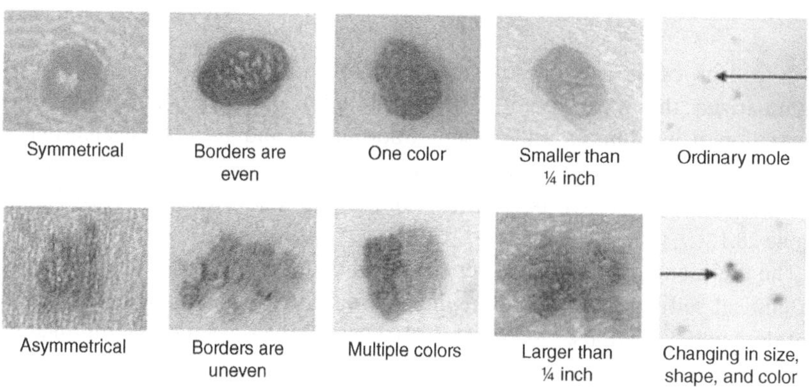

Figure 28.1 Melanoma skin cancer, types, stages, signs, symptoms, and treatment. Source: Skin Cancer MNIST / Kaggle, Inc. / CC BY-NC-SA 4.0.

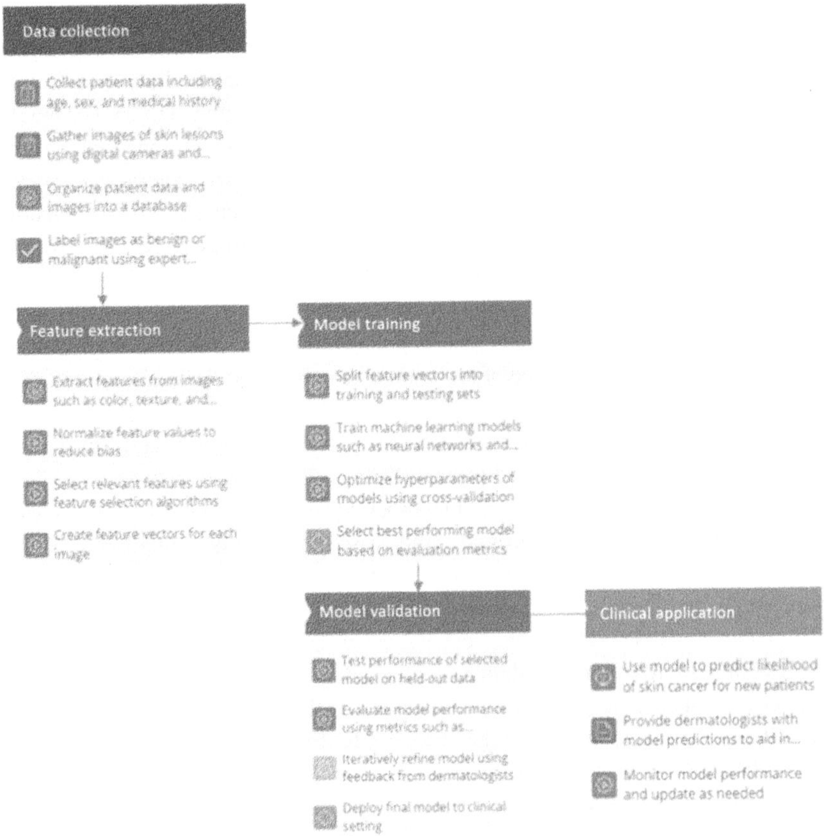

Figure 28.2 Skin cancer detection and classification.

skin cancer categorization, as well as significant hurdles and trouble. We summarized the most recent CNN-based approaches for skin lesion categorization using images and patient information and gave an evaluation of DL-based approaches for prior detection of dermoscopic image analysis. We provide these pertinent polls with information and important insights in Table 28.1.

The traditional method of cancer classification disregards practical limitations in clinical settings. Considerations include data imbalances and limits, different domain adaptations, models, and efficiency. Earlier evaluations summed up techniques for handling frontier problems, but they were incomplete. Some revolutionary solutions, such as pruning, knowledge distillation, and transformer, were not covered.

Table 28.1 Summary of previous reviews on skin cancer classification methods.

References	Title	Venue	Remarks
[6]	Skin Cancer Classification Using Convolutional Neural Networks: Systematic Review	Journal of Medical Internet Research	The study presents a detailed overview of studies on using CNNs to classify skin lesions
[5]	Techniques and algorithms for computer-aided diagnosis of pigmented skin lesions—A review	Biomedical Signal Processing and Control[a)]	This paper gives a review of the recent developments in skin lesion classification using dermoscopic images.
[7]	This paper gives a review of the recent developments in skin lesion classification using dermoscopic images.	data 8	data 9[b)]
[8]	Machine Learning in Dermatology: Current Applications, Opportunities, and Limitations	Dermatology and therapy volume	This paper reviews the fundamentals of machine learning and its wide range of applications in dermatology.
[3]	Artificial intelligence-based image classification methods for diagnosis of skin cancer: Challenges and opportunities	Computers in Biology and Medicine	This review discusses the developments in AI-based methods for skin cancer diagnosis, as well as challenges and future directions to enhance them.

a) The significance of this reference lies in its comprehensive coverage of the methods and algorithms utilized in computer-aided skin cancer diagnosis, highlighting technological progress in this domain.
b) Its significance is in providing insights into how CNNs are applied in medical imaging for improving skin cancer detection and classification.

28.5 Dermatological Images and Datasets

Dermatologists and automated diagnostic systems rely on high-quality images of skin conditions. On the one hand, doctors use high-resolution (HR) photography to diagnose conditions that cannot be seen directly. This is particularly true of telemedicine, doctor visits, and regular clinics. However, to train reliable algorithms, high-quality data must always be used. Deep learning algorithms, in particular, require a significant amount of labeled data to enhance their accuracy. Thus, top-grade dermatologic photos are tough for two clinical analyses and the development of new systems. In this part, we'll look at the three main types of images that are widely used in skin cancer detection, as well as some publicly available statistics. Histopathological images were obtained by scanning and digitizing tissue slides using microscopes (Table 28.2).

They are used to depict the vertical structure and interior properties of sick tissues. Pathological examinations are the "gold standard" for detecting cancer and guiding treatment regimens since they can differentiate between different forms.

28.5.1 Dermatological Images

Skin diseases are diagnosed using three different imaging modalities: clinical examination, dermoscopy, and histology. Clinical photographs are typically taken using devices for remote diagnosis and clinical records.

28.5.2 Clinical Image

These images are created by photographing the disease location directly with the camera. Act as an immunological document for patients and provide valuable insights regarding dermoscopy images. These images for skin cancer classification provide limited morphological details and can result in errors due to imaging settings.

28.5.3 Dermoscopy Images

Dermoscopy is an optical observation device that captures images to assess skin disease characteristics. Dermoscopy is commonly used to diagnose both benign nevi and malignant melanoma. Dermoscopy, sometimes known as a dermatologist's stethoscope, connects the clinical and pathological examinations (Figure 28.3).

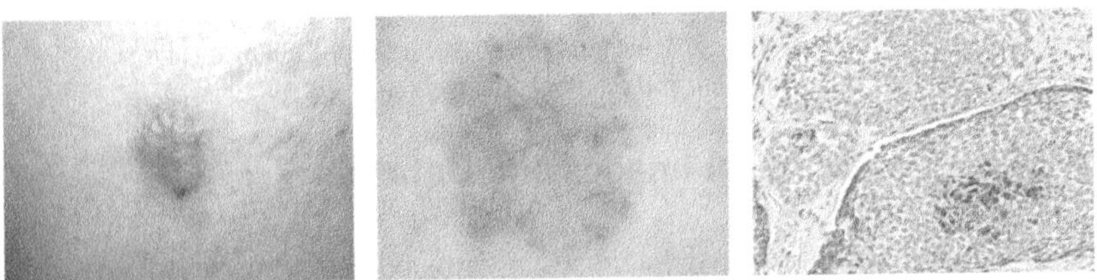

(a) (b) (c)

Figure 28.3 Examples of three types of dermatological images of BCC showing their variances and associations: (a) Clinical picture. (b) Dermoscopic image. (c) Histopathological image. Source: Skin Cancer MNIST / Kaggle, Inc / CC BY-NC-SA 4.0.

Table 28.2 Different methods for solving data imbalance and data limitation.

References	Dataset	Highlights	Limitations
(84) ISIC-2017	By coupling seven GANs to generate seven skin-disease images. At the same time, they improved the efficiency of the model by making the initial layers of GANS share the same parameters.	The model was unable to distinguish the lesion area well when it is mixed with the skin surface, and artifacts such as human hair can also affect the generation of new images.	Accuracy: 0.816
		AUC: 0.88	
(85) ISIC-2018	Proposed a GAN architecture that was customized to the style of skin lesions. At the same time, it can generate higher resolution and more diverse skin disease images by adjusting the progressive growth structure of the generator and discriminator in the GAN network.	The content of the GAN—the generated synthetic dataset was not complicated enough when compared with the original dataset, and it was also not diverse enough.	Accuracy: 0.952
		Sensitivity: 0.832	Specificity: 0.743
(86) ISIC-2018	Utilized conditional generative adversarial networks (CGAN) to extract key information from all layers to generate skin lesion images with different textures and shapes while ensuring the stability of training.	The amount of data used for training was relatively limited.	Accuracy: 0.941
		Precision: 0.915	Recall: 0.799

(Continued)

Table 28.2 (Continued)

References	Dataset	Highlights	Limitations
(87) ISIC Archive	Explored four types of data augmentation methods and a multiple-layer augmentation method in melanoma classification.	The data augmentation methods evaluated in this paper were limited and not validated on a large amount of datasets.	Accuracy: 0.829
(88) HAM10000	They adopted a variety national autoencoder network to get domain-dependent noise vectors. Also, a student-like distribution was employed to increase image diversity, and an auxiliary classifier was used to create images of certain classes.	Due to the specificity of medical images, different image generation models may generate skin disease images that do not belong to the same class.	Accuracy: 0.925

28.6 Datasets

A varied set of dermatological images is required for an accurate categorization of the system. Increasingly sets become available as the need for diagnostic imaging resources in academics increases. In the next part, we present commonly used skin-disease datasets and their accompanying publications for reference.

28.6.1 PH2 Dataset

The PH2 dataset was created by Goyal et al [4] to study classification and segmentation algorithms. The collection includes 200 color dermoscopy photos (768 × 560) of three kinds of skin diseases Common Nevi, Atypical Nevi, and Melanomas. In addition, this includes detailed annotations such as lesion segmentation results and pathological diagnosis. Skin disease diagnostic algorithms are commonly tested using the PH2 dataset. For instance, SegNet was utilized to automatically analyze and segment dermoscopic images in the PH2 dataset, resulting in a 94% accuracy rate

28.6.2 The MED–NODE Dataset

The University Medical Centre Groningen's (UMCG) Department of Dermatology received the MED–NODE Dataset3 contains 170 digital pictures of melanoma and nevi. The MEDNODE system, which uses macroscopic images to identify skin cancer, is created and evaluated (Table 28.3, Figure 28.4).

28.7 Skin Cancer Classification in Typical CNN Frameworks

In the early stages of CNN development, self-building networks were extensively utilized for particular jobs. In one investigation, melanoma was identified using

Table 28.3 Characteristics of different skin-disease datasets.

Dataset	Number of images	Modality of images	Number of lesion types	Image format	Published year
PH	200	Dermoscopic	3	.bmp	2013
MED	170	Macroscopic	2	.jpg	2015
HAM10000	10,015	Dermoscopic	8	.jpg	2018
Derm7pt	2,000	Dermoscopic Structured	15	.jpg data	2018
BCN20000	19424	Dermoscopic	9	.jpg	2019
ISIC	13,000	Dermoscopic	9	.jpg	2016–2020

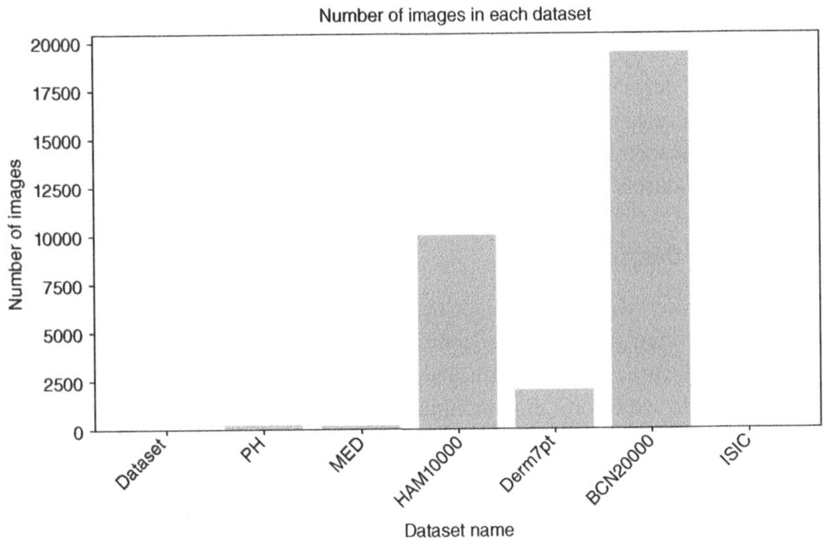

Figure 28.4 Graph 1 different skin-disease datasets and number of images in datasets.

a self-supervised system. Both tagged and unlabeled images were trained using an in-depth belief network and a self-advised support vector machine. Experiments revealed that the proposed technique performed both K-nearest neighbor and support vector machine. Then a rudimentary CNN network was developed to detect melanoma. Every image was preprocess to eliminate noise and artifacts. The processed images were fed into a pretrained CNN to assess whether they were melanoma or benign images. In our test results, it performed better than alternative classification algorithms, VGGNet, GoogleNet, and ResNet showed promising results in classifying skin cancer the most significant work. This is the inceptive a CNN used to train big amount of medical pictures for cancer in skin categorization. These used Inception v3 for building an end-to-end network capable of automatically classifying skin cancer. The model was trained on 129,450 clinical images depicting 2,032 illnesses in the skin.

28.8 Imbalance in Data and Limitations in Disease in Skin Databases

Asymmetry and limits in illness in skin disease databases are significant challenges in cancer categorization assignment skin disease datasets may contain inequitable sample sizes across classes. Most skin disease statistics only include common illnesses such as BCC, SCC, and melanoma. In these datasets, algorithms struggle to accurately classify infrequent skin tumors such as appendiceal carcinomas and cutaneous lymphoma. Generative adversarial networks (GAN) are considered a better alternative since they can produce false data to compensate for data imbalances, both positive and negative. To solve the issue created a style-based GAN that produces higher quality images for skin lesion categorization. The pretrained ResNet 50 model's training set was expanded to include the synthetic images. The study found the style-based GAN varieties in relation to Inception Score, Frechet Inception Distance, precision, and recall. Essentially, the GAN serves as a link between real-world data and personalized training in skin cancer detection. By creating data that resembles real-world movement patterns while providing variances and personalization, AI models can learn more effectively and customize interventions to individual needs, resulting in better patient outcomes. Let "z" be the random vector and "x" be a TS window from the dataset distribution "pX," mathematically speaking. We just take into account the fact that z comes from a uniform distribution with a [1,1] support. Taking "z" as input, the generative model produces TS data, G(z), which also has similar support as "x." Let "G" and "D" be the generating and discriminative models. Write *pG* to represent the distribution of *G*(*z*). Approximating the likelihood that the input TS data is taken from *pX* is the goal of the discriminative model. If *xpX*, then *d*(*x*) = 1, and if *xpG*, then *D*(*x*) = 0. Together, the discriminative and generative models can be trained by resolving.

$$\min \max V(D, G) = E_{X\sim Pd}[\log D(x)] + E_{Z\sim Pz}[\log(1 - D(G(z)))] \quad (28.1)$$

The generator used in the first dataset has five levels. The input layer corresponds to the latent vector "z," which consists of 32 elements. A fully-connected layer with 256 nodes comes next, followed by three more fully-connected layers with 512, 1,024, and 699 nodes in order of precedence. Batch normalization is applied, and a Leaky ReLU activation function is fitted to each layer. The final layer is then molded into a 3 × 233 node structure to fit the incoming data's architecture. In contrast, the discriminator receives input that is either synthetic or real and is first molded into a fully linked layer with 899 nodes. After that, this layer goes through two more fully-connected layers with 512 and 256 nodes, respectively, each batch normalization and leaky ReLU activation functions. The output node is a single node that uses a Sigmoid activation function to determine if the data is synthetic or real.

28.9 ML Techniques for Skin Cancer Diagnosis

A CNN computes local linear combinations of each layer's outputs using weights calculated from the coefficients of several convolutional filters. As a result, when using a CNN to represent IMU data, the time series entries are concatenated at the second layer. Because each entry contains a unique collection of kinematic data, such as skin images, quaternions, and accelerations, this could be problematic.

Random Forest: Five manually created statistic mean, maximum, minimum, standard deviation, and root mean squares that were generated for each of the 78-dimensional windows served as the input for the random forest models. These characteristics record important data for movement identification, like motion energy and window fluctuations.

RNNs: Have the ability to analyze sequential data, such as video frames, with high accuracy to detect movement patterns and forecast future developments.

CNNs: Frequently attain remarkable precision in identifying essential characteristics from pictures or videos allowing impartial evaluation. Although GANs have distinct benefits in terms of data creation, personalization, and understandable feedback, they might not necessarily be more accurate than other well-trained algorithms in all areas of cancer detection. Often, the optimum strategy combines several algorithms to take advantage of each one's unique advantages and produce the greatest possible outcomes. To address the constraints in skin cancer detection studies, this study tells us the help of GANs to create synthetic skin lesion data. GANs have the potential to help AI models analyze varied skin lesion patterns, forecast diagnostic outcomes, and even personalize interventions by supplementing limited and imbalanced datasets. While data normalization improves the acceptability of generated data for GAN training, using class-specific GANs and zero-padding approaches ensures compatibility with deep learning algorithms. This opens the door to more personalized skin cancer detection models and higher diagnosis accuracy, perhaps leading to better patient outcomes. However, ethical constraints, the generalizability of synthetic data to real-world circumstances, and the overall quality of the generated data continue to be persistent obstacles in increasing skin cancer diagnosis through the data augmentation model, which introduces a novel training strategy for both generator and encoder components. In contrast to traditional approaches that tightly couple these components, the discriminator model takes a more relaxed approach. This relaxation allows the generator and encoder to continue training until they can produce a new set of data samples that closely resemble the true distribution of the original data.

Moreover, our proposed model presents a fresh conceptual framework for the trained encoder discriminator duo. This framework can be effectively utilized as a one-class binary classifier. Instead of rigidly categorizing data into two distinct classes, our model's encoder discriminator combination excels at discerning the unique characteristics of a single class. This makes it particularly suitable for anomaly detection and classification tasks where the focus is on identifying deviations from the norm rather than distinguishing between multiple classes. This study aims to investigate and understand a specific subject or problem. It involves a systematic examination of relevant data, literature, or phenomena with the goal of generating insights, making discoveries, or testing hypotheses. The proposed methodology for developing a novel cloud computing system for skin cancer detection using generative AI techniques comprises several key steps. First, the process begins with the collection and preprocessing of data. This involves gathering historical data on skin disease, resolution, sensitivity, and other relevant factors.

In addition, real-time data is integrated through sensors, image sensors, and measurements. Data quality is ensured by addressing missing values, outliers, and performing necessary normalization. Remote sensing data, including images, are also explored for their potential to improve predictions. Next, a robust cloud computing infrastructure is established to support the system's scalability and accessibility. This infrastructure includes setting up data storage solutions and implementing stringent data security measures. This generative model is trained using historical skin data and is carefully fine-tuned for optimal performance. Special attention is given to maintaining meaningful semantic relationships among the features in the generated data. Machine learning (ML) prediction models, including regression and random forests, are developed for skin cancer prediction. These models leverage both the generated synthetic data and real data to create augmented datasets.

Ensemble learning techniques are applied to combine predictions from multiple models, enhancing prediction accuracy. Real-time data integration is a critical aspect, with the cloud-based system continuously updated with data from sensors and other sources. Periodic retraining of prediction models ensures they adapt to changing conditions. Data streaming and event-driven architecture are employed for seamless real-time updates. To make the system user-friendly, a web or mobile application is developed, providing farmers and stakeholders with access to skin cancer predictions. Data is presented through interactive charts, maps, and dashboards for effective visualization. Scalability and performance optimization are achieved by ensuring the system can handle increased data volumes and user loads. Cloud resources are optimized, and auto-scaling mechanisms are implemented to manage varying workloads effectively. Regular model evaluation and feedback collection from users are conducted to improve prediction accuracy and system capabilities. Security measures are maintained to protect data and user privacy, adhering to relevant regulations and standards. User training and support are provided to facilitate effective utilization of the system, accompanied by comprehensive documentation and resources. In addition, ongoing research and innovation efforts are undertaken to stay updated with the latest advancements in generative AI and skin cancer detection techniques, allowing for continuous enhancement of the system's capabilities. Specifically, this aims to generate fake work that is closely similar to real info, while the discriminator strives to differentiate between real and fake samples. In many existing GAN approaches, particularly those applied to natural images, achieving equilibrium requires both components to maintain their capabilities at a similar pace. A standard training strategy is not suitable for numerous application scenarios. Often, maintaining semantic relations within the feature sets in the information formed by the generator is crucial. The data set used for the discriminator differs from those generated by the generator, leading to training instability, characterized by fluctuating generator loss 1.9.

28.10 Conclusion

The collecting of extensive data via wearable sensors is critical. Similar to creating realistic and diverse datasets is critical for developing effective models that assess patients' skin problems. The future conductors of skin cancer diagnosis are algorithms and GANs, which work together to create personalized care symphonies. These technological innovations benefit both individuals and healthcare professionals by enabling data-driven assessments, early intervention, personalized treatment methods, remote monitoring, and ongoing research and development. This collaborative duet between algorithms and GANs is a beacon of hope for those living with skin cancer, with each diagnostic path resonating as a distinct and victorious tune. BiGANs could help to create more realistic and engaging VR settings for skin cancer detection and monitoring. Wearable devices used with BiGANs could improve patient monitoring and performance feedback. Wearable devices that use BiGANs can provide more accurate and personalized insights into skin problems, resulting in more effective diagnosis and treatment methods. The main innovation behind BiGANs is the incorporation of an encoder into the original GAN model. This feature is especially useful in skin cancer detection because it allows for the creation of more semantically rich synthetic datasets. The encoder in the BiGAN model plays a vital role by enabling the learning of latent representations from real data, improving the potential for producing synthetic skin lesion datasets that closely mirror.

References

1 Swann, G. (ed.) (2010). The skin is the body's largest organ. *Journal of Visual Communication in Medicine* 33 (4): 148–149. https://doi.org/10.3109/17453054.2010.525439.

2 Montagna, W. (2012). *The Structure and Function of Skin*. Amsterdam, Netherlands: Elsevier.

3 Stanoszek, L.M., Wang, G.Y., and Harms, P.W. (2017). Histologic mimics of basal cell carcinoma. *Archives of Pathology & Laboratory Medicine* 141: 1490–1502. https://doi.org/10.5858/arpa.2017-0222-RA.

4 Goyal, M., Knackstedt, T., Yan, S., and Hassanpour, S. (2020). Artificial intelligence-based image classification for diagnosis of skin cancer: challenges and opportunities. *Computers in Biology and Medicine* 127: 104065. https://doi.org/10.1016/j.compbiomed.2020.104065.

5 Q. V. Le and M. Tan, *EfficientNet: Rethinking Model Scaling for Convolutional Neural Networks*, Elsevier, 2019.

6 Chen, T. and Guestrin, C. (2016). XGBoost: a scalable tree boosting system. *Proceedings of the 22nd ACM SIGKDD International Conference on Knowledge Discovery and Data Mining*, pp. 785–794, San Francisco, CA.

7 Xie, Q., Luong, M.-T., Hovy, E., and Le, Q.V. (2020). Self-training with noisy student improves imagenet classification. *Proceedings of the 2020 IEEE/CVF Conference on Computer Vision and Pattern Recognition (CVPR)*, pp. 10684–10695, Seattle, WA.

8 ISIC-2019 (2019). ISIC-2019-Skin lesion analysis towards melanoma detection, https://challenge2019.isic-archive.

29

Secure Decentralized ECG Prediction: Balancing Privacy, Performance, and Heterogeneity

Bagesh Kumar[1], Sohan Kumar[1], Yash Vikram Singh Rathore[1], Akash Raj[1], Vanshika Singh Andotra[1], Rishik Gupta[1], and Prakhar Shukla[2]

[1]*Department of Information Technology and Computer Science, Manipal University, Jaipur, India*
[2]*Department of Information Technology, IIIT Allahabad, Allahabad, India*

29.1 Introduction

Electrocardiogram (ECG) analysis is a crucial clinical cardiology method because it gives physicians critical insights into the functioning of the heart and facilitates the identification and evaluation of cardiac problems. It helps in the early identification and treatment of a number of conditions, including heart arrhythmias, myocardial infarction, cardiac hypertrophy and enlargement, and risk stratification in cardiovascular disease [1].

Early identification of arrhythmias, or abnormal heartbeats, which can result in significant consequences including stroke or cardiac arrest, is made possible by ECG analysis. It facilitates the diagnosis of acute myocardial infarction by emphasizing myocardial ischemia or injury. ECG monitoring continually measures heart activity in a variety of clinical contexts, enabling tailored patient care. ECG data is also used in cardiovascular disease risk stratification, which helps physicians identify patients who are more likely to have adverse outcomes. Medical professionals can enhance patient outcomes by tailoring preventive measures based on information such as QT dispersion, T-wave aberrations, and heart rate variability. All things considered, because ECG analysis offers vital information on the electrical activity and operation of the heart, it is essential for the diagnosis and treatment of a variety of cardiac disorders [2].

Significant progress has been made in the processing of complex biomedical data as a result of the marriage of artificial intelligence (AI) with healthcare, especially in the interpretation and use of ECG data. Generative AI appears to offer a data-driven solution to these problems by offering an approach to ECG analysis that is data-driven [3]. Neural networks are used in generative AI to comprehend

Generative Artificial Intelligence for Biomedical and Smart Health Informatics,
First Edition. Edited by Aditya Khamparia and Deepak Gupta.

the underlying structure of ECG signals and generate AI data that closely mimics the original. To increase diagnostic precision, this technique may produce various ECG waveforms, expand on already-existing datasets, and denoise signals. The development of anomaly detection systems, which identify subtle deviations from normal ECG patterns and help in the early diagnosis of arrhythmias, ischemia episodes, and other cardiac problems, is another benefit of generative AI. The most recent developments in generative AI for processing ECG data are examined in this chapter, including the creation of innovative structures, training plans, and assessment techniques. It also looks at the benefits and difficulties of incorporating generative AI into clinical practice, including regulatory compliance, data privacy, and model interpretability. This chapter aims to add to the expanding body of literature on AI-driven healthcare innovation by highlighting the potential of generative AI to transform ECG analysis. It also encourages collaboration between researchers, clinicians, and technologists to improve patient outcomes, diagnostic accuracy, and cardiovascular care delivery [4].

Few difficulties faced by traditional healthcare operations are a lack of data, privacy issues, and limited computational capabilities. Cyberattacks, insider threats, and human mistakes can jeopardize the security and confidentiality of patient data, raising privacy issues. Another major barrier is lack of data, particularly in the case of uncommon or specialist disorders. Large-scale dataset availability is further complicated by fragmented healthcare systems and divided data repositories. Compiling complex medical data becomes significantly more difficult when processing resources are limited. The demand for creative approaches and cutting-edge technologies to solve these problems is rising. Among these include the use of cloud computing and AI, as well as the promotion of ethical data management, improved data security and privacy, and data cooperation and sharing. By putting these technologies into practice, strengthening data governance frameworks, and fostering collaborative collaborations, healthcare organizations may fully leverage data-driven insights to advance medical research, enhance clinical outcomes, and improve services [5].

Federated learning (FL) is a decentralized machine learning paradigm that eliminates the need for centralized data collection by enabling cooperative model training across several devices or organizations. This technology allows medical personnel to study ECG data while maintaining patient confidentiality and privacy. It works by directly placing machine learning models on hardware or local servers, such as hospital servers, wearables, and cloud platforms. FL for ECG analysis includes distributed data sources, cooperative model training, aggregated model updates, and privacy-preserving methods. Since each data source is in charge of its own local data, compliance with data protection regulations like GDPR and HIPAA is guaranteed. FL protects sensitive medical data during model training with privacy-preserving methods such as differential privacy, secure aggregation, and federated averaging [6].

FL for ECG analysis offers several benefits, including improved usage of computational resources, enhanced data security and privacy, and support for collaborative research. FL lessens the risk of data breaches or privacy violations associated with centralized data repositories by storing data locally and performing computations locally. By protecting private patient information and enabling information and resource exchange across medical facilities, research teams, and technology partners, FL promotes collaborative research. FL offers a workable solution for secure and efficient ECG analysis that meets the computing, data privacy, and security needs of the healthcare sector. When technology is integrated into healthcare, there is significant potential for customized treatment, better patient outcomes in cardiovascular care, and higher diagnostic accuracy.

29.2 Parsing ECG Data

29.2.1 Various Methods to Parse ECG Data

The process of removing meaningful information from raw signals before analysis and interpretation is known as ECG data parsing [7]. Among the methods used are deep learning architectures, machine learning, feature extraction, baseline correction, and signal preprocessing. ECG data noise is reduced by signal preprocessing, while baseline wander is minimized, and signal clarity is enhanced via baseline correction. Time-domain features provide information on heart rate variability and cardiac shape by measuring the properties of the ECG waveform over predetermined time intervals. By applying methods like Fourier or wavelet transforms to shift ECG data into the frequency domain, frequency-domain analysis reveals more details about heart rhythms and autonomic systems. Certain waveform components, like the QRS complex, *T* wave, and *P* wave, are influenced by morphological variables in terms of their shape and amplitude.

Machine learning and deep learning are applied to achieve heartbeat categorization, anomaly detection, and therapeutic outcome prediction. To predict clinical outcomes, detect anomalies, and categorize heartbeats, supervised learning techniques such as random forests, convolutional neural networks (CNNs), and support vector machines (SVM) are trained on labeled ECG datasets. Anomaly detection and classification are two examples of unsupervised learning techniques used in the exploratory study of unlabeled ECG data as shown in Figure 29.1. In transfer learning, pretrained models are utilized to extract generic features from large-scale ECG datasets. Then, using smaller, domain-specific datasets, these models are refined to better fit certain therapeutic tasks or patient groups.

Recurrent neural networks (RNNs), generated adversarial networks (GANs), and attention mechanisms are examples of deep learning designs. By enabling

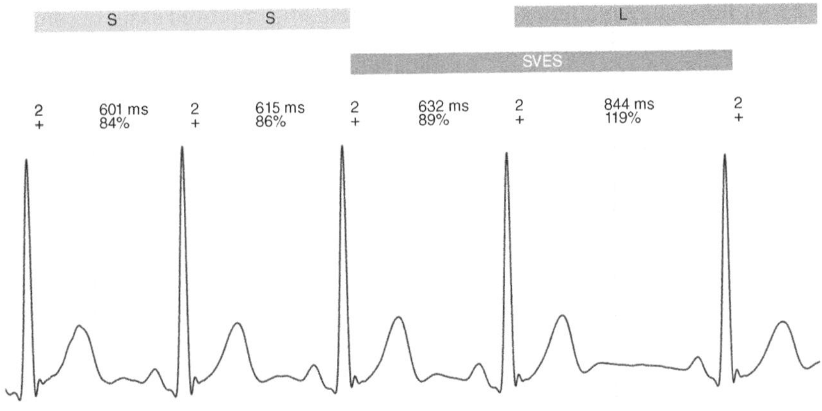

Figure 29.1 Cardiolund ECG parser: It is a medical software for automated rhythm analysis [8].

real-time ECG analysis on wearable technology or local processing units, edge computing frameworks reduce the latency and bandwidth needed for remote monitoring and diagnosis. Continuous monitoring of cardiac activity in an ambulatory situation is made possible by wearable ECG devices with embedded sensors and built-in computing power [9]. This allows for the early diagnosis of cardiac problems such as arrhythmias and ischemia episodes.

29.2.2 Use of Generative AI to Parse ECG Data GANs

GANs, in particular, have shown promise in a number of applications, including the synthesis and interpretation of ECG signals [10]. This is how ECG data is analyzed using generative AI.

Synthetic ECG signals produced by generative models, like GANs, may mimic real-world data distributions quite a bit [11]. By adding these produced signals to the collection of available datasets, data scarcity can be reduced and machine learning models that have been trained on sparse data can be made more resilient. GANs may generate a variety of samples with realistic morphological features that depict variations in cardiac dynamics, heart rate, and arrhythmia patterns by learning the underlying structure of ECG signals from training data.

"Normal" signals serve as a standard for comparison and are generated by GANs that have been trained on regular ECG data. It may be possible to detect an anomaly or abnormality during inference if the learned distribution of normal signals differs significantly from the input ECG signal as shown in Figure 29.2. Therefore, by detecting deviations from predicted patterns in ECG data, GANs

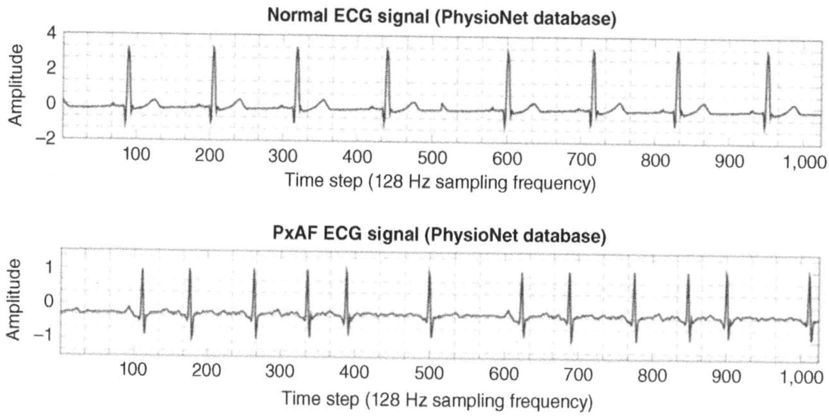

Figure 29.2 (a) A sinus rhythm condition illustration. Variation in heart rate between 60 and 100 beats per minute. (b) The PxAF state. Arrhythmias and changes in the P-wave are examples of heart rate variability [12].

can act as anomaly detectors to aid in the early detection of cardiac arrhythmias, ischemia events, and other cardiac ailments [13].

GANs are an effective way to reduce ECG data noise, which includes baseline drift, muscle artifacts, and electrode motion artifacts. Training a GAN on both clean reference signals and noisy ECG data gives the generator network the capacity to remove noise and recover the original, clean waveform. This method increases signal clarity and accuracy in the analysis tasks of heartbeat segmentation, feature extraction, and arrhythmia classification.

GANs may replicate a wide range of patient demographics, disease states, and treatment outcomes by producing synthetic ECG signals that correlate to certain clinical scenarios or physiological factors. Researchers and medical practitioners can construct bespoke ECG waveforms that indicate specific heart diseases, drug interactions, or cardiac treatments by modifying the generator network's latent variables or input parameters. These artificial scenarios provide important insights into the dynamics of cardiac physiology and pathology and also support hypothesis testing, protocol validation, and medical education [14, 15]. Lost or incomplete ECG data can be recovered with the help of GANs due to transmission issues, anomalies in the signal, or sensor dropout. GANs can predict missing segments or reconstruct distorted parts by comprehending the underlying structure of ECG data. This allows them to preserve continuity for subsequent processing tasks and fill in any gaps. This feature is very useful for remote monitoring applications where accurate ECG data transmission is necessary for prompt diagnosis and intervention.

All things considered, there is a lot of promise for using generative AI, and more especially GANs, to analyze ECG data and address problems like noise contamination, missing data, and lack of data. Scientists and medical practitioners can enhance the quality, diversity, and interpretability of ECG datasets by utilizing AI's generative capabilities. Overall, this will enhance cardiovascular medicine patient care, clinical results, and diagnostic accuracy.

29.3 FL for Decentralized ECG Prediction

29.3.1 Core Principles of FL

FL offers a novel approach to training machine learning models in a collaborative manner, particularly when dealing with sensitive data like patient information. Here's how it works:

- **Local Model:** Training happens on individual devices or local servers at participating institutions (hospitals in the ECG example). This keeps patient data decentralized and avoids the need for a central storage facility [16].
- **Communication of Model Updates:** Instead of sharing raw data, institutions communicate updates to the model itself. These updates can be in the form of gradients (values used to refine the model) or intermediate representations (compressed versions of the model) [17].
- **Privacy-Preserving Aggregation:** A central server collects these model updates from all participants. Through a secure aggregation process, the server improves the overall model without ever requiring access to the raw patient data from any institution [18].

29.3.2 FL Architectures for ECG Analysis

In exploring FL for ECG analysis, two main architectures emerge, each with its strengths and weaknesses: Vertical FL (VFL) and Horizontal FL (HFL) as shown in Figure 29.3.

- **Vertical Federated Learning:** Institutions share preprocessed features extracted from their ECG data. These features could be heart rate variability metrics, frequency domain components, or other relevant characteristics [20].
- **Horizontal Federated Learning:** This approach prioritizes privacy by focusing on sharing model updates. Each institution trains a local model on its own ECG data.

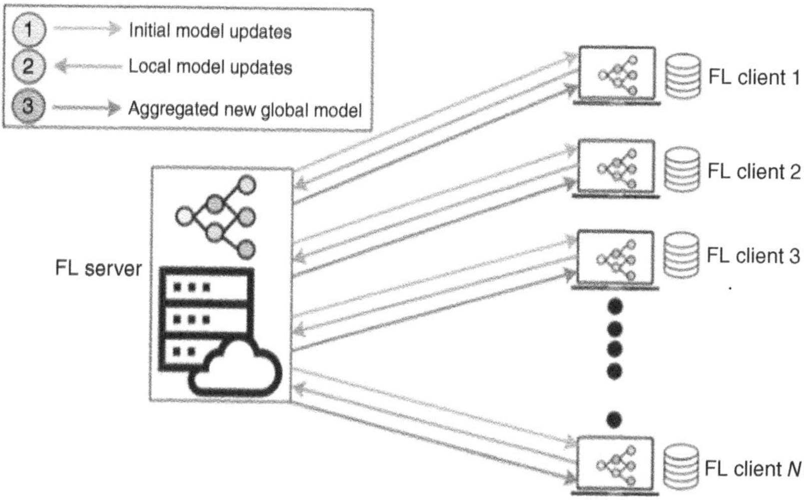

Figure 29.3 This simplified network illustrates FL for ECG analysis. Participating institutions train local models on their ECG data (servers/clients) and share updates (arrows) to improve a central model, all without sharing raw patient data [19].

29.3.2.1 Choosing the Right Architecture

The optimal architecture for a specific ECG analysis project depends on various factors, including:

- **Privacy Requirements:** If preserving patient privacy is paramount, HFL might be the preferred choice.
- **Data Characteristics:** If datasets across institutions have significant variations or require complex feature engineering, VFL might offer advantages.
- **Computational Resources:** If computational resources are limited, HFL might be more feasible due to its simpler communication protocols.

29.4 Security and Privacy in FL

FL presents a promising method for developing private and secure ECG analysis models. Unlike traditional centralized learning, FL trains models cooperatively utilizing distributed data sources maintained by hospitals or individual devices. This preserves patient privacy by removing the requirement to reveal raw ECG data. FL does, however, present certain issues with security and privacy that must be resolved as shown in Figure 29.4 [23].

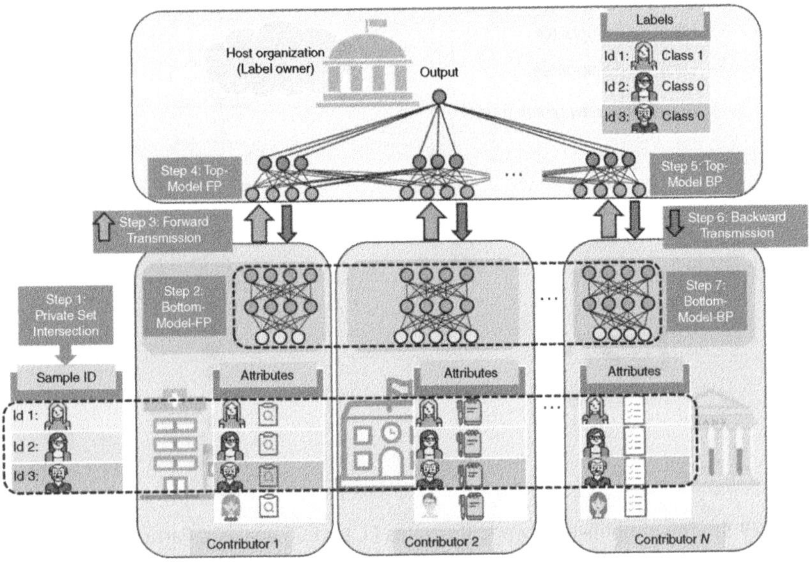

Figure 29.4 An overall workflow for vertical FL. The classic workflow includes the following seven steps: (1) private set intersection; (2) bottom model forward propagation (BM–FP); (3) forward transmission; (4) top model forward propagation (TM–FP); (5) top model backward propagation (TM–BP); (6) backward transmission; (7) bottom model backward propagation (BM–BP). The host is the label owner and the guest is the attribute owner [21, 22].

29.4.1 Privacy Threats

- **Inference Attacks:** Malicious parties may infer sensitive patient data from model updates that are shared during training. Differential privacy is one strategy that may be used to incorporate controlled noise into updates, making it more challenging to reconstruct individual data points from the aggregated model [24].
- **Model Inversion Attacks:** An attacker may be able to link training data or pinpoint particular contributions by breaking down the global model. Secure aggregation techniques and federated averaging techniques can reduce this risk [25].
- **Attacks Using Poisoned Data:** Malicious users may use tampered data to influence the model's output during training. Robust model architectures and anomaly detection methods can help identify and prevent these attacks [26].

29.4.2 Security Threats

- **Central Server Compromise:** An attacker may be able to obtain integrated model updates and maybe even sensitive data if the FL process's central server

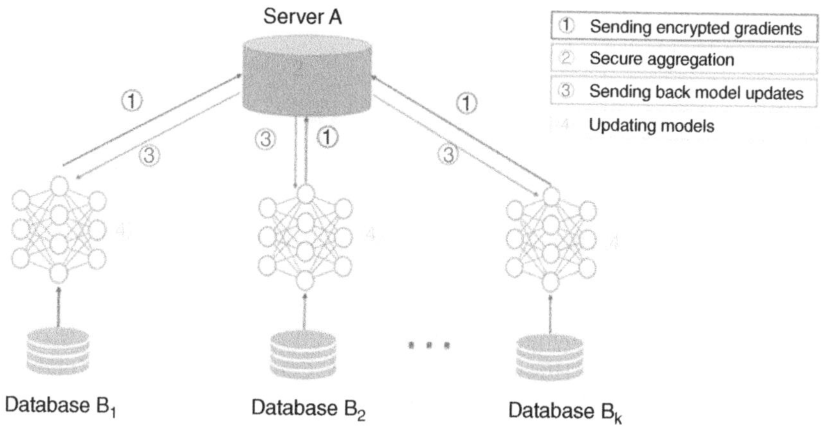

Figure 29.5 Architecture for a horizontal federated learning system [29].

is breached. Encryption methods and secure communication channels are required to safeguard data both in transit and at rest [27].

- **Nonparticipating Device Compromise:** If attackers manage to breach FL-affiliated devices, they may introduce tainted data or interfere with the training procedure. To defend against such attacks, access control and secure device authentication are essential [28].

29.4.3 Methods for Safeguarding Privacy and Security

- **Differential Privacy:** By introducing controlled noise into model updates, differential privacy enhances the statistical complexity of extracting individual data points from the aggregated model.
- **Secure Aggregation:** Using cryptographic techniques, only allowed companies are able to access and implement model changes during training.
- **Federated Averaging:** A widely used method that shares only local model modifications, significantly reducing the likelihood of sensitive data leaks as shown in Figure 29.5.
- **Data Governance:** Explicit rules and laws are needed to regulate data ownership, usage, and access inside the FL system.
- **Openness and Definability:** Mechanisms to understand the model's prediction process are necessary to build trust and ensure appropriate use in healthcare settings.

29.5 Addressing Heterogeneity in ECG Dataset

FL offers a promising approach to train AI models in healthcare while protecting patient privacy. However, data heterogeneity, where data from different hospitals is inconsistent, creates significant challenges. Let's explore these challenges and solution of it with an analogy using ECG data.

29.5.1 Challenges of Heterogeneous Data in FL

Imagine a FL project aiming to develop a model for arrhythmia detection using ECG data from three hospitals.

Hospital A (Large Teaching Hospital): Uses a detailed coding system for ECG abnormalities, including specific codes for various arrhythmias (e.g., atrial fibrillation, ventricular tachycardia). Hospital B (Rural Clinic): Uses a more general coding system, potentially grouping different arrhythmias under a single code ("irregular heartbeat"). Hospital C (Cardiology Center): Focuses on complex arrhythmias and uses highly detailed ECG data points (e.g., QT interval duration) [30, 31].

- **Feature Inconsistency:** The coding systems for ECG abnormalities differ across hospitals. This is similar to Hospital A recording the QT interval in milliseconds (ms) while Hospital B uses seconds (s). The model struggles to understand the relationship between specific ECG features and arrhythmia types across datasets.
- **Data Distribution Shifts:** Hospital C's data might have a higher proportion of ECGs with features indicative of complex arrhythmias. This is like Hospital C focusing on pneumonia cases with heart involvement, while Hospitals A and B have more common pneumonia types. The model could become biased toward identifying these specific arrhythmias, potentially missing other types present in Hospitals A and B.
- **Data Quality Issues:** Hospital B might have missing data points for specific ECG measurements due to limited resources. This is similar to Hospital B having incomplete information on smoking history (a risk factor for pneumonia) in their dataset. Missing data can hinder the model's ability to learn effectively.
- **Class Imbalance:** Hospital B might have fewer ECGs with specific arrhythmias compared to Hospitals A and C. This is similar to Hospital B having fewer pneumonia cases. The model might prioritize learning common ECG patterns from Hospital A and underperform in detecting less frequent arrhythmias, especially ones Hospital B sees less often.

29.5.2 Addressing Data Heterogeneity

While data inconsistencies can hinder FL for pneumonia detection, several approaches can mitigate these challenges:

- **Data Standardization:** Ensure consistent representation of features across hospitals. This could involve adopting common coding systems for diagnoses and medical procedures (e.g., all hospitals using SNOMED CT for standardized medical terminology). Here's an ECG example: Standardize how QT interval (a heart rhythm measurement) is recorded. Hospital A might record it in milliseconds (ms), while Hospital B uses seconds (s). A common standard (e.g., milliseconds) would be agreed upon.

- **Robust Model Architectures:** Utilize model architectures specifically designed to handle data heterogeneity. These models are less susceptible to biases caused by distribution shifts in patient demographics, disease prevalence, or specific data collection practices across hospitals.
- **Weighted Training Data:** To address class imbalances (e.g., fewer pneumonia cases in a rural hospital), consider weighting the contribution of data from different hospitals during the FL process. This can help the model prioritize learning from the less frequent but crucial pneumonia cases.

By implementing these strategies, FL can become a more reliable tool for developing accurate and generalizable AI models for early pneumonia detection, even in the presence of data heterogeneity across healthcare institutions.

29.6 Case Study: Advancing Heart Disease Prediction with Asynchronous Federated Deep Learning

29.6.1 Introduction

In the healthcare sector, accurately predicting heart disease is crucial, and the utilization of deep learning has emerged as a promising method to achieve this goal. This study [9] investigates a pioneering approach called the Asynchronous Federated Deep Learning Approach for Cardiac Prediction (AFLCP). AFLCP integrates a dataset on heart disease with deep neural networks (DNNs) using an asynchronous learning method. By updating DNN parameters asynchronously and employing a temporally weighted aggregation technique, AFLCP aims to improve the accuracy and convergence of the central predictive model. Experimental results demonstrate that AFLCP outperforms conventional techniques in terms of communication cost and model accuracy, highlighting its potential to transform heart disease prediction.

29.6.2 Contributions

1) **Exploration of Communication Techniques:** AFLCP investigates both synchronous and asynchronous communication methods to optimize predictive modeling in healthcare.

2) **Overview of FL Techniques:** The study provides an insightful overview of distributed FL techniques, laying the groundwork for innovative approaches in healthcare analytics.
3) **Introduction of AFLCP:** AFLCP introduces a novel asynchronous FL approach tailored specifically for cardiac prediction, offering a new paradigm in predictive modeling.
4) **Comparison Analysis:** Through rigorous comparison analyses, AFLCP demonstrates superior performance over conventional methods, highlighting its efficacy in predictive accuracy and cost-effectiveness.

29.6.3 Methodology

The methodology employed in this study involves evaluating the AFLCP technique using established metrics such as accuracy, precision, and F1-score. These metrics serve as benchmarks for assessing the correctness and effectiveness of the predictive models. The experimentation is conducted using the TensorFlow Federated (TFF) library on a robust computational setup comprising an Intel Core i7 processor and 16 GB of RAM, ensuring reliability and reproducibility of results.

29.6.4 Results

Experimental results unequivocally demonstrate the superiority of the AFLCP approach over traditional methods. Notably, AFLCP exhibits enhanced performance in terms of communication efficiency and predictive accuracy, validating its efficacy in cardiac disease prediction.

29.6.5 Conclusion

This study presents a groundbreaking privacy-aware solution for predicting heart diseases using asynchronous FL techniques. AFLCP offers a flexible, efficient, and privacy-preserving approach to cardiac prediction, heralding a new era in healthcare analytics. By mitigating concerns regarding data privacy and resource utilization, AFLCP presents a viable framework for widespread adoption in healthcare settings.

29.6.6 Future Directions

Future research endeavors will focus on addressing scalability challenges and expanding the application of AFLCP to predict and treat a myriad of severe illnesses beyond heart disease. Parkinson's disease, diabetes, liver cancer, skin cancer, and breast cancer represent promising avenues for further exploration, underscoring the transformative potential of distributed machine learning techniques in healthcare.

29.7 Conclusion

This chapter explored the exciting intersection of AI and healthcare, specifically focusing on how generative AI and FL can revolutionize ECG analysis. We identified the limitations of traditional methods—data scarcity, privacy concerns, and centralized storage. Generative AI, particularly GANs, offers a powerful solution by creating synthetic signals, improving data quality, and aiding anomaly detection.

FL takes it a step further, enabling collaborative training on diverse datasets while keeping patient data secure. This approach unlocks numerous benefits—better use of computational resources, enhanced data security, and fostering collaborative research. We addressed the challenge of heterogeneous data by proposing solutions such as standardization, robust models, and weighted training. In addition, the AFLCP case study showcased the effectiveness of FL in healthcare analytics.

In essence, this chapter highlights the transformative potential of AI and FL for ECG analysis. This paves the way for a future of personalized diagnosis, remote monitoring, and tailored treatment plans within a decentralized healthcare system. By embracing these advancements and fostering collaboration across disciplines, the healthcare sector can unlock the full potential of AI to improve medical research, patient outcomes, and ultimately, patient care.

References

1 Abdellatif, A.A., Mhaisen, N., Mohamed, A. et al. (2022). Communication-efficient hierarchical federated learning for IoT heterogeneous systems with imbalanced data. *Future Generation Computer Systems* 128: 406–419.

2 Anbalagan, T., Nath, M.K., Vijayalakshmi, D., and Anbalagan, A. (2023). Analysis of various techniques for ECG signal in healthcare, past, present, and future. *Biomedical Engineering Advances* 6: 100089.

3 Antunes, R.S., da Costa, C.A., Küderle, A. et al. (2022). Federated learning for healthcare: systematic review and architecture proposal. *ACM Transactions on Intelligent Systems and Technology (TIST)* 13 (4): 1–23.

4 Arikumar, K.S., Prathiba, S.B., Alazab, M. et al. (2022). FL-PMI: Federated learning-based person movement identification through wearable devices in smart healthcare systems. *Sensors* 22 (4): 1377.

5 Banabilah, S., Aloqaily, M., Alsayed, E. et al. (2022). Federated learning review: fundamentals, enabling technologies, and future applications. *Information Processing & Management* 59 (6): 103061.

6 Berkaya, S.K., Uysal, A.K., Gunal, E.S. et al. (2018). A survey on ECG analysis. *Biomedical Signal Processing and Control* 43: 216–235.

7 Gutierrez, D.M.J., Hassan, H.M., Landi, L. et al. (2022). Application of federated learning techniques for arrhythmia classification using 12-lead ECG signals. *arXiv preprint arXiv:2208.10993.*

8 Kairouz, P., McMahan, H.B., Avent, B. et al. (2021). Advances and open problems in federated learning. *Foundations and Trends® in Machine Learning* 14 (1–2): 1–210.

9 Khan, M., Alsulami, M., Yaqoob, M.M. et al. (2023). Asynchronous federated learning for improved cardiovascular disease prediction using artificial intelligence. *Diagnostics* 13: 2340.

10 Kundroo, M. and Kim, T. (2023). Federated learning with hyper-parameter optimization. *Journal of King Saud University-Computer and Information Sciences* 35 (9): 101740.

11 Li, L., Fan, Y., Tse, M., and Lin, K.-Y. (2020). A review of applications in federated learning. *Computers & Industrial Engineering* 149: 106854.

12 Mishra, A., Dharahas, G., Gite, S. et al. (2022). ECG data analysis with denoising approach and customized CNNs. *Sensors* 22 (5): 1928.

13 Li, Q., He, B., and Song, D. (2021). Model-contrastive federated learning. *Proceedings of the IEEE/CVF Conference on Computer Vision and Pattern Recognition*, 10713–10722.

14 Lin, D., Guo, Y., Sun, H., and Chen, Y. (2022). FedCluster: A federated learning framework for cross-device private ECG classification. *IEEE INFOCOM 2022-IEEE Conference on Computer Communications Workshops (INFOCOM WKSHPS)*, 1–6. IEEE.

15 Mammen, P.M. (2021). Federated learning: opportunities and challenges. *arXiv preprint arXiv:2101.05428.*

16 Pandya, S., Srivastava, G., Jhaveri, R. et al. (2023). Federated learning for smart cities: a comprehensive survey. *Sustainable Energy Technologies and Assessments* 55: 102987.

17 Patel, V.A., Bhattacharya, P., Tanwar, S. et al. (2022). Adoption of federated learning for healthcare informatics: emerging applications and future directions. *IEEE Access* 10: 90792–90826.

18 Rajagopal, S.M., Supriya, M., and Buyya, R. (2023). FedSDM: Federated learning based smart decision making module for ECG data in IoT integrated Edge–Fog–Cloud computing environments. *Internet of Things* 22: 100784.

19 dos Santos Garcia, C., Meincheim, A., Faria Junior, E. R. et al. (2019). Process mining techniques and applications – A systematic mapping study. *Expert Systems with Applications* 133: 260–295. ISSN 0957-4174, https://doi.org/10.1016/j.eswa.2019.05.003.

20 Dasaradharami Reddy, K. and Gadekallu, T.R. (2023). A comprehensive survey on federated learning techniques for healthcare informatics. *Computational Intelligence and Neuroscience* 2023 (1): 8393990.

21 Rieke, N., Hancox, J., Li, W. et al. (2020). The future of digital health with federated learning. *NPJ Digital Medicine* 3 (1): 1–7.

22 Shaik, T., Tao, X., Higgins, N. et al. (2022). FedStack: Personalized activity monitoring using stacked federated learning. *Knowledge-Based Systems* 257: 109929.

23 Wei, K., Li, J., Ma, C. et al. (2022). Vertical federated learning: challenges, methodologies and experiments. *ArXiv*, abs/2202.04309.

24 Xu, M., Du, H., Niyato, D. et al. (2024). Unleashing the power of edge-cloud generative AI in mobile networks: a survey of AIGC services. *IEEE Communications Surveys & Tutorials* 26 (2): 1127–1170.

25 Yang, X., Qi, X., and Zhou, X. (2023). Deep learning technologies for time series abnormality detection in healthcare: a review. *IEEE Access* 11: 117788–117799.

26 Ye, M., Fang, X., Du, B. et al. (2023). Heterogeneous federated learning: state-of-the-art and research challenges. *ACM Computing Surveys* 56 (3): 1–44.

27 Ying, Z., Zhang, G., Pan, Z. et al. (2023). FedECG: A federated semi-supervised learning framework for electrocardiogram abnormalities prediction. *Journal of King Saud University-Computer and Information Sciences* 35 (6): 101568.

28 Yoo, J.H., Jeong, H., Lee, J., and Chung, T.-M. (2021). Federated learning: issues in medical application. *Future Data and Security Engineering: 8th International Conference, FDSE 2021, Virtual Event* (24–26 November 2021), *Proceedings 8*, 3–22. Springer.

29 Sun, L. and Wu, J. (2022). A scalable and transferable federated learning system for classifying healthcare sensor data. *IEEE Journal of Biomedical and Health Informatics* 27 (2): 866–877.

30 Zhang, C., Xie, Y., Bai, H. et al. (2021). A survey on federated learning. *Knowledge-Based Systems* 216: 106775.

31 Zhang, M., Wang, Y., and Luo, T. (2020). Federated learning for arrhythmia detection of non-IID ECG. *2020 IEEE 6th International Conference on Computer and Communications (ICCC)*, 1176–1180. IEEE.

Index

Generative Artificial Intelligence for Biomedical and Smart Health Informatics, First Edition. Edited by Aditya Khamparia and Deepak Gupta.

e

g

h

S

Printed and bound by CPI Group (UK) Ltd, Croydon, CR0 4YY
17/09/2026
14964332-0008